ID0638685

Handbook
of
Orthodontics
for the STUDENT *and* GENERAL PRACTITIONER

ROBERT E. MOYERS, D.D.S., Ph.D.

*Professor of Dentistry (Orthodontics), School of
Dentistry, and Director, Center for Human Growth and Development,
The University of Michigan, Ann Arbor; Consulting Orthodontist,
Mott Children's Health Center, Flint, Michigan*

Handbook
of
Orthodontics
for the STUDENT *and*
GENERAL PRACTITIONER

THIRD EDITION

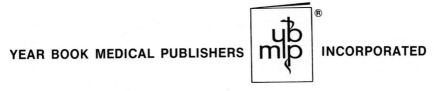

YEAR BOOK MEDICAL PUBLISHERS | ubmp ® | **INCORPORATED**

35 EAST WACKER DRIVE • CHICAGO

Copyright © 1958, 1963 and 1973 by Year Book Medical Publishers, Inc. All rights reserved. No part of this publication may be reproduced, stored in a retrieval system, or transmitted, in any form or by any means, electronic, mechanical, photocopying, recording, or otherwise, without prior written permission from the publisher. Printed in the United States of America.

Second edition, 1963
Reprinted, May 1966
Reprinted, February 1968
Reprinted, January 1969
Reprinted December 1969
Reprinted December 1970
Third edition, 1973
Reprinted, February 1974
Reprinted, November 1975

Library of Congress Catalog Card Number: 74-182004
International Standard Book Number: 0-8151-6002-X

DEDICATION

To my parents, whose many sacrifices made possible my education

Preface to the Third Edition

SINCE THE APPEARANCE of the first edition of this book, many important changes affecting the role of orthodontics within dentistry have taken place. Fluoridation of communal water supplies and the use of caries-preventive measures in routine dental practice have reduced, in a remarkable way, the place of restorative dentistry in the typical dental practice. Affluence in our society and an increased awareness of the benefits of good dental health have caused the general acceptance of dental procedures once sought by only a minority of the people. As public needs have altered, the profession has responded, and the dentist in family practice has sought further training to extend the range of his services. Dentists who a few years ago did but minor periodontic procedures and no orthodontics are now actively involved in clinical therapy in both fields. The practice of dentistry is in a remarkable state of flux: we have moved from patchwork to treatment of the entire masticatory system, from neglect of preventive procedures to entire practices based solely on preventive dentistry and from quiet and almost total avoidance of orthodontics in general practice to the enthusiastic treatment of malocclusion in an increasing number of offices.

As the interest in orthodontics rises, the need for sound sources of knowledge, training and consultation increases. Several fine new textbooks in orthodontics have been published, orthodontic study clubs and associations for the nonspecialist abound and flourish and the position of orthodontics in the undergraduate curriculum has been strengthened. For all these reasons, and more, any book on orthodontics for the student or general practitioner published at this time must be written quite differently than it was only a few years ago.

Dentistry is a profession based primarily on three clinical problems— caries, periodontal disease and malocclusion. Research and modern preventive practice truly have brought dental caries under control for most children in America today. Striking advances in our knowledge of the mechanisms of peridontal disease and advances in clinical practice give rising expectation that periodontal disorders, too, may be either generally prevented or easily controlled. But malocclusion is not a disease process and hence cannot be approached with a dependence on Koch's postulates. Most malocclusions are the result of variability of the growth and development of dental and craniofacial structures and hence complete eradication or true prevention cannot be expected. However, as in the case of caries and periodontal disease, improvements in treatment usually derive from basic research—in this instance, research in growth and development. Growth is the business of the orthodontist: it provides the basis for diagnosis; it is the raw material from which treatment changes are wrought. Only by understanding craniofacial growth and development can we hope to manage the problem of malocclusion. Therefore, this third edition includes much more information on GROWTH AND DEVELOPMENT than previously. The section on DIAGNOSIS likewise has been enlarged to permit a thorough understanding of the factors that produce and sustain malocclusion. As stated in Chapter XII, radiographic cephalometry has literally revolutionized orthodontic diagnosis and treatment. Because of the dramatic advances in this important field, discussion of this subject has been enlarged greatly. The TREATMENT section reflects the expanding desires of the general dentist and student in clinical therapy.

Although this is a third edition, it will be found to be a new book written in response to the needs of a changing field in a changing profession.

Acknowledgments

Nobody really works alone. The ideas in this book have come from many sources, most from colleagues and students with whom I have been associated.

Chapter III was written by Professor James K. Avery. Professor Donald H. Enlow collaborated in writing Chapter IV and Professor W. Stuart Hunter in preparing Chapter XII. I have had a long and profitable association with these three men and am most grateful for their fine contributions. Dr. Ross O. Fisk provided a number of illustrations and useful ideas for Chapter XV. His experience in teaching undergraduate orthodontics at The University of Toronto makes him a valued collaborator. I am indebted to Professor Sigurd Ramfjord for the excellent scheme of occlusal equilibration of the permanent dentition presented in Chapter XVII. The basic approach to the discussion of etiology is derived largely from the works of Professor Rodney Dockrell, Dublin, Ireland.

I asked at least three colleagues to read and criticize each chapter when it was first written. They responded in a most thorough and helpful manner. Some read more than one chapter and some reread chapters as I attempted to incorporate their suggestions. I list their names here so the reader may know of their assistance, but I alone, of course, assume responsibility for all that is written herein. These readers-critics were: Robert G. Aldrich, Major M. Ash, James K. Avery, Melvin Baer, Daniel Balbach, Claude Baril, Harlan Bloomer, James Bosma, Donald H. Enlow, F. Gaynor Evans, Ross O. Fisk, Stanley M. Garn, Ash Hawk, W. Stuart Hunter, Kalevi Koski, Wilton M. Krogman, Takayuki Kuroda, James McNamara, John F. Mortell, William R. Proffit, Michael Riolo, Arthur Storey, Frans P. G. Van der Linden and Donald Woodside.

New drawings and photographs have been prepared by the superb group in Technical Illustration, Harry Willsher, Chief, and Photography, Gerald Davenport, Chief, at The University of Michigan. Mrs. June Bixler has typed most of the manuscript, including many preliminary drafts. Mrs. Louise Pittaway and Mrs. Katherine Ribbens, editors, Center for Human Growth and Development, The University of Michigan, aided in the editing.

Year Book Medical Publishers have given strong support for this book from the original idea to this third edition. Mr. Fred Rogers, Vice-President, has given counsel and encouragement and Mr. Paul Perles has insisted on the highest standards of art, photography and reproduction. Mr. William Keville has played that most difficult role of editor with warm integrity and friendly candor.

Finally, I am grateful to my wife Barbara and daughters Mary and Martha, who have performed such services as doing sketches, checking references and serving as photographer's models. It is fine to be a part of a family that tolerates such time-consuming madnesses as book writing.

All these people—and more—have helped, but errors and omissions that may have occurred are my responsibility. I rely on friendly readers to help me rectify them. Users of the first two editions have made many suggestions. All comments, corrections and criticisms sent to me at the Center for Human Growth and Development, The University of Michigan, 1111 E. Catherine Street, Ann Arbor, Michigan 48104, will be received humbly and gratefully.

ROBERT E. MOYERS

Table of Contents

SECTION 3. TREATMENT

Introduction to the Study and Practice of Orthodontics

> Nothing is known in our profession by guess; and I do not
> believe, that from the first dawn of medical science to the
> present moment, a single correct idea has ever emanated
> from conjecture: it is right therefore, that those who are
> studying their profession should be aware that there is no
> short road to knowledge.—Sir Astley Paston Cooper, in
> *A Treatise on Dislocations and Fractures of the Joints*

A. Problems in studying orthodontics

  1. For the dental student

  2. For the dentist in practice

B. What is orthodontics?

  1. History

  2. Scope

C. The purpose of this book

D. How to use this book

THE COMPLICATED NATURE of dental occlusion, its development, maintenance and correction is the primary reason for the existence of dentistry as a separate healing arts profession. However, we have tended to emphasize in the past the restorative aspects of occlusion rather than its development and correction. The problems of occlusal development and correction are just as much the responsibility and concern of the general practitioner as of the orthodontist; therefore, basic knowledge concerning occlusal development, facial growth and the correction of malocclusion should be part of the training of every dentist. It is not the tradition in many dental schools to spend much time on growth and development or training in the diagnosis and treatment of malocclusion; therefore, some problems arise for the dental student or practicing dentist who wishes to study orthodontics.

A. Problems in Studying Orthodontics

1. FOR THE DENTAL STUDENT

Most undergraduate orthodontic courses consist of a few hours of instruction late in the curriculum, with very little clinical experience. When orthodontic teaching begins, the student's attitudes toward dentistry may have been set by good teaching in other courses in which success is based on other concepts or different clinical goals. For example, good restorative dentistry traditionally has required a higher proportion of technical skills than of biologic knowledge. Orthodontics, perhaps more than any other field of dentistry, is dependent on a thorough working knowledge of the developmental biology of the face. Unwittingly, the dental student may have acquired the idea that dental problems are solved by technics alone. He may think that the only thing separating the several clinical branches of dentistry is variation in technical procedures. Much of clinical dentistry is related to repair or restoration, but orthodontics is carried out primarily by guidance of growth. The strategy and tactics of growth and development are conceptually quite different from replacing lost parts.

Orthodontics, unfortunately, has tended to isolate itself from the mother profession of dentistry and has come to be considered by many a specialty with little role in general practice. As a result, most dentists (including teachers) are frank to admit that they know less about orthodontics than any other branch of clinical dentistry. The teaching of undergraduate orthodontics is difficult, since usually there is little time in the curriculum. Teachers in other departments often have little understanding of orthodontics; consequently, orthodontic concepts are not reinforced and integrated well into general clinical teaching. Finally, the subject does not lend itself well to the semester or quarter module, since the teaching must be spread over months or years while cases are being treated or the child is maturing to the moment when treatment can be begun. All undergraduate orthodontics cannot be taught with a series of lectures and a laboratory confined to one term.

2. FOR THE DENTIST IN PRACTICE

The dentist in practice who has had an inadequate undergraduate orthodontics course, and seeks further training, may be surprised to learn that fewer short courses are offered in orthodontics for the generalist than for most other fields. Scarcely any short course can include clinical experience because of the time necessary to treat a malocclusion. Few articles appear in the dental journals concerning orthodontics for the family dentist and most orthodontic books are written for the specialist. Finally, the attitudes developed finely to ensure success in the other branches of dentistry may handicap the generalist as he begins to study orthodontics; for example, a fine clinical sense of compromise in treatment goals (see Chapter XVI, in which the limiting factors in orthodontic treatment are discussed). The dentist in practice who would learn orthodontics must overcome the lack of good basic undergraduate training, will not find available an extensive literature and will have difficulty in obtaining extensive postgraduate training.

B. What Is Orthodontics?

Orthodontics is that branch of dentistry concerned with the study of the growth of the craniofacial complex, the development of occlusion and the treatment of dentofacial abnormalities.

1. HISTORY

Hippocrates[2] was among the first to comment about craniofacial deformity:

..Οἱ φοξοί οἱ μέν καρῑεραύχενες, ἰσχυροί καί τᾶλλα καί ὀστέοισιν. οἱ δέ κεφαλαλγέες καί ὠτόρρυτοι. Τουτέοισιν ὑπερῷαι κοῖλαι καί ὀδόντες παρηλλαγμένοι."

(Among those individuals with long shaped heads, some have thick necks, strong parts and bones. Others have strongly arched palates, their teeth are irregularly arrayed, crowding one another and they are bothered by headaches and otorrhea.)

Adamandios,[1] writing in the fifth century A.D., noted that "those persons whose lips are pushed out because of cuspid displacement are ill tempered, abusive shouters and defamers":

,,"Οσοι κατά τούς κυνόδοντας κορυφοῦται τά χείλη, κακόθυμοι, ὑβρισταί, κράκται, ἐπεσβόλοι." (Φυσιογνωμικοῖς).

Crude appliances that seemingly were designed to regulate the teeth have been found as archaeologic artifacts in tombs of ancient Egypt, Greece and the Mayans of Mexico. Orthodontics, as we think of it today, however, probably has its roots in France in the eighteenth century, when Pierre Fauchard, that most famous of all dentists, described an orthodontic appliance easily recognized as such by any modern dentist. Other articles concerning the development of the dentition and facial growth were written in the same period, but certainly John Hunter's (1728–1793) natural history of the human teeth is of the most interest to orthodontists.

In the United States in the latter part of the nineteenth century, Kingsley, Farrar, Talbot and Guilford presented pioneer writings on the treatment of malocclusion. Most North Americans maintain that orthodontics, however, really had its origin at the turn of the century, when Edward H. Angle published *A System of Appliances for Correcting Irregularities of the Teeth* and established a school for the training of dentists as orthodontic specialists.

The field developed differently in North America than in Europe. Angle was an intellectual and mechanical genius who dominated the orthodontic scene in the New World more than any one person in Europe. Further, he improvised clever appliances for the precise positioning of the individual teeth, since, from the start, he emphasized the importance of correct occlusion. In Europe, on the other hand, early leaders in the field studied more the role of the craniofacial skeleton in dentofacial anomalies and malocclusion. Perhaps this is the reason that in the United States the field is called orthodontics (from the Greek *orthos,* meaning straight, and *odontos,* meaning tooth), whereas in Europe such terms as dental orthopedics, orthopedie dentofaciale and Gebiss-und Kieferorthopedie are used. Although the terms generally are interchangeable, they reflect differences in emphasis during historical development and they betray differences in the aims of appliance therapy among various countries.

Most dental specialities developed within the profession, gradually evolving their own literature, specialized skills and advanced training programs but maintaining strong ties to the mother profession. In the United States, orthodontic concepts, technics and specialized training, on the other hand, developed largely from within the specialty. Orthodontics in North America from the time of Angle has been a bit more apart from dentistry than any other dental specialty. Therefore, North American concepts of orthodontics, as well as mechanics, are oriented differently than European. The specialty of orthodontics has flourished intellectually, clinically and scientifically and has attracted some of the finest teachers, scientists and clinicians in dentistry to its field, yet orthodontic training in the undergraduate curriculum still is generally superficial. As a result, most dentists really are not well trained in orthodontics. On the other hand, graduate training programs have been strengthened, their scientific base has been broadened and the numbers enrolled have increased until today approximately 10% of all graduating dentists go on to orthodontic specialty training.

2. Scope

Orthodontic therapy is directed to abnormal occlusion of the teeth, growth of the complex of craniofacial bones and function of the orofacial neuromusculature, which alone or in combination may cause any of the following:

a) Impaired mastication.
b) Unfortunate facial aesthetics.
c) Dysfunction of the temporomandibular articulation.
d) Susceptibility to periodontal disease.
e) Susceptibility to dental caries.
f) Impaired speech due to malpositions of the teeth.

Orthodontic therapy involves the three primary tissue systems concerned in dentofacial development, namely, the dentition, the craniofacial skeleton and the facial and jaw musculature (see Chapter V). By means of suitable appliances, the individual teeth can be positioned more favorably to provide better aesthetics, occlusal function, oral health and speech. Correction of the craniofacial skeleton, however, is a different matter, since it is much more difficult to alter the craniofacial skeleton than it is to position teeth. It is possible, however, to direct the growth of the craniofacial skeleton in young children. In older patients, whose facial growth is mostly completed, the teeth are positioned to function better and to camouflage any disharmonies of the facial skeletal pattern. Finally, myotherapy is used to condition and train the neuromusculature as an important part of improved function and aesthetics. Orthodontic treatment may utilize many procedures, although perhaps the most frequent is the precise positioning of the individual teeth with orthodontic appliances. However, appliances for orthopedic correction of the craniofacial skeleton, surgery, myotherapy and even psychotherapy are all used in modern orthodontic practice.

C. The Purpose of This Book

Most books in orthodontics are written for the orthodontic specialist and intended for practitioners with considerable knowledge of the subject. This volume presupposes very little orthodontic background on the part of the reader. It really has two purposes: to serve as an introductory text for dental students and to supply basic orthodontic knowledge for the dentist who does not specialize in orthodontics.

Orthodontics has never occupied a large place in the dental curriculum; therefore, the teacher of orthodontics has the difficult job of presenting a complicated and exciting clinical field in just a few hours. Additionally, the basic science underlying orthodontics—growth and development—usually must be taught in the same orthodontic course also. The new dental graduate soon learns that he is more poorly prepared in orthodontics than in any other clinical field, yet he sees malocclusions every day. Which should he treat? How? Which should he refer? When? Which should he observe for later action? Why? In brief, every dental student and practitioner needs a source of facts concerning growth and orthodontics (1) to augment his formal lectures, (2) to extend his knowledge and (3) to provide a ready reference manual when confronted with clinical problems. Orthodontics is a part of dentistry; therefore, *all* dentists need some orthodontic knowledge if for no other reason than that most malocclusions are diagnosed first by the family dentist, not the orthodontist.

Sometimes it seems that there are two ways in orthodontics, a high road and a low. The high-road treatment is comprehensive, precise, well done and limited by expense to but a few. The high road is supposed to be the way of the specialist. Low-road treatment is thought to be clumsy, utilizing simpler appliances and compromised goals but providing some service for a large proportion of the population and is the way of family dentists. This myth of two quality levels in orthodontics is perpetuated by those who make extravagant or ill-founded claims, for example, "If you use this appliance, you never need to extract teeth"; "The periodontal response is different with this appliance"; "A cephalometric analysis is not necessary with this system"; "This is a general practitioner's appliance," etc. Of course, there is only one way in orthodontics—a way open to all dentists. Some, due to more training and experience, can travel further—that is all. Modern dentists dedicated to the highest standards in all other branches of dentistry do not accept the invitation to lower standards. They prefer to provide their patients with the best possible care, to travel the high road as far as their knowledge and skills will permit.

The purpose of this book is to help each dentist do all the orthodontics he can do and do well, for the biggest orthodontic question facing dentistry is how to extend good orthodontics to all who need it.

D. How to Use This Book

Since this volume is intended to be a handbook rather than an exhaustive text, its plan differs from that of many dental books. It is suggested that one first read the entire book in sequence, studying those portions of most interest. There should be no difficulty in using the book for consultation concerning clinical problems if the arrangement of the subject matter is understood. The book is divided into three sections, GROWTH AND DEVELOPMENT, DIAGNOSIS and TREATMENT, the outline of which can be seen in the Table of Contents. In addition, each chapter's outline is repeated at the beginning of the chapter.

In addition to the References cited at the end of some chapters, there also will be found a list of Suggested Readings. The latter are intended to aid the reader interested in pursuing further the subject under discussion.

Although it is quite true that one cannot move teeth without some sort of appliance, it is equally true that orthodontic treatment cannot be successful without a thorough knowledge of the underlying theory. More malocclusions are mismanaged because of ignorance of the facts of growth and diagnosis than due to lack of knowledge of appliances. Gadgetry is so much fun, but in orthodontics it is useless without basic knowledge. Section 3 will be of little use to the clinician unless he understands Sections 1 and 2 on GROWTH AND DEVELOPMENT and DIAGNOSIS.

When aid with a specific clinical problem is desired, the following procedure is suggested: (1) Locate that portion of Chapter XV where the problem is discussed. (2) While reading, compare the photographs and drawings with your problem. (3) Each section of Chapter XV follows this general order: (a) introduction to the problem, including a discussion of etiology, (b) differential diagnosis, (c) specific steps in treatment, (d) general discussion. As you read this section, make comparisons with the facts you have gathered concerning your case. (4) Refer back to earlier chapters, when it is indicated, for a more detailed discussion of the predisposing conditions of the case. As familiarity with the chapters on GROWTH AND DEVELOPMENT and DIAGNOSIS is gained, such references will be unnecessary. (5) During the discussion of steps in treatment, reference will be made to appliances whose construction is described in Chapter XVII.

Any material that might not be found readily in Chapter XV will be found in other parts of the book. The conditions that underlie a satisfactory plan of treatment are presented, but no attempt is made to describe all the possible methods of therapy for a given problem. Only one procedure, which will give adequate results in the hands of the nonspecialist doing orthodontic work, is described. It will be easy for most readers to think of other satisfactory methods of treatment, and any orthodontist who chances on these pages will know many ways of achieving similar results. The emphasis here, however, is on securing an adequate result with the technical knowledge that is known already or can be learned readily by the family dentist.

No book is a substitute for experience or good training, nor can any set of rules take the place of good judgment or spare one from thinking. Orthodontics, more than any other branch of dentistry, defies distillation to an ever-applicable axiom or procedure.

Ortega y Gasset[3] wrote about the economy of good teaching, that is, the presentation of the least amount of information that will provide the student with an understanding of the subject. Some books are written to impress the reader, some to provide an exhaustive source of material for reference; this book was written to be used in the daily practice of dentistry.

REFERENCES

1. Adamandios: Quoted by Haralabakis, H. N., Presidential Address, Tr. European Orthodont. Soc., pp. 45–47, 1964.
2. Hippocrates: *Epidemics VI,* 1, 2.
3. Ortega y Gasset, J.: *Mission of the University* (London: Routledge & Kegan Paul, Ltd., 1946).

GROWTH AND DEVELOPMENT

Basic Concepts of Growth and Development

Life is change; for when you are through changing, you are through.—BRUCE BARTON

A. Classes of alterations in biologic activities
  1. Short-term physiologic or morphologic alterations
  2. Long-term genetic and evolutionary changes
  3. Developmental events

B. Some definitions
  1. Growth
  2. Development
  3. Maturation

C. Divisions of growth and development
  1. Molecular biology
  2. Developmental biology
  3. Physical growth
  4. Behavioral development

D. Methods of studying physical growth and development
  1. Types of growth data
     a) Opinion
     b) Observations
     c) Ratings and rankings
     d) Quantitative measurements
  2. Methods of gathering growth data
     a) Longitudinal
     b) Cross-sectional
     c) Overlapping or semilongitudinal data
  3. Evaluation of growth data

E. Variables affecting physical growth
  1. Heredity
  2. Nutrition
  3. Illness

ALL OF US have been aware since early childhood that the basic characteristic of life is change. We have watched the short-term biologic activities of animals as they gather food, protect themselves, play and reproduce. We have noticed the slower changes in plants and animals that occur in response to the changing seasons. We have watched ourselves and our friends change as we get older. Biologic scientists make careful study of the various types of alterations in biologic activity.

A. Classes of Alterations in Biologic Activities

1. SHORT-TERM PHYSIOLOGIC OR MORPHOLOGIC ALTERATIONS

The skin may develop a bruise after trauma, the adrenalin titer of our blood rises and falls with changes in our emotions, our body temperature varies according to the time of day and general bodily activities and animal pelts show variations in color and texture with the seasons. All such alterations are sporadic biologic adjustments to changing environmental stimuli. The changes usually are reversible, the organism returning to a state not very different from what it was originally.

2. Long-Term Genetic and Evolutionary Changes

Basic alterations in the genetic make-up of an organism—mutations —may be inherited by offspring. If the mutation changes the organism in such a way that it cannot compete as well in its environment, it may not survive. On the other hand, the mutant may be better fitted for survival than its unchanged neighbors and thus the mutation contributes to the process of natural selection. The summation of the surviving mutations contributes to the evolution of many species. Long-term genetic and evolutionary changes are quite different from the short-term changes mentioned above. Much more time is needed for the new variety to be obvious in its population. Interest in the changes centers not on the individual but on the alterations in the genetic pool within the population. In order to understand the significance of genetic evolutionary changes, population biologists must study large populations within which genetic changes are occurring.

Fig. II-1.—Developmental events in the life cycle of a typical mammal. (After Sussman.[2])

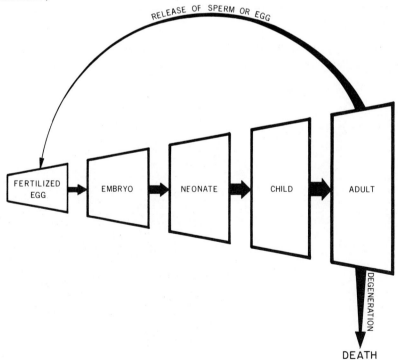

3. DEVELOPMENTAL EVENTS

There are changing biologic activities that occur in a progressive fashion in the life history of every organism and cannot be considered under the two preceding classifications. Let us consider the developmental events in the life cycle of a typical mammal (Fig. II-1). The pace of the changes diagramed is too slow to be included in the first category and far too fast for the second, but there are other important differences: all of the changes are progressive, sequential and irreversible, leaving the organism unalterably changed from its former state. Single cells develop as do unorganized populations of cells, specific organs and individuals. Developmental scientists are concerned with all of the changes in basic structure of an organism from conception to death.

B. Some Definitions

Semantic difficulties are present when the three words growth, development and maturation are considered. Each term carries concepts not present in the others and yet there is overlap (Fig. II-2). Sometimes they are synonyms, sometimes they are not. Their usage varies with the user and the fields of science.

1. GROWTH

Growth may be defined as the normal changes in amount of living substance. Growth is the quantitative aspect of biologic development

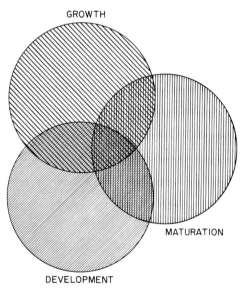

Fig. II-2.—Interaction of growth, development and maturation.

GROWTH

MATURATION

DEVELOPMENT

and is measured in units of increase per units of time, for instance, inches per year, grams per day, and so forth. Growth is the result of biologic processes by means of which living matter normally gets larger. It may be the direct result of cell division or the indirect product of biologic activity, e.g., bones and teeth. Typically, we equate growth with enlargement, but there are instances in which growth results in a normal decrease in size, for example, the thymus gland after puberty. Growth emphasizes the normal dimensional changes during development. Growth may result in increases or decreases in size, change in form or proportion, complexity, texture, and so forth.

2. DEVELOPMENT

Development may be defined as all the normal sequential series of events between fertilization of the ovum and the adult state. Using this definition, there are then three important aspects of development—growth, that is, increase in size, cellular differentiation and morphogenesis, that is, the processes whereby the adult form is achieved. Development brings about a more advanced, effective or complex state. It is the most embracing of the three terms.

3. MATURATION

Maturation means ripening—the stabilization of the adult state brought about by growth and development.

One may ask which term subsumes the expected changes that are seen with aging, i.e., degeneration, senility, etc. For some, it is a part of development. Others include such changes in the concept of maturation. Still others regard the changes of declination seen with old age as apart from growth, development and maturation.

C. Divisions of Growth and Development

Growth and developmental studies do not exist apart from other biologic disciplines or their technics. Studies of developmental events require the knowledge and methods of gross and microscopic anatomy, psychology, biochemistry, physiology, genetics, anthropology, etc. There are, however, four large divisions within the broad field of growth and development.

1. MOLECULAR BIOLOGY

During the 1920s and 1930s, physical scientists developed a fantastic array of exciting concepts and very precise new instrumentation, for example, the electron microscope. During the same time, the field of biochemistry was making equally important advances in concept and precise methods. When it became possible to work out the detailed roles of specific molecules in living systems by means of these new tools of biochemistry and biophysics (the study of physical phenomena in living processes), an exciting new era in biology began. We are in the midst of a biologic revolution that ultimately may be as important for man as the atomic revolution. The discovery of RNA and DNA and the cracking of the genetic code are among the most exciting events in the history of science. A large and amorphous scientific field now called molecular biology includes such fast-developing new disciplines as molecular genetics and biophysics.

2. DEVELOPMENTAL BIOLOGY

Since a fertilized egg starts as a single microscopic cell and eventually, by growth, development and maturation, becomes an adult of millions of cells, the biologists who study this fascinating series of events represent several special areas. The field of developmental biology includes workers from cellular biology, embryology, reproductive biology, perinatal biology and other fields.

3. PHYSICAL GROWTH

The field of physical growth is really the study of organ and body growth and includes analysis of such problems as morphogenesis, height and weight, growth rates, retarded growth, metabolic disturbances in growth, developmental physical fitness, pubescence, and so forth. Developmental scientists working in physical growth include pediatricians, anthropologists, endocrinologists, nutritionists and dentists. Dentistry can take some pride in the fact that research orthodontists probably have contributed more to the knowledge of the postnatal growth of the head and face than any other single discipline. Chapters III, IV, V and VI relate the physical growth of the head and face.

4. BEHAVIORAL DEVELOPMENT

As the child grows physically, he develops patterns of interaction with his environment, i.e., behavior. Behavior appears in typical sequences during development just as the physical attributes of the body appear in an expected pattern. Scientists studying behavioral development include embryologists, developmental psychologists, psychiatrists, physiologists, physiologic psychologists, geneticists, etc.

Previously we viewed these large divisions of growth and development as a linear spectrum from the molecule to the behaving adult individual, but the exciting new breakthroughs in molecular biology cause us to view these divisions in a more circular pattern. The molecular aspects of brain activity, for example, may provide the answers to how we think, reason, remember and forget.

D. Methods of Studying Physical Growth and Development

Clinical orthodontics is concerned mostly with the postnatal physical growth of the head and face. Therefore, a brief mention of the methods of studying physical growth is in order.

1. TYPES OF GROWTH DATA

a) Opinion

When Aunt Tillie says "My, how Johnny has grown. I do believe he's going to be taller than his father," no one really takes her seriously, for this is but a friendly lay opinion of growth prediction that is based on no quantitative data and is intended primarily as flattery. However, opinion does creep into our textbooks and scientific journals, where it is not so easily labeled as opinion, since one has a right to expect substantiated facts in such places. Opinion is, at best, a clever guess based on experience. Much scientific knowledge began as an intuitive hunch made by a careful observer, so opinions are not to be derided. However, they are the crudest form of scientific knowledge and are not to be accepted when better data are available. They should always be designated for what they are—one man's biased guess.

b) Observations

Observations are useful for studying all-or-none phenomena, for example, congenital absence of teeth. Observations also are used in a limited way when more quantitative data are not possible, for example, "In cursory visual examination of 67 Eskimo children ranging between 6 and 11 years, not one case of Class II malocclusion was observed."

c) Ratings and Rankings

Certain data are difficult to quantify and thus are compared to conventional rating scales. Such scales may be based on developmental stages, on typical forms or patterns or on standard color charts. The method is used for the evaluation of breast development, the pubic and axillary hair patterns, ear shape, eye color, fingerprints, etc. Whereas ratings make use of comparisons with conventional accepted scales or classifications, rankings array data in ordered sequences according to value. Thus, one reads such statements in the literature as "When the 10 tallest boys were compared to the 10 shortest boys in the sample it was found . . ."

d) Quantitative Measurements

Science is concerned with quantitation. Indeed, if one cannot express an idea or a fact as a meaningful quantity, he scarcely has begun to think about it in a scientific way. Quantitation minimizes misunderstanding and permits the testing of hypotheses by other workers. Any scientist has the right to be skeptical of another's opinion, no matter how renowned the holder of that opinion, until it can be reduced to numbers for testing and further study.

(1) *Direct data.* Direct growth data are measurements taken on the living child or cadaver by means of calipers, scales, measuring tapes, etc.

(2) *Indirect growth measurements* are those taken from images or reproductions of the actual person, for example, measurements made from photographs, dental casts or cephalograms.

(3) *Derived data.* These data are obtained by comparing two other measurements. When we say that the mandible grew 2 mm. between ages 7 and 8, the 2 mm. have not actually been measured; rather, the mandibular length at 7 years has been subtracted from the mandibular length at 8 years and the increment thus derived.

2. METHODS OF GATHERING GROWTH DATA

a) Longitudinal: Measurements made of the same person or group at regular intervals through time.

(1) *Advantages of the longitudinal method*

Variability in development among individuals within the group is thrown into perspective.

The specific pattern of an individual as he develops can be studied, permitting serial comparisons with himself.

Temporary temporal problems in sampling are smoothed out with time and an unusual event or a mistake in measuring at a given time is seen more easily and corrections made more properly.

(2) *Disadvantages of the longitudinal method*

Time. If one wishes to study the growth of the human face from birth to adulthood by means of longitudinal data, it will take him a lifetime to gather the data.

Expense. Longitudinal studies necessitate the maintenance of laboratories, research personnel and data storage for a long time and thus are costly.

Attrition. The parents of children in longitudinal studies change their places of residence or lose interest in the study and some children die. The result is a gradual diminution in sample size. The attrition in a typical longitudinal study often reaches 50% in 15 years.

b) Cross-sectional: A different individual or a different sample is studied at different periods. Thus, one may measure a group of 7-year-old boys and on the same day, at the same school, measure a group of 8-year-old boys. Changes between 7 and 8 years of age in boys at that school are thus assumed after study of the data obtained.

(1) *Advantages of the cross-sectional method*

Speed.
Cost.
Sample size.

It is much easier to get large samples by the cross-sectional method, and thus the statistical treatment of the data sometimes is made easier.
The method allows repeating of studies more readily.
The method is used for cadavers, skeletons and archaeologic data.

(2) *Disadvantages of the cross-sectional method*

It must always be assumed that the groups being measured and compared are similar.
Cross-sectional group averages tend to obscure individual variations. This is particularly obfuscating when studying the timing of developmental events, for example, the onset of pubescence or the adolescent growth spurt.

c) Overlapping or semilongitudinal data: The two methods are combined by some workers to seek the advantages of each. In this way, one might compress 15 years of study into 3 years of gathering data, each subsample including children studied for the same number of years but started at different ages. For example, subsample A may go from 3 to 6 years of age, subsample B from 4 to 7, subsample C from 5 to 8, etc.

3. EVALUATION OF GROWTH DATA

The evaluation of growth data is one of the most complicated and fascinating branches of statistics. Many facts of growth lie hidden in clinicians' or scientists' crude hunches and can be bared for further study only by careful and imaginative statistical dissection. Those who deride statistical studies of growth and clinical data usually are totally ignorant of the possibilities of modern statistical methods. Although the statistical treatment of biologic data is beyond the scope of this book, it must be mentioned that, in my opinion, an introductory working knowledge of statistics is a necessity for every physician and dentist; otherwise, the reader of scientific journals has no way of evaluating the significance of the findings presented.

E. Variables Affecting Physical Growth

Variability may be seen in the rate, timing or character of growth as well as the achieved or ultimate size.

1. HEREDITY

Genetic studies of physical growth make use of twin and family data. Differences between monozygotic and dizygotic twins are assumed to be differences due to environment. There is genetic control of size of parts to a great extent, of the rate of growth and of the onset of growth events, e.g., menarche, dental calcification or the eruption of teeth. Chapter IV includes a discussion of the genetic aspects of craniofacial growth and Chapter VI includes a discussion of the genetic aspects of dentitional growth.

2. Nutrition

Malnutrition during childhood delays growth, and the adolescent spurt in growth, "catch-up growth," appears when a favorable nutritional regimen is supplied early enough. "Catch-up" growth does not always restore the individual to the size he would have been with no malnutrition, and "catch-up" growth is not so dramatic when severe and prolonged malnutrition has been experienced. Malnutrition may affect size of parts, body proportions, body chemistry and the quality and texture of certain tissues, for example, bone and teeth.

3. Illness

Systemic disease has an effect on child growth, but the plasticity of the human organism during growth is so great that the clinician must differentiate between minor illnesses and major illnesses. The usual minor childhood illnesses ordinarily cannot be shown to have much effect on physical growth. On the other hand, serious prolonged and debilitating illnesses have a marked effect on growth. The pediatrician is concerned not only with the diseases that may kill or maim the child but with those that affect the growth process as well. Some of the effects of disease on facial growth are discussed in Chapter IV.

4. Race

The physical anthropologist studying the racial aspects of growth has a problem in the definition of race as well as in the separation of socioeconomic from racial factors. With the precise control of all variables other than race, it can be shown that there are racial differences of some significance in birth weight, height and weight, growth rate and the onset of various maturational indicators, e.g., menarche, ossification of bones, dental calcification and tooth eruption.

5. Climate and Seasonal Effect on Growth

There is a general tendency for those living in cold climates to have a greater proportion of adipose tissue, and much has been made of the skeletal variations associated with variations in climate. There are seasonal variations in the amount of growth rate of children and in the weights of newborn babies.

6. Adult Physique

There are correlations between the adult physique and earlier developmental events; for example, tall women tend to mature later as well as having variations in the rate of growth with differing somatotypes.

7. SOCIOECONOMIC FACTORS

This category obviously includes some overlapping with factors mentioned previously, e.g., nutrition; yet, there are discrete differences. Children living in favorable socioeconomic conditions tend to be larger, display different types of growth (e.g., height-weight ratios) and to show variation in the timing of growth, when compared to disadvantaged children. Some of the causes of these differences are obvious and some of the implications are interesting. As our society becomes more affluent, how long will we get bigger and mature earlier? Are such changes really an improvement? It is interesting to note that many of the positive relationships are associated with socioeconomic "class" and not family income.

8. EXERCISE

A strong case for the beneficial effects of exercise on growth has not been made in a quantitative fashion. Although it may be useful for the development of motor skills, for fitness and general well-being, those children who exercise strenuously and regularly have not been shown to grow more favorably.

9. FAMILY SIZE AND BIRTH ORDER

There are differences in the size of individuals, in their maturational level of achievement and in their intelligence that can be correlated with the size of the family from which they came. First-born children tend to weigh less at birth and ultimately achieve less stature and a higher I.Q.

10. SECULAR TRENDS

Size and maturational changes can be shown to be occurring with time that, as yet, have not been well explained. Fifteen-year-old boys are approximately 5 inches taller than 15-year-old boys were 50 years ago. The average age at onset of menarche has steadily become earlier throughout the entire world. Both of these facts are true when race, socioeconomic level, nutrition, climate, etc. have been carefully controlled. Such changes are called secular trends in growth, and, although thoroughly and meticulously studied, no really satisfactory explanation has yet been offered for these very interesting findings.

F. Pattern

1. DEFINITION

In developmental biology, pattern means a series of developmental phases in invariant order. The developmental pattern may be typical for an individual, his family, subspecies, species, etc. In facial growth, the word pattern usually means that we tend to look like we did earlier, like other members of our family and other members of the same racial or ethnic group. Such comments as "Johnny has always been tall for his age" and "All the Joneses erupt their teeth early" express concepts of individual and family pattern.

2. CONTRIBUTIONS TO PATTERN

Pattern, of course, is based on the genetic apparatus and its typical interactions with the environment. A number of factors contribute to pattern:

a) Differential growth rates.
b) Varying gradients of growth: Law of Developmental Direction, that is, there is a tendency, most obvious during prenatal growth, for the body to grow cephalically before caudally, medially before laterally and dorsally before ventrally.
c) Evolutionary trends, for example, man is in the process of losing certain of his teeth; in a few million years, he may have no third molars, maxillary lateral incisors or mandibular second bicuspids.

3. CLINICAL IMPLICATIONS

There is much glib talk about "facial pattern." The concept of pattern is extremely important in orthodontics, but it is not easily quantitated and care must be taken to avoid adopting specific clinical procedures based on loosely defined ideas of "pattern." Treatment can be no more accurate than the idea on which the therapy is based, and the idea of facial pattern as it usually is discussed is most subjective.

G. Variability

Infinite variability is the law of nature. Because of the infinite number of genetic possibilities, no two individuals (except perhaps identical twins) are ever exactly alike. Variations in response to environment cause increasing differences between similar individuals with time. Variability may be demonstrated in many ways. In physical growth, it usually is done by statistical comparisons to a large population of individuals of similar age, sex and racial background. Such comparisons usually evoke the question "What is normal?"

1. CONCEPTS OF NORMALITY

There are a number of different ways to discuss normality, but all carry the connotation of the typical or expected for the group.

a) Statistical—In statistics, there are specific mathematical ways for portraying the central tendency of a group or population; for example, the *mean* (an average of values), the *median* (that value midway between the greatest and smallest measurement, i.e., an average of position) and the *mode* (the most frequent measurement, i.e., an average of popularity or frequency).

b) Evolutionary—All forms of life today have passed the critical test of survival. Bizarre and abnormal forms, unable to cope, have been lost.

c) Functional—It is normal for most biologic forms to establish effective homeostasis with the environment in order to adapt and survive.

d) Aesthetics—Often we forget the role that culture plays in determining what within a given group is considered normal. The feet of baby girls have been bound to produce warped, distorted growth, wooden plates have been inserted into the lips of females, scarring of of the face has been practiced, and so forth. What one would consider normal for the feet, the lips or the facial musculature would, of course, be affected, in these instances, by the particular cultural concepts of aesthetics.

e) Clinical—In dentistry, too often we have equated the term "normal" with ideal. Almost every textbook of dentistry includes a picture of "normal occlusion," showing a perfect intercuspation of 32 permanent teeth. The probabilities of such an intercuspation appearing in an individual are very small and thus, from a statistical standpoint, very abnormal. Normal must not be equated with the ideal or the desired, nor is normal appropriate as a goal of treatment for an individual. Rather, it should be thought of as the central tendency for the group. Normal measurements are not necessarily found in any one individual of the group.

There are obvious conflicts among these various concepts of normality. The semantic difficulties must not interfere with the clear thinking needed for understanding growth or planning treatment.

2. AGE EQUIVALENCE

Because individuals develop in different patterns, producing variability, all individuals of a given chronologic age are neither necessarily of the same size nor the same stage of maturation and development. A problem is thus posed for the clinician and the developmental scientist, viz., how does one compare individuals of the same chronologic age but varying stages of biologic development? A number of "developmental ages" have been suggested as a method of meeting this problem. Thus, one hears of skeletal age (SA), usually based on the carpal calcification, dental age (DA), based on the number of teeth calcified or erupted, chronologic age (CA), expressed as years and months from birth, mental age (MA), based on the mental maturity of the individual, and so forth. Thus, a 7-year-old boy (CA) may have a dental age (DA) of 6 and a mental age (MA) of 8, etc. For the study of a given problem in growth, it often is better to compare individuals at the same stage of biologic development rather than at the same chronologic age.

3. SIGNIFICANCE OF VARIABILITY

The significance of variation from the norm for the group in which an individual is found can be understood only if the individual's present status is thought of in terms of his progress toward *his own* goal rather than rigidly comparing him to the group's progress toward *its* goal. It thus becomes necessary to appraise the growth of the individual and to compare him to his own pattern in the light of his familial tendency and the larger group to which he belongs (see Section I, The Evaluation of Physical Growth, below). Gross variation from the central tendency, also may be indicative of pathology or a grossly abnormal pattern of growth that will markedly affect treatment.

H. Timing

The timing of developmental events is largely under genetic control, yet varied by the nutritional state, disease history, etc., which the developmental scientist is interested in when growth processes are "turned on," for example, pubescence, or when they cease, for example, stature increments. The age of maximum growth increments—the adolescent spurt—is not only of developmental interest but is used as a marker for timing other growth events (Fig. II-3).

There are sex differences in timing of many growth phenomena. Usually, girls precede boys, for example, pubescence, dental calcifica-

Fig. II-3.—Variations in growth rate according to developmental period. (After Björk.[1])

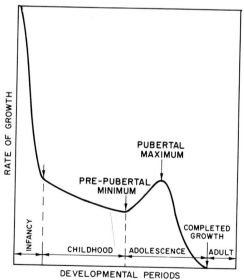

tion, ossification of carpal bones. Further, there are differences related to physique, for example, taller children tend to reach the adolescent spurt later than short-legged, stocky types. The effects of disease on the timing of growth and "catch-up" growth have been mentioned earlier.

Nowhere is timing more critical than in the fusion of facial parts in early prenatal growth (see Chapter III). When dental and facial skeletal growth are not synchronized, some malocclusions are produced and others aggravated. Much of this book deals with the problem of mal-timed developmental events in the face.

I. The Evaluation of Physical Growth

1. *Why assess?*

The clinician is interested in assessing physical growth for the following reasons:
  a) The identification of grossly abnormal growth or even pathologic growth.
  b) The recognition and diagnosis of significant deviations from normal growth.
  c) The planning of therapy.
  d) The determination of the efficacy of therapy.

Unless the clinician has a clear and quantitative assessment of growth at the start of treatment, it will be impossible for him later to evaluate how well any treatment has progressed.

2. *Questions to be asked*

  a) What is the *status* of the patient at the moment? Most of the time, the clinician must base his judgments on a single examination and therefore must determine status of the individual by cross-sectional evaluation alone.

  b) What is the *progress* of growth to date? Sometimes serial records are available and longitudinal comparisons to the patient's own pattern of development can be made.

  c) How does he *compare* with others? Comparison with others of the same age, sex and race is done with derived growth standards, but the abuse of growth standards is a sad and unfortunate story. Most of the mistakes in the use of growth standards are due to two problems in understanding: (1) the choice of the appropriate standard and (2) the nature of biologic variability. Unless the standards have been derived from a population applicable to the problem at hand, it is better not to use standards at all. Indeed, for many problems in facial growth as it relates to clinical practice, appropriate standards are not yet available. Furthermore, to choose one or two mean values from a biased sample and to apply them rigidly to all individuals with no understanding of the entire craniofacial complex and the adaptations and reasons for the variations from the mean is naïve and ridiculous and handicaps planning the treatment.

d) How does he fit the *family pattern?* Only recently have quantitative studies of familial tendency in facial growth appeared in the literature, yet much can be learned by studying records of siblings and parents. Most orthodontists believe that they can treat the second child in a family better because of what they learned from treating the first.

e) What will he do in the *future?* The prediction of craniofacial growth is one of the liveliest topics in the literature today. As yet, one can only predict coarsely the growth of an individual from data derived from populations that have been studied serially. It would be ideal if the dentist studying one cephalogram could make useful quantitative predictions concerning the growth of that patient. Much can be learned, but the estimates are more qualitative description than precise prognostication, more clinical art than science. However; no one should begin orthodontic treatment without estimating to the best of his ability what can be expected in the future. The direction, amount, site and timing of growth affect the treatment and the retention of the results of treatment.

3. *General growth standards*

The evaluation of the physical growth of the total child is a large field of science in itself. Many methods have been devised to appraise height, weight, skeletal development, muscle strength, the onset of pubescence, and so forth. Ingenious and complicated formulae of growth have resulted in many clever graphic methods of portraying growth standards so that the individual may be compared to norms. Such evaluations of physical growth are done daily in pediatric and dental practice (see Chapter VIII), but there is always the danger of oversimplification of the complexity of growth by assuming that any one or two measurements truly reveal the progress of physical growth.

REFERENCES

1. Björk, A.: Prediction of age of maximum puberal growth in body height, Angle Orthodont. 37:134, 1967.
2. Sussman, M.: *Growth and Development.* Foundations of Modern Biology Series (2d ed.; Englewood Cliffs, N.J.: Prentice-Hall, Inc., 1964).

SUGGESTED READINGS

Falkner, F.: *Human Development* (Philadelphia: W. B. Saunders Company, 1966).
Watson, E. H., and Lowrey, G. H.: *Growth and Development of Children* (5th ed.; Chicago: Year Book Medical Publishers, Inc., 1967).

III

Prenatal Facial Growth

JAMES K. AVERY, D.D.S., Ph.D.

Professor of Dentistry, The University of Michigan School of Dentistry, and Professor of Anatomy, The University of Michigan Medical School

> The history of man for the nine months preceding his birth would, probably, be far more interesting and contain events of greater moment than all the three score and ten years that follow it.—SAMUEL TAYLOR COLERIDGE, *Miscellanies, Aesthetic, and Literary*

A. Period of organization of the face

   1. The branchial arches
   2. Development of the perioral region
   3. Changes in facial proportions
   4. Origin of facial malformations

B. Development of oral structures

   1. Development of the tongue
   2. Elevation of the palatal shelves
   3. Factors in normal palatal development
   4. Fusion of the palatal shelves
   5. Tooth development
   6. Salivary gland development

C. Differentiation of supporting structures

   1. Development of the chondrocranium
   2. Development of the maxillary complex
   3. Development of the bony palate
   4. Mandible and temporomandibular joint
   5. Facial muscles
   6. Muscles of mastication

D. The fetal period—third to ninth month

   1. Craniofacial changes
   2. Radiographic changes

A. Period of Organization of the Face

1. THE BRANCHIAL ARCHES

Differentiation of the human face takes place early in prenatal life, specifically between the fifth and seventh weeks after fertilization occurs. During this short period, a number of important events occur that determine the formation of the human face.

In the fourth week after conception, the future face and neck region located under the forebrain of the human embryo become segmented (Fig. III-1, *A*). Five branchial arches are formed, appearing as rounded tubular enlargements, and are bounded by clefts and grooves that help define each arch. They are numbered beginning anteriorly. The mid and lower facial regions develop, in part, from the first two, named the mandibular and hyoid arches. The third also contributes to the base of the tongue. Within each of these branchial arches arise skeletal, muscular, vascular, connective tissue, epithelial and neural elements that develop into the systems supplying the face and neck. Most of the structures of the adult face thus develop from the first and second branchial arches and from tissues surrounding the forebrain. In the early period of development, i.e., the fourth week, it is difficult to distinguish the primary craniofacial features of the human embryo from those of other mammals (Fig. III-1, *A*).

The human face is first characterized by an invagination or dimple in the surface ectoderm layer appearing just below the forebrain. As this pit deepens, it forms the outline of the oral cavity (Fig. III-2, *A*). The

Fig. III-1.—Human embryos at 5 weeks (**A**) and at 7 weeks (**B**). This is the morphologic appearance of the human face during the 2-week time period during which the face develops.

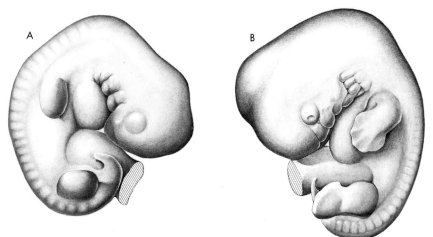

tissue masses immediately surrounding this oral pit will form the human face. In the fourth week, the posterior boundary of the oral pit comes into contact with the developing foregut. As the ectodermal oral plate meets the entodermal lining of the gut, the membranes disintegrate, and continuity between the oral cavity and the gastrointestinal tract is first gained. At 5 weeks (Fig. III-1, *A*), the "face" appears crowded between the rapidly growing forebrain and by the heart, which occupies much of the chest cavity at this stage. The nonfunctioning, developing lungs are still quite small, composed mainly of conducting bronchi, until the respiratory bronchioles begin to form in the fourth month. As the lungs do not function in respiration until after birth, the oxygen needs are supplied from the placenta through the umbilical veins to the heart. The heart, however, must function at a very early age. It becomes conspicuous by its size in the third week and initiates a beat in the fourth week of embryonic life.[11] During the prenatal period, the heart not only pumps blood throughout the body of the embryo but also conducts blood to, through and from the placental system back to this heart. The heart is proportionately much larger at this time than it will be in the adult body and, therefore, requires much space for its proper development. The growth of the heart affects the development of the face, not only because of the importance of the blood supply to its development but also because the face during its early period of rapid growth and organization is crowded between the enlarging forebrain and the pulsating heart. Even at this early stage, the growth pattern of the face is downward and forward as it grows out from between these two organs. Important related occurrences are the flexures that occur during the fourth week in the region of the future neck. The brain flexes ventrally, then dorsally and, as a result, the head becomes more erect.

2. DEVELOPMENT OF THE PERIORAL REGION

The "face" at the fifth week is about as thick as the sheet of paper from which you are reading, and the whole face is only about 1½ mm. wide. At this time, the oral pit is bounded above by the frontal area and below by the mandibular arch, which appears shovel shaped (Fig. III-2, *B*). A midline groove is apparent, disappearing during the sixth week. At this time, two small, oval, raised areas appear just above the lateral aspects of the future mouth. In the next 48 hours, the centers of these raised areas become depressions as the tissues around them continue to grow anteriorly (Fig. III-2, *C*). The depressions deepen into pits that will become the future nostrils and the masses surrounding them—the bridge and the sides of the external nose. The tissue between the nasal pits is termed the medial nasal process and those lateral to the pits are called lateral nasal processes. These tissues originate from the superficial epithelial and connective tissues of the frontal area as they all grow downward and forward (Fig. III-2, *C*). The raised anterior

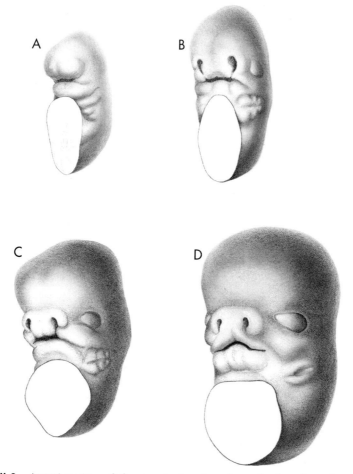

Fig. III-2.—Anterior view of the developing face from the fourth to the eighth prenatal week. The remainder of the body was removed to reveal the face. At 4 weeks (**A**), the future face is indicated by the bulging forebrain and the first branchial arch immediately below it. By 6 weeks (**B**), the oral slit is noted with nasal pits appearing above it. The eyes appear on the sides of the head. The mandibular arch bounds the oral slit below. At 6½ weeks (**C**), the eyes are nearer the front of the face. The nose is defined and the developing ears appear at the corners of the mouth. At 8 weeks (**D**), the masses comprising the face have fused together to bound the oral cavity and the forebrain has begun its forward growth, leaving the ears behind.

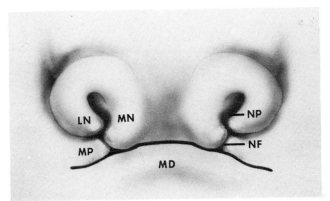

Fig. III-3.—The development of the upper lip. The maxillary processes (*MP*) fuse with the medial nasal processes (*MN*) to form the floor of the nostril. The lateral nasal processes (*LN*) enlarge to form the sides of the nose. The slit below the nostrils is the nasal fin (*NF*) and is the potential cleft lip site. The mandible (*MD*) is below the oral pit. NP = nasal pit.

edges of these pits form the shape of minute horseshoes, with the open sides below (Fig. III-3). As they grow forward, the inferior ends of the horseshoes come into contact (Fig. III-4). The distance between these two nasal pits does not increase during this important period of development, although the pits themselves increase in both height and length.[14]

Since the tissue underlying each nostril represents the first separation of the nasal cavity from the oral cavity, it has been designated the primary palate by some authors.[11] The mode of formation of these pits is important, since a failure in any of the steps in their development may

Fig. III-4.—Frontal section of the upper face showing the nasal pits (*NP*) and forming nasal fins (*NF*). *LN* = lateral nasal processes; *MN* = medial nasal processes; *MP* = maxillary processes; *MD* = mandible.

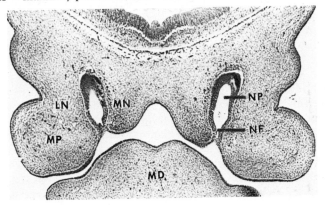

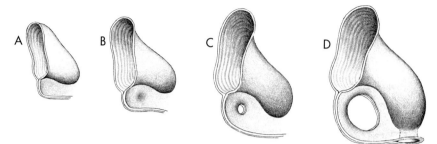

Fig. III-5.—The development of the floor of the nostril and the nasal fin below it. **A** and **B**, as the nostril elongates, the epithelium of the maxillary and medial nasal processes fuse together and an opening appears through which connective tissue of the lip grows. **C**, as the tissue of the lip is unified, it forms the primary palate, which is a small mass of tissue bounded by the oral cavity below and the nostril above. **D**, posteriorly, the nasal pit opens into the roof of the oral cavity by splitting of the two sheets of epithelium.

result in a cleft lip. These steps in fusion of the lip are illustrated in Figure III-5. Step 1 can be defined as the contact between the medial border of the maxillary process and the lateral border of the medial nasal process. The two epithelial-covered processes together form a lamina termed the "nasal fin" (Figs. III-3–III-5). As soon as contact and adhesion of two epithelial sheets occurs, they become fused into a single sheet and then degeneration of this sheet occurs, resulting in connective tissue penetration through the sheet (Fig. III-5, *B* and *C*). This area of penetration expands rapidly and the nasal fin is eliminated except at its anterior and posterior limits. In this way, the lip is unified and separation of the floor of the pits in the form of a cleft is prevented. The tissue underlying the nasal pit is termed the primary palate since it does form a bridge separating the primitive nasal cavity and oral cavity. At the posterior limits of the epithelial fin, the same two epithelial sheets split apart, producing an opening between the nasal pits and the roof of the oral cavity[13] (Fig. III-5, *D*). This posterior opening of the nasal pit is termed the internal nares and is the posterior limit of the primary palate. Later, the nasal cavities enlarge posteriorly to form a space overlying the entire oral cavity. The oral and nasal cavities are then separated by the secondary palatal shelves. These shelves are termed the "secondary palate," as they are secondary to the primary palate and close this anterior nasal opening, causing the resulting nasal cavity to open posteriorly in the nasopharynx (see Fig. III-10). The failure of any of these rather complex developmental steps to occur in sequence and at the approximate interval of time may be, in part, the reason why these congenital defects are some of the most common today. One in every 800 births results in either cleft lip, cleft palate or the combined defect.

In summary, lip development is a three-stage process, the first being contact of the two epithelial sheets covering the adjacent processes, the second, fusion of the epithelium into a single sheet and, finally, a penetration of this sheet by connective tissue of the lip growing through it. The developing eyelids are an example of two epithelial laminae that come into tight contact but do not fuse or undergo connective tissue penetration. They simply remain closed, with their surfaces fused, until the seventh prenatal month, at which time they open, exposing the eyes.

In the sixth week, the upper face appears flat and broad, with the nasal pits positioned on the lateral corners of the face. The distance between the nasal pits represents approximately 90% of the width of the face. Lateral to this region are the maxillary processes, which appear at this stage as triangular or wedge-shaped masses located at the superior lateral aspects of the oral cavity (see Fig. III-3). At 6 weeks, the mandibular arch appears broad and flat and comprises the lower border of the oral cavity. In the midline, a slight constriction still can be seen, and laterally the auricle of the ear will arise from six small hillocks of tissue that appear to circumscribe the branchial cleft positioned between the mandibular and hyoid arches (see Fig. III-1, *A* and *B*). Three of the hillocks arise from the mandibular arch and the three below the cleft arise from the hyoid arch. The first branchial slit later will become the external auditory canal (see Fig. III-2, *C* and *D*).

3. CHANGES IN FACIAL PROPORTIONS

Three or 4 days later, at 6½ weeks, the facial proportions appear to have changed greatly, due to an increase in dimension laterally to the nasal pits. There has been, in this short span of time, an expansion of the anterior region of the brain, causing the lateral maxillary regions to move to the front of the face. Thus, the eyes and adjacent cheek tissues are rotated 90 degrees from the sides to the front of the face because of this differential growth. The medial nasal area now makes up only the relatively small medial segment of the upper lip. The medial nasal tissue interposes between the maxillary wedges at this stage and will become the site of the future philtrum of the upper lip* (see Fig. III-2, *D*).

Early in the seventh week, the face appears recognizably human as a result of the frontal location of the eyes, differentiation of the nose and enlargement of the mandible (see Fig. III-2, *D*). Later, as the face increases in height, the nostrils will no longer be on the same horizontal plane as the eyes. At the seventh week, the furrows separating the

---

*The medial nasal process does not occur in the rabbit, which has a shallow cleft at the midline, hence the term "harelip." It is a misnomer, however, to define the human cleft as a "harelip," since a cleft rarely occurs in the midline; rather, it appears laterally between the medial nasal and maxillary processes. The rare midline cleft occurs when the globular and medial nasal processes do not merge properly (see Fig. III-4).

mandibular, maxillary and nasal areas are less marked. The external ears are now visible, having differentiated from the auricular hillocks. It is of interest that such complex structures as our external ears can arise from six small and initially uniform enlargements. The ear will appear well differentiated by the sixteenth prenatal week.[11]

4. ORIGIN OF FACIAL MALFORMATIONS

The movement of the lateral portions of the face to the front results in furrows in the tissue masses between the optic and oral regions. These furrows mark the lines where oblique clefts of the face may occur. The furrow between the lateral nasal process and the eye marks the anterior boundary of the maxillary processes, and the nasolacrimal system develops beneath this furrow. Abnormal merging of the maxillary and lateral nasal processes may occur and a lip cleft that would already be present at this stage may thus continue laterally as an oro-naso-optic cleft. Again, failure of merging at the corners of the mouth between the maxillary and mandibular tissues produces a macrostomia or enlarged mouth. The sixth and a half prenatal week is an important age in human facial development, for at this time all of the areas of potential malformation of the external face are apparent (see Fig. III-2, *C*).

B. Development of Oral Structures

1. DEVELOPMENT OF THE TONGUE

The tongue musculature originates from the occipital myotomes at the beginning of the fourth week.[1] As it grows anteriorly into the floor of the mouth, it carries forward its nerve and blood supply from more posterior regions and develops into an oral part (the body) and into a pharyngeal part (the base). The body arises, in part, from contributions of the first branchial arch, and the base arises from the second, third and fourth arches. The body of the tongue is indicated by three primodia, the paired lateral lingual swellings and a centrally located tuberculum impar (Fig. III-6, *A*). At the fifth week, the base of the tongue is indicated by a median elevation, the copula. Between the copula and the tuberculum impar a small pit appears, termed the foramen caecum, which gives origin to the thyroid gland tissue. During the sixth and seventh weeks, the lateral lingual swellings enlarge and relatively reduce the size of the tuberculum impar. A furrow appears along the lateral borders of the tongue, separating it from the developing alveolar ridges (Fig. III-6, *B*). The two lateral lingual swellings then merge and the body of the tongue appears as a more unified structure (Fig. III-6, *C*). The tongue grows so rapidly that it pushes into the nasal cavity above and between the two palatine shelves (Fig. III-7, *B*), and by the eighth and a half or ninth week the muscles of the body of the tongue appear clearly differentiated (Fig. III-7, *C*). Thus, the oral and nasal cavities

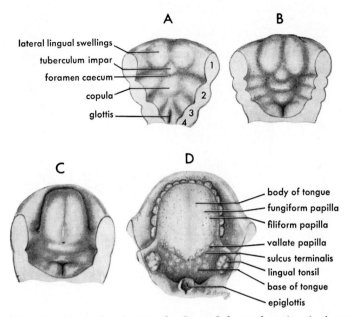

A

B

lateral lingual swellings
tuberculum impar
foramen caecum
copula
glottis

1
2
3
4

C

D

body of tongue
fungiform papilla
filiform papilla
vallate papilla
sulcus terminalis
lingual tonsil
base of tongue
epiglottis

Fig. III-6.—The tongue develops in the floor of the oral cavity. At 4 weeks (**A**), the tongue is composed of small swellings. The numbers refer to the four branchial arches. At 5 weeks (**B**), the body and base of the tongue increase in size. At 6½ weeks (**C**), the body is merged into a single mass and the base develops from the copula. The postnatal tongue (**D**) appears broad and flat, with surface specializations of papillae on the body and lymph nodules on the base. (From Steele, P., *Dimensions of Dental Hygiene* [Philadelphia: Lea & Febiger, 1966], p. 287.)

originate from the single stomodeal cavity and become separated as the palatal shelves elevate and grow between them.

2. ELEVATION OF THE PALATAL SHELVES

As the enlarging tongue pushes dorsally into the nasal cavity, the less-differentiated palatal shelves, because of limited space, are forced downward to the floor of the mouth along either side of the tongue (Fig. III-7, *B*). The next critical step in palatal development results in the movement of the palatal shelves from a vertical position beside the tongue to a horizontal position overlying the tongue. This change in position probably involves movement of both the tongue and palatal shelves (Fig. III-8). As the shelves roll over the tongue posteroanteriorly, the tongue may glide anteriorly to offer less resistance to the shelf movement.[15] Closure of the palatal shelves over the tongue separates the oral and nasal cavities (Fig. III-7, *C* and *D*). The tongue may press upward against the palatal shelves, helping to bring them into closer

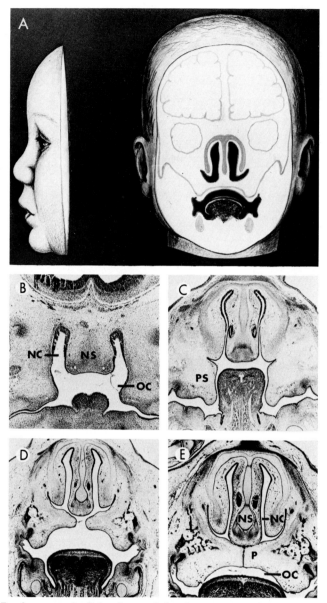

Fig. III-7.—A, removal of the front of the face reveals the relationship of the developing tongue to the palate. At 6 weeks (**B**), the tongue is a small mass of undifferentiated tissue. At 7 weeks (**C**), the enlarged and differentiated tongue extends up into the nasal cavities. The palatal shelves (*PS*) are beside the tongue. At 8½ weeks (**D**), the palatal shelves appear above the tongue. At 10 weeks (**E**), the palatal shelves fuse together to delimit the nasal and oral cavities. (From Shapiro, M. [ed.], *The Scientific Bases of Dentistry* [Philadelphia: W. B. Saunders Company, 1966], p. 77.)

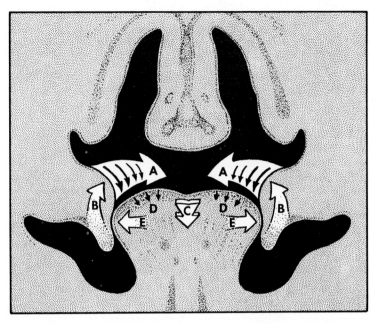

Fig. III-8.—This diagram indicates the movements of the palatal shelves and tongue during palate closure. The tongue moves anteriorly (*C*), depressing downward (*D*) and laterally (*E*) as the palatal shelves slide from *B* to *A* over the tongue.

approximation to facilitate their contact in the midline. These movements of palatal closure may be quite rapid, possibly occurring with about the same speed as when one swallows (Fig. III-8). The process occurs between the eighth and ninth weeks after conception in the human, when, as investigators have shown, the para-oral structures of the human respond to stimulation.[7] It is possible that the nerve supply to the tongue and cheeks is thus sufficiently developed to provide some neuromuscular guidance to this intricate function.

3. Factors in Normal Palatal Development

Other activities, such as bringing the head to an erect position, may be related to the elevation of the palatal shelves.[16] As the head elevates, the neck becomes recognizable and the face is no longer pressed against the thoracic cavity, due partially to settling of the heart more inferiorly in the thorax. At this time, spontaneous movements of the head, elevation of the lower jaw, opening of the mouth and movement of the tongue occur for the first time[7] (see Chapter V). Deficiencies of oxygen, various foodstuffs or vitamins have been reported experimentally to cause

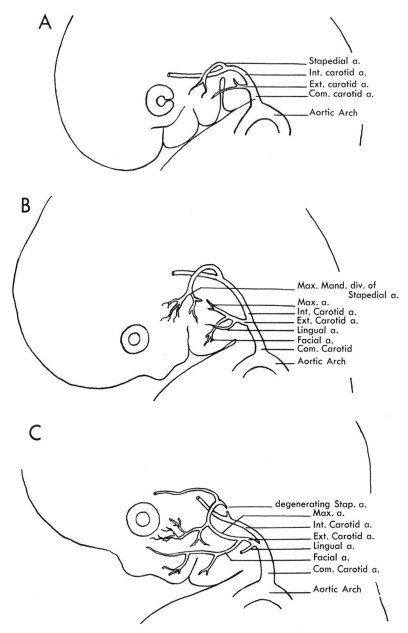

A
Stapedial a.
Int. carotid a.
Ext. carotid a.
Com. carotid a.
Aortic Arch

B
Max. Mand. div. of
Stapedial a.
Max. a.
Int. Carotid a.
Ext. Carotid a.
Lingual a.
Facial a.
Com. Carotid
Aortic Arch

C
degenerating Stap. a.
Max. a.
Int. Carotid a.
Ext. Carotid a.
Lingual a.
Facial a.
Com. Carotid a.
Aortic Arch

Fig. III-9.—Three stages of shift in blood supply from the internal to the external carotid. At 6 weeks (**A**), the flood supply to the face is from the stapedial branch of the internal carotid. At 6½ weeks (**B**), the stapedial has expanded into the maxillary and mandibular divisions. At 7 weeks (**C**), the stapedial detaches from the internal carotid and its terminal branches join the maxillary artery of the external carotid. This shift occurs during the vital stages of face and palate development. (After D. H. Padget.[10])

cleft lip and palate and other types of facial defects in mice and rats.[17] On the other hand, excesses of certain endocrine substances, a number of drugs and irradiation will have teratogenic effects on the developing face and palate, as shown in the embryos of experimental animals.[17] In regard to vascularity, which, of course, controls the amount of oxygen and nutritional elements, the face and palate seem unique in development. There is a most important shift in circulation in this region during the critical time period of the seventh and eighth weeks.[10] The vessels of the branchial arches give rise to the external and internal carotid arteries, which provide the vascular supply to the face and palate when the first and second branchial arch vessels begin to disappear. During the sixth week, the stapedial artery arising from the internal carotid supplies most of the midfacial region (Fig. III-9, *A* and *B*). Then, during the seventh week, the stapedial artery severs its contact with the internal carotid. At the same time, its branches to the maxilla and mandible become attached and confluent with the adjacent facial branches of the external carotid (Fig. III-9, *B* and *C*). If, for any reason, this important shift of the blood supply of the face and palate from the internal to the external carotid is delayed, the effect on the developing tissues undoubtedly would be notable. It is a coincidence that this important shift occurs at this critical time in the palatofacial development.

4. Fusion of the Palatal Shelves

By 8½ prenatal weeks, the palatal shelves appear above the tongue and in near contact with each other (see Fig. III-7, *C*). Then, during the ninth and tenth weeks, they come into contact and fusion begins (Figs. III-7, *D* and III-10, *C*). First, the epithelial coverings of the shelves join to form a single layer of cells. Next, degeneration occurs as the connective tissue of the shelves penetrates this midline epithelial barrier and intermingles across the area (see Fig. III-7, *D*). Thus, the process is similar to that occurring in the lip. In a few cases, the two shelves have been reported to separate after initial fusion, with resulting epithelially covered connective tissue bands stretching across the palate between the shelves.[5] As bone forms in the palate, the area along the midline anteroposteriorly will become a suture where important expansive growth of the palate occurs. The entire palate does not contact and fuse at the same time. Initial contact occurs in the central region of the secondary palate just posterior to the anterior or primary palatine process and closure continues both anteriorly and posteriorly from this point (Fig. III-10, *C*). After initial contact and fusion, further closure occurs by a process of "merging," which results in the medial space between the two processes being eliminated (Fig. III-10, *D*). The anterior palatine foramen and a suture between the premaxilla and the palatal processes of the maxilla remain in the postnatal period as evidence of the early existence of the primary and secondary palate (Fig. III-10, *C* and *D*).

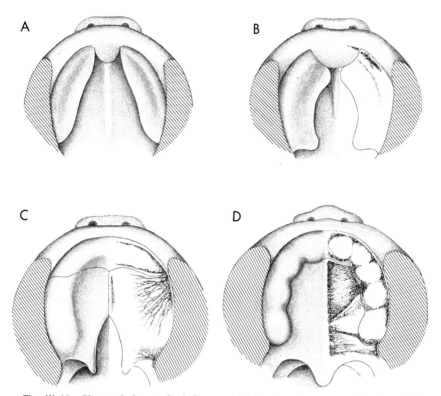

Fig. III-10.—View of the roof of the mouth showing closure and fusion of the palate. Bony development is shown on the right side of the palate. At 8 weeks (**A**), the shelves are horizontal and grow toward the midline. At 9 weeks (**B**), the shelves are in near contact and the premaxillary-maxillary ossification centers appear. At 10 weeks (**C**), the palate has fused and ossification centers of the premaxilla-maxilla grow medially. At 14 weeks (**D**), the premaxillary bone supports the cuspids and first molars and the palatine bone supports the second molars.

5. TOOTH DEVELOPMENT

By the seventh week, the epithelial labial lamina becomes apparent along the perimeter of the maxillary and mandibular processes (Fig. III-11). This wedge of epithelial cells penetrates the underlying connective tissue to separate the tissue of the future alveolar ridge from the lip. At the same time, a second lamina, lingual to the labial lamina, appears and grows into the alveolar ridge. This is the dental lamina, which, at regular intervals, will give rise to the epithelial enamel organs (Fig. III-11). These organs, along with adjacent dental papillae of connective tissue origin, rapidly differentiate to form the enamel and dentin of the teeth. As the developing crowns enlarge and the roots elongate,

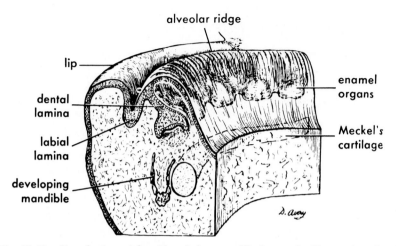

Fig. III-11.—Developing right side of the mandibular arch, illustrating the division of the tissue of the lip and jaw by the developing labial lamina. The dental lamina, tooth germs and Meckel's cartilage are shown. (From Steele, P., *Dimensions of Dental Hygiene* [Philadelphia: Lea & Febiger, 1966], p. 280.)

the jaws increase in anterior and lateral dimension, as well as height, to provide space for the teeth and growing alveolar processes.

6. SALIVARY GLAND DEVELOPMENT

The parotid and submandibular salivary glands appear in the connective tissue of the developing cheek in the sixth week. The third set of major salivary glands, the sublingual, appears in the eighth week. All of the major, as well as minor, salivary glands follow the same pattern of development in which proliferation of epithelial cells initially occurs from the oral mucosa, followed by growth of a solid cord of cells into the underlying connective tissue. This cord of cells then continues to proliferate, growing toward the region of future gland location. At this site, the epithelial cords branch repeatedly and the twig-like ends of the cords form berry-like secretory acini. Gradually, the entire system of epithelial cords becomes hollow and forms the duct system of the gland.[14] The site of origin of each major gland, as revealed by the initial epithelial growth, thus later will be the orifice of the main duct of the gland, ejecting its secretion to the oral cavity. The connective tissue adjacent to the developing glands grows around them, encapsulates them and grows into the glands to subdivide them into lobules (see Fig. III-15). This organization is complete by the third month, and the differentiation of the terminally located acinal cells and canalization of the ducts occurs at about the sixth prenatal month. The acini of the mucous glands become functional during the sixth month, whereas the serous glands become functional by birth.[11]

C. Differentiation of Supporting Structures

1. DEVELOPMENT OF THE CHONDROCRANIUM

The skeletal elements that form the skull develop initially in support of the brain, yet others appear very early in the rapidly developing face as well. The brain is given support by cartilages forming along its base, the chondrocranial elements, whereas the flat bones of the skull, the neurocranial elements, surround the brain. The chondrocranium also is important to the growing face and supports both areas through the development of a bar of cartilage extending uninterrupted along the midline from the anterior nasal region to the foramen magnum (Fig. III-12). The cartilage septum may function in anterior facial growth as well as in support. Its early fibrous attachment to the premaxilla has been demonstrated.[8] According to Scott,[12] it doubles its length from the tenth to the fourteenth prenatal week, trebles it by 17 weeks and is six times as large by 36 weeks. Anteriorly, this cartilage forms a capsule related to the olfactory nerve endings—the nasal capsule. More posteriorly, the cartilage supports the pituitary, laterally the otic capsules develop around the middle and internal ear structures and most posteriorly it forms the occipital cartilages around the foramen magnum. These cartilages establish the cranial base as early as the eighth week and will be transformed mostly into bone, with the future ethmoid bone arising from the nasal capsule and parts of the sphenoid,

Fig. III-12 (left).—Sagittal view of the cartilaginous cranial base at 9 weeks. The bar of cartilage extends uninterrupted posteriorly from the foramen magnum (FM) anteriorly to the tip of the nasal septum. The location of the sella turcica (ST) is seen.

Fig. III-13 (right).—Sagittal view of the cartilaginous cranial base showing the positional relationship of the ethmoid (*E*), the vomer (*V*), the sphenoid (*SP*) and the basioccipital (*BO*) bones. The dotted lines containing (*SE*) and (*SO*) indicate the sites of the future spheno-ethmoidal and spheno-occipital synchondrosis.

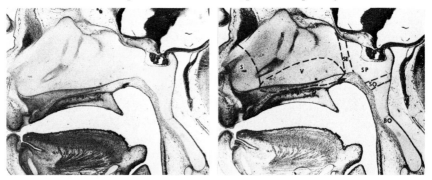

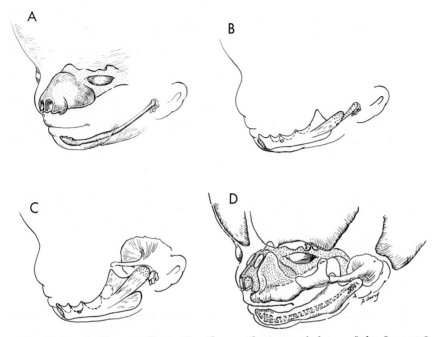

Fig. III-14.—A, diagram illustrating the cartilaginous skeleton of the face at 9 weeks. The nasal capsule represents the maxillary skeleton and Meckel's cartilage represents the mandibular skeleton at this age. **B,** diagram of the mandible at 16 weeks, illustrating the developing body of the mandible and condyle. Meckel's cartilage still persists. **C,** diagram of the mandible at 24 weeks. The coronoid process is evident, as is the appearance of the temporomandibular joint. **D,** diagram of the skeleton of the face at 30 weeks. The membrane bones of the nasomaxillary complex develop externally to the endochondral bones, replacing the cartilages of the middle of the face.

temporal and occipital from the more posterior cartilage. As each of these bones develops, cartilage centers remain between them, forming the cranial base synchondroses (Fig. III-13). These centers will provide for further growth and expansion of the cranial base. The anteriorly located nasal capsule is a large and important cartilage to the developing face and consists of a medial septum component, the mesethmoid, and two lateral cartilage wings (Fig. III-14, *A*).

2. DEVELOPMENT OF THE MAXILLARY COMPLEX

Until bone formation occurs, the nasal capsule is the only skeletal support of the upper face. Lateral and inferior to the cranial base cartilages, ossification centers appear in support of these parts of the face as it begins to develop in width during the prenatal period (Fig. III-14,

B and *C*). The nasal, premaxillary, maxillary, lacrimal, zygomatic, palatine and temporal ossification centers appear and expand until they appear as bones separated only by sutures (Fig. III-14, *D*).

3. DEVELOPMENT OF THE BONY PALATE

The bones of the palate arise from several ossification centers. In the eighth week, bilaterally located bony centers in the anterior palate give rise to the premaxilla and maxilla; they may arise in common but then develop medially in an independent fashion (see Fig. III-10, *B* and *C*). The premaxillary bone supports the maxillary incisor teeth, whereas the maxillary bone supports the cuspid and molar teeth. Posteriorly, the horizontal plates of the palatine bone grow medially from single bilateral ossification centers (see Fig. III-10, *C*). By the fourteenth week, the bony palate is well established, with a midline suture extending its length between the premaxillary, maxillary and palatine bones. A bilateral suture also appears between the palatal aspects of the premaxilla and the maxilla (see Fig. III-10, *D*).

4. MANDIBLE AND TEMPOROMANDIBULAR JOINT

The lower part of the face is supported by a rod-shaped bar known as Meckel's cartilage (Fig. III-14, *A*). This bar extends from near the midline of the mandibular arch posteriorly into the otic capsule, where the two posterior elements later become the malleus and incus bones of the middle ear (Fig. III-14, *A*). These two bones function in the articulation of the mandible in lower animals and are known as the articular and quadrate.[4] There is some evidence in man that the malleus and incus function to provide a movable joint until the mandibular condyle develops in relation to the glenoid fossa of the temporal bone (Fig. III-15). Thus, from approximately the eighth to the eighteenth week, this joint may function in jaw movement until an anterior shift in temporomandibular articulation occurs. Then, these two cartilages ossify and function as middle ear bones. The bony mandible develops laterally to Meckel's cartilage as a thin, flat, rectangular bar, except for a small region near its anterior extremity, where the cartilage ossifies and is fused to the mandible. Since the body of the mandible is attached to Meckel's cartilage, it could function and be carried forward in growth until regression of this cartilage, at which time the condyle becomes functional. The condyle arises independently initially as a carrot-shaped cartilage, and is enclosed by the developing bone of the posterior part of the mandible (see Fig. III-14, *B*). The condylar cartilage is transformed rapidly into bone except at its proximal end, where it forms an articulation with the temporal bone in the glenoid fossa (see Fig. III-14, *C*). This cartilaginous head of the condyle, enveloped in a fibrous covering that is continuous with the joint capsule, persists and

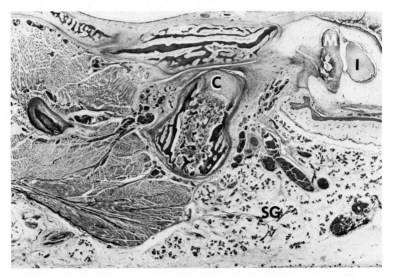

Fig. III-15.—Sagittal section through the developing temporomandibular joint and middle ear at 16 weeks. Note the forming upper and lower compartments of the joint and the ossifying condyle, middle ear bones, developing muscles and salivary glands. C = condyle; I = incus; SG = salivary glands.

Fig. III-16.—Diagram of the postnatal temporomandibular joint, illustrating the dense fibrous articular disk with the adjacent superior and inferior articular spaces. Underlying the fibrous covering of the condyle is a band of hyaline cartilage, below which is the developing bone of the condyle. (From Steele, P., *Dimensions of Dental Hygiene* [Philadelphia: Lea & Febiger, 1966], p. 316.)

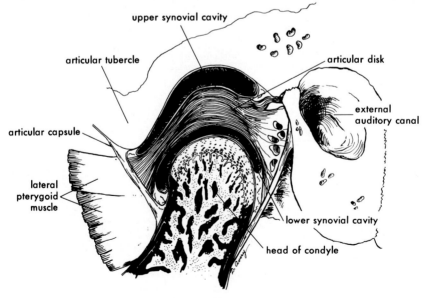

functions as a growth center until about the twenty-fifth year of post-natal life. The two condylar heads function similarly to the epiphysis of long bones. The cartilage farthest from the condylar head gradually is superseded by bone (Fig. III-16). The condylar head is separated from the temporal bone by a thin disk of connective tissue, which appears as a result of two clefts in the fibrous tissue that form the upper and lower compartments of the joint cavity. Gradually, this disk thickens, as does the bone forming the joint cavity, until the complete joint is developed (Fig. III-16).

Bone forms rapidly along the superior surface of the body of the mandible between the developing teeth. As the bony mandible continues to grow during the prenatal period, fibrous connective tissue and what is known as symphyseal cartilage unite the two halves of the mandible and it serves as a growth site until the first year after birth, by which time it is calcified. The angle of the mandible by birth is about 130 degrees with the condyle, thus nearly in a line with the body, whereas the large coronoid process projects above the head of the condyle (see Fig. III-14, *D*).

5. FACIAL MUSCLES

The facial muscle mass, termed the subcutaneous colli, appears in the fourth week in the ventral lateral portion of the hyoid arch just beneath the surface of the skin. Gradually, in the fifth week, it spreads

Fig. III-17 (left).—Diagram of the developing facial muscles at 9 weeks. This sheet of muscle grows cranially from the hyoid arch and splits at the ear into the anterior and posterior auricular parts. Deep and superficial facial muscles arise from this mass.

Fig. III-18 (right).—Diagram of the developing masticatory muscles at 9 weeks. These muscles develop in the mandibular arch before the skeletal elements on which they insert.

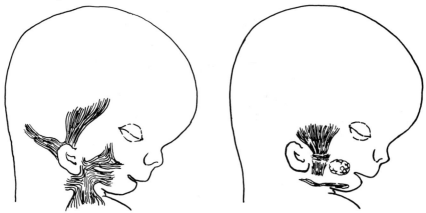

out, unfolding as the head elevates from the chest wall.[2] This muscle mass fans out and stylohyoid, digastric and stapedial muscle masses appear. The seventh nerve travels along with the facial muscle,[3] which now migrates up the side of the neck and over the face and cranium to meet the sheet of muscle from the opposite side. During the fifth to ninth weeks, the muscles of the human face differentiate and become functional to some extent, since stimulation of the perioral region in this latter period may result in reflexogenic responses, such as neck flexion and head turning.[6] The ear causes the muscle to split into the anterior and posterior auricular parts. The advancing sheet then separates into a superficial and a deep layer in the seventh week. The superficial fibers form the spread of the platysma muscle over the mandible to the cheek, forehead and temporal region (Fig. III-17). The sphincter colli is the deep layer and gives rise to several muscles, including the occipitalis. Degeneration of intermediate parts gives rise to the anterior, superior and postauricular, frontalis and occipitalis muscles. Between the seventh and ninth weeks, the superficial and deeper muscles differentiate rapidly. The sphincter colli also forms the orbicularis, the caninus and incisivus labii superioris muscles as the fibers of the more superficial platysma facei attach to the mandible. The quadratus labii inferioris and mentalis muscles of the lower face appear in the eighth to ninth week but are not well defined until the thirteenth week. At this time, the orbicularis oculi and the buccinator muscles appear from the deep fibers of the sphincter colli, whereas the triangularis and platysma arise from the superficial facei. Overlying the buccinator muscle, the buccal fat pad develops (Fig. III-18). It enlarges significantly during prenatal life, extending deep between the masseter and temporalis muscles. It functions in sucking and causes the cheek to appear plump in the newborn. By the fourteenth week, all the facial muscles are in their definitive positions and the young muscle fibers are differentiating.

6. MUSCLES OF MASTICATION

At this same time, the muscles of mastication are developing in the mesenchyme of the mandibular arch. These muscles begin differentiation in the seventh week and nerve fibers are apparent in them by the eighth week. Although the muscles of mastication develop at first in close relationship to Meckel's cartilage and the cranial base cartilages, they are independent and only later attach to the bony skeleton (Fig. III-18). The temporalis muscle begins lateral development in the eighth week, occupying the space anterior to the otic capsule. As the temporal bone begins to ossify in the thirteenth week, the muscle attaches along a broad front. At about this time, the masseter muscle begins attachment to the zygomatic arch as it undergoes lateral growth, providing space for muscle development.[11] The pterygoid muscles differentiate in the seventh week and early are related to the cartilages of the cranial base and condyle (see Fig. III-15). Later, as the bony skull appears and increases in width and length, these muscles expand rapidly. Typical fetal histologic structure of the muscles of mastication appears by the twenty-second week.

D. The Fetal Period—Third to Ninth Month

1. CRANIOFACIAL CHANGES

By the third month, the face assumes a more human appearance. The eyes are now directed forward and the eyelids have grown together and are fused. The head is erect and the bridge of the nose becomes somewhat more prominent. As the face grows downward and forward, the ears appear on a horizontal plane with the eyes instead of at the lower corners of the face, as in the embryonic period. During the fetal period, from the twelfth to the thirty-sixth week, the head increases in length from approximately 18 mm. to 120 mm., in width from about 12 mm. to 74 mm. and in height from 20 mm. to 100 mm., thus maintaining a fairly constant ratio of width to length but not to height.[9] Prior to the fifth month, the height increase is greatest, whereas width and length increases are proportional. At birth, the cranial vault is proportionally about eight times larger than the face. In the embryonic period, the cranium-to-face ratio may be as high as 40:1, dropping at 4 months to 5:1 because of the differentially more rapid facial growth during the period. The cranium then grows faster in the late prenatal months to attain the 8:1 ratio at birth. Postnatal facial growth will reduce the adult ratio to approximately 2:1.

2. RADIOGRAPHIC CHANGES

The radiographic appearance of the mandible at the beginning of the fetal period is that of a slightly curved bone, but, by the fifteenth week, the condyle, coronoid process and the angle become evident.[9] Radiographically, the incisor teeth in the lower jaw make their appearance in the fifth month and the molar crypts are evident in the sixth month. During the fetal period, the mandible increases in length five times, whereas the intercondylar width increases six times. The gonial angle, which was virtually nonexistent at the beginning of this period, increases to about 130 degrees at birth. Although these increases follow closely the over-all growth of the face, the lower jaw appears retrognathic at birth. The palate increases in length fourfold and the maxillary region about fivefold (Fig. III-19). At the beginning of the fetal period, the frontal bones are apparent. The nasal bones appear at 3 months and the first signs of cranial base bone appear at 10½ weeks. The sella turcica is clearly visible at 4½ months and attains its characteristic shape at 5 months. The spheno-ethmoidal and spheno-occipital synchondroses are evident at 6 months (Fig. III-19).

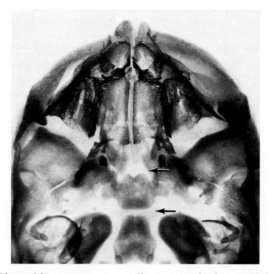

Fig. III-19.—Cleared human specimen illustrating the bones of the cranial base at 21 weeks. The synchondroses of the cranial base are indicated by arrows. Premaxillary, maxillary and palatine processes can be seen forming the palate.

Fig. III-20.—The cranium at birth. Note the fontanelles, one at each corner of the parietal bones. (From Caffey, J., *Pediatric X-ray Diagnosis* [6th ed.; Chicago: Year Book Medical Publishers, Inc., 1972].)

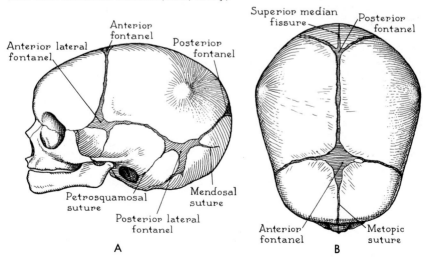

At birth, the intervening connective tissue that separates the bones of the cranial vault is still wide. At six sites located at each corner of the parietal bones they form the fontanelles (Fig. III-20). Synchondroses between the ethmoid, sphenoid and occipital bones are still actively growing at birth. The skull contains 45 separate bones at birth, which will be reduced by fusions and consolidations to 22 in the adult. For example, the frontal bones at birth are still paired and separated by the metopic suture. Similarly, the paired halves of the mandible are separated by the symphyseal suture. The occipital is in four parts, with synchondroses between them, and the tympanic annulus is still separate from the temporal bone. Some of these sutures, such as the midline mandibular suture, disappear shortly after birth. The maxillary mid-palatal suture, however, does not close until the sixth to seventh year, although it may be orthopedically activated until the late teens (see Chapter XV).

REFERENCES

1. Bates, M. N.: Early hypoglossae musculature, Am. J. Anat. 83:329, 1948.
2. Gasser, R. F.: The development of the facial muscles in man, Am. J. Anat. 120:257, 1967.
3. Gasser, R. F.: The development of the facial nerve in man, Ann. Otol., Rhin. & Laryng. 76:37, 1967.
4. Gerrie, J.: The phylogeny of the mammalian tympanic cavity and auditory ossicles, J. Laryng. & Otol. 62:339, 1948.
5. Hayward, J. R., and Avery, J. K.: A variation in cleft palate, J. Oral Surg. 15:320, 1957.
6. Hooker, D.: *The Prenatal Origin of Behavior.* Porter Lecture Series XVIII, March 12–13, 1951 (Lawrence: University of Kansas Press, 1952), 136 pp.
7. Humphrey, T.: The development of mouth opening and related reflexes involving the oral area of human fetuses, Alabama J. M. Sc. 5:126, 1968.
8. Latham, D. A.: Maxillary development and growth: The septo premaxillary ligament, J. Anat. 107:471, 1970.
9. McNamara, J. A.: Morphogenic pattern formation and development in the human head during the fetal period. (In preparation.)
10. Padget, D. H.: The development of the cranial arteries in the human embryo, Contrib. Embryol. 32:212, 1948.
11. Patten, B. M.: *Human Embryology* (3d ed.; New York: Blakiston Division, McGraw-Hill Book Company, Inc., 1968).
12. Scott, J. H.: *Dento-facial Development and Growth: Facial Growth during the Foetal Life* (New York: Pergamon Press, 1967), p. 79.
13. Srivastava, H. C., and Barry, A.: Personal communication.
14. Streeter, G. L.: Developmental horizons in human embryos. Age groups XI to XXII, Contrib. Embryol. 2:197 and 191, 1951.
15. Trasler, D. G., and Fraser, F. C.: Role of the tongue in producing cleft palate in mice with spontaneous cleft lip, Develop. Biol. 6:45, 1963.
16. Verrusio, A. C.: A mechanism for closure of the secondary palate, Teratology 3:17, 1970.
17. Warkany, J., and Kalter, H.: Congenital malformations, New England J. Med. 265:993 and 1046, 1961.

IV

Growth of the Craniofacial Skeleton

In collaboration with

DONALD H. ENLOW, Ph.D.

Professor and Chairman, Department of Anatomy, University of West Virginia; formerly Professor of Anatomy, The University of Michigan Medical School, and Fellow, Center for Human Growth and Development

> Those who are enamoured of practice without science are like a pilot who goes into a ship without rudder or compass and never has any certainty where he is going.
>
> Practice should always be based upon a sound knowledge of theory.—LEONARDO DA VINCI, *The Notebooks of Leonardo da Vinci*, Vol. II, Chap. XXIX (translated by Edward MacCurdy)

A. Methods of studying bone growth

1. Vital staining
2. Radioisotopes
3. Implants
4. Comparative anatomy
5. Roentgenographic cephalometrics
6. Genetic studies
7. Natural markers

B. Osteogenesis

1. Endochondral bone formation
2. Intramembranous bone formation

C. Mechanisms of bone growth

1. Remodeling
2. Growth movements
3. Directions of growth
4. Soft tissues associated with bone

D. Growth sites

1. The mandibular condyle and posterior border of the ramus
2. The lingual tuberosity
3. The maxillary tuberosity
4. The alveolar process
5. Sutures
6. The nasal septum
7. Surfaces

E. Regional growth

1. The mandible
2. The nasomaxillary complex
3. The cranial base and cranial vault

F. Pattern of facial growth

G. Genetics of Craniofacial Growth

1. Over-all facial dimensions
2. Incremental growth
3. Gross craniofacial deformity
   a) Cleft lip and/or cleft palate
   b) Craniofacial syndromes
4. Soft tissue facial features

H. Racial and ethnic differences in facial growth

I. Role of the musculature and function in craniofacial growth

1. Muscle growth and skeletal growth
2. Muscle migration and attachment
3. Function and bone growth
4. Response of the craniofacial skeleton to variations in function
   a) Regional or local effects
   b) General effects

J. Relationships between craniofacial and body growth

1. Body type and facial form
2. Timing of growth events
3. Assessment of body growth for orthodontic purposes

K. Effects of orthodontic treatment on facial growth

1. Methods of altering craniofacial growth
2. Classes of bony responses to force application
3. Effects on the nasomaxillary complex
4. Effects of orthodontic treatment on the mandible
5. Cranial base
6. Effects of orthodontic treatment on the profile and pattern of facial growth

L. Some comments concerning the various theories of craniofacial growth

1. Controlling factors in craniofacial growth
2. Regulation of skull development
3. Control of craniofacial growth

A. Methods of Studying Bone Growth

THE FACE HAS intrigued scientific men for many years. Often the only human remains found by the archaeologist are fragments of the craniofacial skeleton and a few teeth. From these slender clues the anthropologist has reconstructed satisfactory hypotheses concerning the evolution of the human face. There is a rich and lengthy heritage of exciting and cooperative research among archaeologists, physical anthropologists, anatomists and orthodontic scientists.

For many years, our only knowledge of facial growth was inferred from the study of dried skulls of different ages. Valid conclusions deduced from comparisons of several different specimens are difficult, since, of course, the continued growth of no one individual is ever observed. There is, however, a direct lineal descent from archaeology through physical anthropology to cephalometrics. Today, the modern research worker studying bone growth in the head and face has a wide variety of methods at his disposal.

1. VITAL STAINING*

In 1736, Belchier[8] reported that the bones of animals who had eaten the madder plant were stained a red color. In 1739, Duhamel[23] fed madder to animals and then withheld it for a period prior to sacrifice. As a result, the bones contained a band of red stain followed by an unstained band. This method was used until alizarin, the essential dye of the madder plant, was identified and synthesized. Alizarin red S (alizarin sulfonate), acid alizarin blue BB, trypan blue and other vital dyes are still used extensively in bone research today.[45] The nature of the combination of alizarin with bone is said to be a chelation with a divalent cation on the surface of the crystal. It stains the inorganic fraction of only one generation of bone. On the other hand, Procion compounds, when used as vital dyes, bond with the inorganic phase of bone and thus are not lost during decalcification.[33,81] The antibiotic tetracycline also is used as a vital bone marker, since its administration causes a sufficient upset in the ossification process to leave a band quite visible when viewed under ultraviolet light.[30] The primary value of such vital dyes lies in depicting the pattern of postnatal bone deposition over an extended period in one animal. A series of injections will leave layers of dyed bone alternating with unstained bone. By combining two or more dyes, the usefulness of the method is extended.[20] Since it has been shown[44] that vital staining with alizarin red S and tetracycline inhibits normal growth of the experimental animal, they may not be well suited for study of rates of growth, but the pattern of growth is magnificently revealed by this technic (Fig. IV-1). The method reveals the manner in

---

*For a good survey of current progress of in-vivo staining and marking methods, see Baer and Gavan.[5]

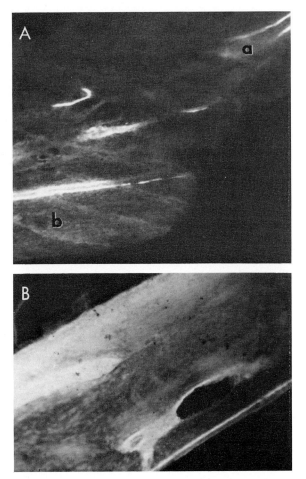

Fig. IV-1.—The use of tetracycline HCl as a vital bone marker in monkeys. **A,** cutaneous resorption: external resorption in nuchal region (*a*); deposition peripheral to nuchal region (*b*). Two fluorescent tetracycline HCl labels are visible. **B,** meningeal depository surface of the anterior cranial floor with contralateral resorption. (**B** courtesy of Dr. Michael Riolo.)

which bone is laid down, the sites of growth, the direction of growth and the relative duration at different sites. It does not, however, provide direct evidence of bone resorption; resorptive activity must be inferred.

2. RADIOISOTOPES

Radioisotopes of certain elements or compounds often are used as in-vivo markers for studying bone growth. Such labeled material is injected and then, after a time, located within the growing bones by means of Geiger counters or by the use of autoradiographic technics. In the latter method, the bones or sections of bones are placed against photographic emulsions that are exposed by emission of the radioactive substance.[22] Salts commonly used for this work are ^{45}Ca and ^{32}P and, in addition, labeled components of proteins such as tritiated proline. Microradiography is another popular method utilized by research workers, primarily for the study of the inorganic matrix and its density. In-vivo isotopes are not used, and thus the technic is to be distinguished from autoradiography. A beam of x-rays at the microscopic level is passed through an undecalcified thin section of bone or tooth that has been placed over a sensitive emulsion. The differential passage of the rays through the different areas of the tissue section is recorded on the film as varying blacks, grays and whites.

3. IMPLANTS

Björk[14] has devised an ingenious method of implanting tiny bits of tantalum into growing bone of animals or human beings. These serve as reference markers during serial cephalometric analysis (see 5, below). The method allows precise orientation of the serial cephalograms and provides information concerning the amount and sites of bone growth (Fig. IV-2).

4. COMPARATIVE ANATOMY

Significant contributions to our knowledge of human facial growth have been provided through comparisons with other species. Not only can experimental work be done more readily on animals but often basic principles common to growth in all species are first recognized and defined by studies in comparative anatomy. Much of our knowledge of the phylogeny of the anatomic components comprising the head has been derived from comparative studies of fossil and present-day species.

5. ROENTGENOGRAPHIC CEPHALOMETRICS

Physical anthropologists and anatomists have carried out many metric studies of the head, using calipers and a number of selected and standardized measurements of both the living and dry skulls. From these methods, a branch of anthropometry evolved that has come to be known as craniometrics or cephalometrics. The reliability of caliper measurements on the living is not high and, of course, intracranial measurements cannot be made. For many years, therefore, workers in several countries sought a method of using cephalometrics in conjunction with x-rays in order that accurate serial measurements of the same growing head might be made. The principal problem was that of design-

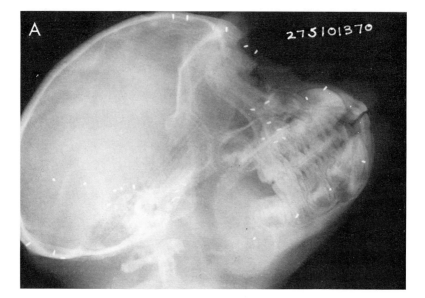

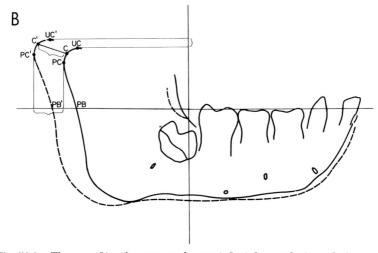

Fig. IV-2.—The use of implants to study craniofacial growth. **A,** cephalogram of a rhesus monkey showing the use of a rather large number of implants.[73] Note specifically the use of implants in the cranial base region. **B,** a method of studying mandibular growth in a rhesus monkey by superimposition over the mandibular implants. Note the change of the landmarks; e.g., *c* to *c'*, *pc* to *pc'*, etc., with growth.

ing a reliable head-positioning device. The first to present such a head positioner or "cephalostat" probably was the Italian, Pacini.[77] But it remained for Broadbent[16] in the United States and Hofrath[42] in Germany to publish, in 1931, the papers that convinced workers that such methods were usable. At the same time, Simon's[93] system of gnathostatics, a method of orienting orthodontic casts to cranial planes, was very popular with orthodontists. So there was a natural evolution and melding of ideas from anthropometrics and gnathostatics into the new field of roentgenographic cephalometrics. Several other early workers, for example, Higley[41] and Margolis,[61] also devised cephalostats during this period. From Higley's instrument have evolved the designs of most modern cephalometers. Soon the methods were standardized and important serial studies of craniofacial growth were under way in many research centers around the world. No other method of study has contributed so much to our knowledge of human craniofacial growth.

Cephalometric methods are used not only for the study of facial growth but also for orthodontic diagnosis, treatment planning and the assessment of therapeutic results. Throughout this book are a number of illustrations that depict modern procedures for cephalometric study of craniofacial growth. Chapter XII, Analysis of the Craniofacial Skeleton, is devoted largely to radiographic cephalometrics. The recent introduction of computerized storage and analysis of cephalometric data has extended the usefulness of the method.[64] Computer graphics permits wider use of data by those without a serial growth sample, allows more economical statistical analysis of vast amounts of data and provides, by interaction between the research worker and the computer, for the promulgation and easier testing of new hypotheses[64, 74] (Fig. IV-3).

6. GENETIC STUDIES

Genetic methods utilizing cephalometrics currently are being used to study parent-child relationships, sibling similarities and twins (see Section G, Genetics of Craniofacial Growth).

7. NATURAL MARKERS

The persistence of certain developmental features of bone has led to their use as natural markers. By means of serial radiography, trabeculae, nutrient canals and lines of arrested growth can be used for reference to study deposition, resorption and remodeling. Israel[52] has supplemented the method by use of a recording microdensitometer.

Enlow[25] has developed and used extensively methods for studying bone deposition, resorption and the process of remodeling in prepared ground sections (Fig. IV-4). By relating the findings to other methods, for example, cephalometrics, vital dyes, and so forth, our knowledge

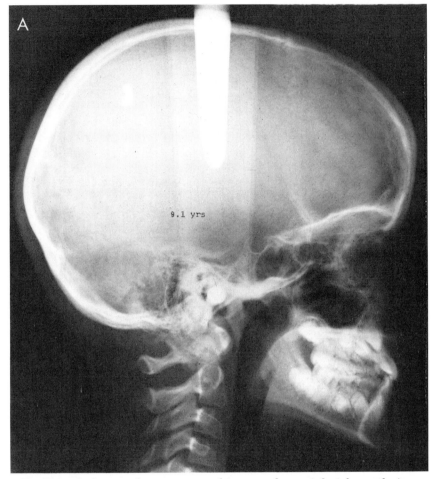

Fig. IV-3.—A, the use of computer graphics to study craniofacial growth. A conventional cephalogram before tracing. (*Continued.*)

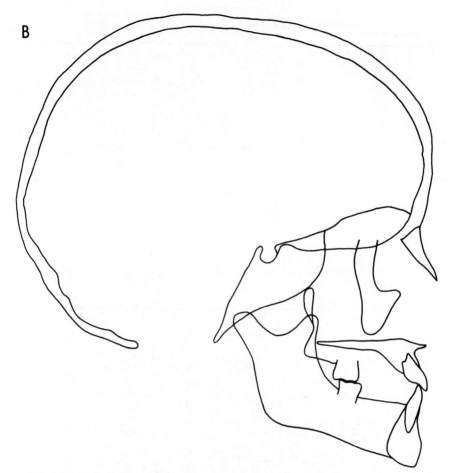

Fig. IV-3 (cont.).—B, a conventional tracing of the cephalogram shown in *A*. (*Continued.*)

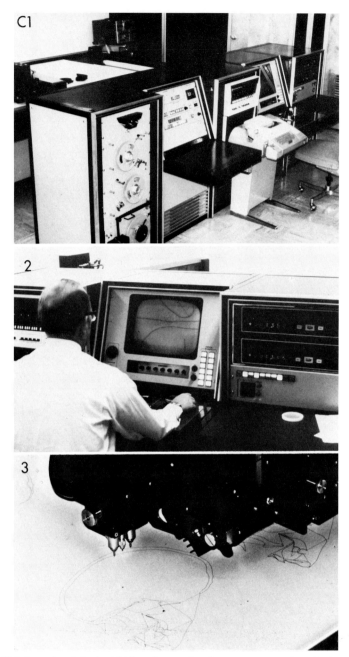

Fig. IV-3 (cont.).—C-1, the Tridea device for direct storage of cephalograms in the computer. Behind the console is a large flat table over which travels a device that reads various shades of white, gray and black and automatically follows the anatomic shadows within the cephalogram. **C-2,** the operator views this tele-

VAR = SN-PALPL A

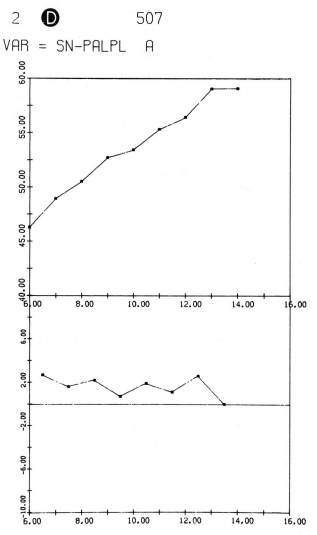

Fig. IV-3 (cont.).—D, an illustration of one way in which stored cephalometric data may be retrieved for analysis. Here, incremental data on one subject and one measurement, the SN-palatal plane angle, are plotted. In the upper chart is plotted the angle as measured at different ages. In the lower plot, one sees the annual increments in this angle. (*Continued.*)

vision tube console where the area being followed by the camera traversing the table and cephalogram is enlarged ten times. The operator monitors the tracing in this fashion, helping the instrument make decisions as to which direction to go when two anatomic shadows cross or merge. **C-3,** after the cephalogram and its anatomic outlines have been stored on tape, the storage is verified by asking the same instrument to draw the outline of the stored anatomic data. Here, the tracing head reproduces on a large sheet of mylar a series of cephalometric tracings that have been stored. (*Continued.*)

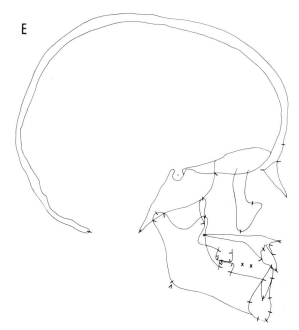

Fig. IV-3 (cont.).—E, a computer plot of data stored from the cephalogram shown in *A.* Compare with the regular handmade tracing shown in *B.*

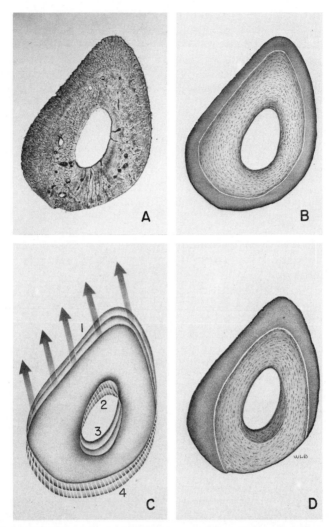

Fig. IV-4.—Enlow's method of studying remodeling from ground bone sections. The sequence of remodeling changes that produced the cortical arrangement seen in photomicrograph **A** is shown schematically in **B, C** and **D.** Prior to the lateral drift, as seen in stage **B,** the cortex is composed of inner (endosteal) and outer (periosteal) zones. Simultaneously, new bone is added at surface *1,* removed from side *2,* added to surface *3* and resorbed on side *4* as shown in **C.** The composite result is a drift movement of this entire region of the bone in the direction indicated by the *arrows* in **C.** The final stage schematized in **D** is comparable with the actual photomicrograph shown in **A.** (From Enlow, D. H.: *Principles of Bone Remodeling* [Springfield, Ill.: Charles C Thomas, Publisher, 1963].)

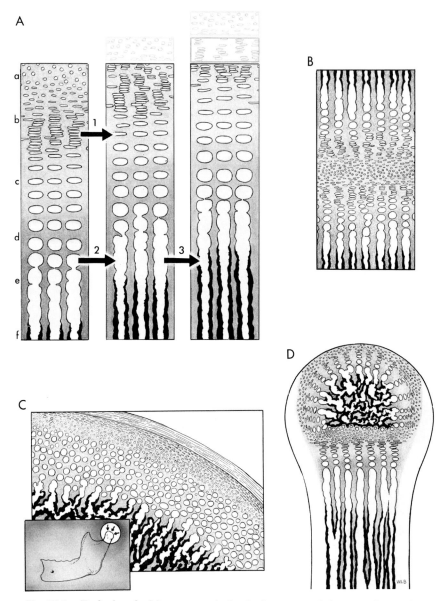

Fig. IV-5.—Endochondral bone growth. In **A,** the zones of the growth cartilage are schematized. Zone *a,* which is termed the reserve cartilage, feeds new cells into zone *b,* the zone of cell division. The cells in this latter zone undergo rapid division in a linear direction, thereby forming longitudinal columns of flattened chondrocytes (isogenous groups). This growth process is responsible for the

of bone growth has been extended greatly. Many of the illustrations in this chapter are based on information derived by these methods of study.

B. Osteogenesis

Bone may form in two connective tissue sites—cartilage and membranous connective tissue. The two basic modes of osteogenesis are named after the site of appearance of bone.

1. ENDOCHONDRAL BONE FORMATION

Endochondral bone formation is a morphogenetic adaptation providing continued production of bone in those special regions that involve relatively high levels of compression. Thus, it is found in the bones associated with movable joints and some parts of the cranial base. During endochondral bone formation, the original mesenchymal tissue first becomes cartilage. Cartilage cells hypertrophy, their matrix becomes calcified, the cells degenerate and osteogenic tissues invade the dying and disintegrating cartilage and replace it (Fig. IV-5). Endochondral bone is not formed directly from cartilage; it invades cartilage and replaces it. Cartilage can grow not only by apposition on its surface but also by proliferation of cells and the intercellular matrix within its substance, thereby expanding the cartilage by interstitial growth as well. The intercellular substance of bone, however, is calcified and thus too hard to permit interstitial growth. The "epiphyseal mechanism" of bone growth (or its equivalent) does not exert a direct regulatory in-

---

elongation of the bone. In succession, the daughter cells undergo hypertrophy (zone *c*), the matrix calcifies (zone *d*) and this calcified matrix becomes partially resorbed and invaded by vessels (zone *e*). Undifferentiated cells carried in by vascular sprouts then provide osteoblasts, which in turn deposit the thin crust of bone on the remnants of the calcified cartilage matrix (zone *f*). This entire process is continuous and repetitive, so that one zone becomes transferred into the next in succession. Note that zone *b* becomes changed directly into zone *c* (*arrow 1*), that zone *d* is transformed into zone *e* (*arrow 2*) and that zone *e* becomes zone *f* (*arrow 3*) as the entire cartilage grows in a linear direction. By this means, the cartilage plate moves toward the top of the illustration as bone replacement follows. In **B,** the growth cartilage of a cranial synchondrosis is schematized. Note that proliferation in bone formation occurs on both sides of the plate in contrast to the epiphyseal plate pictured in **D. C** represents the growth cartilage of the mandibular condyle. A fibrous capsule is present. A zone of chondrocyte proliferation (**B**) occurs just beneath this covering layer. Note that columns of chondrocytes resulting from repeated cell division are poorly represented. A typical long bone epiphysis showing a secondary center, articular cartilage, epiphyseal (growth) plate and medullary endochondral bone is represented in **D.** (*A–D* from Enlow, D. H.: *The Human Face* [New York: Hoeber Medical Division, Harper & Row, Publishers, 1968].

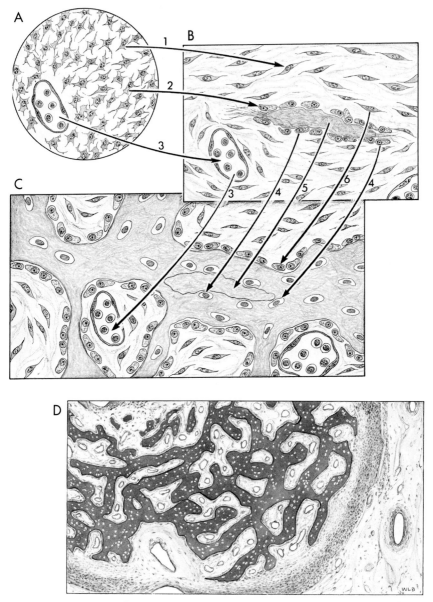

Fig. IV-6.—Intramembranous bone formation. In a center of ossification (**A**), the cells and matrix of the undifferentiated connective tissue (late mesenchyme) undergo a series of changes that produce small spicules of bone. Some cells (*1*) remain relatively undifferentiated but others (*2*) develop into osteoblasts that lay

fluence over the growth changes that occur in all of the other portions of an enlarging bone. Rather, it is concerned essentially with its own local production of bone tissue in those particular areas served by the specialized cartilaginous plate. Growth in the many different regions of a whole bone, however, proceeds in a closely interrelated manner, although the control and coordinating mechanisms are poorly understood at present.

2. INTRAMEMBRANOUS BONE FORMATION

If bone forms in membranous connective tissue, the undifferentiated mesenchymal cells of the connective tissue elaborate osteoid matrix and change to osteoblasts. The matrix or intercellular substance becomes calcified, and bone is the result.

Bone tissues laid down by the periosteum, sutures and the periodontal membrane are all intramembranous in formation (Fig. IV-6). Intramembranous ossification is the predominant mode of growth in the skull, even in composite "endochondral" elements, such as the sphenoid and mandible. The basic modes of formation (or resorption) are similar, regardless of the kind of membrane involved. Intramembranous growth and remodeling apparently can be associated with either "tension" or "pressure," although the nature of relationships and thresholds that occur between different in-vivo forces and the occurrence of deposition and resorption are not now clear (see Section I later in this chapter).

Bone tissue sometimes is classified as "periosteal" or "endosteal" according to its site of formation. Periosteal bone always is of intramembranous origin, but endosteal bone may be either intramembranous or endochondral, depending on site and mode of formation.

---

down the first fibrous bone matrix (osteoid), which subsequently becomes mineralized as in stage **B**. Original blood vessels are retained in close proximity to the formative bony trabeculae (3). As bone deposition by osteoblasts continues, some of these cells are enclosed by their own deposits and thus become osteocytes (4). Some undifferentiated cells develop into new osteoblasts (6), and other remaining osteoblasts undergo cell division to accommodate enlargement of the trabeculae. The outline of an early bone spicule (5) is shown in the enlarged trabeculae for reference. Blood vessels (3) have now become enclosed in the fine cancellous spaces (**C**). These spaces also contain a scattering of fibers, undifferentiated connective tissue cells and osteoblasts. At lower magnification (**D**), the characteristic fine cancellous nature of the cortex is seen. This bone tissue type is widely distributed in the prenatal as well as the young postnatal skeleton. It is a particularly fast-growing variety of bone tissue. Note that the periosteum (also formed from undifferentiated cells in the ossification center) has become arranged into inner (cellular) and outer (fibrous) layers. (From Enlow, D. H.: *The Human Face* [New York: Hoeber Medical Division, Harper & Row Publishers, 1968].)

C. Mechanisms of Bone Growth

The growth of bone, unlike growth processes in most soft tissues, involves a process of direct, cumulative surface deposition. The formation of new bone tissue, however, must be accompanied by an additional process of resorptive removal. The combination of bone additions on one side of a cortical plate and resorption from the other side produces an actual *growth movement* (see Section C-2, below) that provides the progressively increasing dimensions of the whole bone (Fig. IV-7).

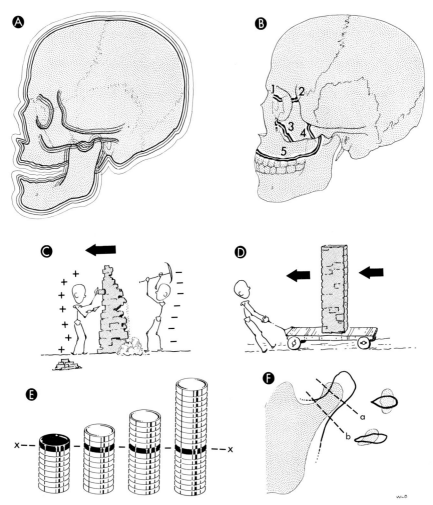

Fig. IV-7.—Diagrammatic representation of the principles of craniofacial growth. Several oversimplified explanations of craniofacial growth have been pre-

Bone growth, however, does not merely involve external deposition in conjunction with internal resorption, as is commonly believed, for complex *remodeling* also is required in order to sustain the configuration of the entire bone as it simultaneously increases in size (Figs. IV-7 and IV-9). Since some regions characteristically undergo more extensive growth than others, the bone would become progressively disproportionate without corresponding remodeling changes. For example, as large amounts of bone are deposited on the posterior margin of the mandibular ramus, the positions of all the other parts of the mandible necessarily become altered with respect to the new dimensions of the enlarged bone (see Fig. IV-9). Furthermore, the many localized areas of the mandible undergo progressive relocation as the entire bone continues to enlarge. Thus, the posterior portion of the corpus becomes relocated into the space previously occupied by the ramus. *Relocation,* the change in relative position of an area, is carried out by the remodeling process (Fig. IV-7). Remodeling produces a continuous, sequential movement and enlargement of all the regional parts in such a manner that the whole bone maintains proportionate configuration during continued differential growth increases.

1. REMODELING

Individual facial bones do not grow as if magnified by a photographic enlarger, for bone cannot increase in size merely by generalized, uni-

---

sented in the literature (see Section L of this chapter). The various bones of the craniofacial skeleton do not enlarge by a process of generalized surface accretion merely following existing contours, as schematized in **A.** Facial growth has been presented as a process occurring largely in facial sutures (*1, 2, 3* and *4* in **B**) and by bone additions to the alveolar margin and maxillary tuberosity (5). This oversimplification, however, does not take into account the extensive and fundamental process of remodeling growth that occurs in virtually all parts of craniofacial bones. A bone may move by two means: it can grow (cortical drift) by selective deposition and resorption (**C**) or it can become displaced (**D**) from one position to another. Relocation is shown by schematized segments (**E**). The black segment at the left occupies the number 1 position. As longitudinal growth (addition of new segments) continues, however, the black segment becomes relocated in a position to number 2, 3, 4, etc. Although its relative position with respect to the other segment constantly changes, note that the black segment itself does not move. It becomes relocated because of growth taking place in other areas. The process of relocation as indicated in **F** underlies most of the remodeling changes that take place during bone growth in the mandible. For example, portions of the condyle become converted by remodeling into the neck. In these superimposed growth stages, sections of *a* and *b* show the local changes in size and shape that occur as the bone enlarges. Remodeling is a process of reshaping and resizing as a consequence of progressive continuous relocation. (From Enlow, D. H.: *The Human Face* [New York: Hoeber Medical Division, Harper & Row, Publishers, 1968].)

form additions on external surfaces. Rather, differential additions and removal take place on the various inner and outer surfaces. Such differential growth activity provides depository increases as well as simultaneous remodeling adjustments throughout the entire bone. As new bone is added in a given area, the relative positions of virtually all the other parts of the bone necessarily become altered, that is, relocated. The factor of relocation, as mentioned previously, is the basis for these widespread changes in all parts of the bone. Selective deposition and resorption (remodeling) of the whole bone serve to (1) alter regional shape in order to conform to progressively new positions and (2) change the dimensions and proportions of each regional part.

2. Growth Movements

Two basic modes of movement are involved during growth—*drift* and *displacement* (see Fig. IV-7). Direct deposition and resorption of bone tissue and characteristic combinations of deposition and resorption occurring in the different bones of the skull result in a growth movement toward the depository surface termed *drift*. Drift occurs in virtually all areas of a growing bone and is not restricted to the major growth "centers." Drift produces generalized enlargement as well as the relocation of the parts involved. Drift takes place simultaneously with displacement but is distinguished from it, as they are basically different modes of growth movement (see Fig. IV-7). *Displacement,* on the other hand, is a movement of the whole bone as a unit. It is a result of the pull or push by different bones and their soft tissues away from one another as they all continue to enlarge. The over-all process of craniofacial enlargement is a composite of drift and displacement. Complex combinations of both processes occur in the many different bones of the skull. Drift and displacement may complement each other (move in the same direction) or they may take place in contrasting directions (Fig. IV-8). These factors greatly complicate meaningful interpretations of growth data and the evaluation of over-all growth patterns, since it often is difficult to determine the relative extent of each in analyses of serial cephalograms. See Chapter XII, Analysis of the Craniofacial Skeleton, for a discussion of this important problem as it relates to diagnostic evaluation of craniofacial form and growth.

3. Directions of Growth

Surfaces oriented toward the actual direction of growth undergo new bone deposition, whereas those surfaces directed away from the course of growth generally are resorptive (see Fig. IV-7). Thus, the posterior border of the ramus is "depository," whereas the anterior edge is "resorptive" (see Fig. IV-10). All of the other surfaces throughout each individual bone demonstrate characteristic, localized patterns of

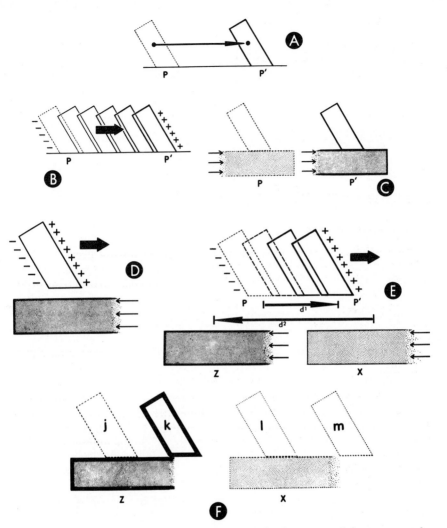

Fig. IV-8.—Cortical drift and the process of displacement. A bone moves by either of two basic processes. In **A,** the model has been positioned from P to P'. It may do this by direct cortical growth (drift) (**B**) or it may be carried by a process of displacement (**C**). These two processes frequently produce movement in divergent directions simultaneously. In **D,** for example, the model itself is growing to the right (*arrow*). The carrier, however, is moving to the left at the same time. In **E,** the model drifts (deposition in conjunction with resorption on contralateral surfaces) from P to P' for a distance designated as d^1. The carrier moves in an opposite course from X to Z for the distance d^2. In **F,** the original relationship prior to these movements is indicated by X and l. The relative position of the model if drift alone occurred would be at m. The carrier, however, has moved from X to Z. If displacement alone occurred, the relative position of the model would be at j. The combination of both drift and displacement, however, results in the final positional relationship seen between Z and k. (From Enlow, D. H.: *The Human Face* [New York: Hoeber Medical Division, Harper & Row, Publishers, 1968].)

addition and removal according to the specific directions of growth involved in each region of the bone.

4. Soft Tissues Associated with Bone

The soft tissue matrix of bone is directly responsible for many of the growth changes that occur in the bone itself. Unlike bone tissue, the covering and lining tissues that enclose bone enlarge primarily by interstitial rather than by appositional growth. The membranes and other soft tissues that deposit bone do not simply "back off" as they lay down new bone beneath them; rather, these soft tissues undergo complex growth changes involving the continued production of new components and remodeling of older components already present. This growth process produces an actual drift of the membrane itself corresponding to the direction of bone movement. The mechanisms of growth and remodeling within the various kinds of membranes, including the periosteum, sutures and the periodontal membrane, are all essentially comparable.

The endosteal and periosteal surfaces of a given bone are characterized by prescribed *growth fields,* each of which has its own growth velocity and is either resorptive or depository in nature, depending on the local growth direction (see Figs. IV-4, IV-7, IV-10, etc.). Growth fields are under the control of overlying soft tissues and function to (1) enlarge the bone as a whole (even though some areas actually may decrease in size because of relocation) and, at the same time, (2) provide relocation by remodeling of all local areas, parts, tuberosities, fossae, crests and so forth. A single growth field can encompass several different parts of several separate bones, all of which take part in a common growth movement even though separated by sutures, synchondroses or condyles.

A growth field moves and expands in coverage as a whole bone enlarges. This progressive movement of the growth field provides relocation and remodeling. As the soft tissue matrix in general expands, the regional effects on the bones that it houses expand correspondingly.

The various factors that influence the control of bone morphogenesis operate in conjunction with the different soft tissues associated directly with the bone. Biomechanical forces, bioelectric potential, heredity, tissue induction, differential cellular sensitivity and response to extrinsic stimuli are all expressed through the action of the soft tissues responsible for the actual production or remodeling of bone. Since function is believed to lead form, the concept of a "functional matrix" is meaningful (see Section I, below). Although this principle does not explain how local control of growth is governed, it provides an effective model for visualizing the events that occur as the different bones and their soft tissue matrices grow in relation to one another.

D. Growth Sites

The enlargement of the craniofacial complex involves a number of special regions that are characterized by particularly marked growth and remodeling changes. These growth sites (sometimes called "centers") represent areas in which differential growth additions bring about major movements associated with continued enlargement.

1. THE MANDIBULAR CONDYLE AND POSTERIOR BORDER OF THE RAMUS

The condyle contributes to the continuing growth of the ramus in a cephaloposterior direction while functioning in movable contact with the cranium. The condylar mechanism is a structural and functional adaptation to these two particular functions; it is not, as often is suggested, a control center that governs the details of growth in the many other parts of the mandible (see Fig. IV-5). The condyle is a "special" growth site in the sense that it combines articulation with regional growth. The additions of new bone provided by the condyle produce one of the dominant growth movements of the mandible as a whole (Fig. IV-9). The posterior border of the ramus, in conjunction with the condyle, also undergoes a major growth movement that follows a posterior and somewhat lateral course (Fig. IV-10). The combination of condylar and ramus growth brings about (1) a backward transposition of the entire ramus (the anterior border is resorptive), thereby permitting a simultaneous elongation of the mandibular body, (2) a displacement of the mandibular corpus in an anterior direction,* (3) a vertical lengthening of the ramus, thereby providing displacement of the mandible inferiorly, and (4) movable articulation during these various growth changes (Fig. IV-9).

2. THE LINGUAL TUBEROSITY

The lingual tuberosity is the site of a marked horizontal elongation of the mandibular body in a posterior direction (Fig. IV-10). The contiguous ramus is positioned, for the most part, laterally to this protuberance, whereas the lingual tuberosity itself lies in direct line with the mandibular arch. As the ramus grows and becomes relocated in a posterior direction, the lingual tuberosity correspondingly grows and moves posteriorly. A remodeling conversion from one to the other takes place as former generations of the backward-shifting ramus become changed into the lengthening and more medially positioned body. The lingual

---

*The actual "force" that produces this displacement is not clear; i.e., is it pushed anteriorly by its own growth enlargement or carried by the growth of soft tissue and other bony elements (Enlow,[25, 26] Moss[71])?

A

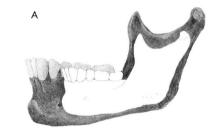

B

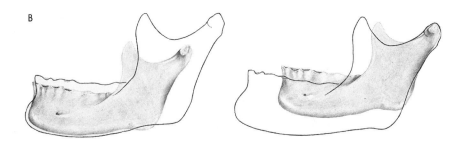

C

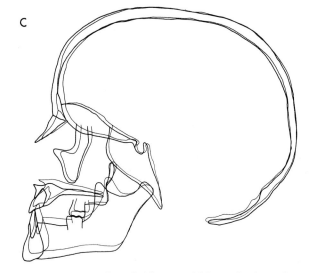

Fig. IV-9.—A, comparison of a child's mandible with that of an adult. This frequently used orientation is very misleading, since the growth does not occur in the amounts indicated at the various sites by this orientation. The child's mandible simply could not become the adult mandible by general over-all growth as this orientation would indicate. **B,** by orienting differently, the effects of growth displacement, remodeling and resorption are better visualized. Here, on the left, a

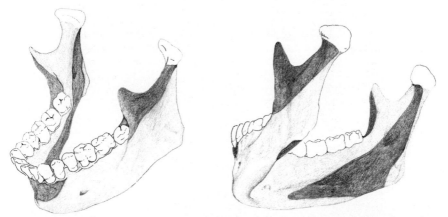

Fig. IV-10.—The distribution of resorptive and depository periosteal surfaces in the human mandible is mapped in these drawings. Periosteal surfaces that undergo progressive removal during growth are indicated in black, outer surfaces that are depository in nature are indicated in light gray.

tuberosity is comparable (in both relative location and growth function) to the maxillary tuberosity (see Fig. IV-14).

3. The Maxillary Tuberosity

Like the lingual tuberosity of the mandible, the maxillary tuberosity is associated with a major growth movement in a posterior direction (see Fig. IV-14). It is responsible for the lengthening of the maxillary body and arch. Unlike the lingual tuberosity, however, a "ramus" is not present and, therefore, complex remodeling conversions from one to the other are not involved.

4. The Alveolar Process

The bony tissue of the alveolar process is very mutable, since it is dependent on the functions of the teeth that it houses. Alveolar bone grows in response to dental eruption, adapts and remodels according to dental needs and resorbs when the teeth are lost.

---

child's mandible without the teeth has been superposed along the mandibular canal. Note the extensive remodeling, deposition and cortical drift necessary to produce the outline of the adult mandible. On the right, the orientation and registration is on the condylar region. Such an orientation dramatizes the displacement of the mandible with growth. **C** shows serial cephalograms superposed on the cranial base. The changes seen at the chin are the summation of all growth changes between the chin and the cranial base, not just mandibular growth and displacement alone.

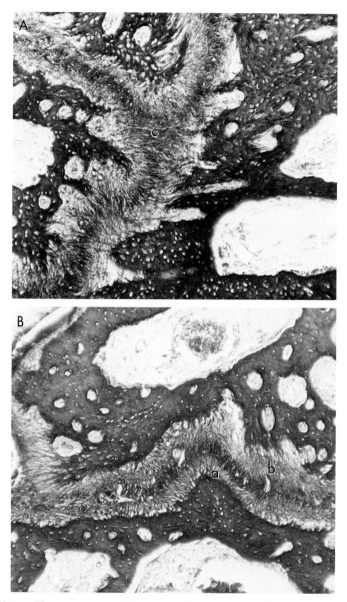

Fig. IV-11.—These sections of the nasal frontal suture from a young, rapidly growing kitten were prepared according to the differential polychrome procedure. All three zones in both **A** and **B** can be seen. The coarse fibers of the border zone (*a*) and the delicate linkage fibrils of the intermediate zone (*b*) are indicated in photomicrograph **B**. The heavy, coarse fiber bundles of the capsular zone (*c*) are labeled in photomicrograph **A**. (From Enlow, D. H.: *The Human Face* [New York: Hoeber Medical Division, Harper & Row, Publishers, 1968].)

5. SUTURES

The bony elements of the middle face are joined with one another and to the cranium by a system of sutural junctions, which also are active sites of growth and progressive adjustments involved in the differential changes occurring among the several bony elements during facial enlargement. Sutures are "tension-adapted" growth regions responding to forces produced by the enlarging soft tissues associated with them (the brain, mucosae, eye, nasal septum, tongue, etc.). Additions of bone within sutures, therefore, do not "push" adjacent elements apart. Rather, as the bones become separated by the enlargement of associated organs, simultaneous deposits of new bone on sutural edges serve to enlarge the bones themselves and to maintain the junctions between them (Figs. IV-11 and IV-12).

6. THE NASAL SEPTUM

Unlike the mandible and cranial base, an endochondral mechanism of growth, as such, is not present in the middle face. However, a process of "pressure-adapted" expansion appears to occur in the forward and downward displacement (not actual growth) of the nasomaxillary complex presumed to be provided by the interstitially enlarging cartilaginous nasal septum. Whether this expanding septum is the sole source of nasomaxillary growth movements or whether it operates in conjunction with other soft tissues is not presently known with certainty.

7. SURFACES

The over-all process of facial enlargement is not restricted to the various major "centers" of growth outlined above, since virtually all inner and outer surfaces of each bone within the facial complex are actively involved in the total growth process (see Figs. IV-10, IV-14 and IV-18). These different endosteal and periosteal surfaces are blanketed by localized growth fields that operate essentially independently but harmoniously with one another. Surface growth activities provide regional increases and remodeling changes that accompany the additions that take place in sutures, synchondroses, condyles, etc. All of the different processes of growth contribute to the over-all pattern of continued enlargement.

E. Regional Growth

Variations in the morphology of a bone are produced by (1) differences in the basic pattern of surface resorption and deposition, (2) the differential extent of deposition and resorption associated with particular fields and (3) the nature of the timing that occurs in the growth activities of different fields.

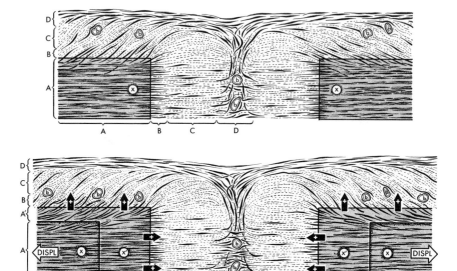

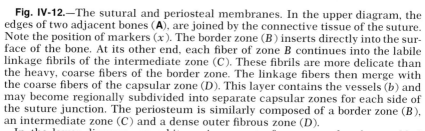

Fig. IV-12.—The sutural and periosteal membranes. In the upper diagram, the edges of two adjacent bones (**A**), are joined by the connective tissue of the suture. Note the position of markers (*x*). The border zone (*B*) inserts directly into the surface of the bone. At its other end, each fiber of zone *B* continues into the labile linkage fibrils of the intermediate zone (*C*). These fibrils are more delicate than the heavy, coarse fibers of the border zone. The linkage fibers then merge with the coarse fibers of the capsular zone (*D*). This layer contains the vessels (*b*) and may become regionally subdivided into separate capsular zones for each side of the suture junction. The periosteum is similarly composed of a border zone (*B*), an intermediate zone (*C*) and a dense outer fibrous zone (*D*).

In the lower diagram, an arbitrary increment of new zone has been added (+ *arrows*) to each sutural bone surface (*A'*). The old bones (*A*) have become displaced away from each other (*DISPL arrows*). Note the changed positions of the markers (*x*). The fibers of the former zone *B* have now become embedded in the new bone (*A'*). A new border zone has formed from the old intermediate zone (*C*). As its fibrils lengthen in a direction away from bone surfaces, they undergo differentiation into coarse, mature collagenous fibers. The bone simultaneously increases in thickness by subperiosteal (and also endosteal) deposition (+ *arrows*). The coarse fibers of the border zone become embedded attachment fibers as the linkage fibrils of the continuous intermediate zone differentiate into the fibers of a new border zone. As the entire periosteum "drifts" in an outward course, the linkage fibrils lengthen in a direction toward zone *D* and increase in number to accommodate the expanded coverage. (From Enlow, D. H.: *The Human Face* [New York: Hoeber Medical Division, Harper & Row, Publishers, 1968].)

1. THE MANDIBLE

The mandible consists of three major parts—the body, the alveolar process and the rami. In the neonate, the body is ill defined, the alveolar process is scarcely present, the rami are proportionately short and the condyles have not yet become well developed. Symphyseal growth still occurs, increasing the width of the mandible. However, by the second year, the symphysis has closed, a feature of man and the other primates.

The mandible is a mixed or composite "endochondral" and "intramembranous" bone. Endochondral growth at the condylar region (and for a short time in other secondary endochondral sites as well) plays an important role in mandibular development. This endochondral growth occurs in conjunction with intramembranous ossification at other growth sites. The mandible may be thought of as a bent tubular bone (the body) to which are added special areas for muscle insertion and tooth attachment (Fig. IV-13). On either end of this bent rod are found the endochondral epiphyseal growth centers of the condyles. The alveolar process does not form until the teeth begin to develop and

Fig. IV-13.—The role of endochondral bone growth in the mandible. One may visualize the mandible as the central portion of a tubular long bone that has been bent so that half of each epiphyseal plate is in either condylar position. This bent tube constitutes the corpus mandibularis, to which are attached areas of bone for muscle insertion and areas for holding the teeth. (Adapted from Symons, N. B. B.: Dent. Rec. 71:41, 1951.)

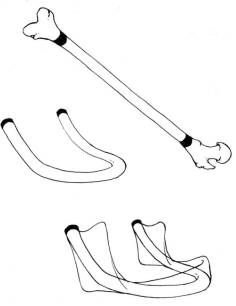

erupt, and it is resorbed when the teeth are lost. Areas of muscle attachment at the coronoid processes and the gonial regions become fully differentiated only in response to the development and functioning of the muscles that insert there. It has been shown experimentally that these regions do not develop well if the muscles are removed very early or if the nerves and vessels serving these muscles are severed.

The mandible appears to "grow" in a forward and downward manner, when visualized in superposed serial cephalometric tracings registered on the cranial base (see Fig. XII-16). Actual growth, however, takes place in a wide variety of regional directions (see Fig. IV-10). The predominant trend of growth generally is superior and posterior, but simultaneous displacement of the whole mandible occurs in an opposite (i.e., anterior and inferior) course, regardless of the many varying regional directions of growth (see Fig. IV-9).

The backward course of generalized mandibular enlargement serves to relocate the ramus in a progressively posterior direction. Thus, former levels occupied by the ramus become converted by remodeling into new parts of the body (see Figs. IV-9 and IV-10). This process provides two growth functions: (1) it produces a lengthening of the mandibular body and (2) it is associated with a movement of the whole mandible forward by simultaneous displacement. The backward movement of the ramus, however, is not simply a process of bone addition on the posterior border with resorption from the anterior margin; rather, the whole ramus becomes involved, including the entire buccal and labial surfaces between the anterior and posterior margins (see Fig. IV-10). These surfaces are oriented in a variety of directions with respect to the generally backward and upward direction of mandibular growth. Thus, the buccal side of the coronoid process is resorptive and the opposite lingual surface is largely depository, since they point away from and toward the superior and posterior direction of growth, respectively. Similarly, the buccal side of the lower ramus is depository, whereas the contralateral lingual side is largely resorptive. The composite of growth changes in all the different regional areas produces a generalized upward and backward movement of the whole ramus as a unit while simultaneously providing proportionate enlargement of the various regions as well (see Fig. IV-10).

The growth movements of the mandible, in general, are complemented by corresponding mutually interrelated changes occurring in the maxilla. A primary function of ramus growth is the continuous positioning of the mandibular arch relative to the complementary growth movements of the overlying maxilla. As the maxillary arch becomes displaced anteriorly, the horizontal growth of the ramus produces a simultaneous displacement of the mandibular arch in equivalent directions and to an approximately equal extent. Similarly, as the maxillary body descends during growth, the mandibular arch correspondingly becomes displaced downward in conjunction with continuing vertical elongation of the ramus.

Although the actual vertical placement of the mandible is determined largely by the growing ramus, vertical growth also occurs on both the superior and inferior sides of the mandibular body (see Fig. IV-10). The deposition of bone on the inferior border of the body is somewhat less and appears to be restricted to adjustments of contours and cortical thickness. Vertical increases on the superior (alveolar) side are related primarily to tooth movements and support. The condylar region generally grows upward and backward, although its direction is related to general patterns of total facial growth. Björk[13] found vertical growth of condyles associated with decreases in gonial angle, more mesial eruption of mandibular teeth and a large amount of compensatory resorption beneath the ramal angle. Condylar growth in a more forward direction is associated with increases in gonial angle and backward eruption of teeth.

Compare these mandibular growth changes with the corresponding maxillary growth changes described below.

2. THE NASOMAXILLARY COMPLEX

The maxilla, like the mandible, *grows* in a complex variety of regional directions (Fig. IV-14), but its predominant course of enlargement is posteriorly and superiorly. *Displacement* takes place in an opposite forward and downward manner (Fig. IV-15). The backward course of maxillary enlargement is produced by progressive surface deposits on the posterior-facing maxillary tuberosity, increasing the horizontal (anteroposterior) dimensions of the alveolar arch by an elongation at

Fig. IV-14.—The distribution of regional depository and resorptive periosteal surfaces in the nasal maxillary complex. Here, the resorptive surfaces are shown in black and the depository surfaces in light gray. The white zones (*t*) are areas in which variation normally occurs in placement of the reversal line between resorptive and repository surfaces.

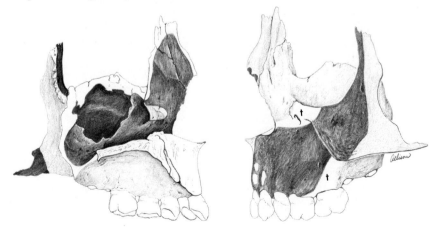

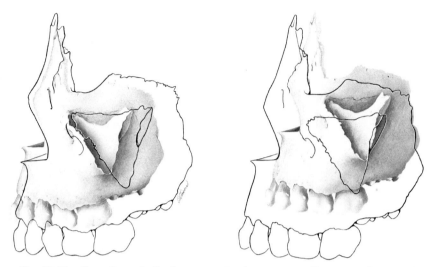

Fig. IV-15.—Growth and displacement in the nasomaxillary complex. In the orientation on the left, the resorption and deposition necessary to produce the adult nasomaxillary complex are clearly shown. Compare with Figure IV-14. On the right, the displacement necessary to achieve the adult nasomaxillary configuration is depicted.

its free (posterior) ends. As this takes place, relocation of the other parts of the maxilla occurs simultaneously. The position of the laterally protruding zygomatic process, for example, becomes constantly moved by a process of remodeling change. If the zygomatic process were to grow in a forward direction, as one might erroneously assume, its relationship relative to the arch as a whole would become disproportionate, since the arch itself grows in a backward direction. The zygomatic process, therefore, maintains a constant relative position by proportionate posterior movements that correspond to the posterior direction of arch elongation. The process of remodeling that carries out this movement combines surface resorption on the anterior face of the malar protrusion with deposition on the opposite posterior side. The resulting backward drift of the whole zygomatic process thus is similar in nature to the posterior movement of the mandibular coronoid process.

Forward of the zygomatic processes, it is noteworthy that the anterior-facing surfaces of the maxillary alveolar arch itself are largely resorptive in character rather than depository (see Fig. IV-14). At first thought, this would appear untenable, since the maxilla itself seemingly "grows" in an anterior direction. The progressive forward protrusion of the upper jaw, however, is a result of displacement rather than of actual growth (see under The Nasal Septum, above). The resorptive nature of the external maxillary surface does not produce an actual regression, although a slight degree of alveolar retraction occurs due to relocation (see Fig.

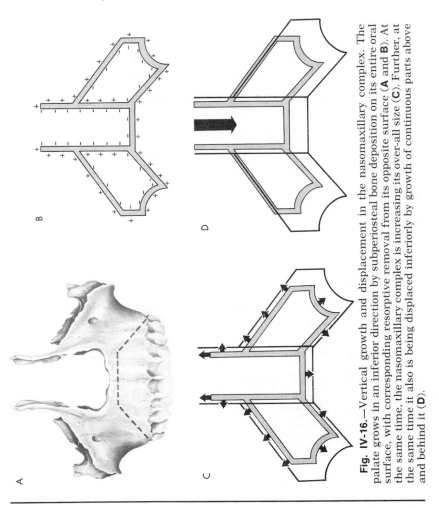

Fig. IV-16.—Vertical growth and displacement in the nasomaxillary complex. The palate grows in an inferior direction by subperiosteal bone deposition on its entire oral surface, with corresponding resorptive removal from its opposite surface (**A** and **B**). At the same time, the nasomaxillary complex is increasing its over-all size (**C**). Further, at the same time it also is being displaced inferiorly by growth of continuous parts above and behind it (**D**).

IV-15). This remodeling pattern is a response to the essentially inferior mode of maxillary arch growth, as described below. The alveolar surface in the anterior portion of the mandibular arch also is characteristically resorptive in nature. In the mandible, however, a distinctive, protruding "chin" is produced by the combination of slight alveolar retraction in conjunction with variable amounts of forward-growing periosteal deposition in the basal region (see Fig. IV-10). A much smaller protuberance, the nasal spine, is formed on the maxilla by a similar remodeling combination.

In Figure IV-14, note that a key growth reversal exists along a line that separates that portion of the maxillary arch located anteriorly to the malar prominence from the region posterior to it. A major change in topographic contour coincides with the ridge that marks this line. Forward of the reversal, the maxillary surface is oriented so that it points away from the downward course of continued growth; therefore, this surface is largely resorptive. The contralateral surfaces on the oral sides of the cortical laminae are depository. The periosteal surface of the cortex posterior to the reversal line, in contrast, faces in a direction toward the inferior and slightly lateral course of growth and thus is depository in type, whereas its contralateral endosteal side is resorptive.

In the maxillary arch, the process of vertical growth involves both orbital and nasal expansion and remodeling. The resulting composite nature of vertical lengthening by the middle face thus requires a degree of downward maxillary arch movement that exceeds the extent of upward growth by the mandibular alveolar arch. The nasal floor descends by a combination of (1) resorption from the superior surface of the bony palate, together with deposition on the inferior side, and (2) a vertical elongation of the frontal and zygomatic processes in association with downward displacement of the whole maxilla (paced presumably by the nasal septum) (Fig. IV-16). The process of inferior displacement also lowers the orbital floor at the same time. However, the extent of downward orbital expansion is considerably less than that of the adjacent nasal chamber. As the floor of the orbit becomes displaced in an inferior manner, simultaneous deposits of bone are laid down on its superior surface, thereby stabilizing the position of the orbit relative to the differential growth movements of the contiguous nasal region and palate. The combined lateral growth movements of the orbits, the nasal walls and the malar region are produced by bone deposition on their lateral-facing surfaces, together with resorption from the various medial-facing surfaces.

The positioning of the maxilla relative to the cranial floor is associated with the growth of the various horizontal and vertical processes of the maxillary, the frontal, the zygomatic and the temporal bones. Similarly, the position of the mandible with respect to the floor of the cranium (and to the overlying maxilla) is associated with the growth of the ramus, which serves as a single morphogenetic counterpart to the composite of these different bony projections in the middle face.

In Figure IV-14 it is noted that the nasal portions of the bony face are characteristically depository on their external surfaces, in contrast to the resorptive nature of the maxillary arch and the malar regions adjacent to them. A progressive forward protrusion of the entire nasal area is thus produced with respect to the remainder of the middle face. The various facial regions, including the nose, the premaxilla, the posterior tuberosity, the forehead, the cheekbones and the orbits, are thus "carried apart" as their contours become expanded in a variety of divergent directions.

3. The Cranial Base and Cranial Vault

The respective modes of growth in the cranial floor and the vault are characterized by several basic differences, since marked differentials in the extent, rate and nature of growth occur between them. The growth of the bones that constitute the calvaria utilizes a suture system in conjunction with relatively small surface deposits on both the ectocranial and endocranial sides. Remodeling adjustments are minor and occur primarily in the areas just adjacent to sutures. Extensive remodeling changes comparable with those found in most other bones of the skull do not take place. Although the calvaria encloses the various hemispheres of the brain, it is noted that all major arteries, veins, nerves and the spinal cord enter or leave by way of the cranial floor. The continued positioning of the foramina associated with them thus is not a factor in the growth of the skull roof. The complex processes of growth in the cranial floor, however, must provide constant stabilization for the passage of these structures. Sutural increases, as a sole growth mechanism, would tend to separate such soft tissue components to a disproportionate extent, owing to the markedly differential degrees of divergence between them and the expansion of the fossae within which they are located (Fig. IV-17).

The cranial floor, unlike the vault, is characterized by complex topo-

Fig. IV-17.—Cranial floor growth. In the cul-de-sac of the cranial floor, the process of sutural growth cannot accommodate the total extent of expansion as seen in *A*. In addition, cortical drift is directly involved (*B*) and, in combination with sutural additions, produces the enlargement of the various fossae.

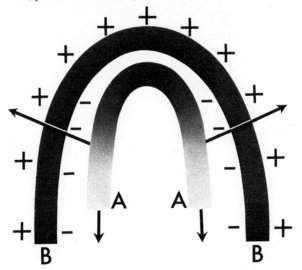

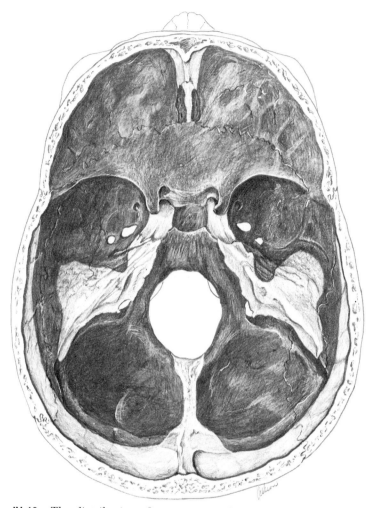

Fig. IV-18.—The distribution of resorptive and depository periosteal surfaces in the cranial floor. Resorptive regions are shown in black and depository areas in gray.

graphic contours. The growing coverage of the even-contoured skull roof is provided largely by sutural increases, which are paced by the expansion of the enclosed brain. In the floor, however, the relatively confined contours of the numerous endocranial fossae cannot be enlarged by sutural increases alone, since the abrupt nature of the curvatures involved and the placement of sutures within them is such that fossa expansion in both lateral and posteroanterior dimensions is not possible solely by this means (Fig. IV-18). In addition to the sutural growth

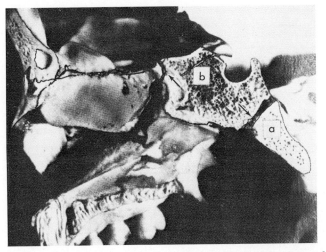

Fig. IV-19.—Growth sites in the cranial base. The sphenoid bone is at *b* and the *left arrow* points to the spheno-ethmoidal synchondrosis. The *right arrow* points to the spheno-occipital synchondrosis. (Adapted from Baume.[6])

present, significant direct cortical drift also takes place in the cranial floor, unlike the calvarium, whereas elongation of the cranial base is provided in part by growth at the synchondroses and direct cortical growth (Fig. IV-19). The process of cortical drift in the cranial floor produces regionally variable degrees of growth movement in a generally ectocranial direction by surface resorption (Fig. IV-20) from the endocranial side, together with proportionate deposition on external surfaces. A reversal line occurs on the endocranial cortical surface that separates the contrasting growth fields of the skull roof from those in the floor (see Fig. IV-19).

Thus, the growth processes that take place in the cranial floor are carried out by a complex balance between sutural growth, elongation at synchondroses and direct, extensive cortical drift and remodeling. This combination provides (1) a differential extent of growth enlargement between the cranial base and the calvaria, (2) a means for the expansion of confined contours in the various endocranial fossa and (3) maintenance of passages and housing for vessels and nerves as well as such appendages as the hypophysis.

The design of the human cranial base and calvaria is adapted to both the upright posture of the body and the development of particularly large cerebral hemispheres. These factors are associated with the placement of the foramen magnum in a midventral position and the presence of a marked flexure in the cranial base. This flexure is produced by the massive forward expansion of the frontal and prefrontal lobes and the backward and downward enlargement of the occipital and

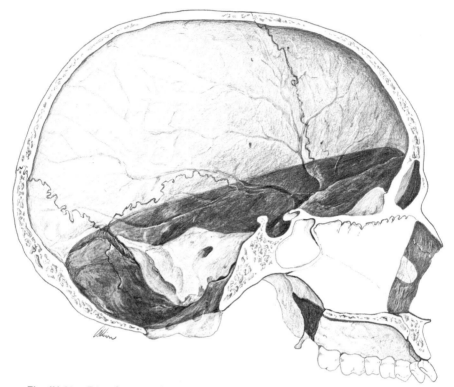

Fig. IV-20.—Distribution of resorptive and depository periosteal surfaces in the cranial vault, cranial base and nasomaxillary complex as seen in a lateral internal view. Resorptive regions are shown in black and depository regions in light gray.

cerebellar lobes relative to the slower-growing ventral brain axis. Correspondingly, cranial base flexure places the foramen magnum in direct alignment with a vertically oriented spinal cord and a forward-pointing alignment of the face and orbits due to man's bipedal posture.

The growth of the cranial base has a direct effect on the placement of the middle face and the mandible. As the anterior cranial fossa and the clivus elongate, the horizontal and vertical dimensions of the underlying space occupied by the enlarging nasomaxillary complex and the ramus increase correspondingly. As the spheno-occipital complex elongates, a related displacement of the entire middle face in an anterior direction necessarily results, producing an enlargement of the adjacent pharyngeal region. Correspondingly, the ramus of the mandible enlarges simultaneously, thereby displacing the mandibular arch anteriorly in conjunction with the forward displacement of the maxilla.

F. Pattern of Facial Growth

Pattern, as the term is used in facial growth, is the visualized expression of all the synchronized mechanisms of growth in the face. Facial growth is rather orderly and consistent; pattern is the word we use to express such orderliness and consistency. The concept of pattern of facial growth is used in three ways: (1) A person tends to have a pattern of facial form and growth similar to others of the same ethnic group. One can, with reasonable accuracy, distinguish cephalometric tracings of some racial groups from those of other races. (2) Members of the same family have similar patterns of facial growth. Although much of what we call family resemblance resides in soft tissue, genetic studies confirm parent, child and sibling similarities. (3) We tend to resemble ourselves at different ages. Thus, if a cephalogram or photograph of a child at 14 years of age is compared with one of the same person taken at age 5, changes produced by growth are readily apparent; however, basic similarities also are observed and the image is recognizable as the same child (Fig. IV-21).

The structural arrangement and the progressive growth of the different craniofacial bones conform to a system of region-to-region "equivalence." Equivalence is an architectural principle based on the counterpart nature of construction among the separate bones. Any bone or some part of that bone is a structural counterpart of some other bone

Figure IV-21.—Pattern of growth: the same individual at two ages.

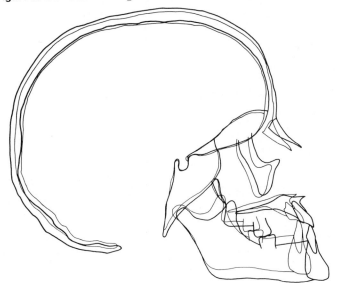

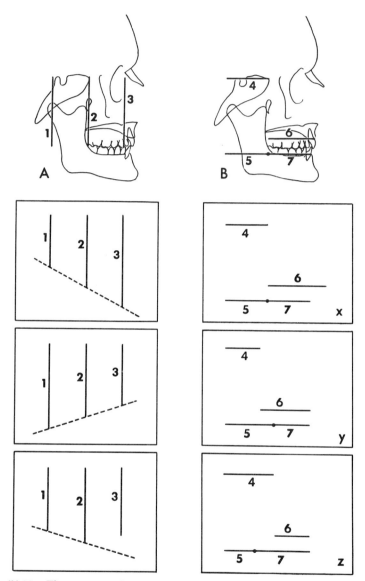

Fig. IV-22.—The concept of equivalent and effective dimensions. When comparing parts of the face cephalometrically, it is important that the dimensions being compared be *equivalent* with each other. Often, traditional cephalometric measurements are compared when they are not equivalent representations. In **A,** for example, if one is to compare facial height anteriorly, posteriorly and in the middle of the head, he must be measuring essentially the same functioning distance each time. In a similar fashion, in **B,** maxillary length as shown by line 6

positioned more or less parallel to it. The feature of bilateral symmetry throughout the body as a whole is a simple example of the equivalent-balance principle. The right side of the mandible is a structural complement of the left, the sizes of both are in approximate balance and, ordinarily, remain so during continued growth. However, the mandible has other equivalent counterparts in the skull. The bony maxillary arch, for example, is a horizontal equivalent of the corpus portion of the mandible extending parallel to it. Similarly, the anterior cranial fossa is an architectural equivalent of the parallel span of the maxilla just below it (Fig. IV-22). The growth of any one such equivalent matches the growth of its counterparts. When evaluating pattern, it is meaningful, therefore, to consider both the form and the growth for an understanding of craniofacial morphology (see Chapter XII, Analysis of the Craniofacial Skeleton).

G. Genetics of Craniofacial Growth

Even a casual observer of familial likeness is convinced that there are important genetic factors in dentofacial development. The problem is to identify the specificity, site, timing and mechanisms of any such genetic controls. Roentgenographic cephalometry lends itself well to quantitative study of the effects on the bony skeleton of any genetic influences on craniofacial growth. Whether genetic mechanisms operate directly through osteogenesis or indirectly through such factors as muscles (see Section I) is not clear at this time. In family-line studies, the variance for a trait is compared in monozygous and dizygous twins. It is assumed that differences between MZ twins are likely nongenetic, whereas DZ twins, although sharing the same prenatal environment, are no more genetically similar than siblings.[59] Indeed, so useful is the cephalogram for genetic studies that Prorok[82] and Hunter[50] have suggested the use of batteries of cephalometric measurements to determine zygosity. Hunter *et al.*[51] have shown a secular change in craniofacial adult dimensions that cannot be explained by genetics alone.

---

is equivalent to line 7 in the mandible. The dimension from the condyle to the chin point is not equivalent to 6 nor the line $5 + 7$ equivalent to 6. By *effective dimensions* is meant those measurements that represent only that portion of the bone that should be measured for a specific determination; thus, in **B,** line 4 is the effective anteroposterior dimension of the cranial base, which is equivalent to the effective anteroposterior depth of the ramus as shown in line 5. Such equivalent dimensions may aggregate in such a way as to compensate for localized imbalances as in *y* and *z* or they may summate to produce or aggravate local imbalances as in *x*. For a more complete discussion of these concepts, see Chapter XII.

1. OVER-ALL FACIAL DIMENSIONS

A number of claims for precise genetic specificity in the dentofacial complex have been made, for example, Hughes and Moore,[46] Moore[67] and Moore and Hughes.[68] Such studies usually have been based solely on subjective observations. Recent quantitative reports are more useful.[36, 48, 50] The problem is complicated by the fact that the genetic expression may influence the size of a part, its shape or the timing of its growth. Therefore, the methods of measuring and the ages studied are critical. Studies of parents and their adult offspring have been shown by Hunter *et al.*[51] to be revealing of the genetic control of facial dimensions. In general, those bodily dimensions measured parallel to the long axis show the strongest genetic component.[50] It is not surprising to learn, then, that facial height dimensions tend to show higher heritability than do measurements of facial depth. Facial breadth (bizygomatic) and mandibular width (bigonial) show a good measure of hereditary variability.[50] The implications of these findings are interesting. First, one should be able to predict facial height or width better than depth and, second, there is support for the idea that nongenetic influences are more likely to affect anteroposterior dimensions, particularly those in the dento-alveolar region.

2. INCREMENTAL GROWTH

The genetic regulation of increments of growth is more difficult to assess and fewer data are available. Meredith[63] was unable to predict growth in nasal height and bigonial width from 8 to 12 years using the data on growth from 5 to 7 years. Hunt[47] found that some midface anteroposterior dimensions had individual predictability but that width and height increments did not. Harvold[37] found low predictability of the maxillomandibular skeletal relationship at 12 years, utilizing serial data from 6 to 9 years.

3. GROSS CRANIOFACIAL DEFORMITY

a) Cleft Lip and/or Cleft Palate

This condition is found approximately once in every 700–800 births in North American and European whites, but is markedly lower in American Negroes and somewhat higher in Japanese.[55] It is very difficult to separate the genetic and teratogenic factors in cleft palate etiology. Cleft lip and/or palate often are part of a more general syndrome; therefore, associated malformations are found with high frequency.[55]

Although there are a number of studies on the inheritance of cleft lip and palate, there still is disagreement on the mode of inheritance. Snodgrasse[94] believes that isolated cleft palate is due to simple recessive heredity with variable expressivity. Fogh-Andersen[27,28] stated that cleft

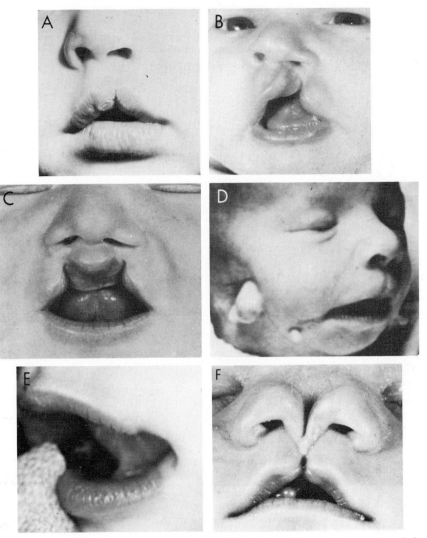

Fig. IV-23.—Some congenital anomalies of the head and face. **A,** incomplete cleft of lip, unilateral. **B,** cleft lip, unilateral. **C,** cleft lip, bilateral. **D,** Pierre Robin syndrome. **E,** macrostomia. **F,** midline cleft.

lip is found more often in males and is inherited as a recessive trait, whereas cleft palate alone is found more frequently in females, in whom it is caused by a dominant character with reduced penetrance. Carter[18] agrees, but holds that cleft lip and/or palate might involve "a major recessive gene." Experimental studies,[29] mostly on mice, suggest that cleft lip and primary palate (anterior to nasopalatine foramen) may be more likely to be mediated genetically, whereas cleft of the secondary palate results more often from teratogens.

Varying opinions are held on the percentage of cleft lip and palate cases that are inherited in humans. Fukuhara and Saito[31] have identified defects in the region that they consider lesser forms of clefting or near misses, so it is not surprising that they hold approximately 50% of the cases to be the result of dominant inheritance.

b) Craniofacial Syndromes

Some craniofacial syndromes are hereditary and some are not, for example, those resulting from rubella; some are part of a generalized syndrome and some are restricted to the head and face.[83] For most syndromes involving the head-face complex, the genetic mechanisms are not yet clear. Some examples of the more common syndromes of the head and face are shown in Figure IV-23.

4. Soft Tissue Facial Features

In probably the most thorough study yet of the genetics of external facial features, Pfannenstiel's[78] primary findings are of interest: (1) chin height, upper and lower lip height and vermilion height are due to multiple genes, (2) a midline depression in the integument of the lower lip ("cleft lip") and a horizontal sulcus mentolabialis are simple dominants, (3) philtrum size and shape are genetically controlled and (4) mouth breadth (when considered as a proportion of lip height, total face height and bigonial width) shows no evidence of genetic mediation.

There is much in the orthodontic literature concerning "endogenous muscle pattern" of the mouth, face and jaws. Endogenous muscle behavior, as contrasted with learned motor activities, presumably would be under some genetic control, but the documentation awaits a method of study.

H. Racial and Ethnic Differences in Facial Growth

The problem of racial and ethnic differences in craniofacial growth is complicated by the difficulty of defining a race or ethnic group. Even a casual reading of the cephalometric literature reveals that the frequency of various facial types reported in the excellent studies of Italians by Maj *et al.*[60] and Muzj[75] demonstrates striking general differences in dentofacial relationships from similar studies of Scandinavians by

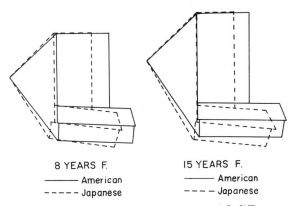

8 YEARS F.   15 YEARS F.
———— American   ———— American
— — — — Japanese   — — — Japanese

Fig. IV-24.—Cephalometric polygons depicting racial differences. (From Kuroda.[57])

Björk,[10] Japanese by Miura *et al.*[65] and Kuroda[57] or North American Negroes by Altemus.[2] Altemus points out that within an ethnic or racial group, examples of almost any of the facial types may appear, but the frequency of a particular type varies from ethnic group to ethnic group. Thus, one sees more mandibular prognathism in Scandinavians and far more retrognathism in Anglo-Saxon samples, although extremes of prognathism and retrognathism are found in both racial groups. North American Negroes display more pronounced bimaxillary protrusion than do North American whites when group means are compared. Many racial groups have been studied, with repeated findings of significant differences in measured means among various ethnic populations (e.g., see Fig. IV-24). Such differences must be taken into account in research studies and when planning orthodontic treatment for an individual patient. Acceptable suggested incisor positions derived by clinicians studying North American Caucasian samples likely will be most inadequate and indeed improper for clinicians treating other racial and ethnic groups. Since the racial differences express themselves in variations in timing as well as in size and form, it has been necessary for research workers and clinicians around the world to identify the typical features as well as the range of measurements normally expected for each group.[74]

I. Role of the Musculature and Function in Craniofacial Growth

Although there is general acceptance of the importance of genetic factors in determining craniofacial form, there is a wide divergence of opinion regarding the role of functional activity.

The classic view holds that the craniofacial skeleton's pattern of growth is determined genetically within fairly rigid limits with respect to size, direction and rate. This view accepts the fact that variations in function occur but, as long as these variations are within normal limits, they have little or no effect on growth and development. Malocclusions, in this view, appear primarily because of inherited variations within the bone and teeth, and the effects of postnatal and environmental factors are of local and minor importance only.

The functional view of facial growth is best and most strongly stated by Moss,[71] whose ideas stem from the work of Van der Klaauw.[97] Moss extended Van der Klaauw's ideas, saying that the growth of the bone itself is secondary, since all growth changes seen in bone reflect the growth and function of the tissue systems associated with the bones. He has given the term "functional matrix" to all of the functional units with which craniofacial skeletal units are associated. He includes in the functional matrix concept the brain, muscles, tendons, glands, vessels, teeth and even empty spaces. Two basic types of matrices are conceived—periosteal, including muscles and teeth, and capsular, volumes enclosed within the skull.[71]

Wolff's law is a well-known principle which states that, in general, the structure and shape of a bone become progressively adapted to the sum of all the changing mechanical forces exerted on it. When these forces attain equilibrium with the physical properties of the bone, growth presumably ceases as such and the morphology of that bone is then in balance with its various mechanical functions. Although this principle is essentially valid, some of the traditional tension-pressure explanations of its operation are oversimplified or incorrect, since many known growth changes do not coincide with the patterns of pressure and tension that have been presumed to produce them.[24] The problems involved have not been resolved.

One of the reasons for the variance in opinions concerning the role of function in craniofacial growth is the present lack of adequate quantified studies in this important area.

1. MUSCLE GROWTH AND SKELETAL GROWTH

During fetal life, skeletal muscle grows by division of muscle cells or differentiation of muscle-forming cells. Sometime during the second trimester, this generalized muscle growth stops and muscle tissues grow from that time on by hypertrophy of individual fibers, the increase in mass of the total muscle resulting as each individual muscle fiber increases in length or width. Increase in mass of a muscle is an index of that muscle's activity; when there is excessive work, it hypertrophies; when there is disuse, it may even atrophy.

Obviously, as the bones to which the muscles are attached grow, the muscles themselves must change their size. Therefore, a relationship exists between the over-all growth of any bone and the muscles attached to that bone. Adjustments between muscle and bone may take place in several ways: (1) they may pace one another evenly, the muscles holding relatively the same relationship to the skeleton with growth; (2) the areas of origin and insertion of the muscles may change due to asynchrony of muscular and skeletal growth. In both of these instances, the muscle migrates over the surface of the enlarging bone and undergoes a process of continual reattachment; (3) muscle fibers may be replaced largely by tendon.

2. Muscle Migration and Attachment

During growth, muscles must migrate to occupy relatively different positions with time. As the skeleton grows, there is a constant adjustment of the attachment relationship between muscle and skeleton, a process complicated by the fact that the outer bone surfaces in regions of muscle attachment frequently are resorptive as well as depository. A phylogenic migration of muscles also occurs. As man assumed a bipedal posture, complex muscle migrations occurred and provided an effective balance of the head over the upright vertebral column.

3. Function and Bone Growth

It is known that disuse and use determine, to some extent, the thickness of the cortical plate of limb bones. For example, arm bones have thicker cortical bone according to the handedness of the individual.[90] Furthermore, there is a decrease in cortical thickness seen during muscular paralysis of the limb muscles. It is important to separate the effects of use and paralysis on the thickness of the bone and the length of the bone. After adult length is achieved, neither disuse nor paralysis affects the length of a bone.[90] Any effects of function on the length of long bones during growth are not yet clearly shown and understood.

4. Response of the Craniofacial Skeleton to Variations in Function

Although much has been written concerning the response of the facial skeleton, few quantitative studies are available and most lack elegance of experimental design. Therefore, the findings, although revealing, are not as conclusive as they might be. Moss's provocative ideas have stimulated much current interest and renewed enthusiasm in this important field.[71, 72]

a) Regional or Local Effects

1) Skeletal regions whose form and size are dependent entirely on function.—Washburn[101] has shown that the removal of the

temporal muscle in experimental animals soon results in the loss of the coronoid process and the linea temporalis. He concluded that these changes in mandibular form were due to the absence of the stimulation of temporal contractions. On the other hand, Castelli and Ramirez[19] show evidence that such changes in form may be due to the loss of vascularization in such experiments.

The alveolar process appears only with the eruption of the teeth and is lost with their extraction.

2) SKELETAL REGIONS THAT DEVELOP MORE FULLY WITH FUNCTION.— In a well-designed experiment, Watt and Williams[102] studied facial growth in two groups of rats—one fed on hard foods and the other on the same diet but softened. The group that required more muscle function to chew the food showed localized thickening and heaviness in the areas of attachment of mandibular muscles. Ahlgren *et al.*,[1] in a combined electromyographic and cephalometric study, demonstrated changes in the gonial angle of the mandible related to bilateral hypertrophy of the masseter muscles in adults.

3) SKELETAL STRUCTURAL ELEMENTS RELATED TO MUSCLE FUNCTION APPARENTLY THROUGH PHYLOGENIC DEVELOPMENT ONLY.—Townsley[96] showed that mechanically determined structures may be present as hereditary features in young bones that have been protected experimentally from muscle contractions and weight bearing. One does not need to invoke Lysenkoism to explain Townsley's findings, for hereditarily determined bony structures may be related to muscular activities associated with phylogenic development of central nervous system complexity.

b) General Effects

1) MOUTH-BREATHING.—For many years, the orthodontic and medical literature has contained descriptive reports of alleged relationships between mouth-breathing and facial growth. The mouth-breather is reported to have narrower nasopharyngeal passages, a higher and narrower palate, maxillary dento-alveolar protrusion, steep mandibular plane, and so forth. Whether the mouth-breathing causes such skeletal variations or the skeletal pattern promotes mouth-breathing is not yet clear. Despite many papers and much clinical interest, the exact relationships, if any, between mouth-breathing and malocclusion are not yet quantitatively well documented. (See Chapter VII, Etiology of Malocclusion.)

2) VARIATIONS IN MASTICATORY FUNCTION.—Variations in masticatory function probably are not sufficient to explain all the characteristic features of ethnic or cultural groups. For example, it often is pointed out that the Eskimo's massive facial features have developed as the result of extensive use of the muscles of mastication. Close examination of such reports does produce evidence that the areas of muscle

attachment in Eskimos are more strongly developed than in many racial groups, but Selmer-Olsen[91] reminded us that the Lapps, living under conditions similar to the Eskimos, have characteristically delicate craniofacial skeletal features. In the same vein, Weidenreich[103] showed that variation in muscle function had a mechanical influence on the superstructures only and not on form and development of the cranium itself.

In the case of the cranium, cranial base and nasomaxillary complex, function features other than muscle apparently play an important role in development, viz., the growth of the brain, the eyeballs, respiratory function, cartilage growth, etc.

The mandible, with its important condylar cartilage, holds a special interest for orthodontists studying the more general effects of variations in function. The mandible has been divided into three elements (Fig. IV-13): (1) a basal or neural element, (2) a tooth-bearing element and

Fig. IV-25.—Effects of altering the functional occlusal position on mandibular growth. In this experiment, 6 monkeys had their occlusal relationships altered by the cementation of gold onlays. The wax patterns were carved so that the only way the monkey could function was to protrude the mandible. In the protruded position only, it achieved balanced intercuspation. **A,** the mean monthly increments of condylar growth before and after the insertion of the experimental appliance. **B,** comparison with control animals: above, the additive effects on condylar growth; below, comparison of mean increments. Note that the growth is not different between experimental and control animals after about the third month.

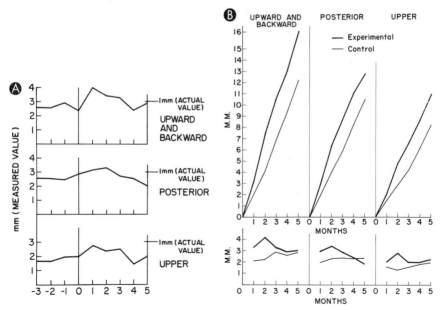

(3) muscle attachment regions. As mentioned earlier, variations in muscle function affect greatly the areas of muscle attachment, and the development and use of the dentition affect the alveolar processes. Concerning these two points there seems little dispute. However, the effect of function on the over-all size of the mandible is debated. Recent reports by Harvold[38] and Moyers *et al.*[73] present evidence that muscle function can have a more general effect on the size and form of the mandible than has been held previously (Fig. IV-25). The findings are important, since they have a direct bearing on the strategy employed to treat malocclusions with a structural disharmony. If the clinician can promote or optimize mandibular growth, for example, during the formative years, it improves the chances of treating well a significant number of common severe clinical problems. Since the evidence shows this to be likely, there has been an increased interest in functional jaw orthopedic appliances.

J. Relationships between Craniofacial and Body Growth

1. BODY TYPE AND FACIAL FORM

Individuals are classified according to their body build. The most common systems of somatotyping classify human beings according to the way their physique combines the features of three basic archetypes —endomorphic, mesomorphic and ectomorphic. Lindegard,[58] using his own modification of Sheldon's three basic types, correlated cephalometric findings with body build. However, most of his correlations were low and insignificant. He did find, though, that some measurements in the head and face increased in size more in proportion to his "sturdiness factor" than to the development of his "length factor." Björk,[12] using Lindegard's method, found that skeletal sturdiness generally was accompanied by large dental arches and large teeth. There also seemed to be a positive relationship between body build and dental eruption, since earlier eruption was associated with skeletal sturdiness. Generally, the reported relationships between body build and dentofacial measurements and indices are rather poor. However, the Italian school enthusiastically maintains that although the various parts of the body present variations in form and dimensions, these variations are not independent but are correlated to produce a harmonic whole. They find high correlations between specific facial types and body types.

Nanda,[76] as well as Pike,[79] found a closer correlation between stature and mandibular growth rates than between stature and maxillary length or total face height.

2. TIMING OF GROWTH EVENTS

Nanda[76] and Björk and Helm[15] have shown that the pubertal spurt in various facial dimensions occurs at different times relative to the pubertal spurt in body height, concluding that the maximum pubertal spurt for most facial measurements occurs slightly later than the general statural spurt. Björk and Helm[15] report that the mandibular condylar spurt appears before a similar increase in sutural growth. The relationship between stature, which is largely a summation of endochondral growth sites, and similar endochondral growth, for example, condyle or cranial base, in the craniofacial complex is thus closer than it is with sutural or periosteal growth.

3. Assessment of Body Growth for Orthodontic Purposes

Although the specific relationships between height and weight and craniofacial measurements do not correlate precisely in the individual child, a recording of height and weight is of use in the general assessment of the growth of the child. For this purpose, the charts of Meredith are a useful record to include in the patient's case history (Fig. IV-26).

A number of workers have studied the correlation between maturation of the hand and wrist bones and dental development and craniofacial growth. To some extent, the usefulness of these correlations for the clinician seems to have been overstated by some. Garn and Rohmann[32] have reported that hand-wrist ossification is useful in detecting growth abnormalities or in extremes of maturation but is not a precise method of measuring developmental progress in normal individuals. Nor are the correlations between the calcification of wrist bones and dental development of use for prognosticative purposes. Winshall[105] concluded that correlations between ossification of carpal bones and dental development, although interesting in corroborating gross delays or advances in timing, could not be relied on for specific individual assessments or predictions.

K. Effects of Orthodontic Treatment on Craniofacial Growth

Angle,[4] who dominated orthodontic thinking in North America during the first part of this century, thought that malocclusions were mainly the result of retardation of the growth of facial bones caused by unfavorable environmental factors. If a full complement of teeth were but placed in ideal occlusion, he believed, function would stimulate the bones to grow to an adequate size. Early treatment was advocated, since the sooner inhibiting factors were removed the better the prognosis. Others, recognizing that all malocclusions were not caused by the functioning environment of the bones, suggested that Angle had misinterpreted and misapplied Wolff's law and that it was not possible to grow bone ad libidum.

Soon after the introduction of roentgenographic cephalometry in the early 1930s, studies were begun to analyze the effect of orthodontic treatment on craniofacial growth. Brodie and his colleagues[17] con-

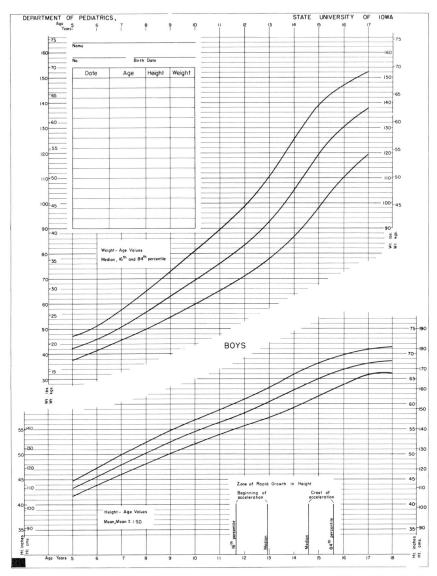

Fig. IV-26.—Height and weight chart, boys 5–18 years of age. (From Meredith.) (*Continued.*)

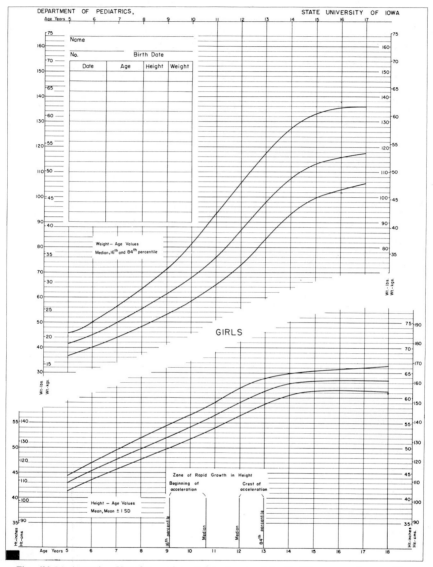

Fig. IV-26 (cont.).—Height and weight chart, girls 5–18 years of age. (From Meredith.) These charts may be obtained from The University of Iowa Bureau of Publications, Iowa City, Iowa.

cluded that Class II treatment had very little effect on facial growth—"the most startling finding was an apparent inability to alter anything but the alveolar process." Papers of this period emphasized the persistence of the morphogenetic pattern of the face and the belief grew, in North America at least, that the facial pattern was constant and unchangeable. Despite a number of papers analyzing the effects of orthodontic treatment, this pessimistic view dominated orthodontic thinking for many years. As late as the mid-1950s, two of our most renowned researchers stated that there was no evidence presented thus far to indicate that orthodontic treatment had any influence outside the alveolar processes.[11, 34] More recently, however, the evidence has begun to accumulate that orthodontic treatment does indeed have a marked effect on craniofacial growth.[4, 7, 35, 40, 43, 53, 54, 56, 66, 80, 85, 104] Our ability to understand this important problem is handicapped by at least three factors: (1) the continuing legacy within the profession and the literature of the earlier more pessimistic views, (2) the lack of satisfactory serial data on untreated malocclusions and (3) the failure to develop more sensitive cephalometric measurements of localized responses to altered conditions and growth.

1. METHODS OF ALTERING CRANIOFACIAL GROWTH

Theoretically, at least, orthodontic treatment might bring about one or more of the following bony responses: (1) change (increase or decrease) in size of a part, (2) an alteration in differential rates of growth, that is, regional growth might be stimulated or retarded, (3) a change in direction of growth, (4) an alteration in the timing of developmental events and (5) changes in shape, i.e., an alteration in proportions without necessarily changing the over-all size of parts.

2. CLASSES OF BONY RESPONSES TO FORCE APPLICATION

a) Responsive Bone

In some regions, any adequate force produces an immediate and direct bony transformation. Genetic control of conformation seems to be minimal or is overcome immediately by orthodontic forces. The best example of responsive bone is the alveolar process.

b) Bone Varying in Response

Some bones seem to respond during active growth but tend to resist orthodontic forces later; the example cited most often is the corpus mandibularis. Baume[6] differentiated between membrane and cartilage bone in this respect, holding that endochondral bone is unresponsive to mechanical stimuli, particularly after growth is completed, in contrast to membranous bone, which responds readily. Baume[6] concluded that "endochondral ossification thus constitutes the mechanism by which the skeleton develops into a genetically predetermined size and form, and these are the growth centers, whereas, growth sites occur in the region of periosteal or sutural bone formation and modeling results in adaptive environmental influence." This view is still maintained by many clinicians but, as we shall see, the evidence is accumulating to show that orthodontic therapy has striking effects on craniofacial growth, both endochondral and intramembranous.

3. EFFECTS ON THE NASOMAXILLARY COMPLEX

Several studies[7, 35, 43, 53, 66, 80, 85, 104] have shown that extra-oral traction with headgear or neck straps can affect the growth of the nasomaxillary complex in one or more of the following ways: (1) inhibition of the normal forward movement of the maxillary teeth, (2) inhibition of the normal downward and forward movement of the maxilla, (3) distal movement of the maxillary dentition, (4) alterations in the cant of the occlusal plane and (5) changes in the direction of the growth of the nasomaxillary complex.

There is no doubt that more extensive changes in the nasomaxillary region occur in young children treated with extra-oral traction; yet, even in the permanent dentition similarly treated, good results often are obtained, although the amount and nature of maxillary response to extra-oral traction seems to be directly related to the remaining growth potential.[104] There is no firm evidence yet that intra-oral elastic forces have any effect outside the dento-alveolar region.

The maxilla is readily responsive to lateral forces as well. It is now standard practice to "split the midpalatal suture," permitting extensive widening of the maxillary apical base[39, 84, 95] (see Chapter XVII). Furthermore, the diverging alveolar processes are altered easily during active periods of vertical growth.

4. EFFECTS OF ORTHODONTIC TREATMENT ON THE MANDIBLE

Functional jaw orthopedics has as one of its goals the controlled promotion of mandibular growth.[3] Although some of the correction achieved with activators and other functional jaw orthopedic appliances is due to directing the eruption of teeth, it now seems clear that in some cases the correction is due primarily to increased growth of the mandible itself. The more recent evidence is compelling and it now seems accepted that under some conditions the rate of mandibular growth, as well as the mandibular growth vector, can be altered.

5. Cranial Base

Thus far, there is little evidence that ordinary orthodontic therapy has much effect on the cranial base. Wieslander[104] found basion significantly more inferiorly and less posteriorly positioned after treatment with cervical traction. The matter has not been studied extensively, perhaps owing to the fact that many assume that no changes are likely to occur in this region. Riolo *et al.*[86] have found changes in the cranial base flexure of rhesus monkeys in response to an experimentally induced more protrusive functional occlusal position of the mandible. The cranial base angle during growth becomes more obtuse but it reverses itself, becoming more acute in response to the new protruded mandibular position.

6. Effects of Orthodontic Treatment on the Profile and Pattern of Facial Growth

The total result of all the previously mentioned changes is a remarkable impact on the convexity of the facial profile. In Class II malocclusion, modern orthodontists routinely reduce the profile convexity in an extensive way. All of the previously mentioned changes summate in the profile. Modern orthodontists have been strangely reticent in documenting the extensive alterations in facial form and pattern that are routinely wrought by their therapy (see Chapter XV).

L. Some Comments Concerning the Various Theories of Craniofacial Growth*

From time to time in the literature there have appeared various theories attempting to explain the intricacies of craniofacial growth by one all-encompassing idea. A number of recent studies have greatly expanded our knowledge of the biology of the skull, enabling us to put these various theories of craniofacial growth into better perspective.

1. Controlling Factors in Craniofacial Growth

The various controlling factors in craniofacial growth have been neatly catalogued by Van Limborgh[99] under the following headings: intrinsic genetic factors, local epigenetic factors, general epigenetic factors, local environmental factors and general environmental factors (Table IV-1). Our ability to classify these factors in no way suggests that the methods by which each operates are fully known.

---

*In writing this section, I have drawn heavily on a splendid paper by Professor Van Limborgh[99] (R.E.M.).

TABLE IV-1.—Controlling Factors in Craniofacial Growth

Intrinsic genetic factors	Genetic factors inherent to the skull tissues
Local epigenetic factors	Genetically determined influences originating from adjacent structures (brain, eyes, etc.)
General epigenetic factors	Genetically determined influences originating from distant structures (sex hormones, etc.)
Local environmental factors	Local nongenetic influences originating from the external environment (local external pressure, muscle forces, etc.)
General environmental factors	General nongenetic influences originating from the external environment (food and oxygen supply, etc.)

2. Regulation of Skull Development

It has been generally held until recently that the embryologic development of the skull is under tight genetic control (Fig. IV-27). However, a number of experiments have proved the interactive relationships between skull development and the presence and state of the primordia of other structures in the head. This may be shown best by examining the development of the eye and the orbit. There will be no orbit if there is no eye primordium. Furthermore, the orbits will develop their normal positions only if the eye primordia are located normally. If there are more or less than the normal number of eye primordia, there will be a corresponding number of orbits.[9, 21, 100] Similar relationships have been established elsewhere in the embryonic skull. Apparently, adjacent structures exert strong morphogenetic influences and, accordingly, Van Limborgh has classified this control of cranial differentiation as local epigenetic[98] (Fig. IV-27). On the basis of our present knowledge, cranial differentiation seems largely controlled by such local epigenetic factors and a few intrinsic genetic factors, with only minor roles assigned to general epigenetic factors and general environmental factors (Fig. IV-27).

3. Control of Craniofacial Growth

Until quite recently, students of facial growth chose among the ideas advanced by Sicher,[92] Scott[87–90] or Moss.[69–72] Let us discuss each briefly.

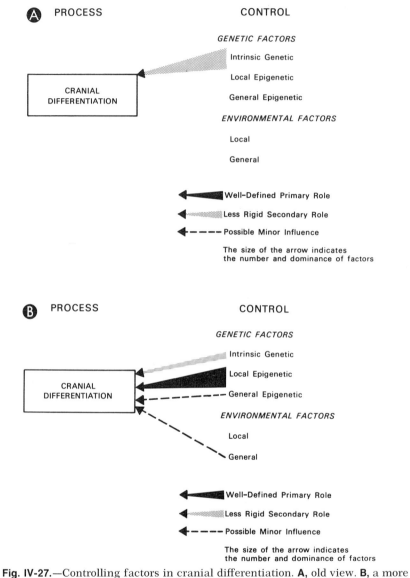

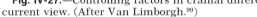

Fig. IV-27.—Controlling factors in cranial differentiation. **A**, old view. **B**, a more current view. (After Van Limborgh.[99])

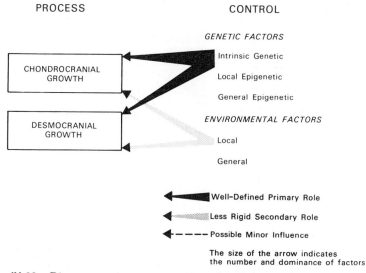

PROCESS

CONTROL

Fig. IV-28.—Diagrammatic representation of Sicher's theory of the control of craniofacial growth. (After Van Limborgh.[99])

a) Sicher's Theory

Sicher[92] held that both the chondrocranium and the desmocranium grow under rather strong genetic control. Only minor remodeling of surface configuration or the internal trabecular structures of the bone tissue would be subject to such local epigenetic factors as the muscles. Under his theory, all of the structures in the head, although genetically attuned to one another, grow without any dependent relationships to one another. Sicher ascribed approximately equal active value to all of the osteogenic tissues, i.e., periosteum, cartilage and sutures. He held further that the paired parallel sutures that attach the facial area to the skull and cranial base regions push the nasomaxillary complex forward to pace its growth with that of the mandible. This particular view assigns a more active role for sutures in the facial region than in the cranial vault. The theory is summarized in Figure IV-28.

b) Scott's Theory

Scott[87, 90] assumed that the primary controlling factors in craniofacial growth are found only in the cartilage and the periosteum and that the sutures are secondary and passive. He viewed the cartilaginous sites throughout the skull as primary centers of growth (Fig. IV-29). Sutural growth may be further altered by local and environmental factors.

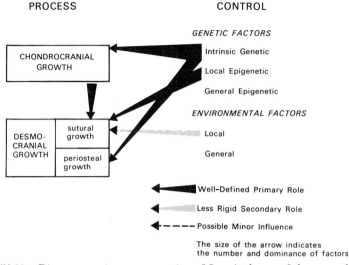

Fig. IV-29.—Diagrammatic representation of Scott's theory of the control of craniofacial growth. (After Van Limborgh.[99])

c) *Moss's Theory*

In recent years, Moss[69-72] has presented his ideas of the functional matrix, which hypothesize that the growth of the skull is quite secondary, being determined largely by the growth and function of functional matrices (in Van Limborgh's terminology, local epigenetic factors). Moss's ideas are based on the theory of functional cranial components originated by Van der Klaauw.[97] According to Van der Klaauw, the skull is made up of units the size, shape and position of which are determined primarily by their functions. Moss's functional matrix refers to adjacent structures related to the presence and functions of Van der Klaauw's functional components. Moss asserts that the growth of the functional components, irrespective of their ossification mechanism, is entirely dependent on the growth and function of the functional matrices. Moss denies any intrinsic regulatory control in the growing bony tissues themselves. Control of the bone growth is by either local epigenetic factors or, additionally, environmental factors (Fig. IV-30).

d) *Van Limborgh's Theory*

Van Limborgh, in a brilliant analytical paper, found all three of the above theories inadequate and attempted to synthesize our present knowledge into a new concept.[99] He questioned Sicher's idea of the independence of skull growth, pointing out that there are no fixed quan-

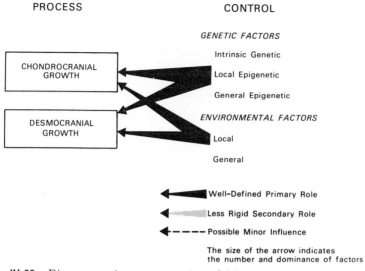

Fig. IV-30.—Diagrammatic representation of Moss's theory of the control of craniofacial growth. (After Van Limborgh.[99])

titative morphologic relationships between specific organs and adjacent skull components of any perfect and decisive relationship. Further, the theory inadequately explains skull growth in such gross deformities as hydrocephalus and the adaptive growth of the skull to alterations in muscle function.

Although supporting Scott's views with respect to the relationship between synchondroses and sutural growth, Van Limborgh challenges his idea that periosteal growth is controlled solely by intrinsic factors. Van Limborgh agrees with Moss that periosteal growth is controlled nearly entirely by influences from adjacent structures and by environmental factors such as muscle forces. He does not agree with Moss's assertions that there is no intrinsic factor in sutural and periosteal tissues, pointing up the difficulties of reconciling Moss's theories with the observed cranial growth in craniostenosis. He further objects to Moss grouping endochondral bone growth simply with intramembranous bone formation, pointing out that in serious malformations, such as hydrocephalus, anencephaly and microcephaly, whereas the desmocranium is markedly altered the chondrocranium remains practically normal. Van Limborgh concludes that none of the three popular theories on the control of bone growth is entirely satisfactory, yet each contains elements of significance that cannot be denied. He summarizes the six essential elements of our current knowledge in Table IV-2, to which we have added a seventh point with respect to the control of mandibu-

TABLE IV-2.—ESSENTIAL ELEMENTS OF OUR CURRENT KNOWLEDGE
OF CRANIOFACIAL GROWTH*

1. Chondrocranial growth is controlled mainly by intrinsic genetic factors
2. Desmocranial growth is controlled by only a few intrinsic genetic factors
3. The growing skull cartilages are growth centers
4. Sutural growth is controlled mainly by influences originating from the skull cartilages and from other adjacent head structures.
5. Periosteal growth is controlled mainly by influences originating from adjacent head structures
6. Sutural and periosteal growth are additionally governed by local nongenetic environmental influences, muscle forces inclusive
7. Mandibular condylar growth is controlled, to some extent, by local nongenetic environmental influences

*Modified from Van Limborgh.[99]

lar condylar growth. His reconciliation of the essentials of our knowledge into a newer concept is shown in Figure IV-31, to which we have added a representation of our knowledge concerning mandibular growth (Fig. IV-32).

To summarize, the differentiation of both the chondrocranium and the desmocranium is controlled by a few intrinsic genetic factors and by many local epigenetic factors that originate from adjacent structures in the head. Intrinsic genetic factors almost exclusively govern the growth of the chondrocranium, whereas desmocranial growth is con-

Fig. IV-31.—Diagrammatic representation of Van Limborgh's concept of the control mechanisms in craniofacial growth. (After Van Limborgh.[99])

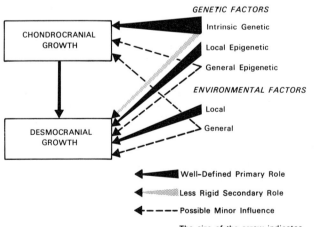

PROCESS   CONTROL

GENETIC FACTORS

CHONDROCRANIAL GROWTH

Intrinsic Genetic

Local Epigenetic

General Epigenetic

ENVIRONMENTAL FACTORS

Local

DESMOCRANIAL GROWTH

General

◄▬▬▬ Well-Defined Primary Role

◄▬▬▬ Less Rigid Secondary Role

◄▬ ▬ ▬ Possible Minor Influence

The size of the arrow indicates
the number and dominance of factors

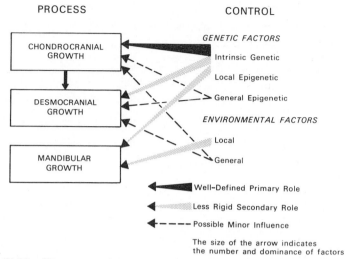

PROCESS   CONTROL

Fig. IV-32.—Diagrammatic representation of control factors in craniofacial growth, including the mandible.

trolled by very few intrinsic genetic factors and many epigenetic factors. In addition, the growth of the desmocranium is influenced by local environmental factors in the form of muscle and occlusal function; general epigenetic and general environmental factors seem to be of rather minor importance. In the mandible, although most of the bone behaves as does the desmocranium, the mandibular condyle, at least, is controlled to some extent by local environmental influences.

REFERENCES

1. Ahlgren, J., Omnell, K. A., Sonesson, B., and Toremalm, N.G.: Bruxism and hypertrophy of the masseter muscle, Pract. oto-rhino-laryng. 31:32, 1969.
2. Altemus, L. A.: A comparison of cephalofacial relationships, Angle Orthodont. 30:223, 1960.
3. Andresen, V., Haeupl, K., and Petrik, L.: *Funktionskieferorthopaedie* (6th ed.; München: J. A. Barth, Publishers, 1957).
4. Angle, E. H.: *Malocclusion of the Teeth* (7th ed.; Philadelphia: S. S. White Dental Mfg. Co., 1907).
5. Baer, M. J., and Gavan, J. A.: Symposium on bone growth as revealed by in vivo markers, Am. J. Phys. Anthropol. 29:155, 1968.
6. Baume, L. J.: Principles of cephalofacial development revealed by experimental biology, Am. J. Orthodont. 47:881, 1961.
7. Baume, L. J., and Derichsweiler, H.: Is the condylar growth center responsive to orthodontic therapy?, Oral Surg. 14:347, 1961.
8. Belchier, J.: An account of the bones of animals being changed to a red color by aliment only, Philosoph. Tr. 39:286, 1736.
9. Bellaires, D. A.: Skull development in chick embryo after ablation of one eye. Nature. London 176:658, 1955.
10. Björk, A.: The face in profile. Svenska tand.-tidsk. 40:No. 5B (supp.) 1947.

11. Björk, A.: Facial growth in man. Studies with the aid of metallic implants, Acta odont. scandinav. 13:9, 1955.

12. Björk, A.: Bite development and body build, Dent. Rec. 75:8, 1955.

13. Björk, A.: Variations in the growth pattern of the human mandible: Longitudinal radiographic study by the implant method, J. D. Res. 42:400, 1963.

14. Björk, A.: The use of metallic implants in the study of facial growth in children: Method and application, Am. J. Phys. Anthropol. 29:243, 1968.

15. Björk, A., and Helm, S.: Prediction of maximum puberal growth in body height, Angle Orthodont. 37:134, 1967.

16. Broadbent, B. H.: A new x-ray technique and its application to orthodontia, Angle Orthodont. 1:45, 1931.

17. Brodie, A. G., Downs, W. B., Goldstein, A., and Myer, E.: Cephalometric appraisal of orthodontic results, Angle Orthodont. 8:261, 1938.

18. Carter, C. O.: The Genetics of Common Malformations, in Fishbein, M. (ed.), *Congenital Malformations*, Proceedings Second International Conference on Congenital Malformations (New York: Medical Congress, Ltd., 1964), pp. 306–313.

19. Castelli, W. A., Ramirez, P. C., and Burdi, A. R.: The effect of experimental surgery on mandibular growth in Syrian hamsters, J. D. Res. 50:356, 1971.

20. Cleall, J. F., Wilson, G. W., and Garnett, D. S.: Normal craniofacial skeletal growth of the rat, Am. J. Phys. Anthropol. 20:225, 1968.

21. Coulombre, A. J., and Crelin, E. S.: The role of the developing eye in the morphogenesis of the avian skull, Am. J. Phys. Anthropol. 16:25, 1958.

22. Dixon, A. D., and Hoyte, D. A. N.: A comparison of autoradiographic and alizarin techniques in the study of bone growth, Anat. Rec. 145:101, 1963.

23. Duhamel, H. L.: Sur une racine qui a la faculté de teindre en rouge les os des animaux vivants, Mém. Acad. Roy. Sc. (Paris), 1–13, 1739.

24. Enlow, D. H.: Wolff's law and the factor of architectonic circumstance, Am. J. Orthodont. 54:803, 1968.

25. Enlow, D. H.: *The Human Face* (New York: Hoeber Medical Division, Harper & Row, Publishers, 1968).

26. Enlow, D. H.: Growth of the face in relation to the cranial base, Tr. European Orthodont. Soc. 44:321, 1968.

27. Fogh-Andersen, P.: *Inheritance of Cleft Lip and Cleft Palate* (Copenhagen: Arnold Busck, 1942).

28. Fogh-Andersen, P.: Inheritance Patterns for Cleft Lip and Cleft Palate, in Pruzansky, S. (ed.). *Congenital Anomalies of the Face and Associated Structures* (Springfield, Ill.: Charles C Thomas, Publisher, 1961), pp. 123–133.

29. Fraser, F. C.: Experimental Induction of Cleft Palate, in Pruzansky, S. (ed.), *Congenital Anomalies of the Face and Associated Structures* (Springfield, Ill.: Charles C Thomas, Publisher, 1961), pp. 188–197.

30. Frost, H. M.: Tetracycline bone labeling in anatomy, Am. J. Phys. Anthropol. 29:183, 1968.

31. Fukuhara, T., and Saito, S.: Genetic considerations on the dysplasia of the nasopalatal segments as a "formes frustes" radiologically found in parents of cleft children, Jap. J. Human Genet. 7:234, 1962.

32. Garn, S. M., and Rohmann, C. G.: The number of hand-wrist centers, Am. J. Phys. Anthropol. 18:293, 1960.

33. Goland, P. P., and Grand, N. G.: Chloro-s-triazines as markers and fixatives for the study of growth in teeth and bones, Am. J. Phys. Anthropol. 29:201, 1968.

34. Graber, T. M.: Extraoral force—facts and fallacies. Am. J. Orthodont. 41:490, 1955.

35. Hanes, R. A.: Bony profile changes resulting from cervical traction compared with those resulting from intermaxillary elastics, Am. J. Orthodont. 45:353, 1959.

36. Harris, J. E.: Craniofacial growth and malocclusion: A multivariate approach to the study of the skeletal contribution to Class II malocclusion, Tr. European Orthodont. Soc. 41:103, 1965.

37. Harvold, E. P.: Some biologic aspects of orthodontic treatment in the transitional dentition, Am. J. Orthodont. 49:1, 1963.

38. Harvold, E. P.: The role of function in the etiology and treatment of malocclusion, Am. J. Orthodont. 54:883, 1968.

39. Hass, R.: Rapid expansion of the maxillary dental arch and nasal cavity by opening the midpalatal suture, Angle Orthodont. 31:73, 1961.

40. Hausser, E.: Cephalometric examination of treated cases with Class II malocclusions, Tr. European Orthodont. Soc. 38:260, 1962.

41. Higley, L. B.: A new and scientific method of producing temporomandibular articulation radiograms, Internat. J. Orthodont. & Oral Surg. 22:983, 1936.
42. Hofrath, H.: Die Bedeutung der Röntgenfern- und Abstandsaufnahme für die Diagnostik der Kieferanomalien, Fortschr. Orthodont. 1:232, 1931.
43. Holdaway, R. A.: Changes in relationship of points A and B during orthodontic treatment, Am. J. Orthodont. 42:176, 1956.
44. Hoyte, D. A. N.: Alizarin as an indicator of bone growth, J. Anat. 94:432, 1960.
45. Hoyte, D. A. N.: Alizarin red in the study of the apposition and resorption of bone, Am. J. Phys. Anthropol. 29:157, 1968.
46. Hughes, B. O., and Moore, G. R.: Heredity, growth and the dentofacial complex, Angle Orthodont. 11:217, 1941.
47. Hunt, E. E., Jr.: Prediction of increments and genetics of craniofacial growth. Presented as part of a symposium on growth and development of the face, teeth and jaws, J. D. Res. Supp. 44 (2), Jan.–Feb., 1965.
48. Hunt, E. E., Jr.: The Developmental Genetics in Man, in *The Introduction to Quantitative Genetics* (Edinburgh: Oliver & Boyd, 1966).
49. Hunter, W. S.: The Inheritance of Mesiodistal Tooth Diameter in Twins, Ph.D. dissertation, The University of Michigan, June, 1959.
50. Hunter, W. S.: A study of the inheritance of craniofacial characteristics as seen in lateral cephalograms of 72 like-sexed twins, Tr. European Orthodont. Soc. 41:59, 1965.
51. Hunter, W. S., Balbach, D., and Lamphiear, D. E.: The heritability of attained growth in the human face, Am. J. Orthodont, 58 (2): 128, 1970.
52. Israel, H.: Microdensitometric analysis for study of skeletal growth and aging in the living subject, Am. J. Phys. Anthropol. 29:287, 1968.
53. King, E. W.: Cervical anchorage in Class II, Division I treatment, a cephalometric appraisal, Angle Orthodont. 27:98, 1957.
54. Klein, P. L.: An evaluation of cervical traction on the maxilla and the upper first permanent molar, Angle Orthodont. 27:61, 1957.
55. Krogman, W. M.: The role of genetic factors in the human face, jaws and teeth: A review, Eugenics Rev. 59:165, 1967.
56. Kuroda, T., McNamara, J., and Moyers, R. E.: Unpublished data.
57. Kuroda, T.: A longitudinal cephalometric study on the craniofacial development in Japanese children, paper presented at the I.A.D.R., New York, March, 1970.
58. Lindegard, B.: Variations in human body build. A somatometric and x-ray cephalometric investigation on Scandinavian adults, Acta psychiat. et neurol. scandinav., Supp. 86, 1953.
59. Lundstrom, A.: The significance of genetic and nongenetic factors in the profile of the facial skeleton, Am. J. Orthodont. 12:910, 1955.
60. Maj, G., Luzj, C., and Lucchese, P.: A cephalometric appraisal of Class II and Class III malocclusions, Angle Orthodont. 30:26, 1960.
61. Margolis, H. I.: Standardized x-ray cephalographics, Am. J. Orthodont. 26:725, 1940.
62. McNamara, J. A., Jr.: Neuromuscular and skeletal adaptations to altered orofacial function (Ph.D. dissertation, Horace H. Rackham School of Graduate Studies, University of Michigan, Ann Arbor, 1972).
63. Meredith, H. V.: A time series analysis of growth in nose height during childhood, Child Develop. 29:19, 1958.
64. Miller, R. L., Moyers, R. E., and Hunter, W. S.: A computer storage and retrieval system for two-dimensional outlines, J. D. Res. 49(5): 1176, 1970.
65. Miura, F., Inoue, N., and Kazuo, S.: The standards of Steiner's analysis for Japanese, Bull. Tokyo Med. and Dent. Univ. 10:No. 3, 387–395, 1963.
66. Moore, A. W.: Orthodontic treatment factors in Class II malocclusion, Am. J. Orthodont. 45:323, 1959.
67. Moore, G. R.: Heredity as a guide in dentofacial orthopedics, Am. J. Orthodont. 30:549, 1944.
68. Moore, G. R., and Hughes, B. O.: Familial factors in diagnosis, treatment and prognosis of dentofacial disturbances, Am. J. Orthodont. 28:603, 1942.
69. Moss, M. L., and Young, R. W.: A functional approach to craniology, Am. J. Phys. Anthropol. 18:281, 1960.
70. Moss, M. L.: Functional analysis of human mandibular growth, J. Pros. Den. 10:1149, 1960.
71. Moss, M. L.: The Functional Matrix, in Kraus, B., and Riedel, R. (eds.), *Vistas in Orthodontics* (Philadelphia: Lea & Febiger, 1962), pp. 85–98.
72. Moss, M. L., and Salentijn, L.: The primary role of functional matrices in facial growth, Am. J. Orthodont. 55:566, 1969.

73. Moyers, R. E., Elgoyhen, J. C., Riolo, M. L., McNamara, J. A., Jr., and Kuroda, T.: Experimental production of Class III in rhesus monkeys, Tr. European Orthodont. Soc. 46:61, 1970.
74. Moyers, R. E., and Miura, F.: The use of serial cephalograms to study racial differences in development I and II. Read at the VIIIth International Congress of Anthropological and Ethnological Sciences, Tokyo, Japan, September, 1968.
75. Muzj, E.: Individual cephalometric research requires selection on the basis of craniofacial types, Tr. European Orthodont. Soc. 40:399, 1964.
76. Nanda, R. S.: The rates of growth of several facial components measured from serial cephalometric roentgenograms, Am. J. Orthodont. 41:658, 1955.
77. Pacini, A. J.: Roentgen ray anthropometry of the skull, J. Radiol. 42:230, 322 and 418, 1922.
78. Pfannenstiel, D.: *Zur Morphologie und Genetik der Mund und Kinnregion* (Zurich: University of Zurich, 1951).
79. Pike, J. B.: A serial investigation of facial and statural growth in seven- to twelve-year-old children, Angle Orthodont. 38:63, 1968.
80. Poulton, D. R.: Changes in Class II malocclusions with and without occipital headgear therapy, Angle Orthodont. 29:234, 1959.
81. Prescott, G. H., Mitchell, D. F., and Fahmy, H.: Procion dyes as matrix markers in growing bone and teeth, Am. J. Phys. Anthropol. 29:219, 1968.
82. Prorok, E. S.: Lateral cephalometric radiograms as an aid to the determination of monozygosity, Angle Orthodont. 33:35, 1963.
83. Pruzansky, S. (ed.): *Congenital Anomalies of the Face and Associated Structures* (Springfield, Ill.: Charles C Thomas, Publisher, 1961).
84. Pullen, H.: Expansion of the dental arch and opening of the maxillary suture in relationship to the development of the internal and external face, D. Cosmos 54:509, 1912.
85. Ricketts, R. M.: The influence of orthodontic treatment on facial growth and development, Angle Orthodont. 30:103, 1960.
86. Riolo, M., and Elgoyhen, J. C.: Growth and remodeling of the cranial floor: An experimental study. Program and abstracts, 50th General Session, Internat. Assoc. Dent. Res. 457:16, 1972.
87. Scott, J. H.: The cartilage of the nasal septum. A contribution to the study of facial growth, Brit. D. J. 95:37, 1953.
88. Scott, J. H.: Growth at facial sutures, Am. J. Orthodont. 42:381, 1956.
89. Scott, J. H.: The cranial base, Am. J. Phys. Anthropol. 16:319, 1958.
90. Scott, J. H.: *Dento-facial Development and Growth* (Oxford: Pergamon Press, 1967).
91. Selmer-Olsen, R.: An odontometric study on the Norwegian Lapps. Skifter utgitt av det Norske Videnskaps-Akademi Oslo, I. Mat.-Naturv. Klasse, No. 3, 1949.
92. Sicher, H.: *Oral Anatomy* (St. Louis: The C. V. Mosby Company, 1952).
93. Simon, P. W.: *Grundzüge einer systematischen Diagnostik der Gebiss-Anomalien* (Berlin: Meusser, 1922).
94. Snodgrasse, R. M.: Heredity and cephalo-facial growth in cleft lip and/or cleft palate children, Bull. Am. A. Cl. Pal. Rehabil. Monog. Supp. No. 1, 1954.
95. Thorne, N.: Expansion of the maxilla—spreading the midpalatal suture, Am. J. Orthodont. 46:626, 1960.
96. Townsley, W.: The influence of mechanical factors on the development and structure of bone, Am. J. Phys. Anthropol. 6:25, 1948.
97. Van der Klaauw, C. J.: Size and position of functional components of the skull, Arch. neerl. zool. 9:1, 1948–52.
98. Van Limborgh, J.: The regulation of the embryonic development of the skull. Acta morphol. neerl.-scandinav. 7:101, 1968.
99. Van Limborgh, J.: A new view on the control of the morphogenesis of the skull, Acta morphol. neerl.-scandinav. 8:143, 1970.
100. Van Limborgh, J., and Tonneyck-Muller, I.: Das Wachstum von Augen und Augenhöhlen beim Hühnerembryo. I., Acta morphol. neerl.-scandinav. 7:253, 1970; II., Acta morphol. neerl.-scandinav. 8:211, 1970.
101. Washburn, S. L.: The relation of the temporalis muscle to the form of the skull, Anat. Rec. 99:239, 1967.
102. Watt, D. G., and Williams, C. H. M.: The effects of the physical consistency of food on the growth and development of the mandible and the maxilla of the rat, Am. J. Orthodont. 37:895, 1951.

103. Weidenreich, F.: The brain and its role in the phylogenetic transformation of the human skull, Tr. Am. Philosoph. Soc. 31:321, 1940.
104. Wieslander, L.: The effect of orthodontic treatment on the concurrent development of the craniofacial complex, Am. J. Orthodont. 49:15, 1963.
105. Winshall, A.: Application of the Skeletal Age Concept to Facial Growth Prediction, M.S. thesis, The University of Michigan, April, 1967.

SUGGESTED READINGS

Blackwood, H. J. J. (ed.): *Bone and Tooth* (Oxford: Pergamon Press, 1964).
Enlow, D. H.: *Principles of Bone Remodeling* (Springfield, Ill.: Charles C Thomas, Publisher, 1963).
Enlow, D. H.: *The Human Face* (New York: Hoeber Medical Division, Harper & Row, Publishers, 1968).
Frost, H. M.: *Bone Remodeling Dynamics* (Springfield, Ill.: Charles C Thomas, Publisher, 1963).
Graber, T. M.: Craniofacial and Dentitional Development, in Falkner, F. (ed.), *Human Development* (Philadelphia: W. B. Saunders Company, 1966).

V

Maturation of the
Orofacial Musculature

> No muscle uses its power in pushing but always in draw-
> ing to itself the parts that are joined to it . . . the function
> of muscle is to pull and not to push except in the case of the
> genitals and the tongue.—LEONARDO DA VINCI, *Dell' Anat-
> omia*, Fogli B (translated by E. MacCurdy in *The Notebooks
> of Leonardo da Vinci*, Vol. I, Chap. III)

A. Some basic concepts of neuromuscular physiology
1. Physiology of skeletal musculature
2. Reflexes
   a) Conditioned reflexes
   b) Unconditioned reflexes
3. Muscle learning
4. Classes of neuromuscular activities
   a) Unconditioned reflexes
   b) Reflexes appearing with normal growth and development
   c) Conditioned reflexes
   d) Voluntary efforts

B. Development of oropharyngeal functions
1. Prenatal maturation
2. Neonatal oral functions
   a) The mouth as a sensory instrument
   b) Infantile suckling and swallowing
   c) Maintenance of the airway
   d) Infant cry
   e) Gagging
3. Early postnatal development of oral functions
   a) Mastication
   b) Facial expressions
   c) Speech
   d) Mature swallow

C. Neurophysiologic regulation of jaw positions and functions

1. Neurology
   a) Receptors
      1) Muscles
      2) Periodontal ligament
      3) Teeth
      4) Mucosa
      5) Tongue
      6) Temporomandibular joints
   b) Reflexes
2. Unconditioned jaw positions and functions
   a) Posture
   b) Unconscious or reflex swallow
3. Jaw functions that appear with normal growth and development
   a) Mastication
   b) Mature swallow
4. Conditioned jaw positions and functions
   a) Mature swallow
   b) Mastication
   c) Other

D. Physiology of occlusal functions

1. Jaw movements
   a) Border movements
      1) Ideal occlusal position
      2) Retruded contact position
      3) Relationships between the retruded position and the usual occlusal position
   b) Functional movements
      1) Swallowing
      2) Mastication
      3) Mandibular posture
      4) Speech
2. Occlusal homeostasis
   a) Sensory aspects
   b) Forces acting against the teeth
   c) Occlusal forces
   d) Drifting of teeth
   e) Facial growth
3. The "centric" concept from a developmental point of view
   a) Postural position of the mandible
   b) Usual occlusal position
   c) Retruded contact position
   d) Ideal occlusal position
4. Neuromuscular adaptation to occlusal disharmony

E. Some clinical implications

1. The effect of neuromuscular behavior on growth of the craniofacial skeleton
2. Neuromuscular aims in orthodontic therapy
3. The effects of orthodontic treatment on the musculature

A. Some Basic Concepts of Neuromuscular Physiology

1. PHYSIOLOGY OF SKELETAL MUSCULATURE

When a muscle is stimulated, it contracts, usually causing its origin and insertion to approach each other, thereby bringing about movement of the limbs or joints involved. Such a contraction is called isotonic. When there is an increase in tension without a change in length, it is called isometric. Contractions while the teeth are held clenched together are isometric. Muscles are not only contractile, but they also are elastic, for after repeated contractions or stretchings, they return to their original or resting length and maintain this length without further contraction.

Sensory, motor and sympathetic nerves are supplied to muscles. Some sensory nerves terminate as free nerve endings serving as mediators of pain, whereas others supply neuromuscular spindles that are specialized sensory cells found within the muscles. The neuromuscular spindles

Fig. V-1.—Two routes to voluntary muscle. (After Murphy.[44])

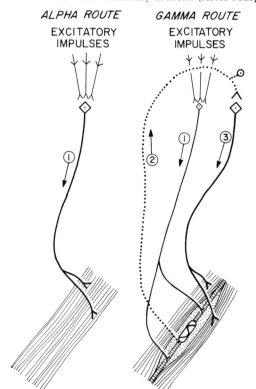

themselves also are supplied with gamma efferent fibers, which carry impulses to the contractile elements of the spindles (Fig. V-1). Motor nerves terminate in the skeletal muscle fibers and sympathetic nerves in the smooth muscle of the blood vessels. Other specialized sensory endings called Golgi tendon organs are located in the tendons.

Before a muscle contracts, it is necessary for an action potential to arrive by means of a motor nerve fiber whose cell is located in the cen-

Fig. V-2.—Neural connections of the muscle spindles in masticatory muscles. The spindle has both afferent and efferent innervations (**A**). As the muscle fibers are stretched (**B**), a misalignment occurs between the extrafusal and intrafusal fibers, depolarizing the annulo-spiral ending in the nuclear bag. An impulse passes centrally through the large afferent crossing the synapse, with the large alpha cell activating it to send an impulse down the alpha efferent fiber to the main muscle fibers, which stimulates the muscle to contract, restoring the alignment between the extrafusal and intrafusal fibers and stopping further contraction. This is the myotatic or stretch reflex. The nuclear bag also can be stretched by contraction of the intrafusal fibers, by impulses that pass down the gamma efferent fibers (**C**). Under these circumstances, the main muscle fibers again are activated; they contract and shorten sufficiently to restore the alignment with the muscle spindle (**D**) and thus render it inactive. See also Figure V-1. (After Murphy.[44])

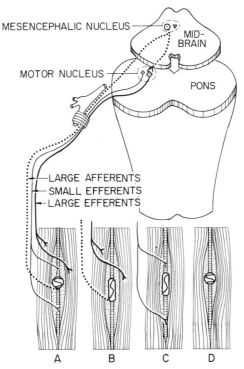

MESENCEPHALIC NUCLEUS

MID-BRAIN

MOTOR NUCLEUS

PONS

LARGE AFFERENTS
SMALL EFFERENTS
LARGE EFFERENTS

A   B   C   D

tral nervous system. Only rarely do all the fibers of a muscle contract simultaneously, since the degree of tension and contraction varies with the number of fibers stimulated and thus called into action. Therefore, there is an asynchrony of motor unit firing (see next paragraph).

Each nerve serves a number of muscle cells, the number varying with the muscle and the delicacy of that muscle's action. Where precise delicate movements are required, each motor fiber serves a smaller number of muscle cells. The nerve cell in the central nervous system, its fiber connecting to the muscle and the muscle cells innervated by that fiber make up the motor unit. The motor unit itself is not in a specific location in the muscle, for its cells often are scattered, but they react together, since they respond to the same impulses.

Neuromuscular spindles within the muscle serve as a kind of feedback mechanism sending sensory information concerning the muscle itself to the central nervous system (Figs. V-2 and V-8). Impulses from the muscles and tendons play a very important role in maintaining normal body posture. Impulses run continually from the spindles of the muscles to the midbrain, where connections are made with motor pathways and the muscles are kept in a constant state of reflex-determined contraction called *tonus*. Tonus serves to maintain body posture; therefore, the muscles with the greatest tonus are those most directly coun-

Fig. V-3.—The reflex arc. **A,** components of a simple monosynaptic reflex arc. **B,** components of a disynaptic reflex arc. (After Ramfjord and Ash.[48])

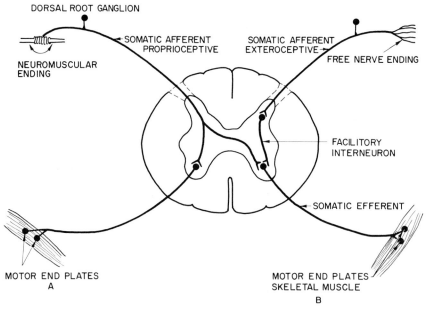

DORSAL ROOT GANGLION

NEUROMUSCULAR ENDING

SOMATIC AFFERENT PROPRIOCEPTIVE

SOMATIC AFFERENT EXTEROCEPTIVE

FREE NERVE ENDING

FACILITORY INTERNEURON

SOMATIC EFFERENT

MOTOR END PLATES
A

MOTOR END PLATES
SKELETAL MUSCLE
B

teracting gravity.[30] When muscles are completely relaxed, there is no electromyographic evidence of motor unit activity. Clemmesen[11] has suggested that resting muscle tone is due to passive elastic tension within the muscle that is quite independent of the reflex stimulation through a motor nerve. Joseph *et al.*[30, 31] have shown that the muscles of mastication never completely rest, due to the continuing force of gravity, for tonus is response to stretch.

When a motor nerve to a muscle is cut, the muscle undergoes atrophy. When a muscle is not used, disuse atrophy sets in, a much slower process than the atrophy resulting from nerve section. The sensory nerves and the connections with the higher centers in the brain also must remain intact if normal neuromuscular function is to prevail.

2. REFLEXES

The basic unit of all integrated neural activity is the reflex arc. Each reflex arc has a receptor, an afferent neuron, at least one synapse (usually more) in a central integrating area, an efferent neuron and an effector organ (Fig. V-3). In both monosynaptic and polysynaptic reflexes, but especially in the latter, activity is modified by facilitation and inhibition.

a) Conditioned Reflexes

A conditioned reflex is an automatic response to a stimulus that previously did not elicit the response. The reflex is acquired by repeatedly pairing the "neutral" stimulus with another stimulus that normally does produce the response. In Pavlov's classic experiments, he noted that dogs normally reflexly salivate when meat is placed in their mouth. By repeatedly sounding a bell prior to placing the meat in the dog's mouth and thus relating the two stimuli in the dog's brain, it was possible later to produce salivation by sounding the bell alone. The basis for much behavior is the formation of conditioned reflexes.

b) Unconditioned Reflexes

At the time of birth, the neonate's central nervous system has already matured sufficiently to perform many integrative processes that are known as "unconditioned reflexes."[24, 26] The baby has appropriate integrative centers in the medulla sufficiently matured to control reflexly blood pressure, respiration, the protective reflexes of coughing and sneezing and to produce limb jerks when he hears a loud sound. As the child grows, the nervous system continues to develop anatomically and to mature physiologically. Basic reflex patterns of muscle activity appear in a scheduled way, e.g., grasping, crawling, climbing, walking. Even though the child may not have been "taught" any of these movements, these primary patterns of (a) unconditioned reflexes and (b) reflexes that normally appear as a part of growth (some say that they are unconditioned and some say that they are conditioned) are the basis for the learning of those patterns of muscle activity that are called conditioned reflexes.

3. MUSCLE LEARNING

During fetal life, motor performance capability appears before sensory control. Gradually, the primitive motor system comes under sensory control of basic functions that must be operable before birth. These endogenous activities are the result of the appearance during prenatal life of unconditioned reflexes concerned with the primitive vital activities typical of the species. Response to environmental stimuli follows and, thus, behavior has two components—endogenous and exogenous. Environment determines the level, timing and coordination of many aspects of behavior after the afferent system is intact and functional. However, endogenous behavior persists, although it may be modified.

We know very little yet of how learning (conditioned reflexes, exogenous behavior, etc.) is coordinated with the primitive phylogenic demands of endogenous behavior (unconditioned reflexes), but it is obvious that learning, training and evaluation have had and can have a marked effect on behavior in higher mammals. In man, many complicated motor activities can be initiated voluntarily that are not possible in most other mammals. Although the dental literature contains many statements concerning our inability to alter "inherited" endogenous orofacial muscle behavior, it is well to remember that (1) our knowledge of the genetic aspects of the jaw and facial muscles is very scant, (2) muscle learning is superposed on preformed patterns of endogenous behavior, (3) learning can modify, suppress, rearrange or facilitate much endogenous behavior and (4) even some primitive endogenous activities can be modified, as is well known to swimming coaches and speech teachers.

It is thought that muscle learning is largely a process of acquiring new conditioned reflexes. In this manner, the various pathways through the brain are gradually developed and imprinted as the baby grows through infancy and childhood into adulthood. These pathways constitute "muscle memory." Thoughts themselves are the result of complex reflexes in the central nervous system. The brain gradually accumulates memory "traces" from both thought and motor activity as a part of the learning process.

Any time a person decides to master a new motor skill, the learning process involves three important stages. First, the brain must have a clear mental image of the task to be mastered. Second, new pathways must be established and the conditioned reflex reinforced by repeated practice of the new skill. Third, control of execution of the new skill must pass, to a great extent, from the higher centers of the brain to the midbrain, brain stem and spinal cord. The first stage involves conscious understanding during slow, meticulous practice of the new motor skill. The second stage involves much concentration as well during repeated practice to reinforce the new pathways. If the third stage is to be reached, cortical reinforcement must be minimized as the new motor skill becomes automatic and more reflexly controlled during execution.

When the piano student reads the sheet of music that has the notes printed as symbolic representations of the music itself, the first stage of learning many new motor tasks is reached. Repeated practice provides the multiple stimuli that aid in coordination and reinforcement of the pathways during the second stage of learning. If the music is to be played properly in recital, the pianist must be able to execute automatically and without hesitation all of the newly learned patterns of muscle behavior without reference to the sheet of music. The same principles of muscle learning are used by athletic coaches, ballet masters and the dentist who would train a patient to learn a new swallowing pattern (see Chapter XV).

4. Classes of Neuromuscular Activities
a) Unconditioned Reflexes

Unconditioned reflexes are present at birth, having appeared as a normal part of the prenatal maturation of the neuromuscular system, a process that does not involve any conditioning or learning. If such maturation has not occurred by birth, the infant may not survive. Such reflexes range from the most simple monosynaptic reflexes, such as tendon jerk, to the very complex reflexes involved in infant nursing; however, they are related mostly to food getting, protection and body regulatory mechanisms.

Among the unconditioned reflexes operable in the oropharyngeal region of the neonate are those of respiration, mandibular posture, tongue posture, infantile swallow, suckling, gagging, vomiting, coughing and sneezing. The infant does not "learn" to cough, for example, for he might choke and die before the learning was completed. In a similar way, he might starve before he "learned" to nurse or die of asphyxiation before he had sufficient "practice" at breathing. Unconditioned reflexes require minimal reinforcement and are very difficult to alter or change by usual conditioning procedures.

b) Reflexes Appearing with Normal Growth and Development

Obviously, no conditioned reflex is capable of being learned until all of the necessary units in the central nervous system and musculature have matured sufficiently to make possible that learning (Piaget's concept of readiness); hence, the arguments concerning certain muscle activities that appear as a normal part of growth and maturation, for example, crawling, walking, grasping and so forth. Does the baby "learn" to grasp and crawl? Was he taught? Would he have acquired these motor skills at a certain age with no teaching or encouragement?

In the orofacial region, the mature swallow and mastication are examples of reflexes that normally appear with growth and development.

c) Conditioned Reflexes

Conditioned reflexes include all reflexes that have been learned, including unwanted "bad habits," e.g., tongue-thrusting and thumbsucking.

d) Voluntary Efforts

Willful acts are under cortical control rather than the lower centers, where reflex activities are integrated.

The infantile swallow of the neonate is an example of an unconditioned reflex. The mature teeth-together swallow, which appears during the first year of life, is an example of a reflex appearing with normal growth and development. The learned teeth-apart swallow caused by a painful tooth is an example of a conditioned reflex swallow, and, of course, voluntary swallows are possible as well.

B. Development of Oropharyngeal Functions

1. PRENATAL MATURATION

During prenatal life, the neuromuscular system does not mature evenly.[24] It is not accidental that the orofacial region matures (in the neurophysiologic sense) ahead of the limb regions, since the mouth is so concerned with a number of vital functions that must be operable by birth, e.g., respiration, nursing and protection of the oropharyngeal airway.[23] In the human fetus, by about the eighth week, generalized uniform reflex movements of the entire body can be elicited by tactile stimulation.[23] Diffuse spontaneous movements in response to as yet unidentified stimuli have been observed as early as 9½ weeks. Localized specific and more peripheral responses cannot be produced before 11 weeks. At this time, stimulation of the nose-mouth region causes lateral body flexion.[23] By 14 weeks, the movements have become much more individualized, so that very delicate activities can be executed.[25] When the mouth area is stimulated, general bodily movements no longer are seen but, instead, facial and orbicular muscle responses are produced. Stimulation of the upper lip causes the mouth to close and, often, deglutition to occur.[23] Respiratory movements of the chest and abdomen are seen first at about 16 weeks. The gag reflex has been demonstrated in a human fetus of 18½ weeks menstrual age.[25] By 25 weeks, respiration is shallow but may support life for a few hours if it is once established. Stimulation of the mouth at 29 weeks menstrual age has elicited sucking, although complete suckling and swallowing is not thought to be developed until at least 32 weeks.[17, 23, 25, 26]

2. Neonatal Oral Functions

a) *The Mouth as a Sensory Instrument*

At birth, the orofacial region is a very active perceptual system. The infant finds the mother's nipple more by tactile than by visual sensation. At birth, the tactile acuity already is more highly developed in the lips and mouth than it is in the fingers (of course, it stays that way throughout life). The infant carries objects to his mouth to aid in the

Fig. V-4.—A, tongue posture in the neonate. Note that while the mandible is in its postural position, the tongue is postured forward and touches the lips while the gum pads are held slightly apart. **B,** variations of adult tongue posture.

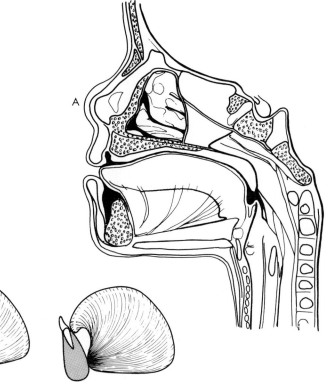

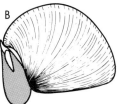

perception of size and texture long before he inserts them into his mouth as a part of teething. The neonate slobbers, drools, chews his toe, sucks his thumb and discovers that gurgling sounds can be made with his mouth.[18] Freudians consider all of this oral eroticism as they do adult smoking, but in the infant it surely is also exploring and exercising the most sensitive perceptual system in the body at that time.

Oral functions in the neonate are guided primarily by local tactile stimuli, particularly those from the lips and the front part of the tongue. At this age, the tongue is guided largely by tactile sensation. The posture of the neonate's tongue is between the gum pads and often far enough forward to rest between the lips, where it can perform its role of sensory guidance more easily (Fig. V-4). The young infant, to a great extent, interprets the world with his mouth, and the integration of oral activities, therefore, is through sensory mechanisms.

The mouth of the infant is used for many purposes. The perceptual functions of the tongue, lips and facial skin are mingled with the sensory functions of taste, smell and jaw position. The neonate's primary relationship to his environment is by means of his mouth, pharynx and larynx. Here, a high concentration of readily available receptors become stimulated and modulate the already matured brain stem coordinations that regulate respiration and nursing and determine head and neck position during breathing and feeding. Bosma[6] calls the mouth a "chambered sensorium" and likens it to the limbs, for example, the upper extremity, which, in the adult human, receives much of its guidance from the cutaneous sensation of the hand. The afferent inputs for the jaw system are the rich sensory resources of the mouth and the temporomandibular articulation. The sensitivity of the tongue and lips is greater than any other body area, and the sensory guidance for oral functioning, including jaw movement, is from a remarkably large area. Furthermore, the sensory inputs are compounded by many dual contacting surfaces, for example, tongue and lips, soft palate and posterior pharyngeal wall and the compartments of the temporomandibular articulation. Obviously, the rate of information input of the oro-jaw system is very high, and the task of integrating, coordinating and interpreting such a vast array of sensory signals requires exceedingly complicated brain mechanisms.[6] Perhaps, in humans, the oral area presents the highest level of sensory-motor integrative functions.

b) Infantile Suckling and Swallowing

One reason why infantile suckling and swallowing have been the subjects of much research is that the effectiveness of these activities is a good indication of the neurologic maturation of premature infants. The infant finds the mother's breast and places the lips around the nipple, effecting a tight seal. "The neck of the teat is first compressed between the upper gum and the tip of the tongue covering the lower gum with a general elevation of the jaw and tongue"[4] as the tongue is "applied against the bulb of the teat from before, backward, indenting the teat and expressing some of its contents."[4] While the milk is being expressed from the breast, supplementary mechanisms within the mouth create a suction (Fig. V-5). The milk now lies in a small reservoir on the dorsum of the tongue but is sealed posteriorly by the opposed soft palate until sufficient increments of milk trigger the next step of the suckle.[6] Peiper[45] and Moyers[41] noted a fairly rigid patterning of suckle-swallow-respiration sequences (Fig. V-6). Thus, the child who suckles twice before swallowing usually follows this rigid pattern, irrespective of the rate of flow of milk. We discovered in our own work[43] that children studied as long as 5 years after weaning, if given a bottle from which to suckle, produced suckling-swallowing-respiratory rhythms similar to those observed when they were infants. Rhythmic elevation and lowering of the jaw provides a sequential change in position of the tongue in coordination with its suckling contractions. The activities of suckling are closely related temporally to the motor functions of positional maintenance of the airway. Electromyographic studies in our laboratory[41] have confirmed visual observations reported in England[22]; that is, that while the mandibular movements are carried out by the muscles of mastication (Vth cranial nerve muscles), the mandible is primarily stabilized during the actual act of swallowing by concomitant contractions of the inframandibular, tongue and facial muscles (VIIth cranial nerve muscles)[41] (Fig. V-7). During the actual time of the infantile swallow, the tongue lies between the gum pads and is in close apposition with the lingual surface of the lips. Characteristic features, then, of the infantile swallow are (1) the jaws are apart, with the tongue between the gum pads, (2) the mandible is stabilized by contractions of the muscles of the VIIth cranial nerve and the interposed tongue and (3) the swallow is initiated, and to a great extent guided, by sensory interchange between the lips and the tongue.

c) *Maintenance of the Airway*

The oro-jaw musculature is responsible for the vital positional relationships that maintain the oropharyngeal airway. While the infant is resting, a rather uniform diameter for the airway is provided by (1) maintaining the mandible anteroposteriorly and (2) stabilizing the tongue and posterior pharyngeal wall relationships. The axial musculature around the vertebra also is concerned. These primitive neonatal protective mechanisms provide the motor background on which are developed, with growth, all of the postural mechanisms of the head and neck region. The physiologic maintenance of the airway is of vital continuing importance from the first day of life.

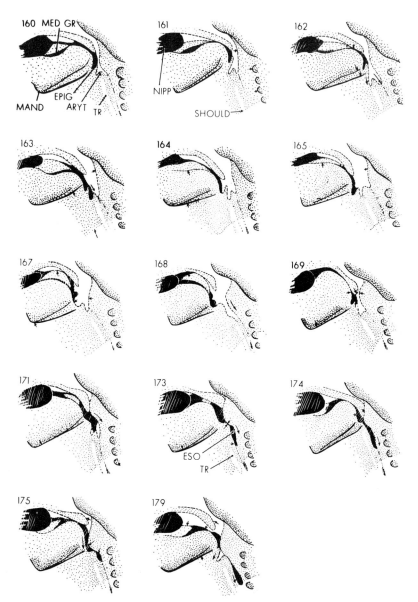

Fig. V-5.—Cineradiographic study of suckle feeding. *EPIG* = epiglottis, *ARYT* = arytenoid mass, *ESO* = esophagus, *TR* = trachea, *NIPP* = nipple, *SHOULD* = shoulder, *MAND* = mandible, *MED GR* = medial groove. Tracings of individual frames taken at 25 frames per second. In the first frame (*160*), the nipple is compressed (note how the barium mixture outlines the anatomic structures). During frames *160–165*, the tongue and mandible are elevated, although the tongue con-

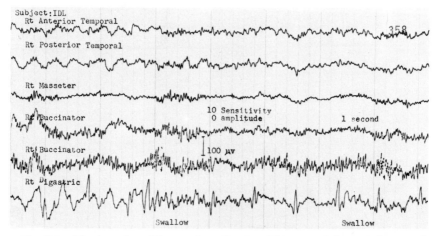

Fig. V-6.—Rhythm of suckling and swallowing. This record shows infant swallows during suckling. It was obtained from a baby a few months of age. Note the greater activity of the buccinator muscle and the minimal activity of the mandibular elevators during swallowing. The slow, gradual, undulating movements shown in the record are those of the mandible rising and falling gently during the nursing process. Fairly rigid rhythm is established between the number of suckles and swallows.

d) Infant Cry

The involvement of the orofacial and jaw musculature in infant crying has been reported in classic studies by Bosma and his co-workers.[7] When the aroused baby is crying, the oral region is unresponsive to local stimulation; the mouth is held wide open and the tongue is separated from the lower lip and from the palate. The steady stabilization of the size of the pharyngeal airway is given up during crying and irregular varying constrictions during expiration of the cry, and large reciprocal expansions during the alternating inspirations are seen.[7]

e) Gagging

Gagging is the reflex refusal to swallow or accept foreign objects in the throat; it is an exaggeration of the protective reflexes guarding the airway and alimentary tract. Gagging is characterized by retching,

---

tinues to be grooved, and the first of the barium bolus is expressed into the pharynx. The pharynx increased in size following the completed swallow. In frames 167–174, the reciprocal phase of the suckle is seen coincident with the pharyngeal phase of the swallow. (After Bosma.[6])

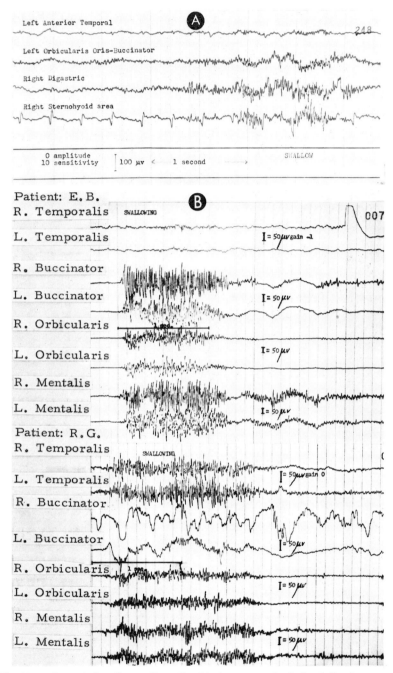

Fig. V-7.—A, an infantile swallow. In this instance, the baby fell asleep at the mother's breast. The swallow recorded is an unconscious swallow of saliva during sleep. Note the dominance of the facial muscles and the minimal activity in the only mandibular elevator sampled. **B,** mature swallows. A comparison of the

C

Left Anterior Temporal

Left Middle Temporal

Left Posterior Temporal

Left Masseter

Right Masseter |50␮v

Right Anterior Temporal

Right Middle Temporal

Right Posterior Temporal

%/₃ D W   1 SEC.

D

Left Anterior Temporal

Left Middle Temporal

Left Posterior Temporal

Left Masseter

Right Masseter |50␮v

Right Anterior Temporal

Right Middle Temporal

Right Posterior Temporal

%/₈ D W   1 SEC.

teeth-together and teeth-apart swallow. The record at the bottom (R. G.) is a typical mature swallow. Note the strong contractions in the temporal muscle. The record at the top (E. B.) is of a child of the same age. Note, however, that this child has a teeth-apart swallow, since there is far greater activity of the facial muscles than there is of the mandibular elevators. Comparison of an unconscious swallow (C) and a volitional swallow of water (D). These records were taken from the same person during the same experimental period.[14]

133

throat spasms, nonproductive vomiting or reflex threat to vomit. The lowest sensory thresholds for gagging in man are found in the faucial pillars, the base of the tongue, the lateral aspects of the soft palate and the posterior pharyngeal wall. Therefore, the nerves involved are the second and third divisions of the Vth, IXth and Xth cranial nerves. Branches of the VIIth, XIth and XIIth cranial nerves may be involved also. Inhibitory fibers for gagging are found in the Xth cranial nerve. A gag center (perhaps a chain of centers) is located in the medulla, close to the centers for vomiting, salivation, cardiac centers, etc., which helps explain the accompanying symptoms of gagging.[12] The elementary gag reflex is present at birth, although its mode of function in later life is greatly altered by the types of visual, acoustic and olfactory stimuli, psychic state and previous experience.[38]

The motor response to gagging propels the contents of the stomach, esophagus and pharynx and closes the nasal passages. Motor elements of the Vth, VIIth, IXth, Xth, XIth and XIIth cranial nerves plus sympathetics and parasympathetics are involved.

The gag reflex displays both temporal and spatial summation, is inhibited by extreme fatigue and depressed by shock or anesthesia. Pain in the region seems to override the gag reflex. For example, when a physician retrieves a bone from the throat, usually no gagging is observed. Clinical control of gagging is based on a thorough knowledge of the psychophysiology involved.[61] For example, hyperventilation produces apnea, which, in turn, suppresses the gagging.

3. EARLY POSTNATAL DEVELOPMENT OF ORAL FUNCTIONS
a) Mastication

The interaction between the rapidly and differentially growing craniofacial skeleton and the maturing neuromuscular system brings about sequential progressive modifications of the elementary oral functions seen in the neonate. Mandibular growth downward and forward is greater at this time than midface growth, giving rise to an increase in oral volume. Maturation of the musculature and definition of the temporomandibular joint helps provide a more stable mandible. Mandibular growth carries the tongue away from the palate and helps provide differential enlargement of the pharynx, maintaining patency of the airway. The soft palate and the tongue commonly are held in apposition, but, as the tongue no longer is lowered by mandibular growth, its functional relationships with the lips are altered—an alteration aided by the vertical development of the alveolar process. At rest, however, the tongue no longer is entirely in generalized apposition with the lips, buccal wall and soft palate. The lips elongate and become more selectively mobile and the tongue develops discrete movements separate from lip and mandibular movements; yet, most of the time, the labial valve mechanism is maintained during rest and feeding so that food is not lost.[6]

The development of speech and mastication as well as facial expression requires a furthering of the independent mobility of the separate parts, whereas in the neonate the lips tightly surround a plunger-like tongue moving in synchrony with gross mandibular movements. Speech, facial expression and mastication require the development of new motor patterns as well as greater autonomy of the motor elements. All of the developmental aspects of these functions are not known, but mastication certainly does not develop gradually from infantile nursing. Rather, it seems, the maturation of the central nervous system permits completely new functions to develop—functions triggered by the eruption of the teeth.

One of the most important factors in the maturation of mastication is the sensory aspect of the newly arriving teeth. The muscles controlling mandibular position are cued by the first occlusal contacts of the antagonistic incisors. Serial electromyographic studies, at very frequent intervals during the arrival of the incisors, have demonstrated conclusively that the very instant the maxillary and mandibular incisors accidentally touch one another, the jaw musculature begins to learn to function in accommodation to the arrival of the teeth.[41] Thus, the closure pattern becomes more precise anteroposteriorly (since incisors arrive first) before it does mediolaterally.

All occlusal functions are learned in stages as the central nervous system and orofacial and jaw musculature mature concomitantly with the development of the dentition. The earliest chewing movements are irregular and poorly coordinated like those during the early stages of learning any motor skill. As the primary dentition is completed, the chewing cycle becomes more stabilized, using more efficiently the individual's occlusal pattern of intercuspation. In the young child, sensory guidance for masticatory movement is provided by the receptors in the temporomandibular articulation, periodontal ligament, tongue, oral mucosa and muscles. Thus, cuspal height, cuspal angle and incisal guidance (which usually is minimal in the primary dentition) play a role in the establishment of chewing patterns in the infant. However, condylar guidance is not important, since the eminentia articularis is ill defined and the temporal (glenoid) fossae are shallow. Rather, it may be supposed that the bone of the eminentia articularis forms where temporomandibular function permits it to develop. In a similar fashion, the plane of occlusion is established by the growth of the alveolar process during eruption of the teeth to heights permitted by function. The individual's pattern of movements during the chewing cycle is the developed integrative pattern of many functional elements. Storey has informally suggested that opening and closing may be unconditioned, whereas the patterns of masticatory movement are conditioned. In the young child, at the time of completion of the primary dentition, masticatory relationships are optimal, since all three systems (bone, teeth and muscle) still show the lability of development and are thus highly adaptive. Cusp height and overbite in the primary dentition are more shallow, bone growth more rapid and adaptive and neuromuscular learning more easily obtained, since patterns of activity are not yet well established. Adaptations to masticatory change are more difficult in later years (see Section C-4-b).

b) Facial Expressions

In a not dissimilar way, most subtle facial expressioning is learned largely by imitation, beginning about the time the gross primitive uses of the VIIth nerve musculature for infantile swallowing are abandoned. However, some human facial expressions are not learned and can be traced back to reflex responses of primitive primates. Similar facial displays have evolved in the four lines of modern primates in which monkey-like forms have developed.[3]

c) Speech

Purposeful speech is different from reflex infant cry. Infant crying is associated with irregular tongue and mandibular positions related to sporadic inspirations and expirations during crying. Speech, on the other hand, is performed on a background of stabilized and learned positions of the mandible, pharynx and tongue. Infant cry usually is a simple displacement of parts accompanied by a single explosive emission, whereas speech can be carried out only by polyphasic and sequential motor activities synchronized closely with breathing.[6, 7] Speech is regular; infant cry is sporadic. Speech requires complicated and sophisticated variations of sensory conditioning elements during learning, whereas infant cry is primitive and not learned.

Speech consists of four parts: (1) language—the knowledge of words used in communicating ideas; (2) voice—sound produced by air passing between the vibrating vocal cords of the larynx; (3) articulation—the movement of the speech organs used in producing a sound i.e., lips, tongue, teeth, mandible, palate and so forth; (4) rhythm—variations of quality, length, timing and stress of a sound, word, phrase or sentence. If there is no impairment of hearing, sight or oral sensation, the child will learn to speak from the speech he hears, reproducing as best he can what he has heard. Speech defects are a loss or disturbance of language, voice, articulation and rhythm or combinations of such losses and disturbances..

At about age 1 month, changes in the quality of infant cry are noticed and are said to indicate developing needs of the child that are expressed in modifications of the reflex infant cry. In another month or two, babbling appears. Open-mouth vowels, e.g., "a," "u," "i," are followed by labial sounds, "p," "b," "m" and guttural sounds, "k," "ch," "g," "ng." Other sounds follow, and a period of acute vocal play and experimentation is entered. Gradually, through hearing association and experimentation, the child adopts the sounds he hears others making and drops those he does not hear. Probably no significance, however, is attached by the child to the sounds at this time. Simple words are learned before short sentences, and the child understands what is said to him some time before he will speak himself. The baby begins with voice and adds articulation, rhythm and language.

d) *Mature Swallow*

During the latter half of the first year of life, several maturational events occur that alter markedly the orofacial musculature's functioning. The arrival of the incisors cues the more precise opening and closing movements of the mandible, compels a more retracted tongue posture and initiates the learning of mastication. As soon as bilateral posterior occlusion is established (usually with the eruption of the first primary molars), true chewing motions are seen to start, and the learning of the mature swallow begins. Gradually, the Vth cranial nerve muscles assume the role of mandibular stabilization during the swallow, and the muscles of facial expression abandon the crude infantile function of suckling and the infantile swallow and begin to learn the more delicate and complicated functions of speech and facial expressions. The transition from infantile to mature swallow takes place over several months, aided by maturation of neuromuscular elements, the appearance of upright head posture and, hence, a change in the direction of gravitational forces on the mandible, the instinctive desire to chew, the necessity to handle textured food, dentitional development and so forth. Most children achieve most features of the mature swallow at 12–15 months. Characteristic features of the mature swallow are (1) the teeth are together (although they may be apart with a liquid bolus), (2) the mandible is stabilized by contractions of the Vth cranial nerve, (3) the tongue tip is held against the palate above and behind the incisors and (4) minimal contractions of the lips are seen during the swallow (see Fig. V-7). Further discussions of the swallow will be found later in this chapter.

C. Neurophysiologic Regulation of Jaw Positions and Functions

Jaw position, like a number of other automatic somatic activities, is largely reflexly controlled, even though it is possible to alter it voluntarily. A surprising number of jaw functions are carried on at the subconscious level, even though conscious control of some of these functions also is possible and sometimes necessary, for example, meaningful speech.

1. NEUROLOGY
a) *Receptors*

Traditionally, the receptors have been described on a morphologic basis and named after the investigator who first described them: Meissner corpuscles have been assigned to the sensation of touch, Ruffini corpuscles to warmth, etc., but it now seems likely that certain receptors respond to several modalities. The receptors in some of the sense organs are specialized, so that they respond to one particular form of energy at a much lower threshold than they respond to others. This form of energy to which the receptor is most sensitive is called its adequate stimulus. Confusion has arisen because there are far more morphologically different types of endings than there are species of sensation, and the morphologic specificity of nerve endings subserving a given sensory modality certainly is in doubt.[21] Receptors may be classified according to the nature of the stimuli: (1) mechanoreceptors, e.g., tactile sense, vibration sense, hearing; (2) thermoreceptors, e.g., heat and cold; etc. Confusion has arisen, too, by classifying receptors according to concepts requiring other parts of the central nervous system for interpretation; for example, proprioception and pain.

1) MUSCLES.—The muscles of the orofacial region are well supplied with encapsulated mechanoreceptors and with free endings. Most important of all are the muscle spindles, mechanoreceptors whose structure and behavior in masticatory muscles are no different than elsewhere in the body. These receptors and the other mechanoreceptors found in the fascial sheaths of the masticatory muscles and in tendons display different rates of discharge in response to alterations in muscle tension induced either by stretch or by contraction. Muscle spindles lie between the main muscle fibers and parallel to them (see Fig. V-1). The spindle has both afferent and efferent innervations (see Fig. V-2). Although the spindles form only a small proportion of the muscle's mass in most muscles in the orofacial region, there are more nerve fibers innervating the spindles than the main muscle fibers, an indication of the spindle's importance. There are two separate routes to voluntary muscle, the alpha and the gamma (see Fig. V-1). In the alpha route, impulses from the higher centers focus on the alpha cell in the motor nucleus. Impulses from the alpha cell go directly to the main muscle fibers. When the gamma route is used, impulses from higher centers focus on the gamma cell in the motor nucleus. When this cell fires, impulses pass peripherally down the small gamma efferent nerve fibers to the intrafusal fibers in the spindle (see Fig. V-1), which pull on the nuclear bag. This excites the receptor activating its afferent fiber, which, in turn, excites the appropriate alpha efferent fibers, leading to contraction in the main muscle fibers. Muscle spindles that subserve the stretch reflex (see Fig. V-2) are abundant in mandibular elevators and less frequent in depressors.[44] Murphy[44] suggests that the resistance of a food bolus reflexly invokes the gamma route to the elevators (Fig. V-8). The intrafusal fibers set the nuclear bags to a predetermined tension, the tensed spindles activating the main muscle fibers.[44] Crushing the bolus shortens the elevators, bringing the extrafusal fibers into alignment with the preset spindles and, as a result, afferent impulses from the spindle stop, thereby halting the contraction.[44] The amount and extent

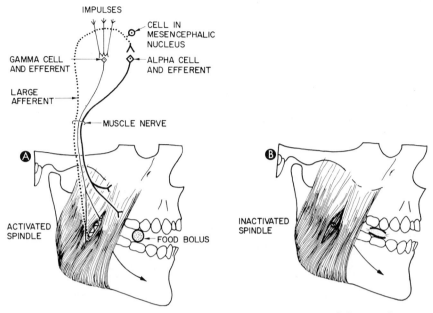

Fig. V-8.—Murphy's[44] postulated mechanism of shortening/inhibition of prime movers as a protective mechanism in mastication. Another explanation involves the elongation of spindles in the lateral pterygoid muscle.

of muscular contraction necessary to crush the bolus has been "programed" by the nervous system before the contraction begins. An adequate discussion of muscle spindle physiology is outside the realm of this book. If Figures V-1, V-2 and V-8 are insufficient for basic understanding, the reader should refer to the Suggested Readings list at the end of the chapter.

2) PERIODONTAL LIGAMENT.—Encapsulated mechanoreceptors, as well as dense plexuses of unmyelinated nerve fibers, are found in the periodontal ligament.[21] The mechanoreceptors are stimulated by displacement of the tooth within the alveolar socket. These receptors transduce forces as light as 0.7 Gm.[37] The unmyelinated nerve fibers constitute the pain receptor system.

3) TEETH.—The dental pulp is well supplied with sensory organs, primarily pain receptors, that ordinarily are not stimulated during normal function. The intradental receptors, as far as is known, play no role in the reflex regulation of jaw position and function.[21] In pathologic circumstances, however, their stimulation results in a controlled overriding of normal reflex jaw control systems as a protective mechanism for the traumatized tooth.

4) MUCOSA.—The mucosa of the oral region, including the palate, faucial pillars, tongue and sublingual region, is supplied with receptors

of numerous forms, including encapsulated and nonencapsulated organized endings, fibrillar extension, nerve networks, free nerve endings and branched terminations.[21] Generally, the frequency of nerve ending occurrence is higher in the front than in the rear of the mouth. The relationships between mucosal receptors and oral sensation are only now becoming clear. However, the accumulating evidence challenges strongly the long-held concept that there are specific receptors for the modalities of heat, cold, touch and pain.

5) Tongue.—The tongue is said to be the most sensitive body surface. The frequency of innervation per unit of area is greater on the dorsal surface than on the inferior and greater anteriorly than posteriorly. The receptors of the tongue mucosa are similar to those of the palate and gingiva; however, the tongue, particularly the anterior two-thirds of the dorsum, exhibits a rough mucosa due to the lingual papillae. Some sort of nerve ending occurs in each lingual papilla on the tongue's dorsum. The tongue is highly thermal sensitive and profoundly sensitive to tactile stimuli.

6) Temporomandibular joints.—There is in each jaw joint a dense population of encapsulated mechanoreceptors responding to variations in the tension of different parts of the joint capsule.[20] A heavy innervation of unmyelinated nerve fibers arranged in dense plexuses in the fibers' capsule and at the posterior articular fat pad constitute the pain receptor system of the joint.[20] The mechanoreceptors in the temporomandibular articulations are similar to those that have been shown in other joints of the body and coordinate the reflexes of the muscles operating over the jaw joints in a fashion similar to that which has been demonstrated for the limbs, spine and elsewhere.[20] There is one very important difference, however: the jaw articulations are both attached to the same bone and, therefore, one of the joints cannot be moved without affecting the other. Recent research has shown that the mechanoreceptors in the jaw joints are the primary contributors to our perception of jaw position during posture and of the direction and rate of jaw movements during normal jaw functions.[20, 59] Previously, the perception of mandibular position had been thought to arise primarily from the muscles. If the teeth occlude or bite an object, the receptors of the periodontal ligament must be considered. However, discrimination of size of objects between the teeth is almost entirely a function of the temporomandibular joint receptors.[49, 55] Severe malocclusion appears to provide pathologic changes in the joints, which, in turn, impair the joint receptors, although muscle dysfunction alone does not affect the sensory innervation.[49, 55]

The four types of receptors found in the temporomandibular joints, their morphology, location and physiologic characteristics are given in Table V-1. Type I receptors contribute to the regulation of the tone of the muscles of mastication and thus are responsible for the continuing variations seen in mandibular posture.[20] The varying discharges from Type I receptors in different parts of both joint capsules contribute

TABLE V-1.—RECEPTORS IN THE TEMPOROMANDIBULAR JOINTS*

TYPE NUMBER (GREENFIELD AND WYKE)	DESCRIPTION (THILANDER)	LOCATION IN JOINT	NERVE FIBERS	ROLE
I	Thinly encapsulated	Fibrous capsule, posteriorly and laterally	Myelinated 6-9 μ	Mechanoreceptor Low threshold Slow adaptation
II	Thickly encapsulated	Fibrous capsule, posteriorly and laterally Articular fat pad	Myelinated 8-12 μ	Mechanoreceptor Low threshold Rapid adaptation
III	Encapsulated Golgi tendon organs	Lateral capsular ligament (superficial)	Myelinated up to 17 μ	Mechanoreceptors High threshold (activated at extreme positions only) Slow adaptation
IV	Free endings, plexuses	Generally in capsule, posterior fat pad and walls of vessels	Myelinated and nonmyelinated 5 μ	Pain High threshold Nonadapting

*From Greenfield and Wyke.[20]

to the reflex reciprocal coordination, facilitation and inhibition of tonus in all the muscles around the jaw region. Likewise, these discharges help make us aware of jaw position, direction and rate of movement.[59] It seems likely, too, that their discharges combine with those of the periodontal ligament, mucosal and tongue receptors to provide what the brain interprets as occlusal sensation. Type II receptors, more numerous in the temporomandibular joints than in most other skeletal joints, function as rapidly adapting mechanoreceptors of low threshold that discharge very briefly only during the onset of joint movement.[20] Type III receptors in the temporomandibular joints are restricted to the lateral ligament of each joint and the accessory ligaments, e.g., the stylomandibular ligament.[20, 59] Type III receptors may be considered analogous to Golgi tendon organs, since they ordinarily are inactive and discharge only when the joint has been displaced to an extreme degree, whereupon they protectively inhibit motor unit activity in the principal movers of the joint. Type IV receptors provide the system of sensory reception that later is interpreted in the brain as pain.[20] They are found in dense networks throughout the fibrous capsule of the joint, in the walls of blood vessels and in the articular fat pads posterior to the condyle of the mandible. Normally inactive, they are provoked only by abnormal irritation of the articular tissues. When stimulated, they

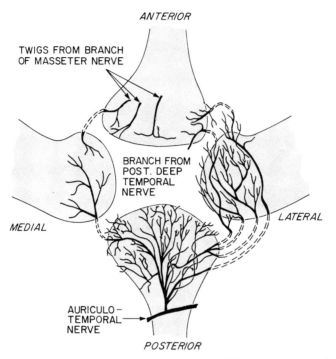

Fig. V-9.—Innervation of the human temporomandibular joint capsule. (Adapted from Thilander[59] and Storey.[55])

alter the reflex postural position of the mandible, the chewing cycle or other functional movements. It is of some clinical interest that pain receptor endings are absent from synovial and meniscal tissues in the adult joint.

Detailed age changes in the neurology of the temporomandibular joints await further investigation—investigation that will be of particular interest to orthodontists.

Impulses arising from the four types of receptors in the temporomandibular joints travel to the brain stem by articular nerves solely of trigeminal origin—auriculotemporal, masseteric and deep temporal nerves (Fig. V-9).

b) Reflexes

Several studies of jaw reflexes have been reported in the literature.[20, 49, 59, 60] Greenfield and Wyke[20] recorded simultaneous bilateral electromyograms from bipolar needle electrodes inserted into the temporalis, masseter and pterygoid muscles of anesthetized cats whose mandible had been freed surgically, so that all movement of the mandible affected only the tissues of the temporomandibular joint. In all of several varied experiments, movements of the operated on experimental side affected only the tissues of the ipsilateral joint. Normally, there is a brief discharge of motor units, which is a rapidly adapting onset response; this is followed, as the jaw movement continues, by a more marked discharge that increases gradually and persists while the mouth is held open. Since striated muscles contain no rapidly adapting mechanoreceptors, it is assumed that the initial response at the onset of movement is due to the reflex discharge of Type II mechanoreceptors, which are numerous in the temporomandibular joint capsule. The later and more prolonged motor unit discharge probably represents the myotactic reflex response to stretch of muscle spindles from the mandibular elevators. Apparently, any response from slowly adapting reflexes of articular origin, that is, Type I receptors, is overridden or inhibited. Kawamura and Majima[32] have recorded, from the sensory and motor nuclei of the trigeminal nerve within the cat brain stem nerve, potentials arriving in response to manipulation of the isolated mandibular condyle. The injection of a local anesthetic into either or both of the temporomandibular joints in normal human subjects results in a marked impairment in the accuracy of voluntary jaw and occlusal movements.[59] Moyers,[40] Ramfjord and Ash[48] and others have shown that occlusal interferences reflexly alter chewing movements and mandibular closing and opening movement patterns, particularly when the occlusal disharmonies are present in the unconscious swallowing position of the mandible (see Section D-4, later in this chapter).

2. UNCONDITIONED JAW POSITIONS AND FUNCTIONS

Most research on the neurophysiologic regulation of jaw positions and functions has been done on the adult and there has been a tendency to transfer prosthodontically oriented concepts based on sound adult clinical practice to children. During development, before all of the parts of the system have appeared and while growth is dominant, it is hazardous to maintain the same clinical assumptions so useful to an understanding of the adult. Functional occlusal homeostasis in an edentulous 70-year-old requiring complete prosthesis or a semiedentulous adult with periodontal disease is different than in a growing 6-year-old with a Class II malocclusion and an active thumb-sucking habit. Our knowledge concerning the developmental aspects of orofacial and jaw neurophysiology is most incomplete at this time, although much research is under way. We must remember that many of our attitudes are the victims of our experience with degenerating occlusions in the adult, and the critical clinical factors that obtain under those circumstances may not be present in the child or may have different relative significance during development.

a) Posture

It is impossible to separate completely postural adjustments from voluntary movements in any rigid way, but it is possible and useful to identify a series of postural reflexes that serve to maintain the body in an upright balanced position, thus providing the constant adjustment necessary to maintain a stable background for voluntary activity[15] (Table V-2). These neuromuscular adjustments include maintained static reflexes involving sustained contraction of the musculature and dynamic short-term phasic reflexes involving transient movement. All are integrated in the central nervous system and are effected largely through extrapyramidal motor pathways.[15]

The postural mechanisms for the vertebrae and the head at least partly determine mandibular posture. The mandibular postural range includes the starting positions for most reflex mandibular movements, the resting positions of the mandible and so forth. Because the functions are so vital and the mechanisms so primitive, we may think of the basic aspects of posture as unconditioned; however, a glance at Table V-2 reveals that the posture observed is the summation and integration of a number of reflexes operating at that moment.

The primary function of jaw posture is maintenance of the airway, but some confusion has arisen from equating the clinical "rest position" of the mandible with mandibular posture. Such terms as "postural rest position" and "physiologic rest position" also seem obfuscating, since a number of postural positions for any joint in the body may be seen at different times. The term "rest position" as used by dentists is a semi-standardized location of one of innumerable possible postural positions for the mandible. "Freeway space" is the vertical interocclusal difference between "rest position" and the usual occlusal position ("centric occlusion"). Rest position is relatively reproducible if the conditions for registering it are standardized. However, there are significant differences in mandibular posture with age,[57] after removal of teeth,[57] after insertion of dentures[58] and after the correction of malocclusion.[50] There also is a strong suggestion that the clinically determined rest position alters after the equilibration of the occlusion when gross occlusal disturbances have been present.[48] The many new research findings in temporomandibular neurophysiology seem to make necessary a complete re-evaluation of many of our clinical concepts of mandibular posture (rest position). Further knowledge will obviate some of the apparent discrepancies between clinical practice and neurophysiologic principles. Our present ignorance of this extremely complex problem makes such explanations as those given here very tentative.

Garnick and Ramfjord[16] found that the interocclusal distance averaged 1.7 mm. when determined by the clinical rest position. On the other hand, when the interocclusal distance was determined electromyographically on the basis of minimal muscle activity, the average dis-

TABLE V-2.—Determinants of Mandibular Posture*

Reflex	Stimulus and Receptor	Response	Center
Stretch reflexes	Stretch. Muscle spindles	Contraction of muscle	Segmental spinal Cord
Positive support-ing (magnet) re-action	Contact with sole or palm. Pro-prioceptorsin distal flexors	Foot extended to support body	
Negative support-ing reaction	Stretch. Proprio-ceptors in ex-tensors	Release of pos-itive support-ing reaction	Cord
Tonic labyrin-thine reflexes	Gravity. Otolithic organs	Extensor rig-idity	Medulla
Tonic neck re-flexes	Head turned (neck proprioceptors): (1) To side (2) Up (3) Down	Change in pat-tern of rig-idity: (1) Flexion of limbs on side to which head is turned (2) Hind legs flex (3) Forelegs flex	Medulla
Labyrinthine righting re-flexes	Gravity. Otolithic organs	Head kept level	Midbrain
Neck-righting reflexes	Stretch of neck muscles. Spindles	Righting of tho-rax and shoul-ders, then pel-vis	Midbrain
Body-on-head righting reflex	Pressure on side of body. Exterocept-ors	Righting of head	Midbrain
Body-on-body righting re-flexes	Pressure on side of body. Exterocept-ors	Righting of body even when head held sideways	Midbrain
Optical righting reflexes	Visual cues	Righting of head. Stretch reflexes	Cortex
Stretch reflexes (mandibular ele-vators)	Stretch. Muscle spindles	Contraction of muscle	Pons

*After Ganong.[15]

tance was 3.29 mm., with an additional resting range of 11 mm.[16] Obviously, if the clinically determined rest position of the mandible frequently is found outside the range of minimal muscle activity of the mandibular elevators, the physiologic determinants of the two mandibular positions must be different. Since the clinical resting posi-tion is really a volitional activity, studies of it may have less relevance to the postural position than was once thought. The mandibular position of minimal muscle activity is more sensitive to input from occlusal interferences, pain and temporomandibular sensory influences. The exact role of fusimotor activity, particularly as it relates to receptors in and around the temporomandibular joints, is, as yet, not completely understood, but it obviously is far more important than previously supposed. Nor is our knowledge complete concerning the developmental aspects of the maintenance and regulation of mandibular posture.

b) *Unconscious or Reflex Swallow*

Although, in the fetus, swallowing can be elicited by tactile stimulation of the face and lips and, in the infant, swallowing can be triggered by tactile stimulation of the lips or tongue tip, in the adult it is prompted most easily by mechanical stimulation of the faucial pillars and posterior pharyngeal walls (innervation supplied by the IXth and Xth cranial nerves).[54] For the area innervated by the pharyngeal branches of the vagus nerve, both touch and pressure provide adequate stimuli, since both superficial and deep receptors are involved.[54]

A discrete, bilaterally represented population of cells in the medial reticular formation of the medulla provides the central organization of swallowing. The swallowing center lies at the level of the facial nucleus.[12]

From the swallowing center, the motor output involves participation of both intrinsic and extrinsic swallowing muscles. The intrinsic muscles always participate in a rigid temporal pattern in an all-or-none fashion and do not appear to be susceptible to proprioceptive feedback or conditioning,[13] a very important restriction for clinicians who would attempt to alter the reflex swallow by training methods. On the other hand, the extrinsic swallowing muscles (e.g., temporal, masseter and digastric muscles) may or may not participate in the synergy of swallowing, are sensitive to sensory feedback and are readily conditioned. As was pointed out earlier, the mandibular elevators do not participate in the reflex human infantile swallow but do participate in the reflex human adult swallow.

3. Jaw Functions That Appear with Normal Growth and Development
a) *Mastication*

See Section B-3-a for a discussion of the development of mastication.

b) *Mature Swallow*

In addition to the reflex mature swallow (see Section B-3-d), other patterns of swallowing quite different from those seen in the neonate make their appearance with growth, development and maturation. Swallowing varies according to the size, nature and texture of the bolus, head and body posture, fatigue, hunger and so forth. The unconscious (reflex) swallow of saliva resists conditioning more than do unconscious swallows during mastication. Unconscious swallowing is far more difficult to condition than is voluntary swallowing. For these reasons, command swallows of water or food are poor criteria for the efficacy of treatment of abnormal swallowing. Similarly, occlusal patterns created by restorative or prosthetic dentistry may be accommodated by the neuromusculature during mastication or voluntary jaw movements under the dentist's control or direction and yet may not be accepted during unconscious swallowing. The role of the unconscious swallow in occlusal trauma often is neglected.

4. CONDITIONED JAW POSITIONS AND FUNCTIONS
a) Mature Swallow

See Section C-3-b for a brief discussion of the implications of conditioning and maturation on the mature swallow.

b) Mastication

Section B-3-a discusses the establishment of reflex mastication.

All elements in the masticatory system are not equally capable of adaptation. Masticatory reflexes can adapt more easily than can those of the unconscious reflex swallow. Each time a tooth position changes, a tooth is lost or an occlusal disharmony appears, learning of new masticatory patterns must occur. Some occlusal interferences reflexly prompt protective adaptive changes in the patterns of jaw movements to avoid the interfering point during function. Balancing interferences have been shown by Ramfjord and Ash[48] and Schaerer *et al.*[51] to produce avoidance responses more readily, whereas working bite interferences are accepted more passively. Conditioning may take place rather quickly, so that functional movements soon are altered automatically. However, the patterns of occlusal avoidance that have been established may create other dysfunctions and impose imbalances on other elements within the masticatory system that cannot compensate so readily, for example, a periodontal lesion resulting from occlusal trauma or temporomandibular joint pain.

c) Other

All learned functions involving mandibular position (e.g., speech, facial expression) can be conditioned or altered by new experiences or training. It should be remembered that for such complicated neuromuscular activities there are many and varied sensory inputs that are perceived by the brain on a background of memory. Volition alone is but one link in a many-stranded cable.

D. Physiology of Occlusal Functions

1. JAW MOVEMENTS

a) Border Movements

Posselt[46] demonstrated the reproducibility of border mandibular movements (Fig. V-10). With Posselt's gnathiothesiometer, one can record any position of the mandible and measure distances between any positions recorded. All function takes place within the limits of the border movements. Figure V-10, A illustrates the border positions of the man-

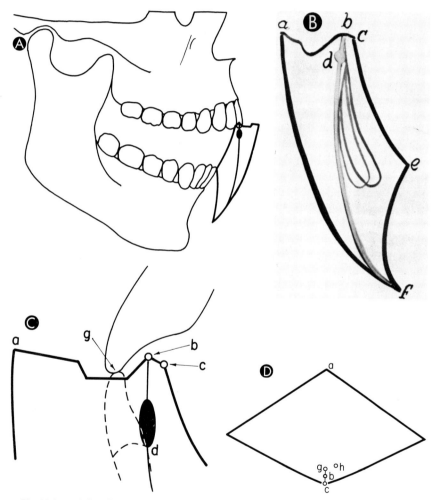

Fig. V-10.—A, border movements of the mandible as recorded in a sagittal plane. (After Posselt[46] and Ramfjord and Ash.[48]) **B,** the envelope of jaw movements. The dark outer line indicates the border jaw positions. All functional movements

dible when recorded from the mandibular incisor and projected to the sagittal plane. Similar drawings may be made for any other part of the mandible and in other planes as well. Two of the border positions are of clinical import—the retruded contact position (see Section D-3) and the ideal occlusal position.

1) IDEAL OCCLUSAL POSITION.—In the neonate, the only mandibular position that can be located at all reliably is the postural position, since consistency in mandibular posture is necessary for maintenance of the airway. Border movements of the mandible are difficult to record reliably at this early age because of immaturity of the joint structures and ligaments, but they become more precisely defined with growth and maturation.

Sillman[53] was the first to observe that the infant develops an occlusal sense with the eruption of the primary teeth. This occlusal sense is the result of the formation of reflexes regulating mandibular movements after antagonistic teeth have begun to touch one another. Thus, occlusal reflexes and relationships originate during the development of the dentition.[41] As the teeth erupt and begin to find intercuspation, afferent impulses are transmitted to the muscles controlling the position of the mandible. In the midbrain, afferent impulses from periodontal receptors are integrated with stimuli from the temporomandibular articulation, tongue, mucosa, higher centers, etc. Although these other sources of afferent input may be present earlier, integration and the formation of occlusal reflexes cannot take place until occlusal contacts begin.

When all the primary teeth have erupted, a position of occlusion has been learned that provides a maximum of occlusal contact and a minimum of torque, stress and strain on the roots and the temporomandibular articulation.[41] The mandible's position during this rather ideal occlusal relationship may be termed the *ideal occlusal position* (see Fig. V-8).

---

take place within the envelope described by these lines: *f-a*, the protrusive path of opening and closure; *f-d-b*, the reflex path of jaw closure; *f*, the extreme open position of the mandible; *a*, the most protruded occlusal position; *c*, the most retruded occlusal position; *b*, the ideal occlusal position; *d*, the postural area of the mandible. The biphasic curve *f-e-c* represents the most retruded path of closure. At *e*, the condyles return to the glenoid fossae. The two loops symbolize chewing strokes. (Adapted from Posselt.[46]) **C**, an enlargement of the occlusal portion of the envelope of jaw positions. Note that point *g* indicates an occlusal position that is not synonymous with the reflex closure path of the mandible (*b*). **D**, a cross section of the envelope of jaw positions. Note that the reflex occlusal position (*b*) is ahead of the most retruded occlusal position (*c*); most cusp-dictated occlusal positions (the so-called centric occlusion) lie a bit ahead of the reflex occlusal position. Eccentric occlusal positions, that is, sliding positions into occlusion dictated by cuspal interferences, are symbolized in this diagram by *g* and *h*. In position *g* there is mediolateral but not anteroposterior balance. In position *h* there is neither.

The ideal occlusal position in the infant seems to coincide with the *unconscious swallowing position of the mandible* and is forward of the most retruded mandibular position. Therefore, during eruption and development, the teeth are guided into occlusion by, and achieve occlusion within limits imposed by, this congenital reflex—a most important clinical point. At this early age, the *intercuspal position* and the *ideal occlusal position* are the same; later in life, they often are made different. It seems that the mandibular position during the unconscious swallow prior to the eruption of the teeth is not as precise as it is after intercuspation has been achieved, perhaps because the muscles alone cannot establish so precise a mandibular position. However, intercuspation of the teeth aids in the integration of the many afferent stimuli reaching the brain, and rather quickly a precise occlusal position demonstrating maximal occlusal contact during the unconscious swallow is achieved.

The anterior limits of the ideal occlusal position are defined first, since the primary incisors erupt first, restricting the mandible's movement in this direction. Later, teeth in the lateral segments, with their cuspal inclined planes, aid in the localization of the mediolateral limits of the ideal occlusal position.

Slight opening of the mandible may cause the firing of afferent impulses from the muscles, whereas anteroposterior or mediolateral shifts of the mandible cause afferent impulses from the muscles, the periodontal ligaments (when the teeth are touching) and the temporomandibular articulation. The mechanoreceptors of the temporomandibular articulation and the periodontal ligaments generally have lower thresholds than the receptors of the ligaments. There also are directional variations in the thresholds of the periodontal mechanoreceptors. Tactile thresholds for axial loading are approximately double those for tangential loading, but discrimination is about the same for the two. Moderate changes in the functioning length of a muscle are tolerated better than the slightest shifting of the mandible while the teeth are in occlusion, which helps to explain the more precise limits of the ideal occlusal position anteroposteriorly and mediolaterally. This may be a partial explanation, too, for the reason that there is more latitude in "opening bites" than there is in changing the occlusal position forward, backward or to the side.

The ideal occlusal position is established during a period of great adaptability of developing bones, erupting teeth and maturing neuromusculature. Since the ideal occlusal position coincides with the position of the mandible in the unconscious swallow, the occlusion is stabilized repeatedly by this primitive reflex operating at the unconscious level. Such an ideal relationship of tooth, bone, muscle and the resultant occlusal homeostasis is the aim of all occlusal therapy. Although these ideal conditions appear naturally as a part of growth in the child, they are more difficult to achieve in the adolescent and the adult. Once they have been lost, they must be regained to achieve continuing occlusal homeostasis. Good therapy is more than acquiring a good static relationship; events must be kept going.

2) RETRUDED CONTACT POSITION.—When the mandible is held by the patient's muscles or manually by the dentist in its most retruded superior position (see Fig. V-10), the mandible can be opened with a hinge movement (see Fig. V-10). The rotational axis for this hinge movement usually is found in or near the condyles, and the position of the mandible has many names in dentistry, for example, centric relation, hinge axis position, retruded occlusal position, ligamentous position, etc. We have chosen for this discussion Posselt's term *retruded contact position*.[46] The clinical significance of this position is discussed in Section D-3, The "Centric" Concept from a Developmental Point of View.

Boucher and Jacoby[8] recorded retruded contact positions under general anesthesia and curare different from those in the same patients under normal conditions. However, Ingervall[27] found no differences in children before and during general anesthesia with and without simultaneous administration of a muscle relaxant.

3) RELATIONSHIPS BETWEEN THE RETRUDED POSITION AND THE USUAL OCCLUSAL POSITION.—Ingervall[27] determined, with cross-sectional data, that 10-year-old girls and adults showed the same mean anteroposterior difference between the retruded contact position and the usual occlusal (intercuspal) position (see Section D-3-b). Eleven-year-old children, however, showed slightly larger mean differences than did adults. Furthermore, the mean difference between the two positions was significantly larger in 5-year-old girls than it was in 10-year-old girls.[27] No one has yet reported serial studies of such jaw relationships, nor have children younger than 5 years of age been studied. Children with both Angle Class II, Division 1 and Angle Class II, Division 2 malocclusions showed significantly larger differences between the two positions than did children with normal occlusion.[27] Almost all children showed some difference between the two positions.

b) Functional Movements

1) SWALLOWING.—Recent studies using intra-oral telemetry have shown that unconscious swallowing occurs forward of the retruded contact position.[19] Perhaps the unconscious swallow in the adult coincides with what was earlier the ideal occlusal position in the young child. Serial studies of the ideal occlusal position and the unconscious swallow are not yet available (see Section C-2-b). Since volitional swallows may be made in any position, care must be taken in the interpretation of research papers on swallowing and mandibular position. All investigators do not differentiate between unconscious, volitional and command swallows, nor do they always mention the amount and substance being swallowed.

2) MASTICATION.—The scientific literature contains many studies

of masticatory movements; however, few are well controlled and documented. Even fewer have included children as subjects. Ahlgren[1] has reported a definitive analysis of the mechanisms of mastication in children. He found that each child has a characteristic chewing pattern, although there are wide variations in chewing movements for the same child. The chewing pattern varies according to the material of the bolus. Tooth contact during mastication occurs in the intercuspal position in almost all children. There usually is a gliding occlusal contact during closing and opening of the masticatory stroke. Ahlgren[1] could establish no relationship between the tooth contact patterns and the occlusion of the teeth, although, in general, children with malocclusions have more complicated chewing patterns. The contraction patterns of the mandibular elevators occur rhythmically in mastication, showing a period of contraction during the closing phase, followed by a period of relaxation during the opening phase of chewing. No significant difference in amplitude pattern of the EMG, coordination patterns or total electrical activity of the muscle could be shown among the various occlusion groups.[1]

3) MANDIBULAR POSTURE.—See Section C-2-a.

4) SPEECH.—Although there are many studies on the relationships of parts during speech, the position of the mandible during various speech functions has not been studied in a manner that would permit comparisons with studies similar to those made by Posselt.[46] However, it is assumed that all speech functions take place inside the border envelope.

2. OCCLUSAL HOMEOSTASIS

In recent years, students of occlusion have abandoned the more mechanistic models of occlusion, preferring now to view the occlusion as the relatively stabilized result of varied and discontinuous dynamic forces operating against the teeth. Occlusal stability, at any moment, is the result of all the summated forces acting against the teeth. Many sophisticated modern studies have measured such forces; still, it is not yet possible to describe precisely in summation all the forces and counterforces that produce occlusal equilibrium.

a) Sensory Aspects

Mechanoreceptors within the periodontal ligament, temporomandibular joint and other parts of the masticatory system provide an exceedingly sensitive feedback mechanism for regulating forces against the teeth. It has been shown that the average person can detect foreign bodies between the teeth as small as 20 microns[56] and that forces as light as 600 milligrams or even smaller can be detected by some individuals.[37]

b) Forces Acting Against the Teeth

Each individual tooth is positioned between sets of contracting muscles; those of the tongue on the one side and those of the lips and cheeks on the other.[47] It has been held, for some time, that as long as the *total* pressure acting against the teeth is balanced throughout time, the position of the tooth is stabilized. It also has been believed that whenever there is a radical change, throughout time, in the muscular environment around the tooth, the tooth will be moved through the bone until balance again is achieved. Weinstein *et al.*[62] supported this contention by enlarging the crowns of posterior teeth on one side only, thus increasing the force of the buccal action against the crown of the tooth, whereupon the tooth nicely was moved lingually until buccolingual balance again was achieved. On the other hand, Lear and Moorrees,[35] using sophisticated sensory monitors throughout an entire 24-hour period, could not find support for the assumption that dental arch form reflected the influences of the surrounding buccolingual musculature. The two studies are not completely incompatible. Arch form itself, as Scott[52] and Burdi and Lillie[9] have shown, is determined early in fetal life, and the form of the basal arch does not change much throughout life; therefore, a stabilizing influence is provided by the bony support for the teeth. Unfortunately, methods have not yet been developed to monitor simultaneously *all* of the forces acting against the teeth. Even in Lear *et al.*'s[34] sophisticated study, they did not measure the occlusal forces or the anterior component of force. The forces of mastication transmitted by the musculature through the inclined planes of the cusps of the teeth and into the roots and surrounding bone probably have a significant role in determining and stabilizing tooth position (see Chapter VI). Most normal forces are within ranges tolerated by the bone or counteracted by other forces against the teeth. Gross upsets in such a stabilizing system occur; for example, tongue-thrusting, digital sucking or orthodontic appliances, bringing movement of teeth and deformation of the alveolar process, until balance again is achieved in a new relationship of parts. As Lear and Moorrees[35] have stated, "The enigma of the relationship between dental arch form and muscle function remains." Its resolution will be difficult because of the many complex variables involved. Furthermore, the relationship between force and bony response, although assumed to be linear in most experiments, is not really known. There are many lovely and inviting theories and models to explain tooth position and dental arch form; however, this fascinatingly complicated matter will not be understood until (1) the level and nature of force thresholds and gradients necessary for bony responses are known, (2) the factors of direction, duration and rate of force application are perceived and (3) systems are available for monitoring *all* of the many forces involved simply, reliably and continually.

c) Occlusal Forces

A number of physiologic forces determine the tooth's position occlusally, including active physiologic eruption, passive eruption, the occlusal force during swallowing, the force of mastication and so forth. The force of mastication shows some variability among individuals and throughout time in the same individual. It also varies according to the substance being chewed and, of course, is altered by fatigue. The occlusal force during swallowing is greatest when swallowing occurs with the teeth together and without a reflex alteration in the original unconscious swallowing position. Occlusal interferences in or near the unconscious swallowing position tend to diminish reflexly the force during the swallow. Since reflex swallowing occurs so frequently, it acts as a dominant mechanism determining the tooth's position. Lear et al.[36] reported that young adults swallowed an average of 585 times each day (range 233–1,008), whereas children swallowed more frequently (range 800–1,200 swallows per day). The reflex mature swallow is one of the most important factors in occlusal homeostasis. The average adult has been found to be able to exert masticatory force of approximately 3–12 kg.,[2] although forces more than three times this high have been recorded in Eskimos.[29] Learning and the nature of the food chewed determine, to some extent, the strength of the forces used during mastication. Continual monitoring of the forces of mastication is carried out by sensory receptors in the periodontal ligament and temporomandibular articulation. Larger forces are tolerated along the axis of the tooth than in other directions, and the slightest bit of hard, unyielding foreign substance, for example, a tiny grain of sand, is detected instantly and the muscle contraction stopped.

d) Drifting of Teeth

In Chapter VI, attention is called to the various factors that determine the tooth's anteroposterior position within the arch. Migration of teeth is a continual process that has been well documented experimentally in animals[33] and in implant studies in humans.[5] Two components must be clearly differentiated: (1) the mesial drifting tendency that may occur beneath the gums before intra-oral emergence and (2) the anterior component of force, which is the mesial result of the functional forces of occlusion (see Section VI-D-2-h). The theory that migration may be due to erupting posterior teeth seems untenable, since migration occurs prior to contact of the crowns of erupting molars and after all teeth are erupted. Other theories hold that migration is due to action of the buccinator muscle and "deposition of bone beneath the gum periosteum."[52]

e) Facial Growth

The differential anteroposterior growth of the mandible and maxilla plays an important role in occlusal homeostasis. The midface achieves adult dimensions earlier in life than does the mandible. Thus, as the mandible continues to grow more forward during the second decade of life, adaptation in angulation and position of teeth must occur if occlusal homeostasis is to be maintained. Mandibular incisors behind the maxillary incisors typically are tipped more lingually during the second decade as the mandible grows forward even though the maxilla has nearly stopped. The result is a normal increase in the amount of mandibular incisal crowding, crowding that may be attributed to nonskeletal factors, for example, eruption of third molars (see Chapter VI). At the same time, occlusal adaptations posteriorly must occur also to accommodate the differential skeletal growth.

3. THE "CENTRIC" CONCEPT FROM A DEVELOPMENTAL POINT OF VIEW

Probably no other term in dental terminology has more interpretations than the word centric. In the noun form, it has a variety of meanings, and the confusion is compounded when the word is used as an adjective. Most of the problems in understanding the term centric are semantic in origin, for we have not always defined well the concepts with which we work. Further, when we read, we often assume that the writer is using the words exactly as we use them. When there is so much variability of concept and insistence on the same terminology for different concepts, confusion is bound to occur.

Both postural and occlusal positions of the mandible may be registered by reference to bony or dental landmarks—any landmarks on the mandible. Such references are of use in recording positions for research or clinical purposes but do not define the terms. Description of a method of recording an occlusal position of the mandible is not a definition, nor is a description of the position of an anatomic part, for example, the condyle, of particular use as a definition. One might say, for example, that Ann Arbor is 40 miles from Detroit, Michigan, which helps to locate it but does not define it; to do so, it might be described as a small, beautiful, thriving university city.

Because the term centric has been used in so many ways by so many workers, it is purposely avoided in the following discussion. Reference is made to Figure V-10 and synonyms for each of the positions are given, many of which include the word centric.

a) *Postural Position of the Mandible (see Section C-2-a)*

A variety of postural positions may be exhibited by the mandible; therefore, a postural range rather than a single postural position for each person is seen.[16] Any postural position is the result of all the physiologic postural determinants operable at the moment the examination is done (Fig. V-11). It has been shown repeatedly in recent years, contrary to previous concepts, that postural positions of the mandible are

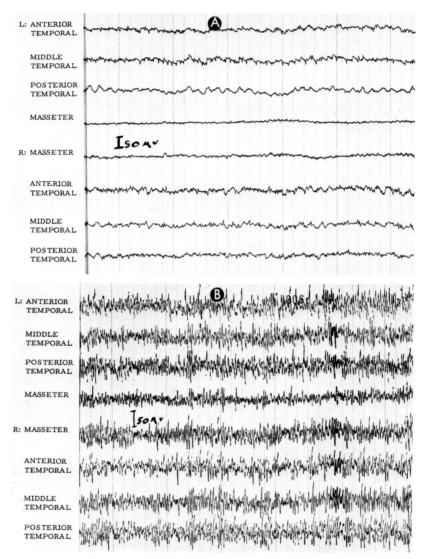

Fig. V-11.—A, electromyograms of the postural position of the mandible. Note the relative quiet and balance of all the muscles supporting the mandible. **B,** electromyograms of the wide-open position of the mandible (*f* in Fig. V-10, B). The increase in muscle activity is indicative of the stretch of the muscles. (*Continued.*)

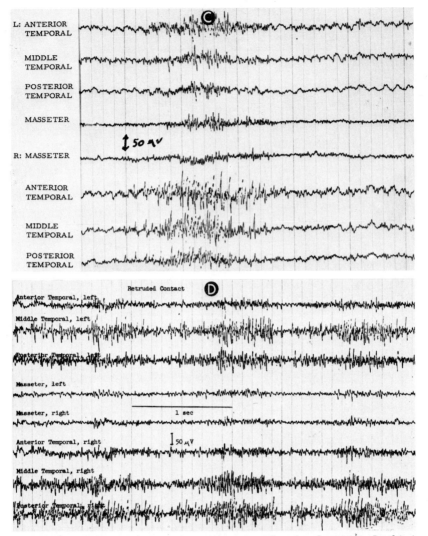

Fig. V-11 (cont.).—C, biting in the patient's usual occlusal position. In this instance, the usual occlusal position is an eccentric position; hence, the imbalances in the different channels of the electromyographic record. At the extreme left is seen the patient's postural position. **D,** the retruded contact position or retruded occlusal position. In this instance, the subject is holding his mandible in the most retruded occlusal position and opening and closing in this jaw relationship. Note the increased activity of the middle and posterior temporal fibers. This activity is necessary, since they are the only muscles that can retrude the mandible. When the dentist places his hand on the patient's chin to establish the retruded occlusal position, this hyperactivity of the posterior fibers is inhibited, since the dentist's arm muscles now hold the mandible in retrusion. (*Continued.*)

Fig. V-11 (cont.).—**E,** the protrusive occlusal position. Note the activity in the anterior temporal fibers and the masseter muscles. Most of the protrusive effort is carried out by the pterygoid muscles, which are not included in this record. **F,** tapping in occlusion after occlusal equilibration. All of the records (Fig. V-11, *A-F*) are of the same subject. Note how different the electromyographic record of the occlusal position is after the occlusal interferences have been removed. Compare *F* with *C.*

more difficult to locate reliably than are occlusal or border positions. Such terms as the physiologic resting position, postural rest position, rest position and so forth are commonly used synonyms. The term postural position is preferred because it is more accurate physiologically and is consistent with general usage in other parts of the body.

b) Usual Occlusal Position (see Section D-1-a)

The position of the mandible as determined by maximal intercuspation of the teeth is termed the "usual occlusal position." Common synonyms are centric occlusion, habitual occlusion, habitual centric, intercuspal position, tooth position, acquired centric, etc. The usual occlusal position is the occlusal position a patient is most likely to use. It quickly may be changed to another usual occlusal position by alterations in the occlusal anatomy of the teeth, drifting of teeth or by pain overriding the determining reflexes (see Fig. V-11).

c) Retruded Contact Position (see Section D-1-a)

The retruded contact position is the most retruded occlusal position of the mandible from which opening and lateral movements can be performed. When the mandible is held in the retruded contact position by the patient's musculature or by the dentist, the incisors trace an arc as the mandible opens on a hinge movement (see Fig. V-10); the axis for this movement usually is within the condylar area. As mentioned before, this position also is called centric relation, hinge axis position, retruded occlusal position and ligamentous position, because the posterior functional range of the mandible is held to be determined by the ligaments. The retruded contact position is an important clinical position, since it is necessary for dentists to record reliably an occlusal position that can be transferred accurately from the patient to the articulator. Furthermore, it is necessary to have an occlusal position of reliability as a starting point to which the patient can return consistently during occlusal equilibration. In adults, the distance between the retruded contact position and the usual occlusal position was found to be 1.25 mm.[46] This distance is greater in normal 10- and 11-year-olds and significantly greater in children with Angle Class II malocclusions.[27]

Sometimes one hears the retruded contact position (centric relation) defined as the most retruded *unstrained* position of the condyle within the temporal fossae from which lateral movements can be made. This definition, although widely used, is a paradox in itself. Since there is only one unstrained position, it is redundant to mention "most retruded." If the most retruded concept is important, it is confusing to mention unstrained, since, despite all definitions to the contrary, the most retruded occlusal position is, of necessity, a position of muscle imbalance. The posterior fibers of the temporal muscle alone can hold the mandible in the retruded contact position, and to do so they must contract in an imbalanced manner, i.e., more than other parts of the temporal muscle (see Fig. V-11). If the dentist is holding the mandible in the retruded contact position, the strain is in the dentist's arm not in the posterior fibers of the patient's temporal muscle. While the temporal muscle is relaxing to permit the dentist to register the retruded contact position, no function can take place. The instant function takes place in the retruded contact position, muscle imbalance must recur.

d) Ideal Occlusal Position

The ideal occlusal position is the attitude of the mandible determined by the unconscious swallowing reflex (see Sections C-2-b and D-1-a). (This definition assumes that there are no occlusal interferences, pain or other sensory input that might cause reflex avoidance of the ideal occlusal position.) This reflex is one of the two most primitive of the reflexes determining mandibular position and was one of the first acquired. Further, it is the only occlusal position showing muscle balance (see Fig. V-11). The aim of all occlusal correction, whether orthodontic, restorative, prosthetic or periodontic, is to cause the patient's usual occlusal position to coincide with the ideal occlusal position. If there is an occlusal interference during the unconscious swallow, the patient may reflexly avoid the interfering cusp, and the desired coincidence of usual and ideal occlusal positions does not occur.

It is almost impossible to register clinically the position of the mandible in an unconscious movement; therefore, it is necessary for the clinician to devise another strategy. Ramfjord and Ash[48] and others have pointed out the usefulness of the retruded contact position in registering occlusal interferences. Since the ideal occlusal position appears most frequently between the retruded contact position and the usual occlusal position, when occlusal interferences are removed by equilibration between the retruded contact position and the usual occlusal position (freedom in centric, long centric, etc.), the dentist is, in reality, accommodating the occlusion to the unconscious swallowing position of the mandible. The practical usefulness of the retruded contact position (centric relation) is due to its proximity to the position taken during the unconscious swallow. The dentist records the retruded position because it is reliable; he equilibrates to remove interferences, thus including within the occlusal pattern the ideal occlusal position even though he cannot register it as surely as he can the retruded position.

4. NEUROMUSCULAR ADAPTATION TO OCCLUSAL DISHARMONY

Impaired masticatory function or occlusal disharmony gives rise to adaptive changes of clinical significance. As each primary tooth is lost, it is followed by a permanent successor different in size and conformation. During the mixed dentition stage, occlusal interferences are many, causing the muscles to learn repeatedly new patterns of mandibular closure in order to avoid interfering teeth.[42] At this time, the muscles often adopt occlusal positions that do not coincide with the ideal occlusal position. Such occlusal positions often are spoken of as "acquired" or "accommodative centrics."

No repeatedly used position of occlusal contact that fails to coincide with the ideal occlusal position is ever acquired by chance. Many are neuromuscular avoidance reflexes, the learning of which was prompted by occlusal interferences. New positions of occlusal contact begin as expedient processes for avoiding tooth interferences and providing better function than the ideal position offers at the moment. The continued presence of the occlusal disharmony, as in the case of a severe malocclusion, may cause the new reflex pathways to be used repeatedly, resulting in an acquired occlusal position so practiced that it resembles the ideal occlusal position. The earlier in life an eccentric occlusion is adopted and held the more difficult it is later to locate the more harmonious ideal occlusal position and to restore normal masticatory function. Here is a most forceful argument for occlusal equilibration of the primary dentition and for early orthodontic treatment of functional malocclusions.

No orthodontic correction will retain well unless the occlusion finally obtained harmonizes with the patient's musculature. Orthodontic correction and occlusal equilibration have a dramatic effect on the reflexes controlling mandibular position (see Figs. XVII-92–XVII-101). Removal of the occlusal interferences causes loss of the stimuli that have forced the muscles to maintain an eccentric occlusion. Once these upsetting stimuli no longer appear, the more basic reflex—the ideal occlusal position reflex—is again dominant. During the presence of tooth interferences, it is biased or suppressed. A fundamental aim of all types of occlusal correction is to substitute the ideal occlusal position for disharmonious eccentric occlusal positions, which are less stable and may contribute to disease or dysfunction.

E. Some Clinical Implications

1. THE EFFECT OF NEUROMUSCULAR BEHAVIOR ON GROWTH OF THE CRANIOFACIAL SKELETON

This subject is discussed in Chapter IV.

2. NEUROMUSCULAR AIMS IN ORTHODONTIC THERAPY

Although the orthodontist's appliances often are directed at attaining better tooth positions within a more balanced craniofacial skeleton, the influences of such therapy on the neuromusculature should not be forgotten. The primary neuromuscular aims in orthodontic therapy are (1) to obliterate all neuromuscular reflexes affecting adversely the dentition or craniofacial skeleton (e.g., thumb-sucking, functional crossbites, mouth-breathing, etc.) and (2) to create an ideal intercuspal relationship so placed within the craniofacial skeleton that it is repeatedly stabilized reflexly by the unconscious swallow. The clinician removes disharmonious influences on tooth position on the assumption that balanced neuromuscular behavior is more advantageous and he utilizes the primitive reflex positions of the mandible to stabilize his therapeutic result.

3. The Effects of Orthodontic Treatment on the Musculature

Ransjo and Thilander[49] found that severe malocclusion provoked pathologic changes in the temporomandibular articulation, which, in turn, impaired the joint receptors, causing orthodontic patients to have a less precise determination of mandibular position than subjects with normal occlusion. After orthodontic treatment, however, there was a *statistically significant reduction* in the range of mandibular position and an improvement in the determination of mandibular position. It is interesting to speculate on the significance of temporomandibular receptors functioning as a conditioned stimulus for avoidance reflexes when there are occlusal interferences. Were more known concerning this possibility, light might be shed on such problems as the role of occlusal interferences in the etiology of malocclusion, relapse after orthodontic therapy, retention and so forth.

Jacob[28] demonstrated that occlusal equilibration on treated orthodontic patients changed a significant number of teeth-apart swallows to teeth-together swallows. Thus, orthodontic treatment, including occlusal equilibration, conditioned swallowing reflexes, which, in turn, helped stabilize the orthodontic treatment. Eggleston and Ekleberry's[14] and Campisciano and Sheba's[10] studies of mandibular positions before, during and after orthodontic therapy, revealed a significant reduction in the occlusal slide from retruded contact position to the usual occlusal position after occlusal equilibration. The "slide into occlusion" was not lost spontaneously during the retention period without equilibration. In a longitudinal study of relapse, Moyers[39] reported occlusal disharmonies to be a most important cause of most relapses in an anteroposterior direction. Furthermore, it was reported that those cases in which the occlusal correction permitted no reflex slides during unconscious swallowing were the most stable 4 years after retention.[39] Other adaptive muscular changes following orthodontic therapy may include altered lip posture, tongue posture, mandibular posture, chewing stroke and method of breathing.

REFERENCES

1. Ahlgren, J.: Mechanism of mastication, Acta odont. scandinav. 24 (supp. 44):1, 1966.
2. Anderson, D. J.: Mastication, in *Handbook of Physiology*, Section 6, Vol. IV (Baltimore: The Williams & Wilkins Company, 1968), pp. 1811–1820.
3. Andrew, R. J.: Evolution of facial expression, Science 142:1034, 1963.

4. Ardran, G. M., Kemp, F. H., and Lind, J.: A cineradiographic study of bottle feeding, Brit. J. Radiol. 31:11, 1958.
5. Björk, A.: Variations in the growth pattern of the growing mandible, J. Dent. Res. 42:400, 1963.
6. Bosma, J. F. (ed.): *Symposium on Oral Sensation and Perception* (Springfield, Ill.: Charles C Thomas, Publisher, 1967).
7. Bosma, J. F., Truby, H. M., and Lind, J.: Cry motions of the newborn infant, Acta paediat. scandinav. Supp. 163:61, 1965.
8. Boucher, L. J., and Jacoby, J.: Posterior border movements of the human mandible, J. Pros. Dent. 11:836, 1961.
9. Burdi, A. R., and Lillie, J. H.: A catenary analysis of the maxillary dental arch during human embryogenesis, Anat. Rec. 154:13, 1966.
10. Campisciano, U. A., and Shiba, S.: A Study of the Effects of Occlusal Equilibration on Orthodontic Retention. Thesis, University of Michigan School of Dentistry, Ann Arbor, 1962, 62 pp.
11. Clemmesen, S.: Some studies on muscle tone, Proc. Roy. Soc. Med. 44:637, 1951.
12. Doty, R. W.: Neural Organization of Deglutition, in *Handbook of Physiology,* Section 6, Vol. IV (Baltimore: The Williams & Wilkins Company, 1968), pp. 1861–1902.
13. Doty, R. W., and Bosma, J. F.: An electromyographic analysis of reflex deglutition, J. Neurophysiol. 19:44, 1956.
14. Eggleston, W. B., Jr., and Ekleberry, J. W.: An Electromyographic and Functional Evaluation of Treated Orthodontic Cases. Thesis, University of Michigan School of Dentistry, Ann Arbor, 1961, 56 pp.
15. Ganong, W. F.: *Review of Medical Physiology* (Los Altos, Calif.: Lange Medical Publications, 1963).
16. Garnick, J. J., and Ramfjord, S. P.: Rest position, J. Pros. Dent. 12:895, 1962.
17. Gesell, A. L., and Amatruda, C.: *Embryology of Behavior; the Beginnings of the Human Mind* (New York: Harper, 1945).
18. Gibson, J. F.: The Mouth as an Organ for Laying Hold on the Environment, in Bosma, J. F. (ed.), *Symposium on Oral Sensation and Perception* (Springfield, Ill.: Charles C Thomas, Publisher, 1967), pp. 111–136.
19. Glickman, I., Pameyer, J. H. N., Roeber, F. W., and Brion, M. A. M.: Functional occlusion as revealed by miniaturized radio transmitters, Dent. Clin. North America 13(3): 667, 1969.
20. Greenfield, B. E., and Wyke, B.: Reflex innervation of the temporomandibular joint, Nature, London 211:940, 1966.
21. Grossman, R. C., and Hattis, B. F.: Oral Mucosal Sensory Innervation and Sensory Experience: A Review, in Bosma, J. F. (ed.), *Symposium on Oral Sensation and Perception* (Springfield, Ill.: Charles C Thomas, Publisher, 1967), pp. 5–62.
22. Gwynne-Evans, E.: Organization of the oro-facial muscles in relation to breathing and feeding, Brit. D. J. 91:135, 1951.
23. Hooker, D.: Fetal Behavior, in *Interrelationship of Mind and Body* (Association for Research in Nervous and Mental Disease) (Baltimore: The Williams & Wilkins Company, 1939), Vol. 19, pp. 237–243.
24. Hooker, D.: *The Origin of Overt Behavior* (Ann Arbor: The University of Michigan Press, 1944).
25. Humphrey, T.: Development of mouth opening and related reflexes involving oral area of human fetuses, Alabama J. M. Sc. 5:126, 1968.
26. Humphrey, T. J.: Some correlations between the appearance of human fetal reflexes and the development of the nervous system, Prog. Brain Res. 4:93, 1964.
27. Ingervall, B.: Studies of mandibular positions in children, Odont. Rev. 19:1 (supp. 15), 1968.
28. Jacob, J. T.: An Electromyographic Study of Orthodontic Retention Patients before and after Occlusal Equilibration. Thesis, University of Michigan School of Dentistry, Ann Arbor, 1960, 41 pp.
29. Jenkins, G. N.: *The Physiology of the Mouth* (Oxford: Blackwell Scientific Publications, 1953).
30. Joseph, J.: *Man's Posture; Electromyographic Studies* (Springfield, Ill.: Charles C Thomas, Publisher, 1960).
31. Joseph, J., Nightingale, A., and Williams, P. L.: Detailed study of electric potentials recorded over some postural muscles while relaxed and standing, J. Physiol. 127:617, 1955.
32. Kawamura, Y., and Majima, T.: Temporomandibular joint's sensory mechanisms controlling activities of the jaw muscles, J. Dent. Res. 43:150, 1964.

33. Latham, R. A., and Scott, J. H.: Mesial movement of the teeth in the Rhesus monkey, Tr. European Orthodont. Soc. 36:199, 1960.
34. Lear, C. S. C., Catz, J., Grossman, R. C., Flanagan, J. B., and Moorrees, C. F. A.: Measurement of lateral muscle forces on the dental arches, Arch. Oral Biol. 10:669, 1965.
35. Lear, C. S. C., and Moorrees, C. F. A.: Buccolingual muscle force and dental arch form, Am. J. Orthodont. 56:379, 1969.
36. Lear, C. S. C., Flanagan, J. B., and Moorrees, C. F. A.: Frequency of deglutition in man, Arch. Oral Biol. 10:83, 1965.
37. Lee, J.: A study of the pressoreceptive thresholds of human teeth. Thesis, University of Michigan School of Dentistry, Ann Arbor, 1965, 40 pp.
38. Miller, H. C., Proud, G. O., and Behile, F. C.: Variations in gag, cough, and swallow reflexes and tone of vocal cords as determined by direct laryngoscopy in newborn infants, Yale J. Biol. & Med. 24:284, 1952.
39. Moyers, R. E.: Clinical procedures to obviate post-treatment relapse. Taped slide sequence No. 211, American Association of Orthodontists, St. Louis, 1970.
40. Moyers, R. E.: An electromyographic analysis of certain muscles involved in temporomandibular movement, Am. J. Orthodont. 36:481, 1950.
41. Moyers, R. E.: The infantile swallow, Tr. European Orthodont. Soc. 40:180, 1964.
42. Moyers, R. E.: Temporomandibular muscle contraction patterns in Angle Class II, Division I malocclusions: An electromyographic analysis, Am. J. Orthodont. 35:837, 1949.
43. Moyers, R. E.: Unpublished data.
44. Murphy, T. R.: Shortening/inhibition of prime movers: A safety factor in mastication, Brit. D. J. 123:578, 1967.
45. Peiper, A.: *Cerebral Function in Infancy and Childhood* (Philadelphia: J. B. Lippincott Company, 1964).
46. Posselt, U.: *Physiology of Occlusion and Rehabilitation* (Philadelphia: F. A. Davis Company, 1962).
47. Proffit, W. R., Kydd, W. L., Wilskie, G. H., and Taylor, D. T.: Intraoral pressures in a young adult group, J. Dent. Res. 43:555, 1964.
48. Ramfjord, S. P., and Ash, M. M., Jr.: *Occlusion* (Philadelphia: W. B. Saunders Company, 1966).
49. Ransjo, K., and Thilander, B.: Perception of mandibular position in cases of temporomandibular joint disorders, Odont. Tskr. 71:134, 1963.
50. Ricketts, R. M.: A study of changes in temporomandibular relations associated with the treatment of Class II malocclusion (Angle), Am. J. Orthodont. 38:918, 1952.
51. Schaerer, P., Stallard, R. E., and Zander, H. A.: Occlusal interferences and mastication: An electromyographic study, J. Pros. Dent. 17:438, 1967.
52. Scott, J. H.: *Dento-facial Development and Growth* (Oxford: Pergamon Press, 1967).
53. Sillman, J. H.: An analysis and discussion of oral changes as related to dental occlusion, Am. J. Orthodont. 39:246, 1953.
54. Storey, A. T.: Extra-trigeminal Sensory Systems Related to Oral Function, in Bosma, J. F. (ed.), *Symposium on Oral Sensation and Perception* (Springfield, Ill.: Charles C Thomas, Publisher, 1967), pp. 84–97.
55. Storey, A. T.: Sensory functions of temporomandibular joint, J. Canad. D. A. 34:294, 1968.
56. Surila, H. S., and Laine, P.: The tactile sensibility of the parodontium to slight axial loadings of the teeth, Acta odont. scandinav. 21:415, 1963.
57. Tallgren, A.: Changes in adult face height due to aging, wear and loss of teeth, and prosthetic treatment, Acta odont. scandinav. 15:1 (Supp. 24), 1957.
58. Tallgren, A.: An electromyographic study of the behavior of certain facial and jaw muscles in long-term complete denture wearers, Odont. Tskr. 71:425, 1963.
59. Thilander, B.: Innervation of the temporomandibular joint capsule in man; an anatomic investigation and a neurophysiologic study of the perception of mandibular position, Tr. Roy. Schools Dent. Stockholm and Umea 7:9, 1961.
60. Thilander, B.: Innervation of the temporomandibular disc in man, Acta odont. scandinav. 22:151, 1964.
61. Tschiassny, K.: Gagging, Ann. Otol., Rhin. & Laryng. 66:1173, 1957.
62. Weinstein, S., Haack, D. C., Morris, L. Y., Snyder, B. B., and Attaway, H. E.: On an equilibrium theory of tooth position. Angle Orthodont. 33:1, 1963.

Suggested Readings

Ahlgren, J.: Mechanism of mastication, Acta odont. scandinav. 24 (supp. 44):1, 1966.
Anderson, D. J.: Periodontal Sensory Mechanisms, in Melcher, A. R., and Bowen, W. H. (eds.), *Biology of the Periodontium* (New York: Academic Press, 1969).

Atwood, D. A.: A critique of research of the rest position of the mandible, J. Pros. Dent. 16:848, 1966.

Bosma, J. F.: Oral and pharyngeal development and function, J. Dent. Res. 42:375, 1963.

Bosma, J. F. (ed.): *Symposium on Oral Sensation and Perception* (Springfield, Ill.: Charles C Thomas, Publisher, 1967).

Bosma, J. F. (ed.): *Second Symposium on Oral Sensation and Perception* (Springfield, Ill.: Charles C Thomas, Publisher, 1970).

Casey, K. L., and Melzack, R.: Neural Mechanisms of Pain: A Conceptual Model, in Way, E. L., *New Concepts in Pain and Its Clinical Management* (Philadelphia: F. A. Davis Company, 1967).

Cleall, J. F.: Deglutition: A study of form and function, Am. J. Orthodont. 51:566, 1965.

Dahlberg, B.: The masticatory effect, Acta med. scandinav., Supp. 139, 1942; also The masticatory habits, J. Dent. Res. 25:67, 1946.

Faigenblum, M. J.: Retching, its causes and management in prosthetic practice, Brit. D. J. 125:485, 1968.

Greenfield, B. E., and Wyke, B.: Reflex innervation of the temporomandibular joint, Nature, London 211:940, 1966.

Ingervall, B.: Studies of mandibular positions in children, Odont. Rev. 19:1 (supp. 15), 1968.

Jacobs, R. M.: Muscle equilibrium: Fact or fancy?, Angle Orthodont. 39:11, 1969.

Kawamura, Y.: Recent concepts of the physiology of mastication, Advances Oral Biol. 1:77, 1963.

Kawamura, Y.: Neurophysiologic background of occlusion, J. Am. Soc. Periodontists 5:175, 1967.

Kawamura, Y.: Mandibular Movement: Normal Anatomy and Physiology and Clinical Dysfunction, in Schwartz, L., and Chayes, C. M. (eds.), *Facial Pain and Mandibular Dysfunction* (Philadelphia: W. B. Saunders Company, 1968), Chap. 6.

Lear, C. S. C., and Moorrees, C. F. A.: Buccolingual muscle force and dental arch form, Am. J. Orthodont. 56:379, 1969.

Møller, E.: The chewing apparatus. An electromyographic study of the action of the muscles of mastication and its correlation to facial morphology, Acta physiol. scandinav., Vol. 69, Supp. 280, 1966.

Moyers, R. E.: The Role of Musculature in Orthodontic Diagnosis and Treatment Planning, in Kraus, B. S., and Reidel, R. A. (eds.), *Vistas in Orthodontics* (Philadelphia: Lea & Febiger, 1962).

Nevakari, K.: An analysis of the mandibular movement from rest to occlusal position. A roentgenographic-cephalometric investigation, Acta odont. scandinav., Vol. 14, Supp. 19, 1956.

Parmeijer, J. H. N., Glickman, I., Roeber, F. W., and Brion, M. A. M.: Functional occlusion as revealed by miniaturized radio transmitters, Dent. Clin. North America, July, 1969, p. 667.

Posselt, U., and Thilander, B.: Influence of innervation of the temporomandibular joint capsule on mandibular border movements, Acta odont. scandinav. 23:601, 1965.

Posselt, U.: *Physiology of Occlusion and Rehabilitation* (2d. ed.; Oxford: Blackwell Scientific Publications, 1968).

Proffit, W. R., Kydd, W. L., Wilskie, G. H., and Taylor, D. T.: Intraoral pressures in a young adult group, J. Dent. Res. 43:555, 1964.

Ramfjord, S. P., and Ash, M. M., Jr.: *Occlusion* (Philadelphia: W. B. Saunders Company, 1966), Chaps. 1–4, pp. 1–96.

Ricketts, R. M.: Respiratory obstruction syndrome, Am. J. Orthodont. 54:495, 1968.

Schaerer, P., Stallard, R. E., and Zander, H. A.: Occlusal interferences and mastication: An electromyographic study, J. Pros. Dent. 17:438, 1967.

Stern, R. H.: Dental occlusion: An evaluation of the canine function theory, J. Southern California D. A. 30:348, 1962.

Storey, A. T.: Physiology of a changing vertical dimension, J. Pros. Dent. 12:912, 1962.

Storey, A. T.: Sensory functions of the temporomandibular joint, J. Canad. D. A. 34:294, 1968.

Subtelny, J. D.: Malocclusions, orthodontic corrections and orofacial muscle adaptation, Angle Orthodont. 40:170, 1970.

Tschiassny, K.: Gagging, Ann. Otol., Rhin. & Laryng. 66:1173, 1957.

VI

Development of the Dentition and the Occlusion

> Adam and Eve had many advantages, but the principal one was that they escaped teething.—MARK TWAIN, *The Tragedy of Pudd'nhead Wilson*, Chapter 4, Pudd'nhead Wilson's Calendar.

A. The mouth of the neonate

B. Development of the primary teeth

　1. Calcification
　2. Eruption
　3. Size and shape of primary teeth
　4. Anomalies
　5. Primary tooth resorption
　6. Ankylosis of primary teeth

C. Development of the primary occlusion

D. Development of the permanent teeth

　1. Calcification
　2. Eruption
　　a) Interrelationships between calcification and eruption
　　b) Factors regulating and affecting eruption
　　c) Timing and variability of eruption
　　d) Sex differences
　　e) Sequence of eruption
　　f) Eruption and bodily growth
　　g) Ectopic development
　　h) Factors determining the tooth's position during eruption

E. The permanent dentition

　1. Size of teeth
　2. Number of teeth
　　a) Missing teeth
　　b) Supernumerary teeth

F. Dimensional changes in the dental arches

1. Width
2. Length
3. Circumference or perimeter
4. Dimensional changes during orthodontic therapy
5. Overbite and overjet

G. The mixed dentition period

1. Uses of the dental arch perimeter
2. Occlusal changes in the mixed dentition
3. First molar eruption
   a) Mandible
   b) Maxilla
4. Incisor eruption
   a) Mandible
   b) Maxilla
5. Cuspid and bicuspid eruption
   a) Mandible
   b) Maxilla
6. Second molar eruption

H. Dentitional and occlusal development in the young adult

1. Third molar development
2. Dimensional changes
3. Occlusal changes
4. Resorption of permanent teeth
5. Arrangement of the teeth in the jaws

I. Clinical implications

1. Normal versus ideal occlusion
2. Models of occlusion
3. Occlusal adaptive mechanisms

A. The Mouth of the Neonate

AT BIRTH, the alveolar processes are covered by gum pads, which soon are segmented to indicate the sites of the developing teeth (Fig. VI-1).[13, 79] The gums are firm, as in an edentulous mouth. The maxillary arch is horseshoe shaped and the gum pads tend to extend buccally and labially beyond those in the mandible; furthermore, the mandibular arch is posterior to the maxillary arch when the gum pads contact.[70] In the anterior region, the gum pads usually are separated, whereas in the back they touch, although in no way has a "bite" or jaw relationship yet been established.[76] The basic form of the arches is determined by at least the fourth month of intrauterine life by the developing tooth germs and the growing basal bone, the tongue adapting to the space provided for it.[72] When teeth are erupted and muscles are functioning, the arch formed by the crowns of the teeth often is altered by muscular activities,

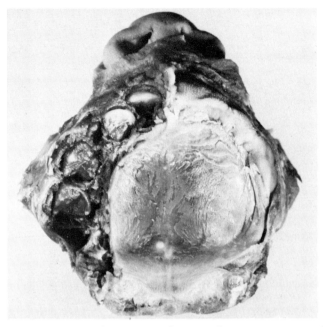

Fig. VI-1.—Neonatal maxillary gum pads. Note the segmentations of the gum pads and how they correspond to the developing primary teeth. (Courtesy of Dr. James McNamara.)

although the original arch form is not determined by the muscles. As the primary teeth are formed, the alveolar processes develop vertically and the anterior intermaxillary space is lost in most children. At this time, too, the infantile swallow is given up for the mature swallowing pattern (see Chapter V).

Occasionally, a child will be born with an incisor or two already present in the mouth, thus causing discomfort to the mother during breast feeding. Neonatal teeth should not be removed unless they are certainly supernumeraries.

B. Development of the Primary Teeth

1. CALCIFICATION

The sequence of initial calcification of the primary teeth is central incisors (14 weeks), first molars (15½ weeks), lateral incisors (16 weeks), canines (17 weeks) and second molars (18 weeks); however, since the primary teeth develop at different rates, this sequence is not maintained in other subsequent developmental characteristics.[49] The crowns of the teeth continue to grow in width until there is coalescence of the calcifying cusp, at which time most of the crown diameter of the tooth

TABLE VI-1.—Usual Sequence of Eruption of Primary Teeth*

$$\frac{\quad}{A}, \quad \frac{A,}{\quad} \quad \frac{B,}{\quad} \quad \frac{\quad}{B} \quad \frac{D,}{D} \quad \frac{C,}{C} \quad \frac{\quad}{E} \quad \frac{E}{\quad}$$

*After Meredith.[58]

has been determined. There are few genetic studies of calcification of primary teeth, but there is evidence that genetic control is exercised in some manner over crown morphology, the rate and sequence of growth, pattern of calcification and mineral content. Prenatal dental development is characterized by at least as much sexual dimorphism, developmental variability, bilateral asymmetry and sequence variability as has been reported in the postnatal development of the deciduous and permanent dentitions. The male is systematically ahead of the female for all teeth.[31] As in permanent tooth eruption, there is a tidy and systematic decreasing gradient of mandibular precedence. For the central incisors, the mandibular tooth is advanced over its maxillary opponent in more than 90% of cases. This drops to 80% for the lateral incisor, 68% for the cuspid, 62% for the first primary molar and 43% for the second primary molar.[31] Needless to say, sex differences and sequence differences in prenatal dental variability help to explain sex differences in congenital dental defects as well as the greater dimensional and morphologic variability of the more distal tooth in each class.

2. Eruption

Eruption, that is, movement of the tooth toward the occlusal plane, begins in a variable fashion but not until root formation has begun. The usual sequence of appearance in the mouth is shown in Table VI-1. The precise time of arrival of each tooth in the mouth is not too important unless it deviates greatly from the averages (Table VI-2). There are no significant sexual differences in primary tooth emergence.

Hatton,[42] in a study of primary tooth eruption in twins, has shown no left-to-right differences in eruption or differences in eruption between monozygous pairs. She estimates the effect of heredity on eruption of primary teeth at 78% and the effect of environment at 22%.

TABLE VI-2.—Eruption of Primary Teeth*

6 mo.—One-third have 1 or more teeth
9 mo.—Mean: 3 teeth; 80% have between 1 and 6 teeth
12 mo.—Mean: 6 teeth; 50% have between 4 and 8 teeth
18 mo.—Mean: 12 teeth; 85% have between 9 and 16 teeth
24 mo.—Mean: 16 teeth; 60% have between 15 and 18 teeth
30 mo.—Mean: 19 teeth; 70% have all primary teeth

*From Hatton.[42]

The primary dentition develops quite independently of other morphologic processes; for example, there is little relationship between primary tooth development and skeletal maturation.[17] Variations in eruption times and sequence have been reported for different populations, and there likely are racial and socioeconomic differences, but variations in research methods are obscure and definitive studies are not yet available.

3. SIZE AND SHAPE OF PRIMARY TEETH

Good data on the size of primary teeth are available (Table VI-3). Each male tooth is larger, especially the cuspids. Primary tooth size and its mineral mass are largely inherited.

4. ANOMALIES

Anomalies of crown development are seen less frequently in the primary than in the permanent dentition and it is rarer for primary teeth to be congenitally missing.

5. PRIMARY TOOTH RESORPTION

It is common to suppose that the eruption of the permanent tooth is the sole factor causing primary tooth resorption; this may not be the case, since the primary tooth, at least in dogs, resorbs even in the absence of the permanent successor.[67] The basic pattern of primary tooth resorption is hastened by inflammation and occlusal trauma; it is delayed by splinting (as when a space-maintainer is attached to the crown) and the absence of a permanent successor.[67]

TABLE VI-3A.—CROWN SIZES OF PRIMARY TEETH OF BOYS*

MAXILLARY DENTITION

Tooth	No.	Mean (mm.)	Standard Deviation	5%	15%	Percentiles (mm.) 50%	85%	95%
A	154	6.42	0.44	5.70	5.97	6.43	6.93	7.11
B	158	5.28	0.41	4.63	4.82	5.32	5.74	5.93
C	170	6.81	0.41	6.16	6.41	6.83	7.24	7.41
D	169	6.78	0.55	5.90	6.24	6.75	7.38	7.72
E	173	8.80	0.57	7.94	8.21	8.82	9.41	9.65
			MANDIBULAR DENTITION					
A	142	4.04	0.32	3.53	3.71	4.00	4.40	4.57
B	161	4.64	0.46	3.94	4.18	4.63	5.11	5.34
C	165	5.81	0.41	5.14	5.43	5.84	6.24	6.46
D	164	7.88	0.50	7.12	7.45	7.92	8.32	8.66
E	170	9.79	0.56	8.92	9.22	9.82	10.36	10.70

*Data from a study of Michigan children. Courtesy of Center for Human Growth and Development, The University of Michigan.

6. ANKYLOSIS OF PRIMARY TEETH

Primary teeth, particularly molars, may become ankylosed (fused) to the alveolar process and their eruption prevented. Although permanent teeth can become ankylosed too, primary teeth are more likely to be involved and lower teeth twice as often as upper.[5] There is little evidence that ankylosis is a random phenomenon nor is it due to trauma or excessive pressure, although this often is said to be the cause.[5] The etiologic picture is not yet clear, but the majority of ankylosed primary teeth are observed in the late primary and the mixed dentition. The condition often is bilateral and a posterior open bite appears as the occlusal level of the ankylosed teeth fails to keep up with the vertical development of adjacent teeth. Ankylosed teeth often are referred to as "submerged teeth"—an unfortunate misnomer, since they do not submerge. Treatment of this condition is described in Chapter XV.

C. Development of the Primary Occlusion

The neuromuscular regulation of jaw relationship is important to the development of primary occlusion (see Chapter V). Interdentation occurs sequentially, beginning in the front as the incisors erupt. As other new teeth appear, the muscles learn to effect the necessary functional occlusal movements. There is less variability in occlusal relationships in the primary than in the permanent dentition, since the primary occlusion is being established during more labile periods of developmental adaptation and the teeth are guided into their occlusal position by the functional matrix of muscles during very active growth of the facial skeleton.

TABLE VI-3*B*.—CROWN SIZES OF PRIMARY TEETH OF GIRLS*

MAXILLARY DENTITION

Tooth	No.	Mean (mm.)	Standard Deviation	5%	15%	Percentiles (mm.) 50%	85%	95%
A	147	6.51	0.42	5.81	6.09	6.53	6.90	7.11
B	147	5.33	0.41	4.69	4.92	5.34	5.72	6.04
C	159	6.64	0.37	5.93	6.31	6.62	7.04	7.25
D	157	6.67	0.49	5.78	6.22	6.70	7.18	7.45
E	165	8.68	0.53	7.83	8.13	8.65	9.24	9.54

MANDIBULAR DENTITION

Tooth	No.	Mean (mm.)	Standard Deviation	5%	15%	Percentiles (mm.) 50%	85%	95%
A	131	4.08	0.31	3.54	3.72	4.09	4.40	4.60
B	149	4.71	0.40	4.08	4.25	4.74	5.15	5.38
C	157	5.72	0.43	5.27	5.41	5.75	6.03	6.33
D	158	7.79	0.49	7.08	7.38	7.79	8.27	8.45
E	166	9.65	0.61	8.84	9.21	9.65	10.21	10.48

*Data from a study of Michigan children. Courtesy of Center for Human Growth and Development, The University of Michigan.

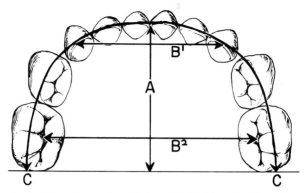

Fig. VI-2.—Arch dimensions. *A*, arch length. *B*¹, bicanine diameter. *B*², bimolar diameter. *C–C*, arch perimeter or arch circumference.

Fig. VI-3.—A, the two primary second molars in occlusion. Note that although there is a Class I molar relationship of the mesial surfaces (left), there is a flush terminal plane on the distal. **B,** primary and permanent tooth size relationships in the lateral segment of the dental arch. The average leeway space in the madibular arch is greater than in the maxillary arch. This large difference in leeway space between the two arches is a factor that permits the late mesial shift of the mandibular first permanent molar in some instances. Note that the figures shown are mean values. When development of a tooth size–arch space problem is expected during the mixed dentition, it is important to compute actual tooth size–space relationships for that particular mouth. Mean values are of interest but they will not provide the diagnosis for an individual case.

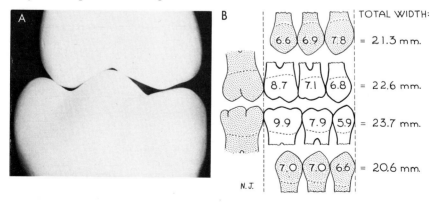

Most primary arches are ovoid and display less variability in conformation than do the permanent (see Fig. VI-36). Usually, there is generalized interdental spacing in the anterior region, which, contrary to popular opinion, does not increase significantly after the primary dentition is completed.[3] In fact, it has been found that the total interdental spacing between the primary teeth decreases continually with age.[2] Although the spacing is most likely to be generalized, there is no pattern of spacing common to all primary dentitions. Somewhat wider spaces found mesial to the maxillary cuspids and distal to the mandibular cuspids are termed primate spaces, since they are particularly prominent in the dentitions of certain lower primates.

At birth, the primary arches are almost wide enough to hold the primary incisors.* Little information is available concerning arch growth during the first few months of life. Apparently, what mandibular arch width increase takes place occurs largely before 9 months of age.[70]

The primary posterior teeth occlude, so that a mandibular cusp articulates just ahead of its corresponding maxillary cusp. The mesiolingual cusp of the maxillary molars occludes in the central fossae of the mandibular molars and the incisors are vertical, with minimal overbite and overjet (see Fig. VI-36). The mandibular second primary molar usually is somewhat wider mesiodistally than the maxillary, giving rise, typically, to a flush terminal plane at the end of the primary dentition (Fig. VI-3)—a point of considerable clinical significance. Interproximal cavities, sucking habits or a disharmonious skeletal pattern may produce a "step" rather than a flush terminal plane. In instances of mandibular hypertrophy, a mesial step develops. When the terminal plane is straight until the arrival of the first permanent molars, the latter are guided into an initial end-to-end relationship (Fig. VI-4) considered "normal" in North America. Among people whose diet includes coarse, rough food, for example, Eskimos, North American Indians and Greek mountaineers,[45] the occlusal surfaces of the primary teeth wear to a great extent. This removal of cuspal interferences permits the mandible, which is growing more at this time than the maxilla, to assume a forward position more easily.[45] Under these circumstances, the result for Greek mountain children at age 5 or 6 often is more an edge-to-edge incisal relationship and a distinct mesial step terminally.[45] When such conditions obtain, the permanent incisors erupt with less overbite and the first permanent molars erupt at once into a firm neutroclusion.

In contrast, children without natural occlusal wear presumably adapt a temporary functional retraction of the mandible during closure, since the relatively greater anteroposterior growth of the mandible produces natural occlusal interferences, usually in the cuspid region. No one has yet studied what effects prolonged functional retraction has on mandibular growth. On the other hand, there is some evidence (and a

---

*The standard measurements of arch dimensions are shown in Figure VI-2.

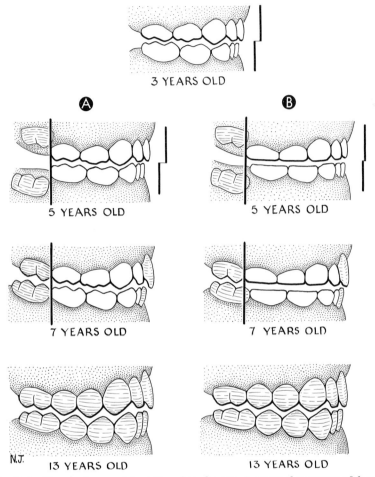

Fig. VI-4.—Two patterns of dentitional exchange. **A,** normal patterns of development during the transitional dentition as described by Broadbent. **B,** more favorable patterns sometimes seen in people living on a diet coarser than that usual to North Americans. We may consider the pattern of transition in **A** to be normal but that in **B** to be more nearly ideal.

whole system of therapy) based on the benefits of functional protraction during growth (see Chapters IV, V, XV and XVII).

D. Development of the Permanent Teeth

1. CALCIFICATION

Although the calcification of the teeth has been studied in many ways, serial radiographic methods are the most practical, since the clinician evaluates his patients' dental development from similar data. Nolla[66] arbitrarily divided the development of each tooth into 10 stages (Fig. VI-5). The mean stages of calcification reached by each tooth for ages 3–17 years are shown in Tables VI-4A and B.[66] The percentages of root lengths and percentages of eruptions achieved at each age are shown in Tables VI-4C to VI-4F. It should be noted that this is an ordinal scale; therefore, it cannot be assumed that the quantitative amounts of tooth material laid down during one stage are the same as during another. Important stages to remember are Stage 2—initial calcification, Stage 6—the time most teeth begin eruptive movements and Stage 8—the stage at which most teeth pierce the alveolar crest. Intra-oral emergence occurs later. Mean times of intra-oral emergence are shown in Figure VI-6.

Girls are more advanced in calcification of permanent teeth than are boys at each stage and more so in the later stages. Sex differences for tooth calcification are less than for bone development. Since girls are well ahead of boys by 10 years of age, the differences cannot be the result of the timing of the secretion of sex hormone.[27]

The variability in calcification of the permanent teeth is much greater than usually is assumed, probably because the most popular "standards" of tooth development distributed to the dental profession were derived from very small samples indeed. In truth, the variability of tooth development is similar to that for eruption, sexual maturity and other similar growth indicators.[28]

There are widely reported racial and ethnic differences in calcification that must be differentiated clearly from socioeconomic and nutritional differences. It is important, therefore, to choose appropriate standards for use in clinical practice.

Tooth calcification correlates positively in a rough way with height, weight, body fat and ossification of the wrist bones, but such correlations rarely are significant; therefore, their clinical usefulness is as yet limited.[54]

2. ERUPTION

a) Interrelationships Between Calcification and Eruption

Eruption is the developmental process that moves a tooth from its crypt position through the alveolar process into the oral cavity and to

TABLE VI-4A.—Norms for Maturation of Permanent Teeth for Boys (Nolla[66])

(Mean stage of calcification for each tooth is shown in terms of the 10 stages of calcification)

Maxillary Teeth (Growth Stage)

Age, Yr.	1|1	2|2	3|3	4|4	5|5	6|6	7|7	8|8
3	4.3	3.4	3.0	2.0	1.0	4.2	1.0	—
4	5.4	4.5	3.9	3.0	2.0	5.3	2.0	—
5	6.4	5.5	4.8	4.0	3.0	6.4	3.0	—
6	7.3	6.4	5.6	4.9	4.0	7.4	4.0	—
7	8.2	7.2	6.3	5.7	4.9	8.2	5.0	—
8	8.8	8.0	7.0	6.5	5.8	8.9	5.8	1.0
9	9.4	8.7	7.7	7.2	6.6	9.4	6.5	1.8
10	9.7	9.3	8.4	7.9	7.3	9.7	7.2	2.3
11	9.95	9.7	8.8	8.6	8.0	9.8	7.8	3.0
12	—	9.95	9.2	9.2	8.7	—	8.3	4.0
13	—	—	9.6	9.6	9.3	—	8.8	4.9
14	—	—	9.8	9.8	9.6	—	9.3	5.9
15	—	—	9.9	9.9	9.9	—	9.6	6.6
16½	—	—	—	—	—	—	10.0	7.7
17	—	—	—	—	—	—	—	8.0

Mandibular Teeth (Growth Stage)

Age, Yr.	1|1	2|2	3|3	4|4	5|5	6|6	7|7	8|8
3	5.2	4.5	3.2	2.6	1.1	5.0	0.7	—
4	6.5	5.7	4.2	3.5	2.2	6.2	2.0	—
5	7.5	6.8	5.1	4.4	3.3	7.0	3.0	—
6	8.2	7.7	5.9	5.2	4.3	7.7	4.0	—
7	8.8	8.5	6.7	6.0	5.3	8.4	5.0	0.8
8	9.3	9.1	7.4	6.8	6.2	9.0	5.9	1.4
9	9.7	9.5	8.0	7.5	7.0	9.5	6.7	1.8
10	10.0	9.8	8.6	8.2	7.7	9.8	7.4	2.0
11	—	—	9.1	8.8	8.3	9.9	7.9	2.7
12	—	—	9.6	9.4	8.9	—	8.4	3.5
13	—	—	9.8	9.7	9.4	—	8.9	4.5
14	—	—	—	10.0	9.7	—	9.3	5.3
15	—	—	—	—	10.0	—	9.7	6.2
16½	—	—	—	—	—	—	10.0	7.3
17	—	—	—	—	—	—	—	7.6

Note: See Figure XI-8 for another way of presenting similar data for clinical use.

TABLE VI-4B.—NORMS FOR MATURATION OF PERMANENT TEETH FOR GIRLS (NOLLA[66])

(Mean stage of calcification for each tooth is shown in terms of the 10 stages of calcification)

MANDIBULAR TEETH (GROWTH STAGE)

AGE, YR.	1|1	2|2	3|3	4|4	5|5	6|6	7|7	8|8
3	5.3	4.7	3.4	2.9	1.7	5.0	1.6	—
4	6.6	6.0	4.4	3.9	2.8	6.2	2.8	—
5	7.6	7.2	5.4	4.9	3.8	7.3	3.9	—
6	8.5	8.1	6.3	5.8	4.8	8.1	5.0	—
7	9.3	8.9	7.2	6.7	5.7	8.7	5.9	1.8
8	9.8	9.5	8.0	7.5	6.6	9.3	6.7	2.1
9	10.0	9.9	8.7	8.3	7.4	9.7	7.4	2.3
10	—	10.0	9.2	8.9	8.1	10.0	8.1	3.2
11	—	—	9.7	9.4	8.6	—	8.6	3.7
12	—	—	10.0	9.7	9.1	—	9.1	4.7
13	—	—	—	10.0	9.4	—	9.5	5.8
14	—	—	—	—	9.7	—	9.7	6.5
15	—	—	—	—	10.0	—	9.8	6.9
16	—	—	—	—	—	—	10.0	7.5
17	—	—	—	—	—	—	—	8.0

MAXILLARY TEETH (GROWTH STAGE)

AGE, YR.	1|1	2|2	3|3	4|4	5|5	6|6	7|7	8|8
3	4.3	3.7	3.3	2.6	2.0	4.5	1.8	—
4	5.4	4.8	4.3	3.6	3.0	5.7	2.8	—
5	6.5	5.8	5.3	4.6	4.0	6.9	3.8	—
6	7.4	6.7	6.2	5.6	4.9	7.9	4.7	—
7	8.3	7.6	7.0	6.5	5.8	8.7	5.6	—
8	9.0	8.4	7.8	7.3	6.6	9.3	6.5	2.1
9	9.6	9.1	8.5	8.1	7.4	9.7	7.2	2.4
10	10.0	9.6	9.1	8.7	8.1	10.0	7.9	3.2
11	—	10.0	9.5	9.3	8.7	—	8.5	4.3
12	—	—	9.8	9.7	9.3	—	9.0	5.4
13	—	—	10.0	10.0	9.7	—	9.5	6.2
14	—	—	—	—	10.0	—	9.7	6.8
15	—	—	—	—	—	—	9.8	7.3
16	—	—	—	—	—	—	10.0	8.0
17	—	—	—	—	—	—	—	8 7

NOTE: See Figure XI-8 for another way of presenting similar data for clinical use.

TABLE VI-4C.—Percentages of Ultimate Root Length by Ages in Boys

AGE	CANINE		FIRST PREMOLAR		SECOND PREMOLAR		FIRST MOLAR		SECOND MOLAR	
	Mean	Standard Deviation	Mean	Standard Deviation	Mean	Standard Deviation	Mean	Standard Deviation	Mean	Standard Deviation
5 yrs	3.75	5.16					26.37	8.78		
6 yrs	9.38	5.36					53.25	17.78		
7 yrs	19.10	7.97	1.58	7.31			68.45	16.86		
8 yrs	32.41	11.39	12.89	9.60	4.92	9.81	78.00	10.84	7.34	10.03
9 yrs	44.91	15.03	27.91	15.61	17.61	16.86	86.99	7.60	17.35	13.82
10 yrs	60.90	15.06	44.17	18.77	30.34	16.86	90.85	6.87	34.08	17.51
11 yrs	76.56	12.44	59.96	20.13	47.61	24.12	92.34	5.76	54.09	20.94
12 yrs	87.32	9.01	78.62	16.07	63.92	23.20	94.63	3.79	68.13	20.23
13 yrs	95.59	4.82	91.52	8.59	83.16	18.84	96.71	2.74	88.49	14.15
14 yrs	96.81	5.59	97.31	5.14	93.38	10.12	96.74	3.19	95.51	6.95
15 yrs	97.13	3.02	96.07	7.94	97.71	4.19	98.21	2.41	97.65	2.74
16 yrs	98.99	2.01	99.73	.54	100.00	0.00	95.67	6.99	99.19	1.61

Note: The data in Tables VI-4C to VI-4F are from the same patients. Courtesy, Center for Human Growth and Development, The University of Michigan.
N = 28.

TABLE VI-4D.—PERCENTAGES OF ULTIMATE ROOT LENGTH BY AGES IN GIRLS*

AGE	CANINE		FIRST PREMOLAR		SECOND PREMOLAR		FIRST MOLAR		SECOND MOLAR	
	Mean	Standard Deviation	Mean	Standard Deviation	Mean	Standard Deviation	Mean	Standard Deviation	Mean	Standard Deviation
5 yrs	8.15	5.44					35.86	14.79		
6 yrs	16.64	13.30					49.30	16.54		
7 yrs	27.78	12.43	8.27	7.83	1.92	10.30	69.73	9.60	4.58	9.84
8 yrs	43.95	13.83	22.19	11.13	13.56	14.32	78.73	9.71	15.28	12.41
9 yrs	62.50	13.36	37.61	15.65	25.76	18.22	87.11	7.95	31.36	19.99
10 yrs	76.44	15.21	58.71	19.92	41.04	20.94	92.54	6.07	43.18	22.19
11 yrs	89.36	10.24	74.41	17.99	63.32	25.75	95.48	4.08	65.18	22.38
12 yrs	94.55	7.31	87.40	14.34	81.63	21.90	98.32	2.33	85.09	22.46
13 yrs	98.13	4.34	96.63	7.01	92.86	14.98	97.98	2.33	91.29	14.23
14 yrs	97.26	1.91	95.41	6.71	92.19	13.02	98.86	1.22	95.45	5.18
15 yrs	99.60	.72	99.76	.36	98.06	2.74	98.00	2.86	96.69	8.10

*Courtesy of Center for Human Growth and Development, The University of Michigan.
N = 26.

TABLE VI-4*E.*—Percentages of Eruption
Achieved at Each Age by Boys*

Age	Canine	First Premolar	Second Premolar	First Molar	Second Molar
5 yrs	0.00	0.00	0.00	0.00	0.00
6 yrs	.28	0.00	0.00	18.98	0.00
7 yrs	5.21	4.72	4.42	39.70	5.83
8 yrs	12.21	12.23	7.06	52.30	8.62
9 yrs	24.04	20.62	14.07	56.70	14.79
10 yrs	38.21	33.11	21.97	60.30	22.86
11 yrs	61.13	49.93	38.23	65.01	39.01
12 yrs	75.15	64.74	48.64	68.92	51.83
13 yrs	79.85	76.32	68.16	72.08	67.71
14 yrs	88.80	88.51	87.00	84.74	85.96
15 yrs	90.94	92.18	94.02	89.89	91.52
16 yrs	94.58	95.15	95.76	97.58	98.58
17 yrs	100.00	100.00	100.00	100.00	100.00

*Courtesy of Center for Human Growth and Development,
The University of Michigan.
N = 28.

TABLE VI-4*F.*—Percentages of Eruption
Achieved at Each Age by Girls*

Age	Canine	First Premolar	Second Premolar	First Molar	Second Molar
5 yrs	0.00	0.00	0.00	10.08	0.00
6 yrs	5.12	4.66	1.57	38.98	3.78
7 yrs	10.48	7.89	3.46	64.65	8.84
8 yrs	23.79	18.49	10.11	74.80	14.73
9 yrs	45.17	32.10	18.49	78.03	21.82
10 yrs	63.43	51.96	32.54	82.91	33.98
11 yrs	80.38	69.97	53.73	85.83	56.91
12 yrs	90.50	82.84	65.95	86.69	73.85
13 yrs	96.68	97.51	86.38	95.04	91.62
14 yrs	98.73	97.46	92.43	94.96	89.32
15 yrs	100.00	100.00	100.00	100.00	100.00

*Courtesy of Center for Human Growth and Development,
The University of Michigan.
N = 26.

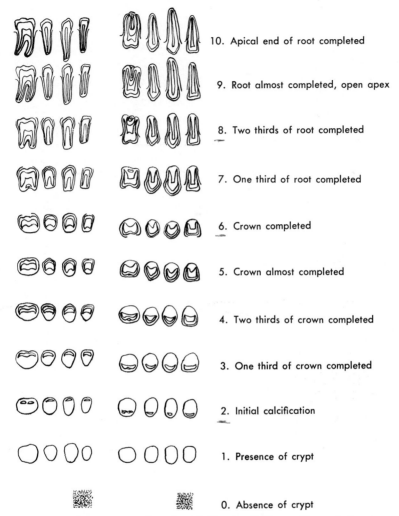

10. Apical end of root completed

9. Root almost completed, open apex

8. Two thirds of root completed

7. One third of root completed

6. Crown completed

5. Crown almost completed

4. Two thirds of crown completed

3. One third of crown completed

2. Initial calcification

1. Presence of crypt

0. Absence of crypt

Fig. VI-5.—Nolla's stages of tooth calcification.[66] The radiograph is compared to the drawings and each tooth is given a developmental score according to the drawing that it most nearly approximates. If the development of the tooth should lie between two stages, half values or plus scores may be used.

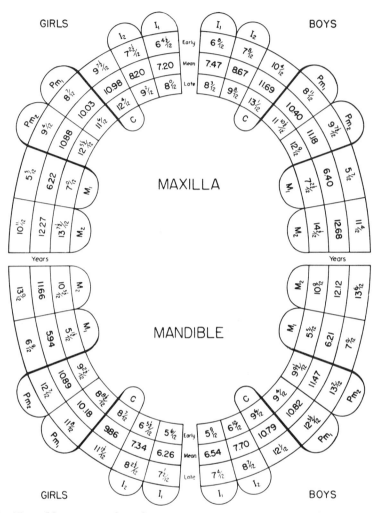

Fig. VI-6.—Mean ages of tooth emergence with plus and minus limits of one standard deviation. (After Hurme.[43])

occlusion with its antagonist. During eruption of succedaneous teeth, many activities occur simultaneously: the primary tooth resorbs, the permanent tooth's root lengthens, the alveolar process increases in height and the permanent tooth moves through the bone (Fig. VI-7). Although all these processes are interrelated, they are more independent than once thought. Shumaker and El Hadary[75] correlated eruption with tooth development and discovered that although mandibular teeth usually do not begin to move occlusally until after Nolla's Stage 6 (crown formation complete), the rate of their eruption does not correlate well

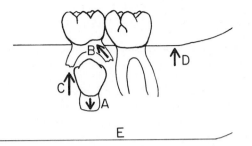

Fig. VI-7.—Developmental processes during eruption. *A*, elongation of the permanent root. *B*, resorption of the primary predecessor. *C*, movement of the permanent tooth occlusally. *D*, growth of the alveolar process. *E*, the inferior border of the mandible, which shows much less growth activity than the other four processes.

with root elongation (Fig. VI-8). From their data may be derived a procedure for predicting emergence of a tooth in the mouth (see Chapter XI-C-3). Bodegam,[8] in an excellent study of eruption in dwarf pigs, noted that no teeth begin to erupt until root formation has begun (see Tables VI-4*C*–VI-4*F*).

Permanent teeth do not begin eruptive movements until after the crown is completed.[64] They pass through the crest of the alveolar process

Fig. VI-8.—A computer plot showing the relationship between root lengthening and eruptive movement of a tooth. In this instance, root lengthening is total tooth length and eruption is *C* (Fig. VI-7). Note that the onset of rapid eruptive movement coincides rather precisely with the completion of crown calcification, about 6 mm., and the beginning of root development.[64]

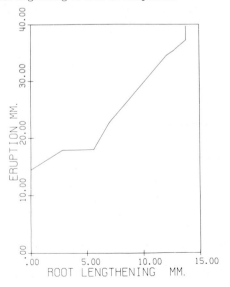

when approximately two-thirds of the root is formed (Stage 8) and pierce the gingival margin when roughly three-fourths of the root is completed (Stage 9) (see Tables VI-4A—VI-4F). It takes from 2 to 5 years for the posterior teeth to reach the alveolar crest following completion of their crowns and from 12 to 20 months to reach occlusion after reaching the alveolar margin.[75] The roots usually are completed a few months after occlusion is attained. The moment of emergence into the oral cavity often is spoken of as the time of eruption. Intra-oral eruption achieves in a few months the first half of the crown's exposure, but its emergence occurs at a progressively slower rate thereafter.[32] Various theories of eruption have been proposed, studied and debated for some time. This is no place to continue such interesting arguments without new data, but some of the research on eruption has clinical significance. Eruptive movements do not correlate well with the amount of root lengthening,[75] and rats' teeth have been shown to erupt when the roots have been destroyed experimentally.[33] Further, it has been suggested that the teeth erupt, allowing the roots to grow, and, therefore, root elongation might better be thought of as a result of eruption rather than one of its causes.[38]

b) Factors Regulating and Affecting Eruption

It is unfortunate and remarkable how little we know in detail concerning some of the factors affecting eruption. Both the sequence and timing of eruption seem to be largely gene determined.[21] Further, there are sequences and timings of eruption that are typical for certain racial groups; for example, Europeans and Americans of European origin tend to erupt their teeth later than American Negroes and Amerinds.[21] What is not known is how genes mediate the basic processes of calcification and eruption.

The nutritional influences on calcification and eruption are relatively much less significant than the genetic, for it is only at the extremes of nutritive variation that the effects on tooth eruption have been shown.[29] This should not be surprising, for it is well known that both calcification and eruption are less responsive to endocrine disturbances than is skeletal development.[29]

Mechanical disturbances can alter the genetic plan of eruption, as can localized pathosis. Periapical lesions as well as pulpotomy of a primary molar[53] will hasten the eruption of the successor premolar (see Fig. VI-13). If the primary tooth is extracted after the permanent successor has begun active eruptive movements (Nolla's Stage 6 or later), the permanent tooth will erupt earlier. If the primary tooth is extracted prior to the onset of permanent eruptive movements (prior to Nolla's Stage 6), the permanent tooth is very likely to be delayed in its eruption, since the alveolar process may re-form atop the successor tooth, making eruption more difficult and slower. The possible effects of extraction of the primary tooth on the eruption of its successor cannot be correlated well with the age of the subject (although invariably this is done in research papers) but can be related to the stage of development of the permanent tooth. It also has been shown that crowding of the permanent teeth affects to a small degree their rate of calcification and eruption.[9]

c) *Timing and Variability of Eruption*

The constant referral to tables showing mean times of eruption often obscures, in my opinion, the wide variability seen in time of intra-oral emergence. For example, the data shown in Figure VI-9 were used by Garn and Rohmann[29] and are from the same study by Hurme as the means and standard deviations shown in Figure VI-6. Note that in 10% of the children the "6-year molar" will erupt either earlier than 4.4 years or later than 7.5 years and 5% of the time the "12-year molar" may appear as late as 14.3 years. Eruption timing tends to appear earlier in American Negro and Indian populations and Asiatics than in Americans of European origin.[21] Moreover, timing of emergence tends to be systematically early or systematically late within lineages.[21] Finally, timing

Fig. VI-9.—Fifth and 95th percentiles (in years) for permanent tooth eruption in boys (*left*) and in girls (*right*). (From Garn and Rohmann.[29])

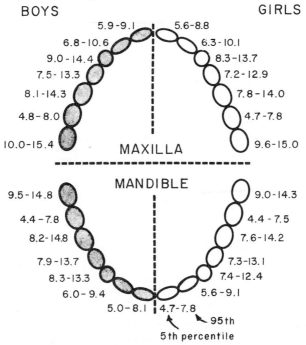

BOYS   GIRLS

5.9-9.1   5.6-8.8
6.8-10.6   6.3-10.1
9.0-14.4   8.3-13.7
7.5-13.3   7.2-12.9
8.1-14.3   7.8-14.0
4.8-8.0   4.7-7.8
10.0-15.4   MAXILLA   9.6-15.0

MANDIBLE
9.5-14.8   9.0-14.3
4.4-7.8   4.4-7.5
8.2-14.8   7.6-14.2
7.9-13.7   7.3-13.1
8.3-13.3   7.4-12.4
6.0-9.4   5.6-9.1
5.0-8.1   4.7-7.8
95th
5th percentile

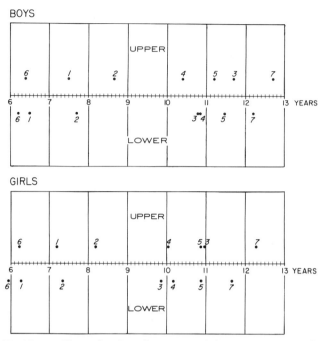

Fig. VI-10.—Normal order of eruption of the permanent teeth.

is correlated within a dentition; that is, those children who erupt any tooth early or late tend to acquire other teeth similarly early or late.[21]

d) *Sex Differences*

Except for third molars, girls erupt their permanent teeth an average of approximately 5 months earlier than do boys[23] (Figs. VI-6, VI-9 and VI-10). The true sex difference in timing of intra-oral emergence is much less than the sex difference in the timing of appearance of most postnatal ossification centers, and the variability of normal eruption timing is small when compared to the normal variability in skeletal development.[29]

e) *Sequence of Eruption*

The apparent sequence of calcification development is not a sure clue to the sequence of emergence into the mouth, since the factors regulating and affecting the rate of eruption vary among the teeth. There is wide variability in the sequence of arrival of teeth in the mouth; some of the variations are important clinically. In the maxilla, the sequences 6-1-2-4-3-5-7 and 6-1-2-4-5-3-7 account for almost half of the cases, whereas in the mandible, the sequences (6-1)-2-3-4-5-7 and

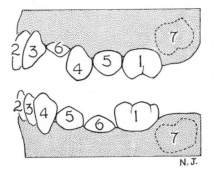

N. J.

Fig. VI-11.—Favorable eruption sequence, the most common of several favorable sequences.

(6-1)-2-4-3-5-7 include more than 40% of all children.[48] Some problems are introduced in comparing various studies and in attempting to predict gingival emergence from the radiograph, since the rate at which the incisors erupt is much faster than that of the molars at the time of immediate emergence into the mouth. If one is seeing a child at 6-month intervals, for example, it may look like the incisor has come in first, whereas, in truth, the molar has preceded it but is moving so slowly that the incisor passes it by. Investigators who have studied eruption sequence at short intervals tend to report the mandibular molars erupting first,[55] whereas those studying eruption at longer intervals tend to note the central incisor erupting first.[48] There seems to be no clinical significance attached to either the 6-1 or 1-6 sequence. On the other hand, the appearance of the second molar ahead of the cuspids or premolars has a strong tendency to shorten the arch perimeter and may create space difficulties.[55] Fortunately, the most common sequence in each arch (viz., maxillary 6-1-2-4-5-3-7 and mandibular 6-1-2-3-4-5-7) is favorable for maintaining the length of the arch during the transitional dentition[55] (Fig. VI-11).

f) Eruption and Bodily Growth

A number of studies have related various indices of bodily maturation and growth with dental development and eruption. Individual differences in the timing of osseous events and individual differences in the timing of dental processes seem to obscure the ready revelation of any common determinants.[59] Studies relating eruption to various somatotypes offer, at best, inconclusive results.

g) Ectopic Development

Ectopic teeth are teeth developing away from their normal position. The most common teeth found in ectopy are the maxillary first permanent molar and the maxillary cuspid. Approximately 3% of North American children may be expected to show ectopically erupting maxillary first permanent molars.[68] Ectopic eruption of maxillary first molars is associated with (1) large primary and permanent teeth, (2) a shorter than average maxillary length, (3) posterior positioning of the maxilla and (4) an atypical angle of eruption of the first molar.[68] Treatment of ectopic eruption is discussed in Chapter XV.

A differentiation should be made between ectopy and impaction. In the latter condition, teeth cannot erupt because of impingement. Third molars and maxillary cuspids may be seen as impacted, even though they began development in normal positions, and hence are not ectopic. In other instances, they may be both ectopic and impacted.

h) Factors Determining the Tooth's Position during Eruption

During eruption, the tooth passes through four distinct stages of development (Fig. VI-12). The factors that determine the tooth's position vary with the stage. At the onset, the position of the tooth germ is thought to be determined largely by genetic mechanisms. During intra-alveolar eruption, the tooth's position is affected also by the presence or absence of adjacent teeth, rate of resorption of the primary teeth, early loss of primary teeth, localized pathologic conditions (Fig. VI-13) and by any factors that alter the growth or conformation of the alveolar process. There is a strong tendency of the teeth to drift mesially even before they appear in the oral cavity. This phenomenon is called the mesial drifting tendency. Once the oral cavity has been entered (intra-oral or preocclusion stage of eruption), the tooth can be moved by the lip, cheek and tongue muscles, by extraneous objects brought into the mouth, for example, thumbs, fingers, pencils, etc., and drift into spaces created by caries or extractions. When the teeth occlude with those of the opposite dental arch (occlusal stage of eruption), a most complicated system of forces determines the position of the tooth (Fig. VI-14). For the first time, the muscles of mastication exert an influence through the interdigitation of the cusps. The upward forces of eruption and alveolar growth are countered by the opposition of the apically directed force

Fig. VI-12.—Stages of eruption. *1*, pre-eruptive; *2*, intra-alveolar; *3*, intra-oral; *4*, occlusal.

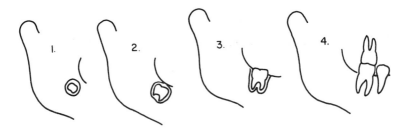

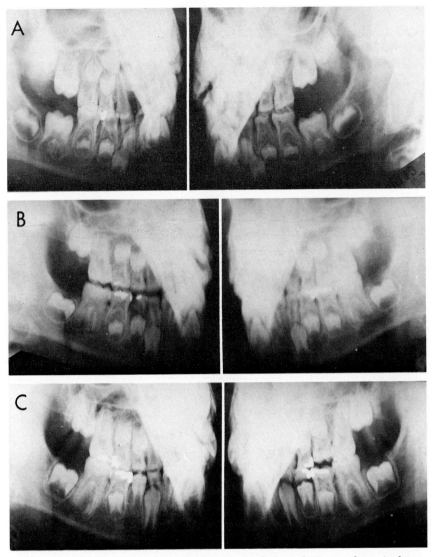

Fig. VI-13.—Alteration in eruption due to a pathologic lesion at the apical area of a primary molar. Compare the eruption of the left and right mandibular first bicuspids. Radiographs were taken at yearly intervals. **A,** 6 years. **B,** 7 years. **C,** 8 years.

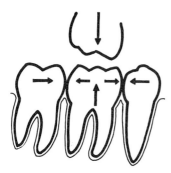

Fig. VI-14.—Direction of forces against a tooth in occlusion.

of occlusion. The periodontal membrane is designed to disseminate the strong forces of chewing to the alveolar bone.

The axial inclination of the permanent teeth is such that some of the forces of chewing produce a mesial result through the contact points of the teeth, the "anterior component of force" (Fig. VI-15). The anterior component of force often is confused with the mesial drifting tendency. The former is the result of muscle forces acting through the intercuspation of the occlusal surfaces, whereas the mesial drifting tendency is an inherent disposition of most teeth to drift mesially even before they are in occlusion. Some clinical problems may be the result of both phenomena. Because of the mesial result, there is a strong tendency of teeth to drift mesially within the alveolar process (Fig. VI-16). The anterior component of force is countered by the approximal contacts of the teeth and by the musculature of the lips and cheeks (Fig. VI-17). As occlusal wear occurs, the anterior component of force is not altered greatly, provided the dental arch is intact and malocclusion is not present. The

Fig. VI-15.—The anterior component of force.

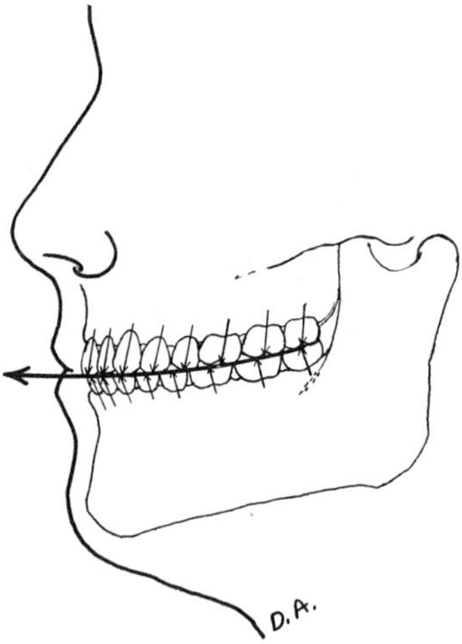

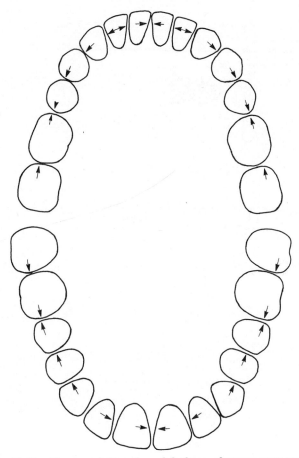

Fig. VI-16.—The usual direction of drifting of permanent teeth.

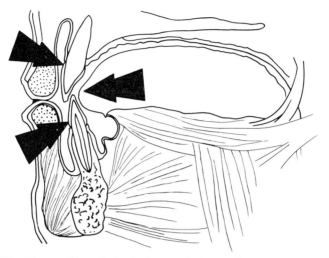

Fig. VI-17.—The position of the incisors relative to the normal lip and tongue posture.

forces of occlusion may, of course, deflect a tooth in another direction if the interdigitation is incorrect. Although occlusal wear decreases the height of the crowns of the teeth, it does not increase the interocclusal distance (freeway space), because alveolar growth compensates nicely throughout most of life. As the crown diminishes in height, the alveolar height increases a like amount. It must be remembered, though, that neither crown nor alveolar height determines the total vertical dimension when the mandible is in its postural position. At the postural position, the vertical dimension is determined by the functioning length of the muscles (Chapter V).

E. The Permanent Dentition

During evolution, several significant changes took place in the teeth and jaws. When *Reptilia* evolved into *Mammalia*, the dentition went from polyphyodont (many sets of teeth) to diphyodont (only two sets of teeth) and it went from homodont (all teeth alike) to heterodont (different types of teeth, i.e., incisors, canines, premolars and molars).[50] There also arose the necessity for teeth and bone to develop somewhat synchronously in order that the function of occlusion could be facilitated. The facial osseous structures also have changed markedly but not quite so radically. Finally, the number of cranial and facial bones has been reduced by loss or fusion and the dental formula has progressed from $\dfrac{5\text{-}1\text{-}4\text{-}7}{4\text{-}1\text{-}4\text{-}7}$ in the mammal-like reptiles to $\dfrac{3\text{-}1\text{-}3\text{-}4}{3\text{-}1\text{-}3\text{-}4}$ as a generalized mammalian pattern to $\dfrac{2\text{-}1\text{-}2\text{-}3}{2\text{-}1\text{-}2\text{-}3}$ as the generalized pattern for primates.

The face of *Homo sapiens*, as Krogman[50] has pointed out so eloquently, is "the battleground upon which this evolutionary war is still being waged."

1. SIZE OF TEETH

In humans, there is strong evidence to support the idea that tooth size is largely determined genetically, although there is experimental proof that extreme environmental variations can alter tooth size in certain animals.[35-37] Marked racial differences exist in the size of teeth, with the Lapps probably having the smallest teeth and Australian aborigines the largest.[22] The sex-size difference averages 4% and is greatest for the maxillary canine and least for incisors (Table VI-5). There

TABLE VI-5.—MESIODISTAL SIZE VARIABILITY AND SEXUAL DIMORPHISM IN THE PERMANENT TEETH[‡]

TOOTH POSITION	MALES			FEMALES			F*	DIMORPHISM[†] %
	No.	MEAN	S.D.	No.	MEAN	S.D.		
				Maxilla				
I₁ Left	297	8·86	0·595	336	8·59	0·554	1·15	3·14
I₁ Right	297	8·83	0·580	336	8·58	0·551	1·11	2·91
I₂ Left	292	6·69	0·612	329	6·57	0·620	−1·03	1·83
I₂ Right	286	6·73	0·569	324	6·61	0·639	−1·26	1·32
C Left	257	7·96	0·450	308	7·61	0·462	−1·05	4·60
C Right	254	7·99	0·436	301	7·65	0·424	1·06	4·44
P₁ Left	265	7·10	0·442	299	6·94	0·429	1·06	2·31
P₁ Right	266	7·09	0·440	296	6·93	0·447	−1·03	2·31
P₂ Left	250	6·76	0·430	281	6·66	0·461	−1·15	1·50
P₂ Right	250	6·78	0·430	280	6·64	0·469	−1·19	2·11
M₁ Left	289	10·12	0·484	329	9·85	0·542	−1·25	2·74
M₁ Right	284	10·14	0·487	323	9·89	0·543	−1·24	2·53
M₂ Left	190	9·97	0·598	225	9·69	0·612	−1·05	2·89
M₂ Right	178	9·99	0·602	218	9·69	0·604	−1·01	3·10
				Mandible				
I₁ Left	297	5·46	0·406	333	5·39	0·398	1·04	1·30
I₁ Right	288	5·44	0·375	322	5·38	0·381	−1·03	1·12
I₂ Left	306	6·05	0·428	329	5·94	0·394	1·18	1·85
I₂ Right	302	6·03	0·412	334	5·91	0·388	1·13	2·03
C Left	282	7·03	0·402	324	6·64	0·388	1·07	5·87
C Right	278	6·97	0·383	323	6·59	0·386	−1·02	5·77
P₁ Left	279	7·24	0·480	309	7·04	0·448	1·15	2·84
P₁ Right	267	7·21	0·467	306	7·02	0·421	1·23	2·71
P₂ Left	235	7·25	0·466	276	7·11	0·506	−1·18	1·97
P₂ Right	240	7·24	0·426	276	7·09	0·514	−1·46	2·12
M₁ Left	284	11·39	0·606	304	11·00	0·647	−1·14	3·55
M₁ Right	271	11·39	0·629	299	10·96	0·682	−1·18	3·92
M₂ Left	163	10·64	0·664	196	10·27	0·664	1·00	3·60
M₂ Right	146	10·69	0·673	190	10·41	0·655	1·06	2·69

*Negative values indicate greater size variance in the female.

[†] $\frac{M}{F} = 1.00$.

[‡]From Garn *et al.*[31a]

is strong evidence of X-linkage in relation to tooth size, since sister-sister correlations are higher than brother-brother and brother-sister.[25] The range of size encountered varies with the tooth and is much larger than most dental anatomy books indicate. Since tooth size is so variable and facial skeletal structures not only vary greatly but also are more subject to varying environmental influences, one frequently encounters in dental practice marked disharmony between the size of the teeth and the bones in which they are placed. Tooth size and bone size seem to be under separate genetic control mechanisms, an unfortunate biologic problem for clinical orthodontic practice.

Butler[12] has discussed the "Field Theory" with respect to dental genetics. "The tooth genes must have a morphogenetic gradient that presides over development, position within a quadrant of like teeth, the shape and size of individual teeth and of a group of like teeth . . ."[50] There also seems to be an over-all patterning for the functional behavior of a tooth within a quadrant, one quadrant and its antimere on the opposite side of the arch and its functional antimere in the opposite arch.[50] What all of this means to the dentist may be summarized in a few sentences. Left-right size correlations are extremely high for individual teeth (average $r = .9$) and even higher if all the teeth in a quadrant are summated.[26] Upper-lower size correlations also are high (average $r = .7$).[26] The more mesial teeth are more genetically stable and display less variability of size.[26]

In studying the relationships among primary and permanent tooth sizes, Moorrees and Reed[63] noted a correlation of $r = .5-.6$ between c, d, e and 3, 4, 5, suggesting an over-all genetic influence over tooth size of both dentitions.

2. NUMBER OF TEETH

a) Missing Teeth

Between 4% and 6% of the population have a congenital absence of some tooth other than third molars.[10, 34, 71] Third molar agenesis occurs approximately 16% of the time in North American whites.[30] Most frequently absent are mandibular second bicuspids, maxillary lateral incisors and maxillary second premolars, in that order.[71] Any tooth may be congenitally missing, although these three account for 85% of all missing teeth (except third molars).[71] Females are more likely to have congenitally missing teeth than are males.[71]

Complete absence of teeth is termed anodontia and incomplete formation of the entire dentition is called oligodontia. The latter condition often is incorrectly labeled "partial anodontia." It is possible that congenital absence of teeth in man today is an expression of phylogenic anisomerism (reduction of the number of teeth by loss or fusion).[50]

The genetics of congenitally missing teeth is quite complex and the mechanisms vary with the tooth. Lasker,[52] in reporting on variability of absence and shape of maxillary lateral incisors, said that the genes responsible likely are different for different conditions even though the anomalies tend to grade into one another. Garn and his group[30] have studied third molars thoroughly and found that agenesis of third molars is related to agenesis of other teeth, delayed calcification of other posterior teeth, different developmental sequences and smaller teeth elsewhere in the mouth. In man, there is an evolutionary tendency to lose teeth and have smaller jaws, but these two trends do not seem to be correlated.

b) *Supernumerary Teeth*

Supernumerary teeth are encountered less frequently than are congenitally missing teeth. They occur more often in the maxilla, particularly in the premaxillary region, than in the mandible. The principal causative factors are said to be (1) heredity, (2) epithelial remnants and (3) gross aberrations in development, such as the supernumeraries seen with cleft palate. They often are classified according to type:

1. Teeth with conical crowns, Black's "enamel droplets." These usually are found at the maxillary midline either singly or in clusters. Often they erupt ectopically and may even be placed upside down and erupt toward the nasal floor.

2. Teeth of normal form and size that are supplemental to those of the regular dentition.

3. Teeth showing variation in size and cuspal form. These may be larger or smaller than normal or the occlusal surface may be deeply pitted. They are recognized by their anatomy, however, and usually are found near their "proper" place in the dental arch.

F. Dimensional Changes in the Dental Arches

Three sets of measurements often are confused: (1) the combined widths of the teeth, (2) the dimensions of the dental arch in which the teeth are arrayed and (3) the dimensions of the mandible or maxilla proper, that is, the so-called basal bone. It may seem paradoxic that during *growth* these values change in different fashions; viz., the widths of the teeth stay the same and the circumference of the dental arch, wherein the teeth are placed, diminishes, whereas the length of the mandibular and maxillary bones themselves increases. The dental arch size and shape are first determined by the cartilaginous skeleton of the fetal maxilla and mandible.[11] A close relationship then develops between the tooth germs and growing jaw bones. Only during the postnatal period do the environmental forces acting against the crowns of the teeth affect the dental arch size and shape. Dental arch size does not correlate well with the sizes of the teeth contained within it. This section discusses the growth changes in the dental arches. Tooth sizes are dealt with in Sections B-3 and E-1 of this chapter. Growth of the bones of the craniofacial complex is treated in Chapters III and IV.

The usual arch dimensions measured are (1) widths at the canines, primary molars (premolars) and first permanent molars, (2) length and (3) circumference (see Fig. VI-2).

1. WIDTH

The intercanine diameter increases only slightly in the mandible, and some of this increase is due to the distal tipping of the primary cuspids into the primate space (Fig. VI-18). Moorrees[61] gives mean values of 1.12 mm. increase between 5 and 18 years when measured at the gingival level and 2.45 mm. when measured at the cusp tip, whereas Sillman[77] reports 3.5 mm. for males only. In the maxilla, the intercanine diameter widens more and the permanent and primary cuspid tips seem to be in the same place; therefore, all of the increase likely is true widening (4.39 mm. at the tip, 1.76 mm. at the gingival level,[61] 5.00 mm. in males[77]). Figure VI-19 diagrams these width changes. Note that in the mandible the only significant increase occurs during the eruption of the incisors when the primary cuspids are moved distally into the primate spaces. Because the maxillary alveolar processes diverge, forming the palatal walls, width increases tend to be timed with periods of vertical alveolar growth, that is, during active eruption of the teeth. Note in Figure VI-19 that the periods of maxillary width increase coincide with the eruption of the incisors and the cuspids and premolars.

Primary molar-premolar width increases are slight in both arches, that is, the mean increase is less than 2 mm., probably because the permanent crowns are narrower than the primary, and the maxillary teeth undergo significant changes in buccolingual axial inclination (see Fig. VI-19).

Maxillary first permanent molar width increases significantly more (Fig. VI-20) than does the intermolar width in the mandible.[47] Although the alveolar process growth is almost vertical in the mandible, the

Fig. VI-18.—The movement of the primary cuspids distally into the primate spaces with the eruption of the permanent mandibular incisors. Note that if one is measuring the diameter between the primary cuspids, a wider diameter is recorded as they are pushed distally on the divergent arch.

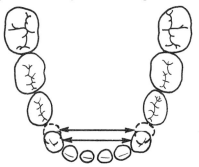

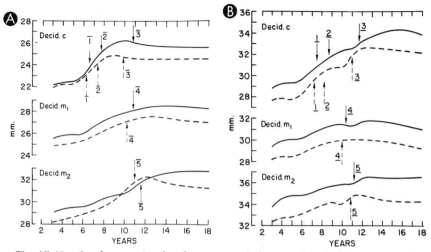

Fig. VI-19.—A, changes in the diameters of the mandibular primary dental arch. ———— males; - - - - females. Note the relationship of the eruption of permanent teeth to alterations in the diameter. **B,** changes in the maxillary diameters of the primary dentition. ———— males; - - - - females. (From Moorrees.[61])

Fig. VI-20.—A, the stability of the mandibular first permanent molar diameter. Note that only slight changes in this diameter occur and those are concomitant with the eruption of the second permanent molar, which presumably frees the first permanent molar to change its axial inclination. **B,** width increases in the maxillary first permanent molar region. The gradual and significant increases in maxillary molar width eventually are countered by the mesial drifting of the first permanent molar to a narrower diameter. (From Moorrees.[61])

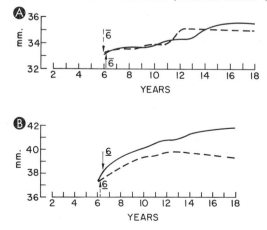

crowns of the first molars erupt tipped somewhat lingually and do not upright until the time of the eruption of the second molars (Fig. VI-20). As they upright, they cause an increase in the bimolar width, but this is not, of course, an increase in the diameter of the mandible itself. Furthermore, both first molars move forward at the time of the late mesial shift to pre-empt any remaining leeway space and thus assume a narrower diameter along the convergent dental arch. The real bony width increase may be a bit more than that recorded when using these drifting dental landmarks.

It is important to note the reasons for the rather marked differences in width increases between the two dental arches. The only postnatal mechanism for widening the basal bony width of the mandible is that of deposition on the lateral borders of the corpus mandibularis. Such deposition occurs, but only in small amounts, and offers little help for the clinician wishing to widen the mandibular dental arch. The maxilla, in sharp contrast, widens with vertical growth simply because the alveolar processes diverge; therefore, more width increase is seen and more can be procured permanently during treatment (see Fig. VI-23). Furthermore, the midpalatal suture can be reopened with "palatal splitting" (see Chapter XV) to acquire surprisingly large amounts of actual widening of the maxilla. There is little correlation between dental arch widths and any facial width measurements; therefore, knowledge of the latter is of no real use in planning orthodontic treatment.

2. LENGTH

Dental arch length is measured at the midline from a point midway between the central incisors to a tangent touching the distal surfaces of the second primary molars or second premolars (see Fig. VI-2). Although often measured and reported, it does not have the clinical importance of the circumference, and any changes in arch length are but coarse reflections of changes in perimeter. Sometimes one-half the circumference is referred to as arch length.

3. CIRCUMFERENCE OR PERIMETER

The most important of the dental arch dimensions is arch circumference or perimeter, which usually is measured from the distal surface of the second primary molar (or mesial surface of the first permanent molar) around the arch over the contact points and incisal edges in a smoothed curve to the distal surface of the second primary molar (or first permanent molar) of the opposite side (see Fig. VI-2). A wide range of variability is seen in circumferential increments and the mandibular and maxillary perimeters behave a bit differently; therefore, they will be discussed separately.

Both Fisk[18] and Moorrees[61] report a mean reduction in mandibular arch circumference during the transitional and early adolescent denti-

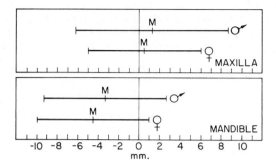

Fig. VI-21.—Changes in the arch perimeters from the primary to the early permanent dentition. Note the large decreases in the mandibular arch perimeter and the relatively stable maxillary arch perimeter. (From Moorrees.[61])

tion of about 5 mm. Such a large decrease is due to (1) the late mesial shift of the first permanent molars as the "leeway space" (q.v. in Section G-2 of this chapter) is pre-empted, (2) the mesial drifting tendency of the posterior teeth throughout all of life, (3) slight amounts of interproximal wear of the teeth and (4) the lingual positioning of the incisors due to differential mandibulomaxillary growth.

The mandibular permanent incisors are thicker labiolingually than the predecessors, yet they usually occupy the same position in the arch. When the mandibular permanent incisors become tipped labially, the arch perimeter may increase a slight amount. In summary, mandibular arch perimeter usually decreases greatly in both sexes (Fig. VI-21) during the transitional and young adult period.

Maxillary arch perimeter, in contrast, typically increases slightly,

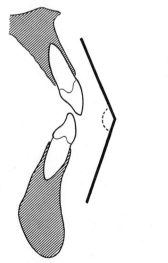

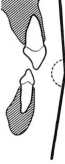

Fig. VI-22.—A comparison of the angulation of the permanent and primary incisors.

N, J.

although it has about an equal chance to either increase or decrease (Fig. VI-21). The very marked difference in angulation of the maxillary permanent incisors, as compared to the primary (Fig. VI-22), and the greater increases in width probably account for the tendency to preserve the circumference in the upper jaw even though the permanent molars are drifting mesially.

4. DIMENSIONAL CHANGES DURING ORTHODONTIC THERAPY

Figure VI-23 summarizes the normal growth changes in both dental arches and compares such changes with changes that can be brought about by orthodontic therapy. It is important to note very carefully that it is far easier to increase dental arch width and length in the maxilla than it is in the mandible. In fact, it is relatively simple to increase the maxillary dental arch width and length, difficult to increase and retain the mandibular dental arch width and nearly impossible to move man-

Fig. VI-23.—Changes in the dentition's dimensions produced by growth and the possibilities for altering dimensions during orthodontic treatment. Of particular clinical interest is the fact that mandibular dental arch dimensions are not increased during growth and ordinarily there is difficulty in changing them with orthodontic treatment. In fact, the mandibular arch perimeter shortens radically during growth.

	PRIMARY DENTITION		MIXED DENTITION	
	GROWTH	TREATMENT	GROWTH	TREATMENT
MANDIBLE WIDTH	O	+	O	O
PERIMETER	O	O	− −	O
MAXILLA WIDTH	+	+	+	+ +
PERIMETER	O	+	O	+ +

O Same   + Mild Increase Occurs or can be Obtained
− − Decreases Greatly   + + Significant Increase Occurs or can be Obtained

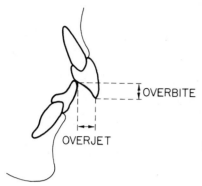

Fig. VI-24.—Overbite and overjet.

dibular molars distally significantly to increase the perimeter and hold that increase. The effects of orthodontic treatment on dental arch dimensions are not to be confused with the effects of orthodontic treatment on craniofacial skeletal dimensions. For a discussion of this subject read Chapter 4, Section K.

5. OVERBITE AND OVERJET

Overbite (vertical overlap of the incisors) and overjet (horizontal overlap, Fig. VI-24) undergo significant changes during the primary and transitional dentitions (see Figs. VI-36–VI-44). During the primary dentition, the overbite decreases a slight amount, although the overjet often is reduced to zero. From the early mixed dentition to late adolescence, the overbite increases (between 9 and 12 years) and then decreases.[19] Overbite is correlated with a number of vertical facial dimensions, notably ramus height,[19] whereas overjet usually is a reflection of the anteroposterior relationships of the maxillary and mandibular denture bases.

G. The Mixed Dentition Period

That period during which both primary and permanent teeth are in the mouth together is known as the mixed dentition. Those permanent teeth that follow into a place in the arch once held by a primary tooth are called successional teeth, e.g., incisors, cuspids and bicuspids. Those permanent teeth that erupt posteriorly to the primary teeth are termed accessional teeth.[3]

From a clinical point of view, there are two very important aspects to the mixed dentition period: (1) the utilization of the arch perimeter and (2) the adaptive changes in occlusion that occur during the transition from one dentition to another.

1. Uses of the Dental Arch Perimeter

Misconceptions regarding the normal changes in and the uses of the dental arch perimeter probably cause more clinical failures in mixed dentition therapy than anything else. In the discussion that follows, concentration will be on the mandible, since it is by far more critical clinically than the maxilla.

For this discussion and that which follows concerning the occlusal changes in the mixed dentition, the following scheme of developmental stages will be used:

Stage I—the completed primary dentition (Figs. VI-25 and VI-26).
Stage II—after the eruption of the permanent central incisors and first permanent molars (Fig. VI-27).
Stage III—after eruption of the permanent lateral incisors (Fig. VI-28).
  a) after eruption of $\bar{2}$ but before the loss of $\bar{c}$.
  b) after the loss of $\bar{c}$.
  c) after the loss of $\bar{D}$ but before the loss of $\bar{E}$.
  d) after the loss of $\bar{E}$ but before the eruption of $\bar{7}$.
Stage IV—after the eruption of $\bar{3}$, $\bar{4}$ and $\bar{5}$ (Fig. VI-29).

All stages may not appear in some cases; for example, Stage III*a*, when the erupting lateral incisor causes the exfoliation of the primary cuspid.

There are three uses of the arch perimeter:

1—alignment of the permanent incisors: they arrive typically crowded (see Fig. VI-28).
2—space for the cuspids and premolars.
3—adjustment of the molar occlusion: the first permanent molars, which erupt end-to-end, must change to a Class I relationship if normal occlusion is to obtain.

Fig. VI-25.—Available space in the primary dental arch.[62] Note that the entire dental perimeter is not occupied by tooth substance in successive illustrations (Figs. VI-25 to VI-30). Study the changing relationships of the teeth to the interdental spaces.

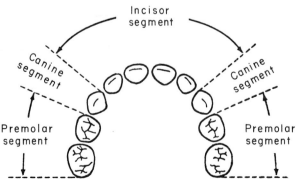

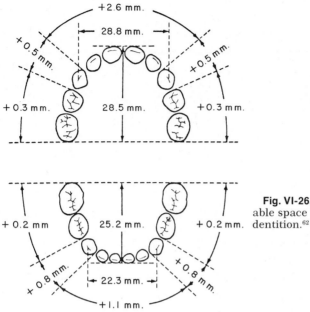

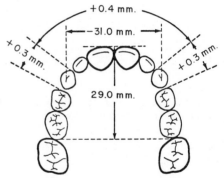

Fig. VI-26.—The mean available space in the primary dentition.[62]

Fig. VI-27.—Changes in the available space after the eruption of the first permanent molar and central incisors.[62]

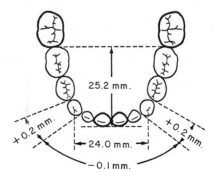

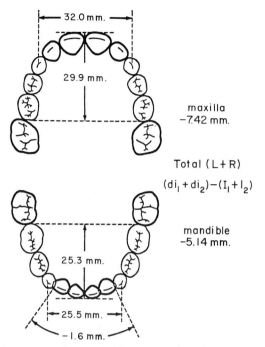

Fig. VI-28.—Changes in the available space after the eruption of the lateral incisors. Note the negative leeway space in the incisal region.[62]

As the larger permanent incisors erupt, they find space in the arch only because (1) the arch width increases slightly, (2) there is some interdental spacing and (3) the primary cuspids are moved distally. Still, there is a typical slight crowding at the end of Stage III (see Fig. VI-28), which usually is not relieved until the primary cuspids are lost. When the incisors then align, they do so at some expense to the posterior space available for cuspid and premolar eruption and molar adjustment. The cuspid and premolars erupt into the normally excessive posterior leeway space. If molar adjustment is to be achieved by dental means, there must be some posterior space left after the arrival of the cuspid and premolars so that a late mesial shift of the first permanent molar may take place. Normally, such a late mesial shift occurs to some extent but there are other mechanisms of occlusal adjustment, which will be discussed in the next section.

Everyone agrees that the mandibular arch perimeter shortens during the mixed dentition, but there are divergent opinions concerning where, how and when that shortening takes place. These differences of opinion are not just interesting theoretical points; the planning of space management is altered significantly according to which of several concepts is accepted as correct by the clinician. For example, Baume[3] has suggested that the primate space and other interdental spacing may be closed from the rear with the eruption of the first permanent molars, whereas Clinch[14] and Maher[56] report the primate space to be closed from the anterior with the eruption of the lateral incisor, which forces the primary cuspid distally.

In the first theory (Baume's early mesial shift), the perimeter is said to shorten to close the primate space; in the alternative theory, the primate space closes without loss of circumference. The leeway space is the difference in size between the primary teeth and their permanent successors. Anteriorly, this is a negative value, even if one includes the interdental spacing around the primary incisors (see Fig. VI-28). Posteriorly, the leeway space is positive, since the combined widths of $\bar{c} + \bar{d} + \bar{e}$ exceed the combined widths of $\bar{3} + \bar{4} + \bar{5}$ (see Fig. VI-3B). However, the total leeway is the most important clinical consideration (Fig.

Fig. VI-29.—Arch dimensions and available space after the eruption of the cuspids and premolars.[62]

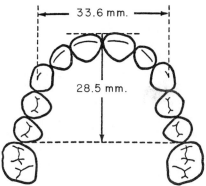
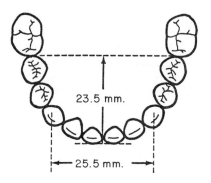

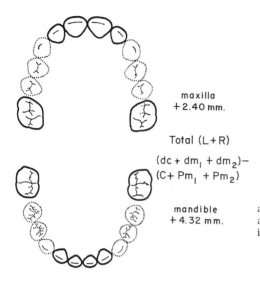

maxilla
+2.40 mm.

Total (L+R)

(dc + dm$_1$ + dm$_2$)−
(C+ Pm$_1$ + Pm$_2$)

mandible
+4.32 mm.

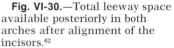

Fig. VI-30.—Total leeway space available posteriorly in both arches after alignment of the incisors.[62]

VI-30). The method of utilization of the leeway space is the key factor in the transitional dentition. If Maher[56] is correct, the perimeter is not shortened during incisor eruption, but if Baume[3] is correct, the perimeter is shortened during incisor eruption because the first permanent molars also are erupting at the same time. Maher[56] compared a series of arch measurements (Fig. VI-31). He found little support for the idea of an early mesial shift (Fig. VI-32). The mean measurement from the infradentale to the primary cuspid increased with the eruption of the incisors, whereas the measurement from the midpoint to the first permanent molar remained the same. The midpoint first permanent molar measurement, however, shortens greatly later with the loss of the primary second molar (the late mesial shift). Moorrees and Chadha's[62] data support this concept, although they did not study and report this matter specifically (Fig. VI-33).

Fig. VI-31.—Maher's method of determining the late mesial shift mechanism.[56]

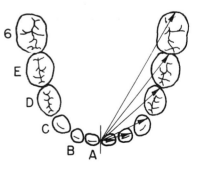

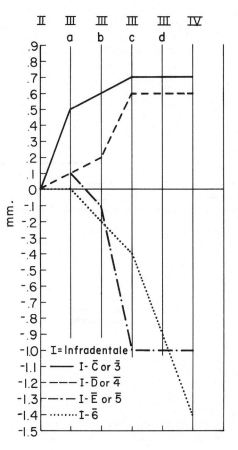

Fig. VI-32.—Changes in the position of the teeth relative to developmental stages in the mixed dentition compared to Figure VI-31. *II,* the completed primary dentition. *III-a,* at the time of the emergence of the lateral incisors. *III-b,* the emergence of the permanent cuspids. *III-c,* the emergence of the first premolar. *III-d,* the emergence of the second premolar.

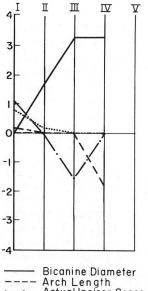

Fig. VI-33.—A summary of mandibular space changes related to arch dimensional changes. (Derived from Moorrees and Chadha.[62])

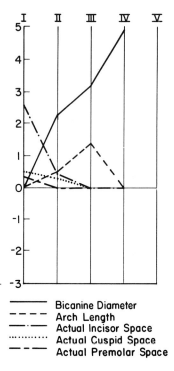

Fig. VI-34.—A summary of maxillary space changes related to arch dimensional changes. (Derived from Moorrees and Chadha.[62])

——————— Bicanine Diameter
– – – – Arch Length
—— · —— Actual Incisor Space
················ Actual Cuspid Space
— – — Actual Premolar Space

In the maxilla, similar accommodative adjustments occur during the mixed dentition, although the matter is less critical, since the upper incisors can alter their inclination to relieve shortages of space in the anterior arch and the upper molars may be orthodontally moved distally to reduce posterior space shortages. Furthermore, the maxillary perimeter does not display such a tendency to shorten as does the mandibular (Fig. VI-34).

2. OCCLUSAL CHANGES IN THE MIXED DENTITION

As noted earlier, the usual flush terminal plane of the primary dentition typically provides an end-to-end relationship of the first permanent molars. The first permanent molars then achieve a Class I relationship by (1) a late mesial shift after the loss of the second primary molar, (2) greater forward growth of the mandible than the maxilla or, most likely, (3) a combination of (1) and (2) (see Fig. VI-35A). Theoretically, one might presume that there are twelve paths through the mixed dentition, since each of the three occlusal classifications on the left side of Figure VI-35 could become one of the four adult classes on the right side. Several theoretical possibilities are not found in actuality. Murray,[65] Micklow[60] and Lamont[51] have done cephalometric studies of the transi-

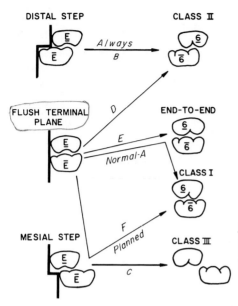

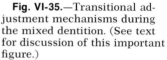

Fig. VI-35.—Transitional adjustment mechanisms during the mixed dentition. (See text for discussion of this important figure.)

tional occlusal adjustment mechanisms and report a number of clinically interesting findings. For example, a distal step in the primary dentition will always result in a Class II occlusion in the permanent dentition (see Fig. VI-35*B*), since it is a reflection of a Class II skeletal pattern—a condition that is not self-corrective with growth. In a similar fashion, mesial steps may become Class III malocclusions (Fig. VI-35*C*); not all, however, since mesial steps may occur by ways other than as a result of mandibular prognathism. Of particular clinical interest are the factors that induce a flush terminal plane to change by ways other than the expected end-to-end and later Class I molar intercuspation. If, for example, a child has a flush terminal plane in the primary dentition, a mild Class II facial skeleton and insufficient arch perimeter space to permit a late mesial shift of the first permanent molars, the occlusion likely will become a Class II by the end of mixed dentition (see Fig. VI-35*D*). If a child has a flush terminal plane, a normal skeletal pattern and no leeway space to permit a late mesial shift in either arch, an end-to-end molar relationship may obtain by the time of the eruption of the premolars (see Fig. VI-35*E*). It is particularly advantageous to obtain a Class I molar relationship prior to the loss of the second primary molars, since all of the arch perimeter can be used for alignment of teeth and none be allotted to molar adjustment. Murray[65] found that four factors contributed to the anteroposterior occlusal adjustments in the transitional dentition: (1) forward growth of the maxilla, (2) maxillary leeway space, (3) forward growth of the mandible and (4) mandibular leeway space. Although there are two adjustment mechanisms, one dental and one skeletal, by far the more important is skeletal growth. In minor skeletal disharmonies with large leeway spaces, dentitional adjustments can be overcome, but no child has enough mandibular leeway space to achieve naturally a Class I molar relationship within a severe Class II facial skeleton; strenuous orthodontic intervention is the only alternative.

Harvold[41] attempted to predict the anterior skeletal profile relationship at 12 years with information available at 9 years. The relationship of the maxilla to the mandible could not be predicted for 12 when it was known at 9, nor could increments of growth be predicted or aid in the prediction. To a large extent, the occlusal relationships are at the mercy of the skeletal growth pattern. It will be learned later that the amount of space in an arch for dental adjustments can be predicted quite accurately, a procedure used routinely when planning mixed dentition treatment, but we are not yet able to predict within practical limits maxillary or mandibular increments, the relative maxillomandibular growth or the final maxillomandibular relationship.

3. First Molar Eruption

In Sections G-3–G-6, the reader should refer to Figures VI-36–VI-44 (a normal cast series), Figures VI-45–VI-53 (serial radiographic views) and Figures VI-54 VI-59 (skull dissections).

a) Mandible

The majority of children erupt the first permanent molar prior to the central incisors, although some children reverse this order (see Fig. VI-10). There seems to be no clinical significance in either sequence. The first permanent molar is guided into its occlusal position during eruption by the distal surface of the second primary molar (see Figs. VI-4 and VI-35). The occlusal relationship that the mandibular first permanent molar initially obtains with its maxillary antagonist is thus determined by the terminal plane relationship of the second primary molars (see Figs. VI-3 and VI-4). Baume[3] holds that the eruption of the mandibular first permanent molar moves both the first and second primary molars forward, closing the primate space from the rear. This concept of an "early mesial shift" may have been an artifact of plaster cast data and is not supported by the work of Maher[56] or the cephalometric studies by Murray,[65] Micklow[60] and Lamont[51] (see Fig. VI-32). On the other hand, the relationship of the permanent molars to each other can be changed by a cavity in the distal surface of either second primary molar.[44] Changes in occlusal relationship that occur during the period of the first molar eruption rarely are caused by that eruption but are more likely to be due to coincidental mandibular growth (Figs. VI-37 and VI-38).

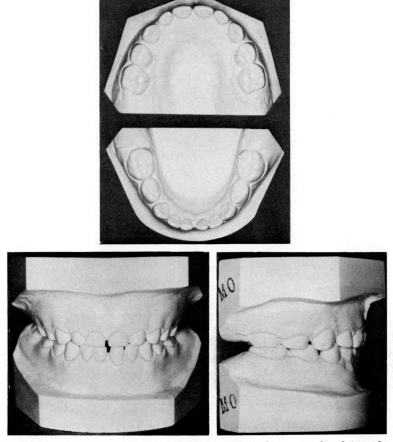

Fig. VI-36.—Primary occlusion at 5 years. Note the generalized interdental spacing, primate spaces (distal to lateral incisors in the maxilla and distal to cuspids in the mandible), moderate overbite and overjet and flush terminal plane. (Figs. VI-36–VI-44 courtesy of Dr. R. R. McIntyre.)

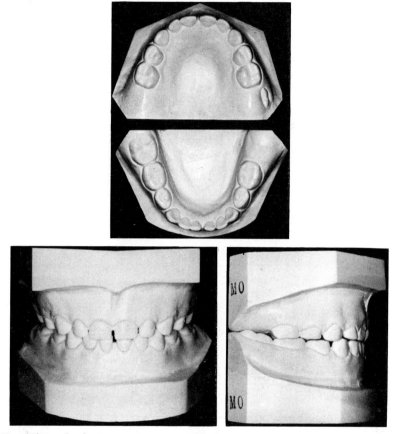

Fig. VI-37.—Occlusion at 6 years. Note diminished overbite and overjet and beginning of a mesial step at the distal surfaces of the primary molars.

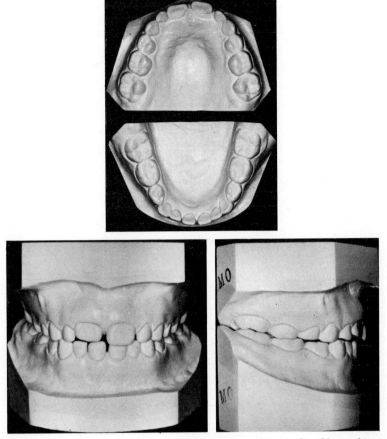

Fig. VI-38.—Occlusion at 7 years. All first molars and central and lateral incisors have erupted. A distinct mesial step has permitted Class I interdigitation of the permanent molars, and the erupting incisors have closed the primate spaces in both arches.

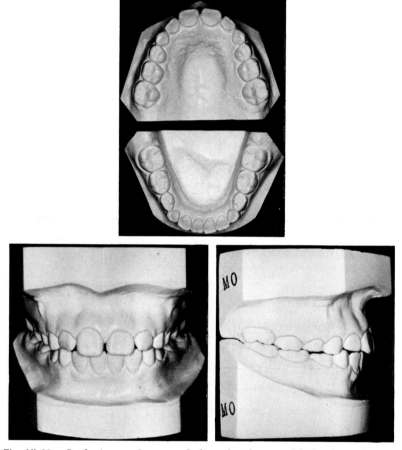

Fig. VI-39.—Occlusion at 8 years. Ordinarily, the mandibular lateral incisors erupt into the line of arch, completing closure of the primate spaces. Note interdental spacing in the maxillary incisor region. The permanent molars have a firm Class I occlusion by this age if a mesial step has been available at the time of their eruption.

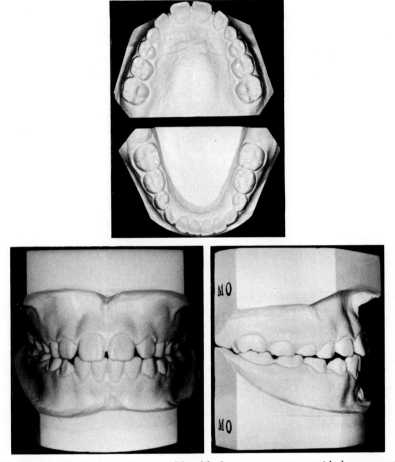

Fig. VI-40.—Occlusion at 9 years. Mandibular permanent cuspids have erupted in this case. Although this is desirable, often the mandibular cuspid and first bicuspid arrive almost simultaneously.

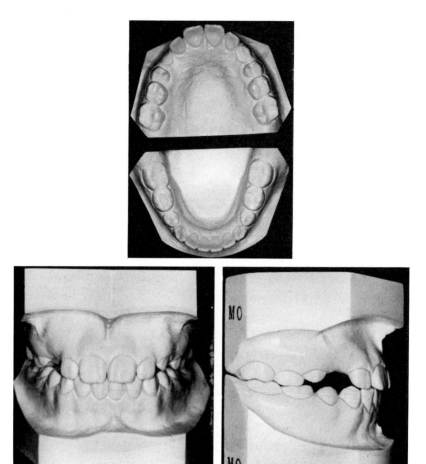

Fig. VI-41.—Occlusion at 10 years. First bicuspids are erupted and maxillary permanent cuspids are appearing. In most mouths, the maxillary second bicuspids erupt before the cuspids.

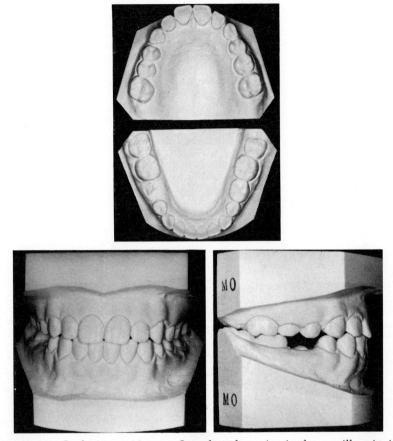

Fig. VI-42.—Occlusion at 11 years. Interdental spacing in the maxillary incisor region has been closed by eruption of the cuspids, and one second bicuspid has appeared in each arch. Eruption of second molars in the mandible at this time is not the most favorable sequence; it is better if they are delayed until all bicuspids have erupted.

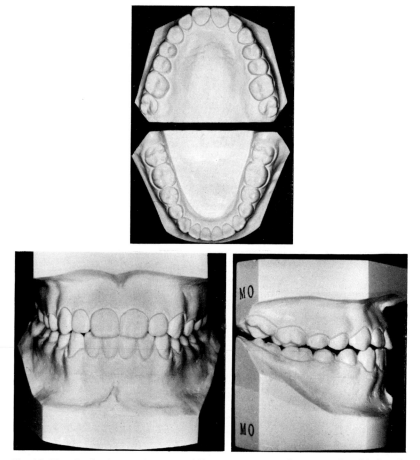

Fig. VI-43.—Occlusion at 12 years. All permanent teeth except the third molars are in position. Note absence of any interdental spacing and the slight tendency to procumbency of the dentition. The procumbency typical of the recently completed dentition seems to diminish soon unless there is gross discrepancy between the size of the teeth and the alveolar perimeter.

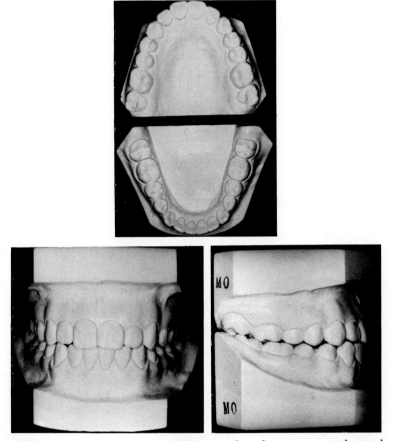

Fig. VI-44.—Occlusion at 13 years. There are few changes except the tendency to less dental procumbency than seen previously.

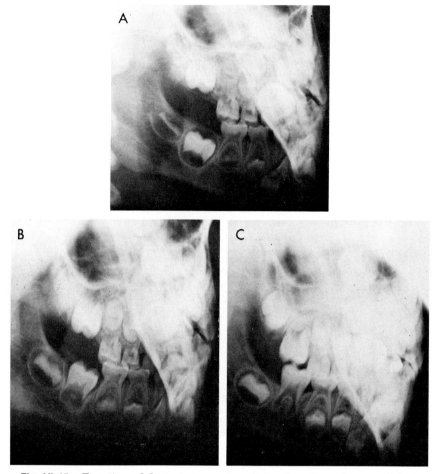

Fig. VI-45.—Eruption of first permanent molars when there is a mesial step on distal surfaces of the deciduous teeth. **A,** age 5. Note distinct mesial step established before eruption of first permanent molars. The mandibular primate space is open. **B,** age 6. The erupting first permanent molars are guided by the distal surfaces of the second primary molars. The mandibular primate space persists. **C,** age 7. Erupting first permanent molars are firmly interdigitated into Class I occlusion without closing the mandibular primate space.

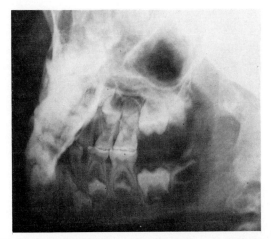

Fig. VI-46.—Dentition at 5 years. Observe the flush terminal plane and compare with Figure VI-45, *A*. Note the sequence of eruption and position of developing permanent teeth. Figures VI-46–VI-53 are serial radiographs of the same child.

Fig. VI-47.—Dentition at 6 years. First permanent molars are ready to pierce the mucosa and enter the mouth. In this series, note how resorption of the anterior border of the ramus frees the mandibular second permanent molar so that it may erupt.

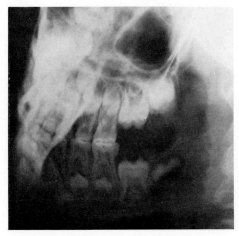

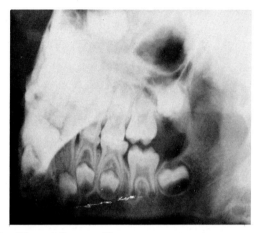

Fig. VI-48.—Dentition at 7 years. The permanent molars seem to be headed for Class II malocclusion, since posterior surfaces of the primary molars present a distinctly distal step. Perhaps the occlusion was not exactly correct when the radiograph was taken or the condition was transitory, because Figure VI-49 shows occlusion at 8 years to be nearer than at age 6 (Fig. VI-47).

Fig. VI-49.—Dentition at 8 years. Note end-to-end molar relationship and positions and sequence of the erupting teeth.

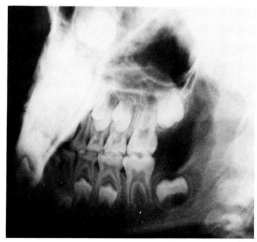

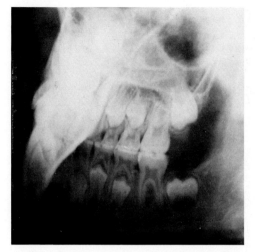

Fig. VI-50.—Dentition at 9 years. Little anteroposterior change is seen, but important changes in vertical position are apparent. At this age, the sequence of eruption should be observed with care. Special caution is required if the second molars advance into the mouth before the last of the cuspids and bicuspids.

Fig. VI-51.—Dentition at 10 years. In this case, the mandibular bicuspid is arriving just before the cuspid; this is not serious if there is space for the cuspid. The maxillary first bicuspid also is just ready to appear in the mouth.

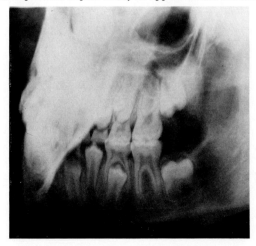

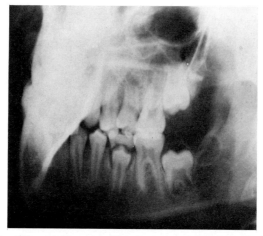

Fig. VI-52.—Dentition at 11 years. This is an unusual view of what is meant by late mesial shift. End-to-end molar relationship has persisted until loss of the mandibular second primary molar allows adjustment into Class I occlusion. The maxillary teeth have tipped forward, and there is interproximal contact of all teeth, while interproximal spacing is still seen in the mandible. Some very mild Class II malocclusions are established at this time because the slight mesial adjustment in the maxillary dental arch, when the last primary tooth is lost, is just enough to cause Class II molar relationship.

Fig. VI-53.—Dentition at 12 years. The permanent teeth have settled into excellent occlusion. Note the mesial step on the distal surface of the first molars, proving that the mandibular first molars have moved mesially more after loss of the primary second molar.

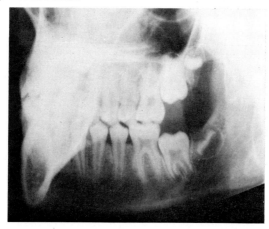

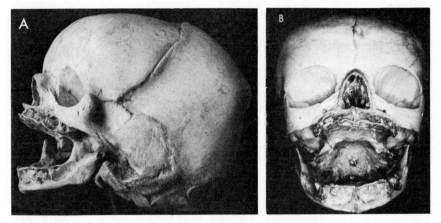

Fig. VI-54.—A, a skull dissection of a neonate. Note the overlap of the parietal and frontal bones. Note, too, the calcifying primary teeth. **B,** front view.

Fig. VI-55.—A, a skull specimen at approximately 8 months of age. The mandibular left second primary molar has been lost from its crypt. Note how advanced is the calcification of the first permanent molars. By this time, one sees rapid alveolar process growth and considerable resorption already on the anterior border of the ramus in anticipation of the eruption of the first permanent molar. **B,** front view. Note the relationship of the calcifying and erupting primary teeth.

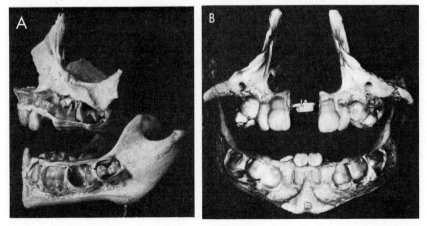

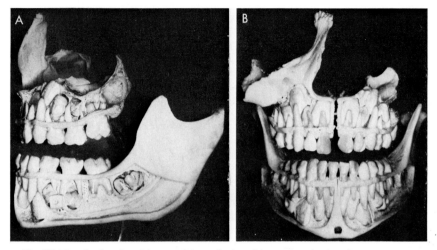

Fig. VI-56.—A, the dentition and its relationship to developing bony structures at approximately 4 years of age. Now the crypt for the second permanent molar is clearly visible and the first permanent molars are moving rapidly toward the plane of occlusion with sufficient space in the line of arch for them. Space has been provided by the resorption at the anterior border of the ramus. **B,** a front view of the same specimen. Note the intimate relationship of the calcifying permanent incisors to the roots of the primary incisors.

Fig. VI-57.—A, the dentition at approximately 6 years. At this time, a very complicated situation exists. Note the presence of all the permanent teeth either lingually to their primary predecessors or directly beneath them as in the molar region. **B,** a front view of the same specimen.

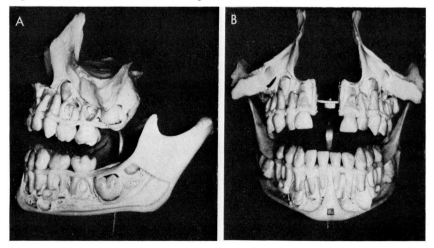

b) *Maxilla*

During formation, the crowns of the maxillary molars face dorsally rather than occlusally. As the maxilla moves forward, space is created posteriorly, permitting appositional enlargement of the maxillary tuberosity. During this rather rapid tuberosity growth, the first permanent molar rotates, and by the time the crown pierces the gingiva, it is facing more occlusally (see Fig. VI-57). Occasionally, the maxillary first permanent molar is found in ectopic eruption (see Section D-2-g of this chapter).

4. INCISOR ERUPTION

a) *Mandible*

The mandibular first permanent molars are followed almost immediately by eruption of the mandibular central incisors. Although the incisors usually follow the first permanent molars in piercing the gingiva, they reach their full clinical crown height sooner. Perhaps this is why, as has already been mentioned, some studies have indicated that the incisors erupt ahead of the molars more frequently than reported in other studies. It has been claimed that the eruption of the central incisors before the permanent molars predisposes to malocclusion. Lo and Moyers[55] found this order of eruption to have little clinical significance. The permanent mandibular incisors develop lingually to the resorbing roots of the primary incisors, forcing the latter labially to be exfoliated (see Fig. VI-56). The lingual eruptive position is no cause for alarm if the primary incisors are resorbing normally. As soon as the primary central incisors have been exfoliated, further eruption and lingual activity moves the permanent incisors labially to their normal balanced position between the internal functional matrix, that is, the tongue and the external functional matrix, the lip and facial musculature (see Fig. VI-17).

The size of the primary teeth, the amount of interdental spacing and the size of the anterior perimeter of the dental arch are factors that determine whether the permanent incisors will erupt crowded. Figure VI-28 shows that normally there is some crowding after the lateral incisors are erupted. The lateral incisors are more likely to be lingually positioned on eruption; yet, as they emerge, they not only push the primary lateral incisors labially but they also move the primary cuspids distally and laterally, closing the primate spaces from the mesial[6] (see Fig. VI-18). When the permanent incisors are disproportionately large for the arch in which they are found, the eruption of the lateral incisor may cause the exfoliation of the primary cuspid. In other instances, such a disharmony of tooth size and arch perimeter will maintain the lateral incisors in their original lingual position. As soon as the lateral incisors emerge into the mouth, a Mixed Dentition Analysis may be made to estimate the amount of arch space available for the permanent teeth and the occlusal adjustments that accompany the transitional dentition period. When the primary cuspids are prematurely lost, the anterior arc is less stable and the incisors may be tipped lingually by hyperactivity of the mentalis muscle, a condition frequently found with Class II, Division 1 malocclusion or thumb-sucking. Lingual tipping of the incisors permits the developing permanent cuspid to slide labially, where it may erupt later in labioversion. This is a sensitive time and a sensitive region. The first symptoms of some malocclusions frequently are diagnosed at the time of eruption of mandibular incisors. Space supervision therapy (q.v., Chapter XV) begins at this time and must be synchronized well with dental development. Good timing is one of the fundamentals of good orthodontic therapy.

b) Maxilla

The maxillary anterior segment is supported by the mandibular anterior arc, which has formed earlier, providing the functional stops against which the maxillary incisors erupt. Usually, the maxillary central incisors erupt just after the mandibular central incisors or concurrently with the mandibular lateral incisors (see Fig. VI-38). The maxillary permanent incisors erupt with a more labial inclination than their predecessors, in accordance with their greater labiolingual thickness and wider diameter. Little variation is seen in eruption of the maxillary central incisor unless one is deflected by abnormal exfoliation

Fig. VI-58.—A, the dentition at approximately 9 years of age. Now one can see the maxillary cuspid erupting at an angle against the root of the lateral incisor. **B,** a front view of the same specimen. Note the hazardous relationship of the cuspids to the roots of the lateral incisors in this projection. Great care and caution must be taken in moving lateral incisors at this stage of development.

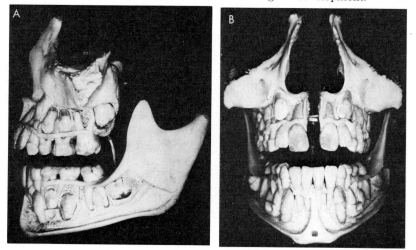

of the primary tooth, a supernumerary tooth or by trauma. The maxillary central incisors erupt with a slight distal inclination and some midline space between them, which space is diminished with eruption of the lateral incisors and closed as the cuspids wedge their way into the arch.

The maxillary lateral incisors, on the other hand, often experience more difficulty in assuming their normal positions, for, as they are erupting, the maxillary cuspids' developing crown lies just labially and distally to their roots (see Fig. VI-58). The cuspid in this position often can cause the lateral incisor's crown to erupt more labially than the central incisor. After the erupting cuspid has changed its course (it often seems to have been deflected by the root of the lateral incisor), the lateral incisor then rights itself and comes into position beside the central incisor. Minor rotations may be seen in the position of both the central and lateral incisor but they usually are corrected as the cuspids erupt (see Figs. VI-40–VI-41). Ordinarily, it is not good practice to attempt alignment of central and lateral incisors while the cuspid crown is atop the root of the lateral incisor, since orthodontic pressure against the lateral incisor's crown may press the root against the erupting cuspid crown and cause root resorption.

5. CUSPID AND BICUSPID ERUPTION

Favorable development of occlusion in this region is largely dependent on three factors: (1) a favorable sequence of eruption, (2) a satisfactory tooth size–available space ratio and (3) the attainment of a normal molar relationship with minimal diminution of the space available for the bicuspids.

a) Mandible

The most favorable eruption sequence in the mandible is cuspid, first bicuspid, second bicuspid and second molar. Fortunately, this also is one of the most frequent sequences. It is useful if the cuspid erupts first, since it tends to maintain the arch perimeter and to prevent lingual tipping of incisors. When the incisors are tipped lingually, they may overerupt, since by lingual tipping they lose their centric stops with the maxillary incisors. In severe Class II malocclusions, mandibular incisors erupt past the plane of occlusion until they find functional stops against the maxillary palatal mucosa. In Class II, such overeruption often occurs without lingual tipping. A complication of this enhancement of the occlusal curve is the movement of the mandibular cuspid during eruption into labioversion, which is far more likely to occur if the first bicuspid precedes it in eruption. It is quite normal for the cuspid to lag behind the first bicuspid during early development, but it moves more rapidly during the latter stages of eruption and usually passes the first bicuspid before breaking through the alveolar crest. Eruption of the cuspid may be hastened by extraction of the primary cuspid while the permanent cuspid is in developmental Stage 7 (see Space Supervision in Chapter XV). Where the tooth size–space available ratio is poor, the cuspid may be stopped in its eruption by the first primary molar or the primary molar may be hastened in its exfoliation.

Only rarely does the first bicuspid experience difficulty in erupting. Bicuspid rotations sometimes occur with uneven resorption of the roots of the primary molars (Fig. VI-60). If such rotations are seen to be developing, it is good practice to construct a space-maintainer, extract the primary molar (no earlier than Stage 7 of the developing bicuspid) and hold space for the erupting tooth.

Since the second bicuspid is the last of the mandibular succedaneous teeth to erupt, there will not be room for it if there has been a shortening of the dental arch perimeter by mesial movement of the first molar, nor will there be room for the second bicuspid if the tooth size–space available ratio is poor. When the second primary molar is lost prematurely, the erupting second molar often helps the first molar move mesially before the second bicuspid can erupt. The eruption of the mandibular second molar out of sequence may be a troublesome problem in space management if it is not detected early enough to maintain the arch perimeter. Before the primary molars are lost, a Mixed Dentition Analysis must be done to determine whether mesial movement of the first permanent molar need be controlled. When the leeway space is in-

Fig. VI-59.—A, a skull dissection of a completed adult dentition at approximately 18 years of age. Note the similarity of position of the developing third molars to that seen for second molars and first molars at earlier ages. **B,** a front view of the same specimen.

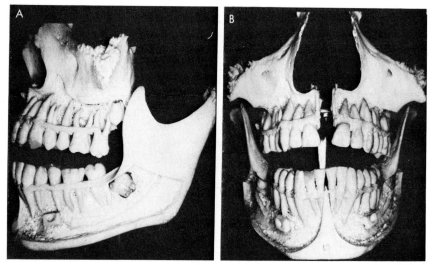

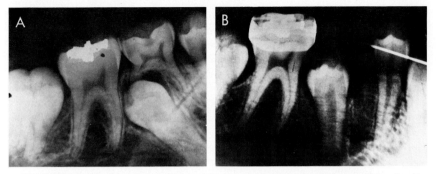

Fig. VI-60.—A, uneven resorption of the second primary molar resulting in displacement of the second premolar—or did the displacement of the second premolar cause the uneven resorption of the primary molar's roots? **B,** the spontaneous correction of the second primary premolar malposition after extraction of the primary predecessor.

sufficient, the first molar must not be allowed to move mesially until the second bicuspid has had a chance at its proper position in the arch.

Mandibular second bicuspids display extreme variation in their calcification and developmental schedule. Therefore, it is difficult to predict the exact time of their emergence in the mouth; besides, they often are congenitally missing. The determination of congenital absence of mandibular second bicuspids must be done carefully because of the wide developmental variability.

b) Maxilla

The sequence of eruption is typically different in the maxilla, being either first bicuspid, second bicuspid and cuspid or first bicuspid, cuspid and second bicuspid. Although the maxillary anterior segment is not prone to collapse lingually, since normally it is supported by the mandibular arch, it is, however, very easily displaced labially by thumbsucking, tongue-thrusting or a hyperactive mentalis muscle. Such displacement of the maxillary anterior segment affects the eruptive pattern of the cuspids and bicuspids. The maxillary first bicuspid usually erupts uneventfully, following the mandibular cuspid and/or the mandibular first bicuspid. Since the maxillary first bicuspid is very nearly the same size as its predecessor, usually neither the primary cuspid nor the primary second molar is displaced by its arrival. The greater mesiodistal width of the second primary molar permits easy eruption of the second bicuspid into its place in the arch. However, this leeway in the second bicuspid region may be necessary to provide space anteriorly for the accommodation of the wider permanent cuspid even though the anterior arc is increasing at this time. A tight situation exists in the maxillary arch, which is emphasized by the tendency to mesial drifting and the hazardous and circuitous eruptive course of the cuspid. There should be an excess of space in the arch when the second bicuspid arrives, the cuspid must follow immediately and the first permanent molar must not be allowed to rotate and tip mesially or the cuspid is likely to be blocked out of the arch in labioversion. The eruption of the second permanent molar ahead of a cuspid or bicuspid is thus as critical in the maxilla as in the mandible.

Davey[15] studied the effects of the loss of maxillary second primary molars on the position of the first permanent molars. He found that the earlier the primary teeth are lost the more mesial drifting of the permanent molar occurs, although timing has no effect on distal drifting of first primary molars or first bicuspids. Cusp height and leeway space affected the molar drift. More molar drifting occurred where the cusps were short and there was a shortage of leeway space. Occlusal relationships, caries and sex showed no effects on drifting.[15]

The maxillary cuspid follows a more difficult and tortuous path of eruption than any other tooth. At the age of 3 years it is high in the maxilla, with its crown directed mesially and somewhat lingually. It moves toward the occlusal plane, gradually uprighting itself until it seems to strike the distal aspect of the lateral incisor root, apparently becoming deflected to a more vertical position. It often erupts into the oral cavity with a marked mesial inclination, appearing high in the alveolar process, a cause for concern on the part of some parents. The cuspid's eruption closes the interdental spacing between the incisors, providing space for the final uprighting of the cuspid. When in its correct occlusal position, it has a slight mesial inclination. Should the arch length become shortened due to interproximal caries or an unfavorable sequence of eruption, the cuspid will have insufficient space for its final positioning. It is then left in labioversion with a decided mesial inclination. This maxillary malocclusion is analogous to the blocking out of a mandibular second bicuspid lingually. If arch length is short in both arches, the upper cuspid and lower second bicuspid arrive malposed because they are typically the last teeth ahead of the first molars to erupt in their respective arches.

6. SECOND MOLAR ERUPTION

Normally, the mandibular second molar arrives in the oral cavity after all the teeth anterior to it. When it precedes a second bicuspid, it may tip the first molar mesially, the sequelae to which have been discussed previously. The mandibular second molar typically erupts into the mouth before the maxillary second molar.

The maxillary second molar also should follow all of the teeth anterior to it into the arch. There is a greater tendency to loss of arch length in the maxilla when the primary teeth are lost prematurely. The eruption of the maxillary second molar ahead of the mandibular second molar is said to be symptomatic of a developing Class II malocclusion.[55] It also is seen with premature loss of maxillary primary molars and sometimes may be seen in skeletal Class II because there is even more space than normal in the maxilla for maxillary second molar development or less space in the shortened mandible for mandibular second molar development.

H. Dentitional and Occlusal Development in the Young Adult

1. THIRD MOLAR DEVELOPMENT

Third molars show no more variability in calcification and eruption than do any other teeth.[23] The third molar is unique among human teeth, since it displays no sexual differences in formation nor is its formation related as closely to somatic growth and sexual maturation as are the other teeth.[23] On the other hand, the third molar shows high constancy with its own pattern of development; that is, early calcifying third molars erupt early and complete their roots early.[23] There is evidence of ethnic differences, since the Finns acquire their third molars later than the Middle American whites studied by Garn *et al.*[23] Haralabakis[40] found Greeks with a mean eruption time of 24 years and Shourie[74] reported some South Indians erupting third molars as early as 13 years. North American Negroes erupt third molars earlier than do whites.[30]

Third molar agenesis occurs 16% of the time in Middle Western American whites.[23] When one or more third molars are missing there is a strong tendency for agenesis of other teeth, delayed formation of other posterior teeth, differences in developmental sequences, reduction in the size of other teeth and even delayed timing and eruptive movements of the third molar in the siblings of affected children.[24, 30] Since the third molar may not begin its calcification until as late as 14 years, the diagnosis of agenesis cannot always be made with certainty in the mixed dentition. However, it should be noted that there is symmetry of development, which aids in the diagnosis when one molar seems to be missing. When a third molar is missing, the clinician should not be surprised to see greater incidence of hypoplastic maxillary lateral incisors, less frequent eruption of second molars before second premolars and smaller than normal teeth.[30]

The question of the role of the third molar in the crowding of mandibular incisors during the late teen-age period has been much debated. A number of simultaneous phenomena confuse the issue: the arch perimeter shortens, the incisor crowding increases, the third molars develop and the mandible grows forward more than the maxilla. Events that occur together do not, of course, necessarily depend on one another. A firm stand cannot yet be taken, but it seems that the evidence leans toward absolving the third molar for the increased crowding.

Vego[78] and Keene[46] found that arches with third molars had more crowding of incisors than those without, but they also found, as did Garn *et al.*,[24] that the rest of the teeth are smaller when the third molars are absent. Bergstrom and Jensen,[4] studying incisor crowding by measurements on casts of subjects with unilateral absence of mandibular third molars, noted more crowding on the side where the third molar was present. Vego[78] and others refer to the "pressure" of third molars against the dental arch—but no one has measured it! Björk *et al.*[7] found incisor crowding correlated better with mandibular increments than with the eruption of third molars. More crowding is seen in males than in females. This observance is probably true because their mandibular increments are greater at this time.[7]

Fuder[20] could not show the mandibular third molar to be a primary cause of the increase in incisal crowding that often coincides with third molar development. He found the first molars farther forward and the incisors more procumbent in individuals with third molars than in those with third molar agenesis. However, he could not show, in his serial study, that the third molars played a primary role in the position of any teeth mesial to it, since the differences in first molar position and incisal procumbency appeared before significant development of the third molar. He suggested, therefore, that the position of the first molar may be a genetic manifestation, just as the third molar agenesis is.

2. DIMENSIONAL CHANGES

Dental arch length and perimeter decrease a surprising amount during the late adolescent and young adult period. Fisk[18] found that the mandibular perimeter decreased 5.0 mm. between 9 and 16 years of age and Knott[47] noted mandibular length shortening 3.0 mm. between 9 and 15 years. The respective maxillary measurements are about half these amounts. During these same periods, maxillary and mandibular arch widths increase 1–2 mm., but these increases are completed in both arches by 12 years. There are only a few studies of arch dimensional changes after age 15 years, but they show a continued shortening of the perimeter.

3. OCCLUSAL CHANGES

Both overbite and overjet decrease throughout the second decade of life, probably due to the relatively greater forward growth of the mandible. Björk *et al.*[6, 7] found that the changes in sagittal relationships of the dentitions could be better related to the growth of the jaws than to dental events; for example, the developmental course of the third molars. Fisk[18] noted that in the majority of his subjects the mandibular molar had a more forward occlusal relationship with age. Such posterior occlusal changes are due to the mesial drifting tendency, slight interproximal wear and, most importantly, the continuing growth of the mandible.

4. Resorption of Permanent Teeth

By the end of the second decade, most persons display idiopathic resorption of one or more teeth. Massler and Malone[57] found that nearly 90% of all teeth show some evidence of resorption by 19 years of age. Although most of the instances were mild and confined to apical blunting, nearly 10% showed between 2 mm. and 4 mm. of root resorption. There is a significant increase in the frequency of the more severe types of resorption with age and an increase in both the number of resorbed teeth and the severity of the resorption when orthodontic treatment has occurred. Teeth that are likely to resorb more rapidly during orthodontic therapy can be predicted quite well by a careful examination of the radiographs[57] prior to therapy. Obviously, there is a general potential for resorption of permanent teeth varying with the person and the tooth—a potential that may be triggered by orthodontic tooth movements.

5. Arrangement of the Teeth in the Jaws

Most reports of occlusion are concerned with the arrangement of the crowns of the teeth; however, Dempster *et al.*[16] have reported an exhaustive study of the relationship of the roots to the craniofacial skeleton. The bicuspid roots are the most nearly perpendicular to the plane of occlusion. The lower incisor cuspid and molar roots are directed obliquely backward. The roots of the maxillary teeth, anterior to the second bicuspid, are directed posteriorly and inward, whereas the roots of the maxillary molars are more vertical than the opposing lower molars.

A number of attempts have been made to describe the dental arc mathematically in an effort to seek a basic or ideal pattern. The line of occlusal contact between the upper and the lower teeth also has been studied many times and often is referred to as the occlusal curve, the occlusal plane (although it is not a plane), the curve of Spee, the compensating curve and so forth. Attempts have been made, in both the natural and artificial dentitions, to relate the occlusal curve to protrusive movements of the jaw. Finally, workers in prosthodontics have extended these ideas into a concept of a three-dimensional spherical curvature involving both the right and left posterior teeth and both mandibular condyles, suggesting that a sphere of 8 inches or 20 cm. in diameter was the "correct" dimension for all occlusal arc designs. Such ideas are based on the conjecture that the roots of the teeth converge to a center. The roots do not converge toward a common center and the occlusal surfaces of the posterior teeth cannot be fully congruent with the surface of any size sphere.[16] As might be expected, there is great variability in the positions of the teeth within the skull. It is obvious that any attempts to reduce all human occlusal patterns to one "ideal" or basic mean pattern are naïve at best and ridiculous at worst.

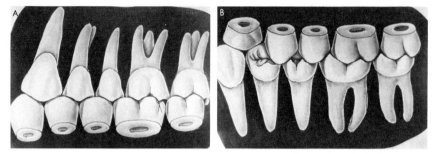

Fig. VI-61.—A, ideal intercuspation, buccal view. **B,** ideal intercuspation, lingual view.

I. Clinical Implications

1. Normal versus Ideal Occlusion

The word "normal" implies variations around an average or mean value, whereas "ideal" connotes a hypothetical concept or goal. There is a particular clinical difference between a "normal occlusion" and an "ideal occlusion." Unfortunately, the word *normal* has been used for years in orthodontics as a synonym for *ideal*, causing both semantic and treatment difficulties. It is perfectly proper to label as normal a mouth in which all of the teeth are present and occluding in a healthy, stable and pleasing manner but with variations in position within measurable normal limits. Perhaps no one has ever seen a perfect or ideal occlusion, but that does not diminish the practical use of the concept, for every dentist treating occlusions must have an ideal pattern in mind even if he never achieves it. Nature herself rarely shows an ideal occlusion. Her best effort usually is within a range of normality. It is perfectly reasonable, when planning orthodontic treatment, to have in mind the image of ideal intercuspation (Fig. VI-61). It also is perfectly proper and practical to accept at the end of treatment an arrangement of the teeth within the jaws in positions that are neither ideal nor normal but may be stable in a particular person's face.

2. Models of Occlusion

Occlusion is said to be the common theme of all branches of dentistry, but the concepts of occlusion that are held by practitioners of the different dental fields tend to be contradictory. The working clinical occlusal hypotheses of one field are not applicable, understood or used in another branch of dentistry. Any one of a number of mental images or models of occlusion may be in a dentist's mind. Some regard human occlusion as a very precise machine, the fit of whose parts must be done with great care. As in any machine, all parts are needed for it to run well.

Such a model does not explain where the energy that runs the machine originates and avoids the important aspect of control of the machine. Another occlusal model suggested is that of teaching a pet a new trick. Such a concept introduces the idea of neuromuscular learning. All tricks cannot be learned by all and some learn better than others. It is the dentist's duty to decide which "tricks" patients should learn for their own benefit. A patient must be taught how to adapt to a new set of dentures, for example, and once the "trick" of handling the dentures is learned the problem is over. The difficulty with this concept is that there are innumerable occlusal "tricks" that cannot be mastered by any patient. No person with a Class II skeletal pattern and occlusion can "learn" to hold his jaw forward in a more favorable Class I occlusal relationship because the conscious cortical control of this new mandibular position is constantly overcome by the more primitive reflexes that tend to maintain the mandible more posteriorly. Tulley, an English orthodontist, has likened the treatment of occlusion to playing a never-ending game of chess with the devil. The dentist sits down after the game has started and is not always able to guess what moves have been made previously. The rules that govern the game have not all been chosen by the clinician, that is, the rules of bone biology, nerve physiology, muscle learning, psychology and so forth. The rules change as the game progresses or conditions alter. The analogy breaks down when one asks "What is winning?" There is no victor; it is enough to keep the game going. Life, after all, is more than the mere maintenance of structures; events must be kept going, functions must be perpetuated.

3. OCCLUSAL ADAPTIVE MECHANISMS

What, then, is good occlusion? What concept or model of occlusion should the dentist have? That of normal? Ideal? Perhaps that occlusion is best which best adapts to its changing functions. Such a concept implies that adaptive mechanisms are present and necessary and that there are feedback mechanisms from the occlusal system that help provide occlusal homeostasis. Any occlusal treatment that lacks functional homeostasis is destined to clinical failure.

A look at Table VI-6 reveals the adaptive mechanisms of the dentition, bone and musculature through various stages of occlusal development and maintenance. In youth, during development, dental eruption, tooth movements and the wear and loss of primary teeth provide the period of greatest dental adaptability. The alveolar process during growth is highly adaptable, as is the craniofacial skeleton. Childhood also is a period of developmental neuromuscular learning. Clinical treatment at this time can take advantage of these responsive adaptive mechanisms.

In the healthy adult, however, most of the dental adaptive mechanisms have been lost except for wear, extrusion of the teeth, the anterior component of force and drifting. The only bony adaptations left are those

TABLE VI-6.—Mechanisms of Adaptation

	Dentition	Bone	Musculature
Developing dentition	Eruption and tooth movement	Growth	Learning, imprinting
Healthy adult dentition	Wear, extrusion, anterior component	Repair	Supportive occlusal reflexes
Deteriorating adult dentition	Reconstructive dentistry	Resorption pathology	Traumatic occlusal reflexes; protective occlusal responses
Edentulous adult	Prosthetic dentistry	Resorption	Loss of sensory input

of repair, since growth is largely over. Protective reflexes are constant adaptations but some such reflexes (see Chapter V) can be destructive. The supportive occlusal reflexes, for example, the unconscious swallow, can be stabilizing to the occlusion of the adult although not adaptive.

If the adult dentition begins to deteriorate, there are no natural means left for dental adaptation and they must be provided by reconstructive dentistry. Pathologic bone loss provides adaptation of a kind but it must not be allowed to proceed and the dentist, during therapy, attempts to restore the conditions providing bone repair. Occlusal equilibration procedures may obliterate potentially destructive reflexes. After disease and tooth loss have occurred, when growth no longer is possible, and when many of the healthy reparative processes have gone, occlusal treatment becomes a very difficult problem if functional homeostasis is to be achieved.

Finally, in the edentulous adult there are no natural dental adaptive mechanisms left and the prosthesis made by the dentist adapts and changes entirely differently than the natural dentition did. Resorption of bone is the most common bony adaptive function now seen, for the neuromusculature shows very diminished conditioning possibilities. Therefore, the prosthetic occlusion usually is established within the bounds of the most primitively controlled neuromuscular restrictions, that is, the mandibulomaxillary relationship determined by the unconscious swallow.

In summary, clinical goals are not necessarily either normal or ideal. Rather, they are pragmatic; that is, they are determined by the conditions of the individual patient. The determining factors are the adaptive mechanisms the clinician can yet best utilize. The goal of occlusal treatment is not just to maintain structures. It is not to meet some hypothetical norm or idea. Rather, it is to keep events going. That occlusion is best which most easily provides continuing functional homeostasis.

REFERENCES

1. Altemus, L. A.: Frequency of the incidence of malocclusion in American Negro children aged twelve to sixteen, Angle Orthodont. 29:189, 1959.
2. Arnold, E.: A Study of the Significance of the Interdental Spacing in the Primary Dentition, Thesis, School of Dentistry, University of Michigan, Ann Arbor, 1954.
3. Baume, L. J.: Physiologic tooth migration and its significance for the development of occlusion: II. The biogenesis of the accessional dentition, J. Dent. Res. 29:331, 1950.
4. Bergstrom, K., and Jensen, R.: The significance of the third molars in the aetiology of crowding; a biometric study of unilateral aplasia of the third molars, Tr. European Orthodont. Soc. 36:84, 1960.
5. Biederman, W.: Etiology and treatment of tooth ankylosis, Am. J. Orthodont. 48:670, 1962.
6. Björk, A.: Estimation of age changes in overjet and sagittal jaw relation, Tr. European Orthodont. Soc. 29:240, 1953.
7. Björk, A., Jensen, E., and Palling, M.: Mandibular growth and third molar impaction, Acta odont. scandinav. 14:231, 1956.
8. Bodegam, J. C.: Experiments on Tooth Eruption in Miniature Pigs. Thesis, University of Nijmegen, 1969.
9. Bradley, R. E.: The relationship between eruption, calcification, and crowding of certain mandibular teeth, Angle Orthodont. 31:230, 1961.
10. Brown, R. V.: Pattern and frequency of congenital absence of teeth, Iowa D. J. 43:60, 1957.
11. Burdi, A. R., and Lillie, J. H.: A catenary analysis of the maxillary dental arch during human embryogenesis, Anat. Rec. 154:13, 1966.
12. Butler, P. M.: Tooth Morphology and Primate Evolution, in Brothwell, D. R. (ed.), *Dental Anthropology* (New York: Pergamon Press, 1963), Vol. V, pp. 1–14.
13. Clinch, L.: Variations in the mutual relationships of the upper and lower gum pads in the newborn child, Brit. Soc. Study Orthodont. Tr., pp. 91–107, 1932.
14. Clinch, L.: An analysis of serial models between three and eight years of age, Dent. Rec. 71:61, 1951.
15. Davey, K. W.: Effect of premature loss of deciduous molars on antero-posterior position of maxillary first permanent molars and other maxillary teeth, J. Canad. D. A. 32:406, 1966; also J. Dent. Child. 34:383, 1967.
16. Dempster, W. T., Adams, W. J., and Duddles, R. A.: Arrangement in the jaws of the roots of the teeth, J.A.D.A. 67:779, 1963.
17. Falkner, F.: Deciduous tooth eruption, Arch. Dis. Childhood 32:386, 1957.
18. Fisk, R. O.: Normal mandibular arch changes between ages 9–16, J. Canad. D. A. 32:652, 1966.
19. Flemming, H. B.: An investigation of the vertical overbite during the eruption of the permanent dentition, Angle Orthodont. 31:53, 1961.
20. Fuder, E. J.: A Study of Changes in the Mandibular Arch during the Second and Third Decade. Thesis, Horace H. Rackham School of Graduate Studies, University of Michigan, Ann Arbor, 1969.
21. Garn, S. M.: The genetics of normal human growth, De Genetica Medica-Paris II, Edizioni Dell Instituto "Gregorio Mendel," Rome, 1962.
22. Garn, S. M., and Lewis, A. B.: Tooth-size, body-size and "giant" fossil man, Am. J. Anthropol. 61:874, 1958.
23. Garn, S. M., Lewis, A. B., and Bonne, B.: Third molar formation and its development course, Angle Orthodont. 32:270, 1962.
24. Garn, S. M., Lewis, A. B., and Kerewsky, R.: Third molar agenesis and variation in size of the remaining teeth, Nature, London 201:839, 1964.
25. Garn, S. M., Lewis, A. B., and Kerewsky, R. S.: X-linked inheritance of tooth size, J. Dent. Res. 44:439, 1965.
26. Garn, S. M., Lewis, A. B., and Kerewsky, R. S.: The meaning of bilateral asymmetry in the permanent dentition, Angle Orthodont. 36:55, 1966.
27. Garn, S. M., Lewis, A. B., Koski, K., and Polacheck, D. L.: The sex difference in tooth calcification, J. Dent. Res. 37:561, 1958.
28. Garn, S. M., Lewis, A. B., and Polacheck, D. L.: Variability of tooth formation, J. Dent. Res. 38:135, 1959.
29. Garn, S. M., and Rohmann, C.: Interaction of nutrition and genetics in the timing of growth, Pediat. Clin. North America 13:353, 1966.
30. Garn, S. M., Lewis, A. B., and Vicinius, T. H.: Third molar polymorphism and its significance to dental genetics, J. Dent. Res. 42:1344, 1963.

31. Garn, S. M., Burdi, A. R., Miller, R. L., and Nagy, J.: Prenatal origins of postnatal dental variability. (Abstract), Am. J. Phys. Anthropol. 33:130, 1970.

31a. Garn, S. M., Lewis, A. B., and Walenga, A. J.: Maximum-confidence values for the human mesiodistal crown dimension of human teeth, Arch. Oral Biol. 13:841, 1968.

32. Giles, N. B., Knott, V., and Meredith, H. V.: Increase in intraoral height of selected permanent teeth during the quadrennium following gingival emergence, Angle Orthodont. 33:195, 1963.

33. Gowgiel, J. M.: Experiments in tooth eruption, J. Dent. Res. 40:736, 1961. (Abstract.)

34. Grahnen, H.: *Hypodontia in the Permanent Dentition; A Clinical and Genetical Investigation* (Lund: Gleerup, 1956) (Odont. Rev. Vol. 7, supp. 3, 1956).

35. Grainger, R. M., and Paynter, K. J.: Relation of nutrition to the morphology and size of rat molar teeth, J. Canad. D. A. 22:519, 1956.

36. Grainger, R. M., and Paynter, K. J.: Influence of nutrition and genetics on morphology and caries susceptibility, J.A.M.A. 177:306, 1961.

37. Grainger, R. M., and Paynter, K. J.: Relationship of morphology and size of teeth to caries, Internat. Dent. J. 12:147, 1962.

38. Gregg, J. M.: Immobilization of the erupting molar in the Syrian hamster, J. Dent. Res. 44:1219, 1965.

39. Griewe, P. W.: Tooth Size and Symmetry in the Human Dentition, M.S. thesis, State University of Iowa, Iowa City, 1949.

40. Haralabakis, H.: Observations on the time of eruption, congenital absence, and impaction of the third molar teeth, Tr. European Orthodont. Soc. 33:308, 1957.

41. Harvold, E. P.: Some biological aspects of orthodontic treatment in the transitional dentition, Am. J. Orthodont. 49:1, 1963.

42. Hatton, M.: A measure of the effects of heredity and environment on eruption of the deciduous teeth, J. Dent. Res. 34:397, 1955.

43. Hurme, V. O.: Ranges of normalcy in the eruption of permanent teeth, J. Dent. Child. 16:11, 1949.

44. Jarvis, A.: The Role of Dental Caries in Space Closure in the Mixed Dentition. Thesis, Faculty of Dentistry, University of Toronto, Canada, 1952.

45. Johns, E. E., and Moyers, R. E.: Unpublished data.

46. Keene, H. J.: Third molar agenesis, spacing and crowding of teeth and tooth size in caries-resistant naval recruits, Am. J. Orthodont. 50:445, 1964.

47. Knott, V.: Size and form of the dental arches in children with good occlusion studied longitudinally from age 9 years to late adolescence, Am. J. Phys. Anthropol. 19:263, 1961.

48. Knott, V., and Meredith, H. V.: Statistics on eruption of the permanent dentition from serial data for North American white children, Angle Orthodont. 36:68, 1966.

49. Kraus, B. S., and Jordan, R. E.: *The Human Dentition Before Birth* (Philadelphia: Lea & Febiger, 1965).

50. Krogman, W. M.: Role of genetic factors in the human face, jaws and teeth: A review, Eugenics Rev. 59:165, 1967.

51. Lamont, I.: Arch Length—Tooth Size and Distoclusion; Their Relationship to A-B Point Differences. Thesis, School of Dentistry, University of Michigan, Ann Arbor, 1964.

52. Lasker, G. W.: Genetic analysis of racial traits of the teeth, Cold Spring Harbor Symp. Quant. Biol. 15:191, 1950.

53. Lauterstien, A. M., Pruzansky, S., and Barber, T. K.: Effect of deciduous mandibular molar pulpotomy on the eruption of succedaneous premolar, J. Dent. Res. 41:1367, 1962.

54. Lewis, A. B., and Garn, S. M.: The relationship between tooth formation and other maturational factors, Angle Orthodont. 30:70, 1960.

55. Lo, R. T., and Moyers, R. E.: Studies in the etiology and prevention of malocclusion. I. The sequence of eruption of the permanent dentition, Am. J. Orthodont. 39:460, 1953.

56. Maher, J. F.: Mandibular Arch Development in the Late Mixed Dentition. Thesis, School of Dentistry, University of Michigan, Ann Arbor, 1955.

57. Massler, M., and Malone, A. J.: Root resorption in human permanent teeth, Am. J. Orthodont. 40:619, 1954.

58. Meredith, H. V.: Order and age of eruption for the deciduous dentition, J. Dent. Res. 25:43, 1946.

59. Meredith, H. V.: Relation between the eruption of selected mandibular teeth and the circumpuberal acceleration in stature, J. Dent. Child. 25:75, 1959.

60. Micklow, J. B.: A Cephalometric and Cast Analysis of the Changes which Occur at the Terminal Plane from the Primary Through the Permanent Dentition. Thesis, School of Dentistry, University of Michigan, Ann Arbor, 1964.

61. Moorrees, C.: *The Dentition of the Growing Child: A Longitudinal Study of Dental*

Development between 3 and 18 Years of Age (Cambridge, Mass.: Harvard University Press, 1959).

62. Moorrees, C., and Chadha, J. M.: Available space for the incisors during dental development—growth study based on physiologic age, Angle Orthodont. 35:12, 1965.
63. Moorrees, C. F. A., and Reed, R. B.: Correlations among crown diameters of human teeth, Arch. Oral Biol. 9:685, 1964.
64. Moyers, R. E., Castelli, P., and Kott, D.: The relationship between tooth development and eruption. Unpublished data.
65. Murray, J. J.: Dynamics of occlusal adjustment; a cephalometric analysis, Alumni Bulletin, School of Dentistry, University of Michigan 61:32, 1959.
66. Nolla, C.: Development of the permanent teeth, J. Dent. Child. 27:254, 1960.
67. Obersztyn, A.: Experimental investigation of factors causing resorption of deciduous teeth, J. Dent. Res. 42:660, 1963.
68. Pulver, F.: The etiology and prevalence of ectopic eruption of the maxillary first permanent molar, J. Dent. Child. 35:138, 1968.
69. Raak, K. D.: The Mesiodistal Diameter of the Deciduous Teeth, M.S. thesis, State University of Iowa, Iowa City, 1950.
70. Richardson, A. S., and Castaldi, C. R.: Dental development during the first two years of life, J. Canad. D. A. 33:418, 1967.
71. Rose, J. S.: A survey of congenitally missing teeth, excluding third molars, in 6000 orthodontic patients, Brit. Soc. Study Orthodont. Tr., pp. 75–82, 1966.
72. Scott, J. H.: What determines the form of the dental arches? Orthodont. Rec. 1:15, 1958.
73. Seipel, C. M.: Variations of tooth position, Svensk tand.-tidsk., Vol. 39, 1946.
74. Shourie, K. L.: Eruption age of teeth in India, Indian J. Med. Res. 43:105, 1946.
75. Shumaker, D. B., and El Hadary, M. S.: Roentgenographic study of eruption, J.A.D.A. 61:535, 1960.
76. Sillman, J. H.: Relationship of maxillary and mandibular gum pads in the newborn infant, Am. J. Orthodont. 24:409, 1938.
77. Sillman, J. H.: Dimensional changes of the dental arches: Longitudinal study from birth to 25 years, Am. J. Orthodont. 50:824, 1964.
78. Vego, L.: A longitudinal study of mandibular arch perimeter, Angle Orthodont. 32:187, 1962.
79. West, C. M.: The development of the gums and their relationship to the deciduous teeth in the human fetus, Contrib. Embryol. 16:25, 1925.
80. Witzky, H. P.: A Longitudinal Cephalometric Evaluation of the Mandibular Dental Arch. Thesis, School of Dentistry, University of Michigan, Ann Arbor, 1961.

VII

Etiology of Malocclusion

Happy is he who has been able to learn the causes of things.—VIRGIL, Georgics, I, line 490.

A. **The orthodontic equation**

B. **Primary etiologic sites**
   1. Neuromuscular system
   2. Bone
   3. Teeth
   4. Soft parts (excluding muscle)

C. **Time**

D. **Causes and clinical entities**
   1. Heredity
   2. Developmental defects of unknown origin
   3. Trauma
      a) Prenatal trauma and birth injuries
         1) Hypoplasia of the mandible
         2) "Vogelgesicht"
         3) Position of the fetus
      b) Postnatal trauma
         1) Fractures of jaws and teeth
         2) Habits
   4. Physical agents
      a) Premature extraction of primary teeth
      b) Nature of food
   5. Habits
      a) Thumb-sucking and finger-sucking
      b) Tongue-thrusting
      c) Lip-sucking and lip-biting
      d) Posture
      e) Nail-biting
      f) Other habits
   6. Disease
      a) Systemic diseases
      b) Endocrine disorders
      c) Local diseases

1) Nasopharyngeal diseases and disturbed respiratory function
2) Gingival and periodontal diseases
3) Tumors
4) Caries
   (a) Premature loss of primary teeth
   (b) Disturbances in sequence of eruption of permanent teeth
   (c) Loss of permanent teeth
7. Malnutrition

E. Summary

THE MAJORITY of malocclusions requiring comprehensive treatment result from one of two conditions: (1) a relative discrepancy between the sizes of the teeth and the sizes of the jaws available to accommodate those teeth and (2) disharmonious facial skeletal patterns. Both of these general conditions are innate to the patient and essentially are genetically determined. There are familial dispositions to large-sized teeth as there are to mandibular prognathism. Since these two problems are so frequent and so serious, it is difficult to write about the etiology of all malocclusions and at the same time maintain perspective for the student or inexperienced clinician.

Etiology of malocclusion often is approached by classifying all "causes" of malocclusion as local factors or systemic factors; perhaps they are termed intrinsic and extrinsic. Such a system is revealing but difficult; for example, one author considers thumb-sucking an extrinsic factor whereas another terms it a local factor. That which is most needed by the reader is the thing most difficult to convey by writing— perspective—for often more space is needed to describe the origins of significant but infrequent problems than is required for the most common severe types of malocclusion.

Little is known concerning all of the initial causes of dentofacial deformity. Confusion is due to the study of etiology from the point of view of the final clinical entity. This approach is difficult because many malocclusions that appear similar, and are classified alike, do not have the same etiologic pattern. It is almost traditional to discuss etiology in this manner; that is, beginning with a clinical classification and working back to the causes. Ideally, the study of etiology should begin with the original cause. Since knowledge in this area is scanty, this discussion of etiology will center on the tissue primarily involved.

The idea of discussing etiology in terms of the primary tissue site was first suggested by Dockrell,[4] was used in earlier editions of this book and later was adopted by such prominent orthodontic scholars as Mayne,[11] Harvold[7] and Moore.[12] Until more real knowledge of the etiology of specific malocclusions is available, it is practical and meaningful to discuss the primary tissue sites in which malocclusions arise.

CAUSES———ACT AT——▸TIMES————ON————▸TISSUES——PRODUCING——▸RESULTS

Fig. VII-1.—The orthodontic equation. (Figs. VII-1–VII-6 from Dockrell.[4])

A. The Orthodontic Equation

The equation shown in Figure VII-1 is a brief expression of the development of any and all dentofacial deformities. A certain original cause acts for a time at a site and produces a result. It is a simplistic expression of Koch's postulates, but it is an oversimplification to assume that Koch's logic applies to developmental problems, e.g., malocclusions, for there are few *specific* causes of precise malocclusions. Tuberculosis may always be caused by *Mycobacterium tuberculosis* but open bite is not always caused by thumb-sucking.

Since we cannot isolate and identify all of the original causes, they may be studied best by grouping them as follows: (1) heredity, (2) developmental causes of unknown origin, (3) trauma, (4) physical agents, (5) habits, (6) disease and (7) malnutrition. It will be seen that there is a certain overlapping of these groups. The duration of operation of these causes and the age at which they are seen are both functions of *time,* and thus may be grouped together under this heading. The primary sites principally involved are: (1) the bones of the facial skeleton, (2) the teeth, (3) the neuromuscular system and (4) the soft parts, excepting muscle. It will be noted that each of the regions involved is made up of a different tissue. Bone, muscle and teeth grow at different rates and in different manners. They adapt to environmental impact in different ways. Regardless of the original cause of a growth variation, it must

Fig. VII-2.—The orthodontic equation elaborated.

CAUSES——ACT AT——▸TIMES————ON————▸TISSUES——PRODUCING——▸RESULTS

SOME PREDISPOSING	PRENATAL OR	SOME PRIMARILY	MAY BE THE FOLLOWING
SOME EXCITING	POSTNATAL	SOME SECONDARILY	OR A COMBINATION OF THESE
1. HEREDITY	1. CONTINUOUS OR INTERMITTENT	1. NEUROMUSCULAR TISSUE	1. MALFUNCTION
2. DEVELOPMENTAL CAUSES OF UNKNOWN ORIGIN	2. MAY ACT AT DIFFERENT AGE LEVELS	2. TEETH	2. MALOCCLUSION
3. TRAUMA		3. BONE AND CARTILAGE	3. OSSEOUS DYSPLASIA
4. PHYSICAL AGENTS		4. SOFT TISSUES—OTHER THAN MUSCLES	
5. HABITS			
6. DISEASE			
7. MALNUTRITION			

be remembered that the place where that cause shows its effect is most important. The difference in tissue response during development is a determining factor in differentiating between many similarly appearing clinical problems. Rarely is one site alone involved; usually others become affected, and we term one the site primarily involved and consider the others as being secondarily concerned. The result is malocclusion, malfunction or osseous dysplasia—more probably a combination of all three. The orthodontic equation thus developed is shown in Figure VII-2. The outline for this chapter is based largely on an elaboration of the parts of Dockrell's equation.

We are now in a position to observe clearly the difference, from the standpoint of etiology, between malocclusion, malfunction and osseous dysplasia. If teeth are involved, malocclusion results; if the neuromuscular system is involved, the result is muscle malfunction; if bones are involved, an osseous dysplasia results. Most clinical problems are a combination of variations from the normal or expected in these three tissue systems. Indeed, malocclusion, in contrast to disease or pathology, may be the result of a combination of minor variations from the normal. Each variation itself is too mild to be classed as "abnormal," but the combination summates to produce a malocclusion. Most malocclusions are simply clinically significant deviations from the expected or normal range of growth.

B. Primary Etiologic Sites

1. NEUROMUSCULAR SYSTEM

The muscle groups that serve most frequently as primary etiologic sites are (1) the muscles of mastication (Vth cranial nerve), (2) the muscles of facial expression (VIIth cranial nerve) and (3) the tongue, but their many elaborate nerve connections are involved as well. These include the various ganglia in and around the facial area; the centers of coordination, integration and inhibition in the midbrain and external cortex; and the many sensory fibers supplying the teeth, oral and pharyngeal mucosa, muscles, tendons and skin.

The neuromuscular system plays its primary role in the etiology of dentofacial deformity by the effects of reflex contractions on the bony skeleton and the dentition. Both bones and teeth are affected by the many functional activities of the orofacial region. The region is a source of enormous and varied sensory input making possible an infinite variety of reflex activities, all of which help determine the skeletal form and the occlusal stability. More complete discussions of the interrelationships between muscle and bone and muscle and teeth will be found in Chapters IV, V and VI.

Figure VII-3 is a scheme depicting the possible roles of the neuromusculature in the etiology of dentofacial deformity. By far the most important part of the diagram are the words "habits" and "contraction

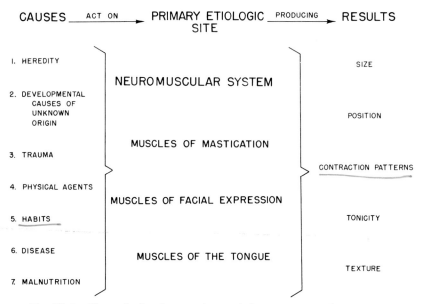

Fig. VII-3.—The orthodontic equation and the neuromuscular system.

patterns." Imbalancing contraction patterns are a part of nearly all malocclusions.

Treatment of clinical problems that have their primary etiologic site in the neuromuscular system must involve conditioning reflexes to bring about a more favorable functional environment for the growing craniofacial skeleton and the developing dentition and occlusion.

2. BONE

Since the bones of the face (particularly the maxilla and mandible) serve as bases for the dental arches, aberrations in their growth may alter occlusal relationships and functioning. Most orthodontic problems of skeletal origin are due to a misfit of bony parts. Osseous dysplasia is far more frequent than grossly abnormal size of a bone. Read Chapter IV carefully for an understanding of the importance of the growth of the craniofacial skeleton. Many of the most common serious malocclusions are skeletal in origin. The cephalometric procedure (see Chapter XII) aids in the identification and localization of regions of osseous disharmony. Figure VII-4 shows how the groups of initial causes, acting on bone as a primary etiologic site, give rise to clinical orthodontic problems.

Treatment of osseous dysplasia must either (1) alter the growing craniofacial skeleton or (2) camouflage its disharmony by moving teeth

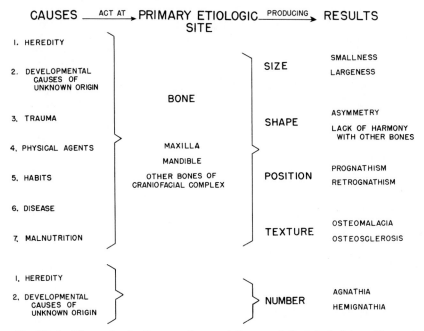

Fig. VII-4.—The orthodontic equation and the craniofacial skeleton. Terms in the right-hand column are names given some of the clinical problems originating in the craniofacial skeleton.

to mask the unfortunate skeletal pattern. Many recent studies have shown that orthodontic therapy has a far more marked effect on the craniofacial skeleton than previously was thought (see Chapter IV, Section K).

3. TEETH

The teeth may be a primary site in the etiology of dentofacial deformity in many varied ways. Gross variations in size and shape are encountered frequently and always are of concern. Decreases or increases in the regular number of teeth will give rise to malocclusion and/or malfunction. The matter of abnormal position is so obvious that it scarcely needs mention. Often forgotten is the possibility that malpositions of teeth can induce malfunction and, hence, indirectly through the malfunction, alter the growth of the bones. One of the most frequent causes of orthodontic problems is teeth that are too large for the arches in which they are found (or arches too small for the teeth they hold). Figure VII-5 shows how clinical problems may result from the action on teeth, as a primary etiologic site, by any of the groups of original causes.

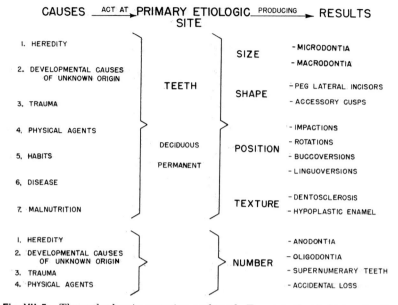

Fig. VII-5.—The orthodontic equation and teeth. Terms in the right-hand column are names given clinical problems that originate in the dentition.

Fig. VII-6.—The orthodontic equation and soft tissues (other than neuromuscular tissue). Terms in the right-hand column are some of those used to describe variations seen in these tissues.

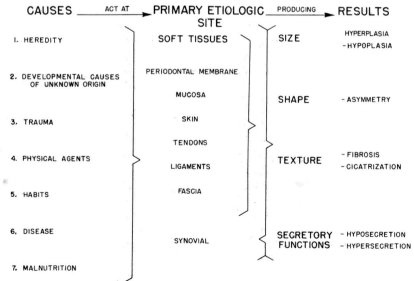

Treatment of malocclusions that originate within the dentition is carried out by moving teeth, which is very different from conditioning reflexes or directing bone growth.

4. SOFT PARTS (EXCLUDING MUSCLE)

The role of the soft tissues, other than neuromuscular, in the etiology of malocclusion is not so clearly discernible, nor is it as important as that of the three sites discussed previously. Any factor that upsets or appreciably alters the physiologic status of any part of the masticatory system may come to be indicted as an etiologic matter of importance (Fig. VII-6).

C. Time

The time factor in the development of malocclusion has two components: the period during which the cause operates and the age at which it is seen. It should be noted that the length of time that a certain cause may be operative is not always continual; in fact, it may cease and recur in an intermittent fashion. From an etiologic point of view, the most useful division of the age component is into those causes active prenatally and those whose effects are noted only after birth. A cause may be either continual or intermittent and it may show its effect either prenatally or postnatally.

D. Causes and Clinical Entities

With the foregoing brief description of the orthodontic equation, we are now in a position to discuss the various groups of causes and their specific clinical manifestations. In some instances, something is known about the effect of a specific cause on the growth pattern of the face but, for the most part, we are forced to generalize and group similar causes for discussion.

1. HEREDITY

Familial resemblances of tooth arrangement and facial contour are well known, for heredity has long been indicted as a chief cause of malocclusion. Aberrations of genetic origin may make their appearance prenatally or they may not be seen until many years after birth, e.g., patterns of tooth eruption. The role of heredity in craniofacial growth and the etiology of dentofacial deformities has been the subject of many research and clinical studies, yet surprisingly little is really known. For a discussion of the genetic aspects of the growth of the craniofacial skeleton read Chapter IV, Section G. The genetics of tooth and occlusal development are described in Chapter VI. Very little is yet understood concerning the part genes play in the maturation of the

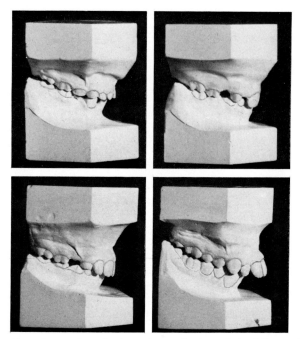

Fig. VII-7.—Genetics and occlusion; the occlusion of 4 siblings. Occlusion is similar enough to look like serial record casts of the same individual.

orofacial musculature (see Chapter V). Interesting familial resemblances are seen frequently (Fig. VII-7), yet the mode of transmission or even the site of gene action is not understood, except for a few cleancut problems, for example, absence of teeth or some gross craniofacial syndromes. Scant though our quantified knowledge may be, all are agreed that heredity plays a major role in the etiology of dentofacial anomalies.

2. Developmental Defects of Unknown Origin

These are largely anomalies originating in failure of an embryonic tissue, or part, to differentiate properly. Most such aberrations, therefore, make their appearance prenatally and are gross defects of a rare or infrequent type. Examples are absence of certain muscles, facial clefts, micrognathia, oligodontia and anodontia.

3. Trauma

Both prenatal trauma to the fetus and postnatal injuries may result in dentofacial deformity.

a) *Prenatal Trauma and Birth Injuries*

1) HYPOPLASIA OF THE MANDIBLE.—This can be caused by intrauterine pressure or trauma during delivery.

2) "VOGELGESICHT."—This is inhibited growth of the mandible due to ankylosis of the temporomandibular joint. The ankylosis may be a developmental defect or may be due to trauma at birth.

3) POSITION OF THE FETUS.—A knee or a leg may press against the face in such a manner as to promote asymmetry of facial growth or to cause retardation of mandibular development.

b) *Postnatal Trauma*

1) FRACTURES OF JAWS AND TEETH.

2) HABITS (see Section D-5, p. 252).—These may produce low-grade trauma that is operative over an extended period.

4. PHYSICAL AGENTS

a) *Premature Extraction of Primary Teeth*

Since this usually is due to caries, it is discussed under Disease (Section D-6, p. 260).

b) *Nature of Food*

It has been shown repeatedly that absence from the diet of rough and coarse food that requires thorough chewing is a factor in the production of maldevelopment of the dental arches. People existing on a primitive fibrous diet stimulate their muscles to work more and thus increase the load of function on the teeth. This type of diet usually produces less caries (less substrate for cariogenic organisms), greater mean arch width and increased wear of the occlusal surfaces of the teeth (Fig. VII-8). The importance of occlusal wear in the transitional denti-

Fig. VII-8.—Occlusal wear of primary teeth. Typical of occlusal wear seen among many people who exist on a primitive, coarse diet. The two pictured are Greek children from the mountain province of Euritania.

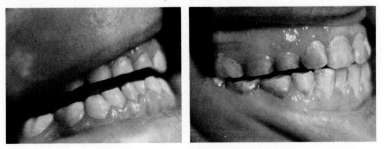

tion is discussed at length in Chapter VI. The evidence seems conclusive that our highly refined, soft, pappy modern diets play a role in the etiology of some malocclusions. Lack of adequate function results in contraction of the dental arches, insufficient occlusal wear and absence of occlusal adjustment normally seen in the maturing dentition. For a discussion of the role of function in the growth of the craniofacial skeleton see Chapter IV, Section I.

5. HABITS

All habits are learned patterns of muscle contraction of a very complex nature. Certain habits serve as stimuli to normal growth of the jaws; for example, normal lip action and proper mastication. The abnormal habits that may interfere with the regular pattern of facial growth must be differentiated from the desired normal habits that are a part of normal oropharyngeal function and thus play an important role in craniofacial growth and occlusal physiology. The habits of concern to us here are those likely to be involved in the etiology of malocclusion. The maturation of the orofacial musculature, in its normative role, is discussed in Chapter V. Deleterious habitual patterns of muscle behavior often are associated with perverted or impeded osseous growth, tooth malpositions, disturbed breathing habits, difficulties in speech, upset balance in the facial musculature and psychologic problems. Therefore, one cannot correct malocclusion without involvement in habits. Bottle-fed babies more frequently display undesirable sucking habits if the bottle has been used as a device to quiet them and induce sleep. After such a child is weaned, he learns to suck his thumb or finger while going to sleep. Many mothers will say that their child never sucks his thumb "except when he goes to bed." Other children learn early that the surest way to attract parental attention is to suck their fingers. Later, the dentist must not forget that the sudden cessation of a habit that has been active for several years may have a tremendous psychologic impact on the child.

a) Thumb-Sucking and Finger-Sucking

Digital sucking is practiced by many children for a variety of reasons; however, if it is not directly involved in the production or maintenance of malocclusion, it probably should not be of primary clinical concern to the dentist. As we shall see, most digital sucking habits begin very early in life and frequently are outgrown by 3 or 4 years of age. Unfortunately, dentists see few children before this time. Often the family physician or pediatrician attending so young a child is unaware of the possible dental complications resulting from these habits. It should be remembered that many children practice digital sucking habits without any evident dentofacial deformity, but it also is true that the digital sucking pressure habit may be a direct cause of a severe malocclusion.

The mechanotherapy for the treatment of the resulting malocclusion may be easy but the psychologic implications of the therapy are less clearly understood and occasionally seem to have been overstated. Therefore, the attention of the dentist often is directed to the thumb-sucker as well as to the malocclusion.

The time of appearance of digital sucking habits has some significance. Those that appear during the very first weeks of life are typically related to feeding problems. The neonate surely is not yet involved in sibling rivalries, and his insecurities are related to such primitive demands as hunger. However, some children do not begin to suck a thumb or finger until it is used as a teething device during the difficult eruption of a primary molar. Still later, some children use digital sucking for the release of emotional tensions with which they are unable to cope, taking solace in regressing to an infantile behavior pattern. All digital sucking habits should be studied for their psychologic implications, for they may be related to hunger, satisfying of the sucking instinct, insecurity or even a desire to attract attention.

Developmental psychologists have produced a number of theories to explain "non-nutritive digital sucking" (as they term it). Most early ideas concerning digital sucking were firmly based on classic Freudian theory. Freud[6] suggested that orality in the infant is related to pregenital organization and the sexual activity is not yet separated from the taking of nourishment. Thus, the object of one activity, thumb-sucking, also is that of another, nursing. A logical development of this theory relates to attempts to stop the thumb-sucking habit, for the Freudian belief holds that an abrupt interference with such a basic mechanism will likely lead to the substitution of such antisocial tendencies as stuttering or masturbation. Digital sucking also has been related to inadequate sucking activity. It was found in a series of studies that there was less thumb-sucking in both animals and humans when fed ad lib than there was when feedings were widely separated. Further, it was learned that, in general, nonthumb-sucking children took a longer time for feeding than was taken by thumb-suckers. In opposition to the theory of inadequate sucking activity is the oral drive theory of Sears and Wise,[15] whose work suggests that the strength of the oral drive is in part a function of how long a child continues to feed by sucking. Thus, it is not the frustration of weaning that produces thumb-sucking but, rather, the oral drive, which has been strengthened by the prolongation of nursing. Sears and Wise's theory is in keeping with a Freudian hypothesis that sucking increases the erotogenesis of the mouth. Benjamin,[1] in an interesting series of experiments with monkeys, found that there was far less thumb-sucking among those whose nutritive sucking experience had been greatly reduced. This theory holds that thumb-sucking is an expression of a need to suck that arises because of the association of sucking with the primary reinforcing aspects of feeding. Another very interesting theory has been proposed by Benjamin, who suggests that thumb-sucking arises very simply from the rooting and placing reflexes common to all mammalian infants.[1] These primitive reflexes are maximal during the first 3 months of life. Her hypothesis was tested by covering infant's hands with mittens the very first few weeks of life so that the thumb was not accidentally involved in the placing reflex.

All thumb-sucking theories are not Freudian in origin, for recently several have suggested that thumb-sucking is one of the earliest examples of neuromuscular learning in the infant and that it follows all the general laws of the learning process. A multidisciplinary research team at the University of Alberta reported that children who sucked their thumbs failed to demonstrate any consistent psychologic differences from a control sample. This team's well-documented results strongly support the theory that digital sucking habits in humans are a simple learned response.[8] They found no support for the psychoanalytic interpretation of thumb-sucking as a symptom of psychologic disturbance. Further proof for their ideas was presented by studying the psychologic effects of orthodontic intervention; typical orthodontic therapy for arresting the habit failed to produce any significant increase in alternative or substitutive undesirable psychologic behavior.

The various theories concerning "non-nutritive digital sucking" are not completely incompatible with one another. Rather, they suggest that the thumb-sucking habit should be viewed by the clinician as a behavioral pattern of multivariate nature. It is quite possible that thumb-sucking may begin for one reason and be sustained at subsequent ages by other factors. Most of the findings reported thus far seem to support best the learning theory, particularly if the learning of digital sucking is associated with unrestricted and prolonged nutritive sucking.

For the clinician, the most important question is, simply, does digital sucking cause malocclusion? Many children who practice digital sucking habits have no evidence of malocclusion; however, Popovich[13] has reported a high association of abnormal sucking habits with the malocclusion sample at the Burlington Orthodontic Research Centre in Ontario, Canada. Cook[2] measured the forces of thumb-sucking, finding three distinctly different patterns of force application during sucking, all utilizing forces sufficiently strong to displace teeth or deform growing bone. It should be remembered that the type of malocclusion that may develop in the thumb-sucker is dependent on a number of variables —the position of the digit, associated orofacial muscle contractions, the position of the mandible during sucking, the facial skeletal pattern, the force applied to the teeth and alveolar process, the frequency and duration of sucking and so forth. An anterior open bite is the most frequent malocclusion (Fig. VII-9). Protraction of the maxillary anterior teeth will be seen particularly if the pollex is held upward against the palate (Fig. VII-10). Mandibular postural retraction may develop if the weight of the hand or arm continually forces the mandible to assume a retruded position in order to practice the habit. Concomitantly, the mandibular incisors may be tipped lingually. When the maxillary incisors have been tipped labially and an open bite has developed, it becomes

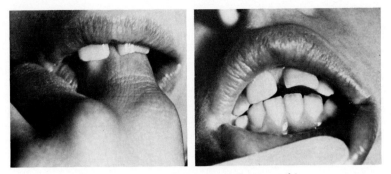

Fig. VII-9.—Malocclusion from finger-sucking.

necessary for the tongue to thrust forward during swallowing in order to effect an anterior seal. During thumb-sucking, buccal wall contractions produce, in some sucking patterns, a negative pressure within the mouth, with resultant narrowing of the maxillary arch (Fig. VII-11). With this upset in the force system in and around the maxillary complex, it often is impossible for the nasal floor to drop vertically to its expected position during growth. Therefore, thumb-suckers may be found to have a narrower nasal floor and a high palatal vault. The maxillary lip becomes hypotonic and the mandibular lip becomes hyperactive, since it must be elevated by contractions of the orbicularis muscle to a position between the malposed incisors during swallowing. These abnormal muscle contractions during sucking and swallowing

Fig. VII-10.—Adaptation of oral and facial musculature to thumb-sucking. Note malposition of tongue, mandible and circumoral muscles.

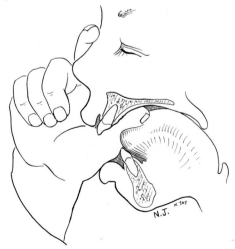

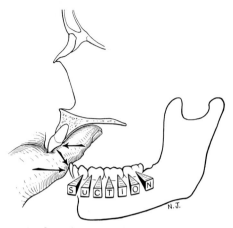

Fig. VII-11.—Direction of application of force to the dentition during thumb-sucking. Maxillary incisors are pushed labially, mandibular incisors lingually, while buccal muscles exert pressure lingually against teeth in the lateral segments of the dental arch.

Fig. VII-12.—The tongue during normal and abnormal swallowing. **A,** normal. Teeth are in light contact, lips closed and dorsum of the tongue elevated to touch the roof of the mouth. Tip of the tongue may be held as shown or lightly in contact with lingual surfaces of mandibular incisors. **B,** abnormal swallowing due to hypertrophied tonsils. As the tongue is retracted, it touches inflamed and swollen tonsils. Pain causes dropping of the mandible, so the tongue can thrust forward away from the pharyngeal region. With the mandible lowered, the lips must be closed forcibly to keep the tongue in the oral cavity. Therefore, there is strong contraction of the mentalis muscle with all tongue-thrusts during swallowing.

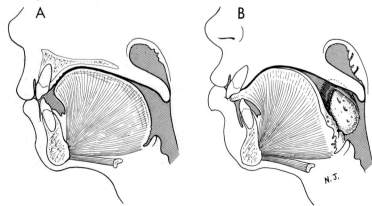

stabilize the deformation. Some malocclusions arising from sucking habits may be self-corrective on cessation of the habit; for example, if the skeletal pattern is normal, the habit is stopped early, the deformity has been mild, there is a teeth-together swallow and the associated neuromuscular habits are of a mild nature. Unfortunately, many thumb-suckers produce malocclusions that require orthodontic therapy. The treatment by the dentist of digital sucking habits is discussed in Chapter XVI.

b) *Tongue-Thrusting*

Tongue-thrust swallows that may be etiologic to malocclusion are of two types: (1) the simple tongue-thrust swallow, which is a tongue-thrust associated with a normal or teeth-together swallow, and (2) the complex tongue-thrust swallow, which is a tongue-thrust associated with a teeth-apart swallow. As has been described in Chapter V, the child normally swallows with the teeth in occlusion, the lips likely closed and the tongue held against the palate behind the anterior teeth (Fig. VII-12). The simple tongue-thrust swallow usually is associated with a history of digital sucking, even though the sucking habit may no longer be practiced, since it is necessary for the tongue to thrust forward through the open bite to maintain an anterior seal with the lips during the swallow. Figure VII-13 is an example of the simple tongue-thrust swallow and its attendant malocclusion. Complex tongue-thrusts, on the other hand, are far more likely to be associated with chronic naso-respiratory distress, mouth-breathing, tonsillitis or pharyngitis (Fig. VII-14). When the tonsils are inflamed, the root of the tongue may encroach on the enlarged faucial pillars (see Fig. VII-12). To avoid this painful encroachment, the mandible reflexly drops, separating the teeth and providing more room for the tongue to be thrust forward during swallowing to a less painful position. Pain and lessening of space in

Fig. VII-13.—Malocclusion caused by an abnormal tongue-thrusting habit during swallowing.

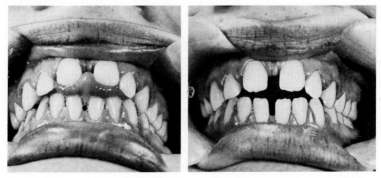

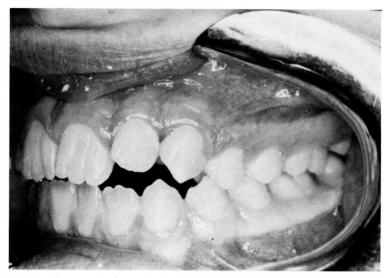

Fig. VII-14.—Intra-oral photograph of a complex tongue-thrust before treatment.

the throat precipitate a new forward tongue posture and swallowing reflex, while the teeth and growing alveolar processes accommodate themselves to the attendant upset in neuromuscular forces. During chronic mouth-breathing, a large freeway space is seen, since dropping the mandible and protruding the tongue provides a more adequate airway. Since maintenance of the airway is a more primitive and demanding reflex than the mature swallow, the latter is conditioned to the necessity for mouth-breathing. The jaws are thus held apart during the swallow in order that the tongue can remain in a protracted position. The prognosis for treatment of these two tongue-thrust types is very different (see Chapter XV).

Other tongue habits that often are confused with tongue-thrust swallow include tongue-sucking, the retained infantile tongue posture and the retained infantile swallow (see Chapter XV).

c) Lip-Sucking and Lip-Biting

Lip-sucking may appear by itself or it may be seen with thumb-sucking. In almost all instances, it is the mandibular lip that is involved in sucking, although biting habits of the maxillary lip are observed as well. When the mandibular lip is repeatedly held beneath the maxillary anterior teeth, the result is labioversion of these teeth, often an open bite and sometimes linguoversion of the mandibular incisors (Fig. VII-15).

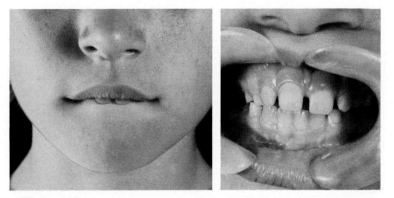

Fig. VII-15.—Malocclusion caused by lip-sucking. Note labioversion of maxillary anterior teeth and anterior open bite.

d) Posture

Persons with faulty body posture frequently demonstrate undesirable mandibular postural positioning as well. Both may be expressions of poor general health. On the other hand, the person who holds himself straight and erect with his head well placed over his spinal column will almost reflexly hold his chin forward in a preferred position. Posture is the summated expression of muscle reflexes and therefore is capable of change and correction (see Chapters V and XV).

e) Nail-Biting

Nail-biting is mentioned frequently as a cause of tooth malpositions. The malocclusion associated with this habit is likely to be of a more localized nature than those seen with some of the other pressure habits mentioned. High-strung, nervous children most often display this habit, and not infrequently their social and psychologic maladjustment is of greater clinical importance than the habit, which is nothing but a symptom of their basic problem.

f) Other Habits

The constant holding of a very young baby supine on a hard, flat surface can mold and shape the head by flattening the occiput or produce facial asymmetry. The significance of pillowing and sleeping on the arm, though, is thought to be greatly exaggerated. The habitual sucking of pencils, pacifiers or other hard objects can be just as deleterious to facial growth as thumb-sucking and finger-sucking.

6. DISEASE

a) Systemic Diseases

Febrile diseases are known to upset the dentitional developmental timetable during infancy and early childhood. For the most part, though, systemic disease is more likely to have an effect on the quality rather than the quantity of craniofacial growth. Malocclusion may be a secondary result of some neuropathies and neuromuscular disorders and it may be one of the sequelae of treatment of such problems as scoliosis by prolonged wearing of casts or appliances for immobilizing the spine. The dentist must seek pediatric consultation when the child with a malocclusion has any systemic problem that might influence the course of orthodontic therapy. No malocclusion is known to be pathognomonic of any usual childhood disease.

b) Endocrine Disorders

Endocrine dysfunction prenatally may be manifest in hypoplasia of the teeth themselves. Postnatally, endocrine disturbances may retard or hasten, but ordinarily they do not distort, the direction of facial growth. They may affect the rate of ossification of the bones, the time of suture closure, the time of eruption of the teeth and the rate of resorption of the primary teeth. The periodontal membrane and gingivae are extremely sensitive to endocrine dysfunction and the teeth thus are affected indirectly. No malocclusion is known to be pathognomonic of any specific endocrine disturbance. It is my opinion that any professional discussion of the effects of endocrinopathies on the child's growth should be presented by a pediatrician.

c) Local Diseases

1) NASOPHARYNGEAL DISEASES AND DISTURBED RESPIRATORY FUNCTION.—Anything that interferes with normal respiratory physiology may affect the growth of the face. Mouth-breathers seem to have a high incidence of malocclusions. No single type of malocclusion is seen regularly, for the initial disorder that led to mouth-breathing may be any one of the following: diverted nasal septum, enlarged turbinates, chronic inflammation and congestion of the nasopharyngeal mucosa, allergy, adenoid hypertrophy, inflammation and hypertrophy of the tonsils or a sucking habit. The typical mouth-breathing syndrome is characterized by contraction of the maxillary denture, labioversion of the maxillary anterior teeth, crowding of the anterior teeth in both arches, hypertrophy and chapping of the lower lip, hypotonicity and apparent shortening of the maxillary lip and frequently marked overbite (Fig. VII-16). The molar relationship may be that of neutroclusion or distoclusion.

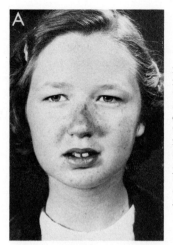

Fig. VII-16.—Malocclusion and mouth-breathing. **A,** face of a mouth-breather. **B,** hypertrophied tonsils, which may result in an alteration in tongue posture, mandibular posture, the action of the tongue during the swallow and the mode of breathing. **C,** hypertrophied adenoid mass. Such enlarged adenoids usually make necessary breathing through the mouth. (**B** and **C** courtesy of Dr. Robert Aldrich.)

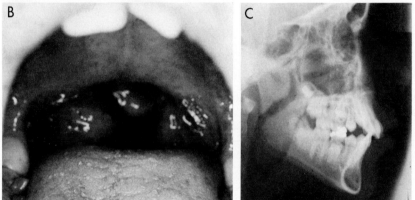

Whether mouth-breathing is due to an anatomic predisposition, a nasal obstruction or an inflammation of the nasal mucosa, the alterations in muscle function are similar. The soft palate is raised to make a nasal seal with the posterior pharyngeal wall, the mandible is dropped to provide a greater oral airway and the tongue is lowered from contact with the palate and is protruded. Secondary effects often noticed include (1) greater freeway space, (2) teeth-apart swallows and (3) a relative increase in buccal wall pressure against maxillary teeth.

Mouth-breathing may be temporary (e.g., during a cold), seasonal (e.g., in association with nasorespiratory allergies) or chronic, as a result of habit of obstruction. Rondon[14] and Eastman[5] have studied the effects of mouth-breathing on the craniofacial morphogenesis, finding small but significant differences in mandibular morphology in chronic mouth-breathers.

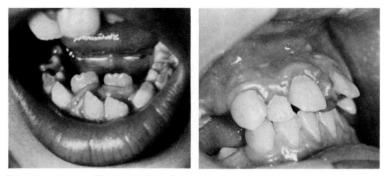

Fig. VII-17 (left).—Hypertrophy of the gingivae and incisal malalignment.
Fig. VII-18 (right).—Fibroma at the maxillary midline causing diastema.

2) GINGIVAL AND PERIODONTAL DISEASES.—Infections and other disorders of the periodontal membrane and gingivae have a direct and highly localized effect on the teeth. They may cause loss of teeth, changes in the closure patterns of the mandible to avoid trauma to sensitive areas, ankylosis of the teeth and other conditions that influence the position of the teeth (Fig. VII-17).

3) TUMORS.—Tumors in the dental area can cause malocclusion (Fig. VII-18). Severe malfunction will result when they are found in the articulatory region.

4) CARIES.—The greatest single cause of localized malocclusion undoubtedly is dental caries. Caries may be responsible for early loss of primary teeth, drifting of permanent teeth, premature eruption of permanent teeth, etc. Although caries is not the sole cause of these conditions, it is responsible for most of them and they will be discussed here.

(a) *Premature loss of primary teeth.*—In this instance, the word "premature" refers to the child's own dental development, *not* to population standards. Specifically, it refers to the stage of development of the permanent tooth that will succeed the lost primary tooth. When a primary tooth is lost before the permanent successor has started to erupt (crown formation completed and root formation begun—Nolla's Stage 6), bone is likely to re-form atop the permanent tooth, delaying its eruption. When its eruption is delayed, more time is available for other teeth to drift into the space that would have been occupied by the delayed tooth (see Chapter VI, Section D, Development of the Permanent Teeth). "Premature loss" means loss so early that the natural maintenance of arch perimeter may be jeopardized. "Early loss" of primary teeth refers to their loss prior to the expected time but without perimeter loss. The definitions of "premature" and "early" loss are dependent on the conditions in one child's mouth; for example, development pattern of permanent teeth, size of teeth, arch perimeter and so forth.

Of importance in this connection is not only the total loss of the primary teeth but partial loss of crown substance to caries as well. Jarvis[9] has shown that interproximal caries plays a most important role in shortening of arch length. Any decrease in the mesiodistal width of a primary molar may result in the forward drifting of the first permanent molar. It has been said that the most important appliance in the field of prophylactic orthodontics is a well-placed fully contoured restoration in a primary molar. If this is true, the next most important appliance must be the space-maintainer inserted to prevent drifting when the entire primary tooth has been lost. There is a tendency to forget that drifting of teeth can take place before and during eruption just as well as after complete eruption into position. This problem of premature loss of primary teeth cannot be met successfully without a knowledge of the drifting tendencies of the teeth and the effects of loss of primary teeth and eruption of permanent teeth on the arch perimeter (see Chapter VI, Section D).

The loss of primary INCISORS ordinarily is not a matter of concern; however, should a primary incisor be lost before the crowns of the permanent incisors are in a position to prevent drifting of the more distally placed primary teeth, malocclusion of the primary denture may result (Fig. VII-19). If a primary incisor is lost before age 4, radiographs should be taken of the developing permanent incisor and the space observed regularly.

Primary CUSPIDS, when lost, may be a matter of greater concern. In the maxilla, the permanent cuspid erupts so late that if the primary cuspid is removed before the central and lateral incisors have been moved together, it may permit permanent spacing of the anterior teeth. Strange as it seems, incisor spacing and labioversion of the cuspid may

Fig. VII-19 (left).—Severe drifting of primary teeth due to loss of the primary incisor. It is best not to assume that loss of primary incisors is inconsequential but rather to judge each problem separately. Very early loss of maxillary incisors can mean trouble.

Fig. VII-20 (right).—Labioversion of maxillary cuspids with spacing between incisors.

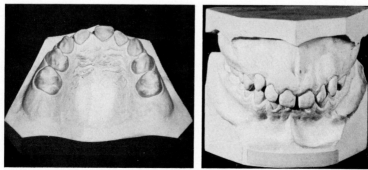

occur in the same case (Fig. VII-20). Primary cuspid loss in the mandible is more frequent and more serious. The untimely loss of these teeth may result in lingual tipping of the four mandibular incisors if there is abnormal activity of the mentalis muscle, an extreme overjet, or teeth-apart swallow. It has been widely recommended that the primary cuspid be extracted to facilitate the alignment of the permanent incisors in the mandible (see Chapter XV, Section C-1, Space Management). Removal of the primary cuspid to achieve incisal alignment sometimes must be correlated with an appliance to prevent lingual tipping of the incisors (see Chapter XV, Section C-1). Many a blocked-out mandibular cuspid owes its position to the ill-planned removal of the primary cuspid, just as many an anterior malalignment is due to the prolonged retention of the same tooth.

The loss of FIRST PRIMARY MOLARS is not thought by some to be of clinical import. This is because the problem does not manifest itself for some time after the tooth's removal. The first bicuspid is not misplaced during its eruption, since it is a bit narrower mesiodistally than is the first primary molar. If the first primary molar is lost very early, the second primary molar may shift forward at the time the first permanent molar is erupting (see Fig. VII-22). If the first primary molar is lost after firm neutroclusion of the first permanent molars is established, there is less likelihood of space loss.

Quantified studies on the effects of the loss of the first primary molar are rare, but the indications seem to be (1) its loss is not as damaging as the loss of the second primary molar, (2) if lost during active eruption of the first premolar, there is little chance of loss of the arch perimeter and (3) if lost prior to the start of eruption of the first premolar, perimeter loss may occur.

The early loss of the SECOND PRIMARY MOLAR will allow the first permanent molar to drift forward at once, even though it is not yet erupted. The second primary molar is wider mesiodistally than its successor, but the difference in their widths is utilized in the anterior part of the arch to provide space for the permanent cuspids. For this reason, in the maxillary denture, the early loss of the second primary molar results not in an impacted or blocked-out second bicuspid but in a cuspid in labioversion. This malposition occurs because the cuspid erupts, in the upper arch, after the first and second bicuspids, which thus have first chance at the available space. In the mandible, where the eruption sequence is different and the second bicuspid is the last of the three teeth to arrive, it is the tooth blocked out of position (Fig. VII-21). Too much emphasis cannot be placed on the importance of the second primary molar during the mixed dentition stage. Loss of crown substance to caries in this tooth may be more serious than the loss of an entire other tooth. It plays an important role in the establishment of occlusal relationships (Chapter VI) and in the maintenance of arch perimeter (Chapter XV, Section C-1).

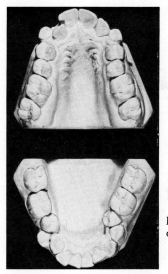

Fig. VII-21.—Blocked-out maxillary permanent cuspids and mandibular second bicuspids.

When TWO OR MORE PRIMARY MOLARS are lost early in the dentition's development there is, in addition to the accumulated effects of drifting already noted, the opportunity for other changes to take place. With the loss of posterior dental support, the mandible may be held in a position to provide some sort of adaptive occlusal function and a resulting accommodative posterior crossbite (Fig. VII-22). These positional crossbites have far-reaching effects on the temporomandibular musculature, the growth of the facial bones and the final positions of the permanent teeth.

Davey,[3] in an extensive study of the loss of maxillary primary molars, concluded that the factors related to migration of the first permanent molar after loss of the second or first and second primary molars were (1) the amount of leeway—more drift occurred in arches with less leeway space, (2) cusp height—high permanent molar cusps inhibit drifting and (3) age when the primary teeth are lost—the greatest loss occurred when the primary molars were lost prior to the eruption of the first permanent molars. Davey also noted that the effects caused by leeway space and cusp height may be cumulative after premature loss of maxillary primary molars. We do not have similar data for the mandible yet, nor do we have similar studies wherein "prematurity" is related to the individual's dental development rather than to the "expected time" according to population norms.

(b) *Disturbances in sequence of eruption of permanent teeth.*—Lo and Moyers[10] have shown that the normal sequence of eruption of the permanent teeth will provide the highest percentage of normal occlu-

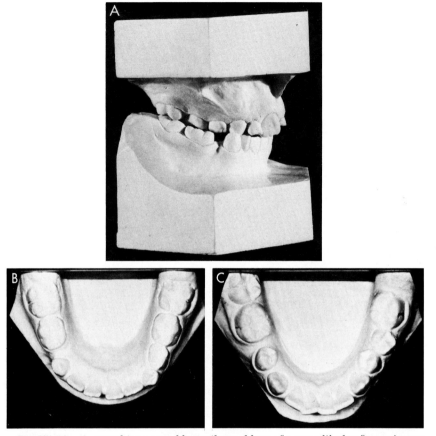

Fig. VII-22.—A, crossbite caused by unilateral loss of a mandibular first primary molar. Loss of the tooth allowed drifting of other teeth, causing tooth interferences, and the muscles shifted the mandible to achieve an adequate occlusal relationship. **B,** effects of premature loss of first primary molar at an early age. **C,** effects of loss of primary second molar prior to the eruption of the first permanent molar. Note the mesial position of the right first molar and earlier eruption of the right second molar. (**B** and **C** courtesy of Dr. Sheldon Rosenstein.)

sions (Table VII-1). Abnormal orders of arrival may permit shifting of the teeth, with resultant space loss. The premature loss of any primary tooth may allow the earlier arrival of its permanent successor or it may delay it, according to the stage of dental development. Periapical pathology of the primary teeth particularly hastens this process due to loss of bone and increased vascularity of the region. In severe cases, the permanent crown may erupt into position before there is sufficient

TABLE VII-1.—VARIATIONS IN SEQUENCES OF ERUPTION*

MAXILLA			MANDIBLE		
SEQUENCE	CASES	%	SEQUENCE	CASES	%
1) 6124537	115	48.72	1) 6123457	108	45.77
2) 6124357	38	16.01	2) 6123475	44	18.64
3) 6124573	28	11.87	3) 6124357	20	8.47
4) 6123457	14	5.93	4) 6123745	14	5.93
5) 6124375	13	5.51	5) 6124537	14	5.93
6) remaining 13			6) remaining 12		
sequences	28	11.87	sequences	36	15.26

*After Lo and Moyers.[10]

root development to stabilize the tooth's position. Tumors and super-numerary teeth may deflect or impede the course of eruption and thus upset the order of arrival. Prolonged retention of primary teeth, either because of failure of the roots to resorb or because of ankylosis of the root with the alveolar process, is another factor that disturbs the sequence of eruption. One of the most important sequences to observe is that of early arrival of the second molar. When this tooth develops ahead of any anterior teeth, it may have a dramatic effect in shortening arch perimeter (see Chapter XV).

(c) *Loss of permanent teeth.*—The loss of a permanent tooth results in a major upset in the physiologic functioning of the dentition, since the break in mesiodistal contacts permits shifting of the teeth. Because of their susceptibility to caries, the first permanent molars are of particular interest. This matter is discussed in some detail in Chapter XV.

7. MALNUTRITION

Malnutrition may affect occlusal development through either systemic or local effects. Although nutritional deficiencies due to inadequate intake are seen seldom in the United States, malnourishment due to malabsorption difficulties are seen everywhere. Malnutrition is more likely to affect the quality of tissues being formed and the rates of calcification than it is the size of parts (although the latter has been demonstrated in animals). Insofar as local effects are concerned, the roles of fluoride intake and refined carbohydrates in caries production are well known. Although there is no malocclusion that is pathognomonic of any typical and common nutritional deficiency, good nutrition plays an important role in growth and the maintenance of good bodily health and oral hygiene.

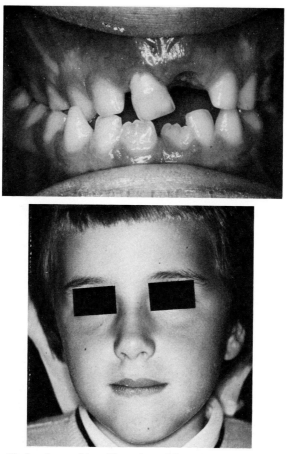

Fig. VII-23.—Skeletal crossbite. Note that although the relationship seems correct on the patient's left side, there is a crossbite involving one half of the dental arch on the right side. The patient also has obvious mandibular prognathism, even at this early age. The patient's face shows that the crossbite is due to an osseous dysplasia rather than to dental or muscular factors.

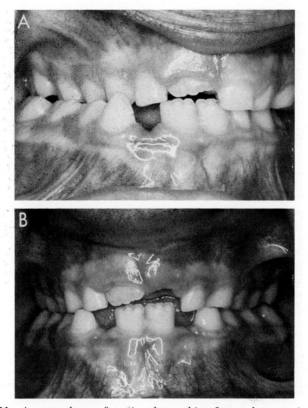

Fig. VII-24.—A muscular or functional crossbite. It can be seen in **A** that the midlines do not coincide and that one half of the mandibular denture is outside the maxillary denture. This patient's dentition was equilibrated very carefully and **B** shows the result when the patient returned to the clinic 1 week later. Note that the removal of the occlusal interferences in the primary teeth enabled the muscles to return the mandible to its proper position and to a proper occlusion. (See Chapter X, Analysis of the Orofacial Musculature.) Treatment of this case consisted of removing the sensory input to an imbalancing eccentric occlusal reflex (see Chapter V). No teeth were moved nor was there time for significant bone growth to occur.

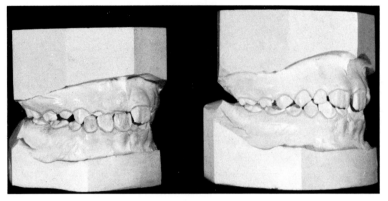

Fig. VII-25.—A dental type crossbite. Note here that the mandibular and maxillary bases are harmonious with each other, that the midlines coincide and that the crossbite is localized in the right incisor region. This crossbite is due to tipping of individual teeth. The adequate result of tipping them back to their proper position is shown at the right. The treatment was done by a simple appliance, applying forces mostly to the teeth out of position. Correction of such cases usually occurs in a few months.

E. Summary

Very few malocclusions have a single specific cause. For example, there is no virus that produces Class II, Division 1 nor an organism that specifically causes crossbite; even thumb-sucking does not always cause the same malocclusion. Rather, the clinical entity we call malocclusion is the result of the interaction of many factors affecting a developing system that has its own growth pattern. However, there is a dominant tendency for some malocclusions to appear within a single tissue system and to affect other tissue systems secondarily as they, in turn, adapt. Most severe types are osseous in origin, on which are superimposed dental and muscular features.

In order to illustrate the idea of a single tissue system involvement at the *start,* three examples of crossbite are shown in Figures VII-23– VII-25. These three problems, although bearing the same name, have disparate origins, one arising in skeletal asymmetry, one a functional shifting of the mandible by the muscles and one a simple tipping of teeth. All are crossbites, yet they are entirely different in their beginnings, their treatment and their prognosis.

Malocclusions originate because of imbalances among the developing systems that form the craniofacial complex, imbalances with which the growing face cannot cope.

REFERENCES

1. Benjamin, L.: Non-nutritive sucking and dental malocclusion in the deciduous and permanent teeth of rhesus monkey, Child Develop. 33:29, 1962.
2. Cook, J.: Intraoral Pressures Involved in Thumb and Finger Sucking. Master's thesis, University of Michigan, Ann Arbor, 1958.
3. Davey, K. W.: Effect of premature loss of primary molars on the anteroposterior position of maxillary first permanent molars and other teeth, J. Dent. Child. 34:383, 1967.
4. Dockrell, R.: Classifying aetiology of malocclusion, Dent. Rec. 72:25, 1952.
5. Eastman, G. A.: Oropharyngeal Muscular Interrelationships in Chronic Nasorespiratory Allergy—Cephalometric Study. Master's thesis, University of Michigan, Ann Arbor, 1963.
6. Freud, S.: *Three Contributions to the Theory of Sex* (3d ed.; New York and Washington: Nervous and Mental Disease Publishing Company, 1919).
7. Harvold, E.: Some biologic aspects of orthodontic treatment in the transitional dentition, Am. J. Orthodont. 49: 1, 1963.
8. Haryett, R., *et al.*: Chronic thumb-sucking: The psychologic effects and the relative effectiveness of various methods of treatment, Am. J. Orthodont. 53:569, 1957.
9. Jarvis, A.: Role of Dental Caries in Space Closure in the Mixed Dentition. Master's thesis, University of Toronto, 1952.
10. Lo, R., and Moyers, R. E.: Sequence of eruption of permanent dentition, Am. J. Orthodont. 39:460, 1953.
11. Mayne, W.: Serial Extraction, in Graber, T. M. (ed.), *Current Orthodontic Concepts and Techniques* (Philadelphia: W. B. Saunders Company, 1969), Chap. 4.
12. Moore, A.: Critique of orthodontic dogma, Angle Orthodont. 39:69, 1969.
13. Popovich, F.: Personal communication: Based on findings at the Burlington Orthodontic Research Centre.
14. Rondon, A. J.: Chronic Upper Respiratory Allergy and Its Relation to Dentofacial Development. Master's thesis, University of Michigan, Ann Arbor, 1956.
15. Sears, R., and Wise, G.: Relation of cup-feeding in infancy to thumb-sucking and the oral drive, Am. J. Orthopsychiat. 20:123, 1950.

Suggested Readings

Davey, K. W.: Effect of premature loss of primary molars on the anteroposterior position of maxillary first permanent molars and other teeth, J. Dent. Child. 34:383, 1967.
Dockrell, R.: Classifying aetiology of malocclusion, Dent. Rec. 72:25, 1952.
Haryett, R., *et al.*: Chronic thumb-sucking: The psychologic effects and the relative effectiveness of various methods of treatment, Am. J. Orthodont. 53:569, 1957.
Moore, A.: Critique of orthodontic dogma, Angle Orthodont. 39:69, 1969.
Sears, R., and Wise, G.: Relation of cup-feeding in infancy to thumb-sucking and the oral drive, Am. J. Orthopsychiat. 20:123, 1950.

DIAGNOSIS

VIII

The Orthodontic Examination

More mistakes are made from want of a proper examination than for any other reason.—DR. RUSSELL JOHN HOWARD, quoted by F. G. St. Clair Strange, in *The Hip,* Chapter 5.

The first step toward cure is to know what the disease is. (Ad sanitatem gradus est novisse morbum.)—LATIN PROVERB

A. Before the examination

B. The cursory examination

1. Consider general health, appearance and attitude
2. Examine the external facial features
   a) Position and posture of lips
   b) Color and texture of lips
   c) Method of breathing
   d) Soft tissue profile
   e) Swallow
3. Analyze the facial form
4. Describe intra-oral features
   a) Gingivae
   b) Faucial pillars and throat
   c) Tongue
   d) Number of teeth
   e) Size of teeth
   f) Sequence and position of erupting teeth
   g) Malposed individual teeth
   h) Occlusal relationships of the teeth
5. Classify the occlusion
6. Evaluate the available space
7. Study the functional occlusal relationship
8. Complete the permanent record
   a) The case history
   b) Record casts
   c) Radiographic record

OFTEN ONE SEES the terms "examination," "diagnosis," "classification" and "treatment planning" used interchangeably. Since each term has its own precise meaning, they should not be substituted for one another. Such misusage is semantic proof of confused thinking!

The *cursory examination* is a procedure for gathering initial data— the compilation of sufficient facts to permit a tentative diagnosis (Fig. VIII-1). *Diagnosis* is the study and interpretation of data concerning a clinical problem in order to determine the presence or absence of abnormality. In orthodontics, the diagnosis establishes or denies the existence and character of dentofacial deformity. Once the presence of an abnormality has been determined, similar abnormalities often are grouped together for convenience in discussion; this process is the *classification*. After the data have been gathered, studied and interpreted and the problem named, the treatment must be planned. *Treatment planning* is strategy; the *treatment* itself is the tactics. A necessary sequential dependence will be seen: we examine, we diagnose, we classify, we plan, we treat. Logic points to this sequence; practice management demands it.

A. Before the Examination

Much has been written concerning the preparation for a dental examination and the psychology of "handling" children in the dental office.

Fig. VIII-1.—Flow chart of the orthodontic examination.

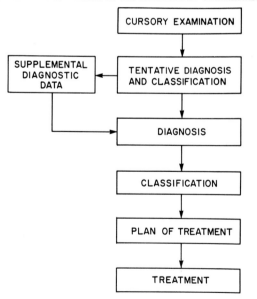

UNIVERSITY OF MICHIGAN   -   SCHOOL OF DENTISTRY
DEPARTMENT OF PEDODONTICS - HEALTH QUESTIONNAIRE

Name _____ Sex_____ Birth Date _____

Address _____

Telephone _____ Date _____

Directions

If your answer is YES to the question asked, place a circle around (YES). If your answer
is NO, encircle (NO).

Please answer all questions. If you wish to qualify an answer, you may write in the
spaces between questions.

Answers to the following questions will be considered confidential.

1. Are you being treated by a physician now?   YES NO

2. Are you taking any medicine now?   YES NO

3. Have you ever been seriously sick or hospitalized?   YES NO

4. Have you ever been told by a physician that you have a heart murmur? YES NO

5. Do you have asthma or hay fever? (Underline which condition)   YES NO

6. Do you ever have hives or skin rash? (Underline which condition)   YES NO

7. Have you ever had convulsions (fits)?   YES NO

8. Have you ever had any of the following diseases?
         Rheumatic Fever   YES NO

         Inflammatory Rheumatism   YES NO

         Jaundice (yellow skin and eyes),   Hepatitis   YES NO

         Diabetes   YES NO

         Tuberculosis   YES NO

         Measles   YES NO

         Scarlet Fever   YES NO

9. Have you ever experienced an unusual reaction (allergy
   or sensitization) to any of the following medicines?
         Aspirin   YES NO

         Penicillin   YES NO

         Sulfonamides (Sulfa)   YES NO

         Ataractics (tranquilizers)   YES NO

         Dental local anesthetics (to put teeth asleep)   YES NO

         Other medicines   YES NO

10. When you scratch or cut yourself, do you stop bleeding promptly?   YES NO

11. Do you brush your teeth at least three times a day?   YES NO

12. Are you using fluoride tablets or drops at this time?   YES NO

_____ Parent's signature

Fig. VIII-2.—A short health questionnaire to be filled out by the patient's parent.

Elaborate parental preparation of the child's mind for a visit to the dentist is to be discouraged lest the child become unduly apprehensive. Most children are naturally relaxed. If they are tense in the dental office, it is important to learn the source of the tension. If the child is anxious while still in the waiting room, it may help to ask the mother to remain outside during the examination. While the dentist is showing the patient to the chair, the assistant may say to the mother, "We have a rule that parents wait outside during the examination. You know how *some* mothers are. Doctor Jones will want to talk with you later." Few mothers fail to respond to this approach. Not all children should be seen alone; this procedure has proved successful in instances in which the child's fears had their origins in the mother's attitude. The mother may complete a health record and questionnaire (Fig. VIII-2) while waiting for the discussion with the dentist.

A child usually will respond casually if he is treated casually. A good relationship will be established with most children by being busy at your work and slightly indifferent to them. Too much attention should be avoided. Often it is the dentist who is nervous, and the child quickly realizes this. The orthodontic examination is not painful and as soon as this is learned, cooperation of most young patients is ensured.

B. The Cursory Examination

The purpose of the cursory examination is to provide the minimal necessary facts on which a tentative diagnosis and classification can be made. The detailed analysis on which treatment planning is based is done later (see Chapters X–XII). The difference between the cursory examination and the detailed analysis–treatment plan is a matter of economics. One cannot afford to do a detailed analysis of every child seen, nor do most require such attention. On the other hand, neither can one afford to undertake extended orthodontic therapy with only the facts acquired in the cursory examination. Considerable clinical skill is required to make quick, correct, initial examinations of the potential orthodontic patient in order to know which patients to treat, which to refer, which to observe and which will require further diagnostic data before such decisions can be made.

The steps to be described provide a satisfactory cursory orthodontic examination easily managed in the office of the typical family dentist. No use is made in the cursory examination of elaborate diagnostic aids, e.g., cephalograms. Such procedures are, however, described in Chapters X–XII. Each step should be in sequence and all observations written down. The orthodontic appraisal of a patient cannot be reduced to such a simple system of notations as those used for charting cavities and planning restorative dentistry. Furthermore, the details of a developing occlusion change so rapidly from one observation to the next that they cannot be remembered. It is helpful to have a recent periapical radio-

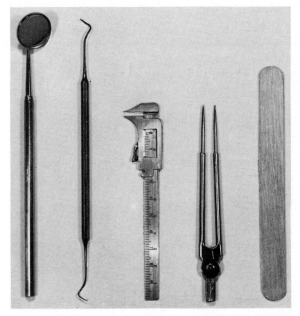

Fig. VIII-3.—Instruments used for the cursory orthodontic examination. Left to right: mouth mirror, explorer, tooth-measuring gauge, dividers and tongue depressor.

graphic survey while making the cursory examination. If such a radiographic survey is not available, securing it becomes part of the examination.

The following instruments should be in place on the bracket table (Fig. VIII-3):

> Mouth mirror
> Explorer
> Gauge for measuring teeth
> Dividers
> Tongue depressor

Step 1. CONSIDER GENERAL HEALTH, APPEARANCE AND ATTITUDE

The first step in any orthodontic examination is to form a general idea of the patient's health status, physical appearance and attitude toward orthodontics. Actually, the examination should begin the moment the patient is first seen. Often it is possible to learn much concerning his general appearance, stature, posture, attitude and the parent-child relationship as he walks into the examination room and seats himself. The child with an extensive medical history or an unfortunate previous dental experience may be unduly apprehensive. First questions serve not only to inform the examiner but to ease the mind of the child. It may be useful for the dentist himself to ask the usual questions necessary for completion of the record card as the child tells his name, age, street address, school, family physician and so forth. An opportunity is given to observe the child's facial features, speech mannerisms, attitude toward you, etc. General questions concerning the child's health and past illnesses may be asked and related to the questionnaire completed by the mother, although, of course, a complete physical examination is the responsibility of the physician. Of particular interest to the dentist are data about allergies and chronic nasorespiratory disorders. Do not hesitate to ask the child any question that seems necessary or pertinent. His answers frequently are more enlightening than those of his parents.

For appraising the child's physical development, the stature and weight charts devised by Meredith (see Fig. IV-26, pp. 102 and 103) are useful. (The relationship between facial and bodily growth is discussed in Chapter IV.) Begin the examination by forming a general impression of the child's health and appearance.

Step 2. EXAMINE THE EXTERNAL FACIAL FEATURES

The patient should be seated in the chair so that his spine is erect and his head is placed well over the vertebral column. The

Fig. VIII-4.—A, improper position of the head for orthodontic examination. **B,** proper position of the head. The Frankfurt plane should be parallel to the floor. Note the difference in the patient's profile in these two views.

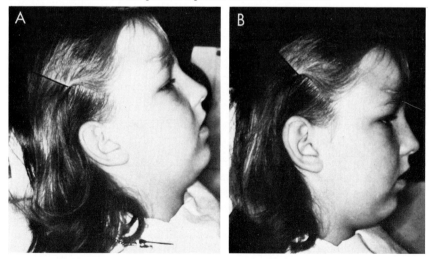

Frankfurt plane should be roughly parallel to the floor. This position in the chair, although not usual for intra-oral dental examinations, is more useful for examining the external facial features, jaw functions and occlusal relationships (Fig. VIII-4).

a) Position and Posture of Lips

Lip posture is best studied during normal head and mandibular posture (Fig. VIII-4). Normally, the lips meet each other in an unstrained relationship at the level of the occlusal plane (Fig. VIII-5). Palpate the lips to ascertain whether they are of equal tonus and muscular development. Study the role of each lip during the unconscious swallow. A detailed analysis of lip function is given in Chapter X; however, in the cursory examination, the lips' posture, relative size and role in swallowing should be noted.

b) Color and Texture of Lips

When one lip is of a color or texture different from the other, there is a reason. If, for example, the lower lip rests beneath the upper incisors during a swallow, it usually is redder, heavier and more likely to be

Fig. VIII-5.—Normal lip posture.

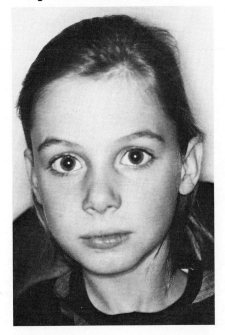

moist and smooth (see Fig. X-2). The less active upper lip more frequently is chapped and lighter in color.

c) Method of Breathing

It is easiest to study the method of breathing while the patient is unaware that he is being observed. The mouth-breather's lips are separated
at rest to allow him to respire, whereas the nasal-breather's lips are
held lightly together. After a general impression of the breathing method
is formed, ask the patient to take a deep breath and then blow it out.
Most children, given such a command, will inspire through the mouth,
although an occasional nasal-breather will inspire through the nose
with the lips lightly closed. Then ask the patient to close his lips and
take a deep breath through his nose. A child who is a normal nasal-
breather has good reflex control of the alar muscles, which control the
size and shape of the external nares. Therefore, the nasal-breather di-
lates the external nares reflexly during inspiration. On the other hand,
although all mouth-breathers (except rare ones with nasal stenosis or
congestion) can breathe through their noses, they usually do not change
the size or shape of the external nares during inspiration (see Fig. X-6).
Occasionally, mouth-breathers actually contract the nares while inspiring. Even the nasal-breather who has temporary nasal congestion
will demonstrate alar contraction reflexly when asked to take a breath
while keeping his lips closed. Unilateral nasal function may be diagnosed by placing a small mirror on the upper lip, which will cloud with
condensed moisture from the nasal breathing, or by use of a cotton
"butterfly" (see Fig. X-7).

d) Soft Tissue Profile

Observation of the superficial facial features at rest and in action
complements greatly our knowledge of the occlusal relationships and
the positions of the teeth. Extreme malpositions of teeth rarely are seen
without accompanying muscle imbalances. The important questions
are "Do the muscles of the lips and face contribute to any tooth malpositions, or are they accommodating to the malpositions?" and "How
might they adapt to any corrective movements of the incisors?" Detailed
analysis of the facial musculature is discussed in Chapter X, but the
role of the facial muscles must be noted in the cursory examination.

e) Swallow

It is important in the cursory examination to learn how the patient
swallows. Observe the patient swallowing unconsciously, noting whether
the lips contract. Then gently place a mouth mirror or tongue depressor
on the lower lip and ask the patient to swallow (Fig. VIII-6). Normal

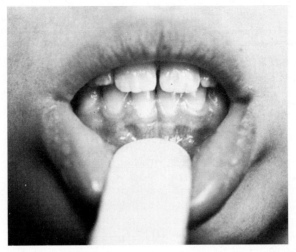

Fig. VIII-6.—Use of a tongue depressor on the lower lip to check the type of swallow.

Fig. VIII-7.—Palpation of the temporal muscle for checking the swallow.

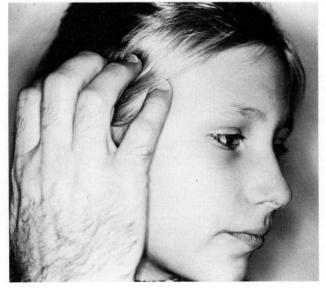

(teeth-together) swallows are completed, whereas teeth-apart swallows are inhibited, since mandibular lips and mentalis contractions are necessary in teeth-apart swallows. Palpate the temporal muscle during command swallows of saliva or a small amount of water (Fig. VIII-7). Teeth-together swallowers must contract this muscle to elevate the mandible and hold the teeth in occlusion; teeth-apart swallowers do not have to contract the mandible muscle. Further methods of analyzing swallowing are given in Chapter X.

Step 3. ANALYZE THE FACIAL FORM

Even though detailed analysis of the craniofacial skeleton is best done in the cephalogram, and a more thorough analysis will be done before actual treatment is begun, an appraisal of the facial form is an absolute necessity for even the shortest examination. (More detailed analyses of the facial skeleton, both cephalometric and noncephalometric, are given in Chapter XII.)

The Facial Form Analysis method outlined below is Mortell's modification of a procedure developed by Cheney. It has been used for several years in the undergraduate orthodontic clinic at The University of Michigan and has proved practical and worthwhile. It is subjective, therefore not quantitative, and is suggested for use only when radiographic cephalometry is not available. The Facial Form Analysis provides, however, a quick systematic evaluation of the relationship of the various parts of the facial skeleton.

The Facial Form Analysis relates the facial parts to two planes, the

Fig. VIII-8.—The planes of the Facial Form Analysis. **A,** lateral view. **B,** frontal view.

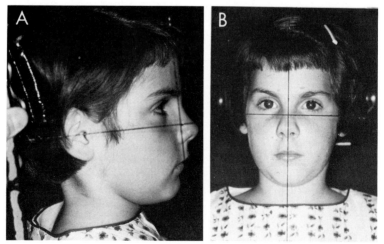

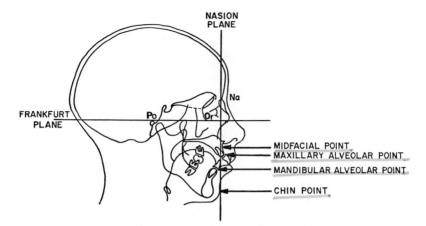

Fig. VIII-9.—Landmarks of the Facial Form Analysis. The midfacial point is analogous to the cephalometric A point and may be estimated by using the ala of the nose. The maxillary alveolar point is analogous to superior prosthion and is found at the interseptal gingival tip between the maxillary central incisors. The mandibular alveolar point, analogous to the cephalometric inferior prosthion, is found at the interseptal gingival tip between the mandibular central incisors. The chin point is the most protrusive point of the skin overlying the chin.

Frankfurt and the Nasion, in the lateral view. The Frankfurt plane (Fig. VIII-8), on the living, joins the tragus (representing the external auditory meatus) and the orbitale (the lowest point in the bony orbit). The Nasion plane (Izard's plane) is erected perpendicularly to the Frankfurt plane and passes through the Nasion point (Fig. VIII-8). The deepest point in the bony profile of the frontonasal curvature is taken on the living as Nasion. The face is related to the midsagittal plane alone in the frontal view. Figure VIII-9 illustrates the landmarks used for recording findings of the Facial Form Analysis. The locations of the landmarks on the patient, as shown for a typical case (Figs. VIII-10 and VIII-11), are marked directly on the form and the soft tissue profile is drawn. To make it easier to visualize the exact placement of the landmarks as they appear in the patient, vertical dotted lines are used to represent the distance between perpendiculars erected to Frankfurt at orbitale and nasion, and that same distance anterior to the Nasion plane. The questions asked are most pertinent and are useful to an understanding of the clinical significance of the relationships noted. The Facial Form Analysis does not provide answers; it simply makes it easier for the clinician to identify any gross malrelationship of parts and to pose the most critical questions that must be asked before treatment is begun.

Clyde K.

Patient's Name, Date

FACIAL FORM ANALYSIS

I. Lateral View

Frankfurt

Midfacial

Maxillary alveolar

Mandibular alveolar

Chin point

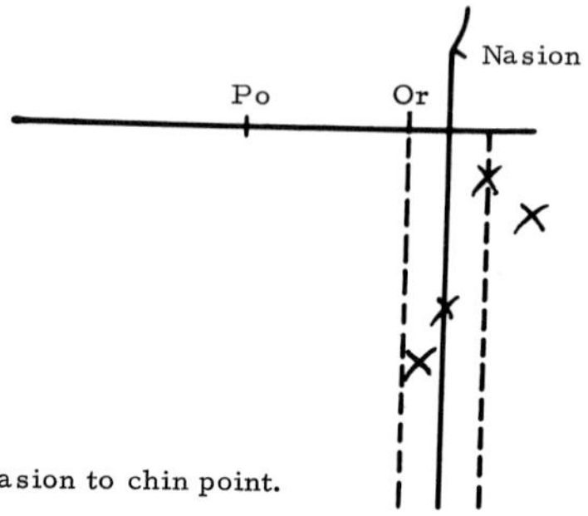

Draw in the profile from Nasion to chin point.

1. What molar relationship is indicated by facial skeleton? *Class II*

2. a. What is the overjet? *9.0* b. What is the overbite? *6.1 mm.*

3. What is the significance of the incisor relationship? *Both upper and lower incisors tipped labially*

4. What is molar relationship? *Cl II* What is the cuspid relationship? *Class II*

5. Is mandible shifted in A-P on closure? Yes __No__

6. Angle between Frankfurt horizontal and occlusal plane; flat, normal, (steep.)

7. Obtusity of gonial angle, less than normal, normal, (greater than normal.)

8. Inclination of maxillary central incisors relative to nasion plane; <u>anteriorly inclined</u>, normal, vertical, posteriorly inclined.

9. Inclination of mandibular central incisors relative to nasion plane; <u>anteriorly inclined</u>, normal, vertical, posteriorly inclined.

Summary: *Severe skeletal class II c̄ extreme incisal labioversion.*

Fig. VIII-10.—An example of a completed Facial Form Analysis, lateral view.

II. Frontal view

Are the following landmarks symmetric?
If not, indicate location.

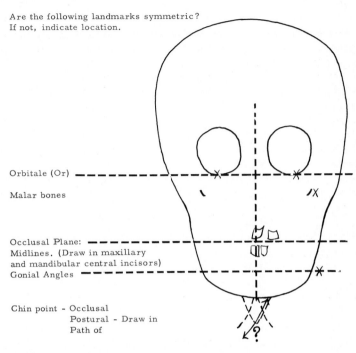

Orbitale (Or)

Malar bones

Occlusal Plane:
Midlines. (Draw in maxillary
and mandibular central incisors)
Gonial Angles

Chin point - Occlusal
     Postural - Draw in
     Path of

Maxillary arch form; tapering, trapezoid, ovoid, "U" - type.
Mandibular arch form; tapering, trapezoid, ovoid, "U" - type.
Summary: *Slight skeletal asymmetry, dental mid-lines harmonious with their bases, but not with each other.*

Fig. VIII-11.—An example of a completed Facial Form Analysis, frontal view.

Step 4. DESCRIBE INTRA-ORAL FEATURES

a) Gingivae

Localized gingival lesions may be symptomatic of traumatogenic occlusion, poor oral hygiene, delayed eruption of permanent teeth, hyperactivity of the mentalis muscle (see Fig. X-5), mouth-breathing, etc. The appearance and health of the gingival tissues is an index of periodontal health.

b) Faucial Pillars and Throat

Oral health is closely related to pharyngeal conditions. Inflamed, hypertrophied or infected tonsils may give rise to alterations in the tongue posture, mandibular posture or swallowing reflexes (see Chapters VII and X).

c) Tongue

Study of tongue activity is difficult because the tongue ordinarily is not clearly visible. Since most tongue functions are synchronized well with the circumoral muscles and the muscles of mastication, abnormal function in one will result in associative or accommodative abnormal function in the others. Abnormal function of the tongue often is first suggested when one notes abnormal functions of the lips. When the lips are parted by a mouth mirror or the cheeks are withdrawn by retractors so that the mouth may be viewed better, normal tongue activity is inhibited and cannot be observed. The diagnostic trick is to examine the tongue in its normal functions without displacement of the lips and cheeks. Much has been written concerning the tongue as a gauge of oral health. From an orthodontic point of view, considerations other than its color and texture are perhaps more important, for example, its relative size, its postural position and its role and positions in several reflex functions.

(1) Study the posture of the tongue while the mandible is in its postural position. Sometimes this can be done if the lips rest apart, or tongue posture can be noted in the lateral cephalogram of mandibular posture. If neither of the procedures is fruitful, gently part the lips after cautioning the patient not to move.

(2) Observe the tongue during various swallowing procedures—the unconscious swallow, the command swallow of saliva, the command swallow of water and the unconscious swallow during chewing. Do not separate the lips to see what the tongue is doing; rather, observe the contractions of the orbicularis oris and mentalis muscles and deduce from their activity the tongue's positions during swallowing. Complete details of the analysis of the swallow are given in Chapter X.

(3) Observe the role of the tongue during mastication.

(4) Observe the role of the tongue during speech. Some have overstated the relationship between speech and malocclusion. Many patients with gross malocclusions have excellent speech because they have great motor skills and can adapt the lips and tongue well to malpositions of the teeth and malrelationships of the jaw. Only a few malocclusions are the result of abnormal tongue function present only during speech. However, observation of abnormal use of the tongue during speech may be of use in analyzing other malfunctions of the tongue (see Chapter X).

d) Number of Teeth

Counting the number of teeth often is forgotten. The examiner must account for 48 teeth—20 deciduous and the 28 permanent teeth, which are developing at the time of the usual orthodontic examination. For this reason, a complete standard periapical or panoramic survey is necessary.

e) Size of Teeth

Like all other biologic forms, teeth come in different sizes. From an orthodontic point of view, their most important measurement is their mesiodistal width. The tooth-measuring gauge (see Fig. VIII-3), or a Boley gauge that has been reduced in size, provides a simple and accurate method of measuring teeth. Table VIII-1 gives the mean mesiodistal widths of various permanent teeth for purposes of comparison. The problem of tooth size and malocclusion is always a relative one, since teeth accommodated nicely in one mouth are crowded in another.

TABLE VIII-1*A*.—MESIODISTAL TOOTH WIDTHS (PERMANENT MALE DENTITION)*

MAXILLARY DENTITION

Tooth	N	Mean (mm.)	Standard Deviation	5%	15%	Percentiles (mm.) 50%	85%	95%
1	164	8.91	0.74	7.98	8.26	8.92	9.65	10.01
2	162	6.99	0.63	5.90	6.36	7.00	7.58	7.90
3	156	7.89	0.63	6.95	7.41	7.98	8.43	8.76
4	155	6.74	0.54	5.92	6.22	6.79	7.24	7.51
5	147	6.69	0.45	5.97	6.33	6.71	7.10	7.40
6	170	10.81	0.70	9.68	10.19	10.83	11.44	11.94
7	119	9.14	1.36	6.07	8.24	9.48	10.23	10.60

MANDIBULAR DENTITION

1	183	5.54	0.35	4.98	5.15	5.52	5.89	6.12
2	159	6.05	0.43	5.39	5.65	6.05	6.42	6.87
3	161	6.98	0.58	6.22	6.52	7.03	7.50	7.67
4	157	6.91	0.70	5.46	6.24	6.97	7.57	7.86
5	141	7.25	0.70	6.41	6.81	7.26	7.63	8.08
6	163	11.18	0.84	9.93	10.59	11.23	11.79	12.19
7	110	9.68	1.08	8.41	8.93	9.71	10.48	11.24

*Courtesy of Center for Human Growth and Development, The University of Michigan.

TABLE VIII-1*B*.—MESIODISTAL TOOTH WIDTHS (PERMANENT FEMALE DENTITION)*

MAXILLARY DENTITION

Tooth	N	Mean (mm.)	Standard Deviation	5%	15%	Percentiles (mm.) 50%	85%	95%
1	123	8.60	0.77	7.41	8.04	8.61	9.30	9.68
2	117	6.85	0.68	5.60	6.21	6.88	7.43	7.95
3	120	7.44	0.50	6.70	7.03	7.48	7.89	8.05
4	121	6.51	0.56	5.57	6.01	6.60	7.01	7.28
5	106	6.48	0.52	5.63	6.02	6.51	6.96	7.37
6	137	10.29	1.01	8.32	9.63	10.34	11.10	11.68
7	79	8.49	1.32	6.76	7.67	8.78	9.54	9.87

MANDIBULAR DENTITION

1	148	5.46	0.64	4.84	5.14	5.43	5.78	5.98
2	123	5.84	0.60	5.29	5.56	5.89	6.26	6.39
3	121	6.56	0.38	6.01	6.21	6.55	6.90	7.27
4	121	6.75	0.74	5.24	6.16	6.84	7.51	7.74
5	106	7.07	0.57	6.26	6.64	7.04	7.48	7.86
6	128	10.61	1.14	8.79	9.86	10.84	11.40	11.91
7	83	9.39	0.69	8.11	8.71	9.43	10.04	10.42

*Courtesy of Center for Human Growth and Development, The University of Michigan.

f) Sequence and Position of Erupting Teeth

There are a variety of eruptive sequences for the permanent dentition (see Chapter VI, Section D-2-e). Some sequences preserve well the arch perimeter, whereas others are early symptoms of developing malocclusions (Fig. VIII-12).

Fig. VIII-12.—Symbolization of the sequence of eruption. **A,** normal sequence. **B,** abnormal sequence.

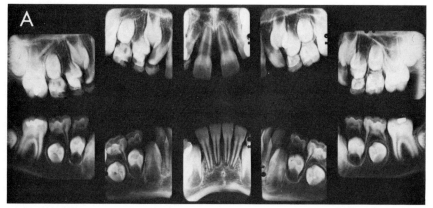

```
      7354216 | 6124537
      7543216 | 6123457
```

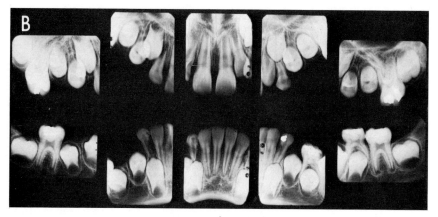

```
        ???   |   ???
      7354216 | 6124573
      3574216 | 6124735
        ???   |   ???
```

g) *Malposed Individual Teeth*

Malpositions of teeth must be determined according to their developmental status not by their ultimate position in the line of the arch. For example, maxillary cuspids usually erupt high in the alveolar process, point mesially and labially and look a bit unsightly to patient and parent. Such a position is normal only if there is adequate space in the arch for the tooth and if the examiner can visualize this position as part of normal eruption. Later, the same position is a malposition.

h) *Occlusal Relationships of the Teeth*

With the mandible in the retruded contact position or the ideal occlusal position (see Chapters X and XII), the occlusal relationships of the teeth should be considered in detail, beginning at one side in the molar region and advancing around the arch to the opposite side. (1) Note the precise intercuspation of each of the posterior teeth, and whether the intercuspation is symmetric. (2) Determine precisely the anteroposterior relationship of the molars and cuspids, and determine any reasons for dissimilarity between their intercuspation. (3) Study the effects of tipped and rotated permanent teeth. (4) The incisor relationships, both vertical and horizontal, should be measured (Fig. VIII-13). (5) Note any lack of occlusal stops as an open bite, and find an explanation for its existence. There are two definitions of open bite in current orthodontic usage.

Fig. VIII-13.—Method of measuring overjet. The Boley gauge is placed against the labial surface of the lower incisor, the sliding portion of the gauge is moved back to touch the labial surface of the upper incisor and the distance is then read off directly.

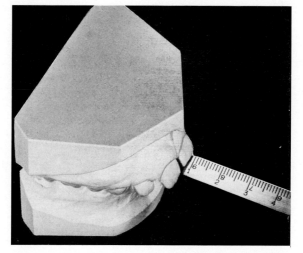

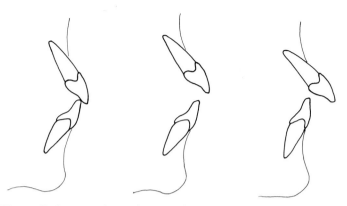

Fig. VIII-14.—Definition of open bite. At the left, the normal incisor relationship showing contact between upper and lower incisors. In the middle, an open bite without overlap of the incisors. At the right, an open bite with overlap of the incisors. Often, only the middle figure is described as an open bite, but the condition at the right also is an open bite, since there are no functional or occlusal stops present. The absence of occlusal contact with antagonistic teeth (functional stops) is proof of an open bite.

The first defines open bite as the absence of incisal overlap (Fig. VIII-14); the second defines open bite as the absence of an occlusal stop (Fig. VIII-14). It is most important to use the latter definition. Some cases, for example, Class II, Division 1, may show incisal overlap and what seems to be an unimportant lack of intermaxillary incisal contact. However, as treatment proceeds, the incisors are retracted and the occlusal plane leveled, the open bite becomes more obvious (Fig. VIII-15). In such instances, incisal retraction encroaches on the tongue's functional

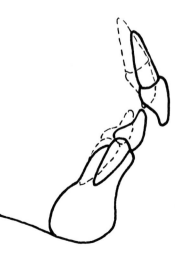

Fig. VIII-15.—Mild open bites, often undiagnosed at the start of treatment, are dramatized during treatment if the incisors are retracted into the functional space of the tongue.

space, dramatizing with treatment a condition that was present but undiagnosed at the start.

Step 5. CLASSIFY THE OCCLUSION

It is not enough to classify the occlusion on the basis of the first permanent molar relationship alone. The skeletal profile must be classified, the cuspid relationship noted, the incisor relationship studied, the position of the dentures to their bases observed and so forth. Study carefully Chapter IX on Classification, for the classification procedure is one of the most misused and misunderstood procedures in orthodontics.

Step 6. EVALUATE THE AVAILABLE SPACE

One of the most important steps in the cursory orthodontic examination is the evaluation of the space available to achieve desired tooth positions and occlusal corrections. Before all of the permanent teeth are present in the mouth, this procedure is called the Mixed Dentition Analysis, details of which will be found in Chapter XI. When the permanent dentition is completed as far as the second molars, space analysis often is more critical and difficult, and the diagnostic setup (see Chapter XI) may be utilized.

Perhaps evaluation of the available space is the most difficult task during the cursory examination, since a quantitative estimate of the amount of space available and needed is necessary. Most parts of the cursory examination are qualitative and subjective judgments; space analysis, even at the start, is based on precise measurements. One may be tempted to make quick, crude estimates by visual observation alone, or by ratings as "very crowded," "moderately crowded," "spaced," etc. Unless one's retinas are calibrated in millimeters, casual inspection is insufficient even for the cursory examination. The Mixed Dentition Analysis described in Chapter XI is intended for use on dental casts. If casts are available, the Mixed Dentition Analysis should be completed on them during the cursory examination. Often, however, a cursory examination is done before record casts are obtained. It is better, under such circumstances, to do a Mixed Dentition Analysis directly in the mouth (Fig. VIII-16) than to make casual guesses that may bias incorrectly all other initial thoughts concerning the case. The Mixed Dentition Analysis obtained directly in the mouth is helpful at this time but must be verified later when casts are available.

Step 7. STUDY THE FUNCTIONAL OCCLUSAL RELATIONSHIP

There is a possible or potential functional element in every malocclusion. The patient's usual occlusal position may be due to occlusal interferences in the undeviated path of closure, that is, in-

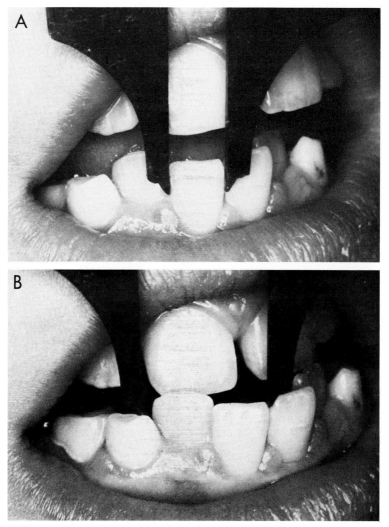

Fig. VIII-16.—The Mixed Dentition Analysis directly in the mouth. **A,** measuring the lower incisor width. **B,** ascertaining the amount of space needed to align two of the lower incisors (see Chapter XI for details of the Mixed Dentition Analysis).

terferences may prompt a reflex shifting of the mandible during closure to an occlusal position dictated by the cusps and forcing an imbalance on the musculature; such malocclusions have been mistermed functional malocclusions (although they more properly should be labeled malfunctional occlusions). Such "slides into centric" (aren't they really slides out of centric?) may be seen at any age, but the functional slides into occlusion in the primary and mixed dentitions are of a grosser nature than those ordinarily seen in the completed permanent dentition.

Fig. VIII-17.—Extra-oral testing for a functional slide into occlusion. Dots are placed at selected points on the midline and the patient is asked to open and close his jaw gently. **A,** the jaw wide open. Note that the dots are now aligned. **B,** the mandible in a postural position. Note that the dots are still aligned. **C,** the teeth in occlusion. In this instance, as the teeth came together, the mandible was guided by cuspal interferences into a functional crossbite and was forced to swing to the left on closure. Note the malalignment of the dots in **C.**

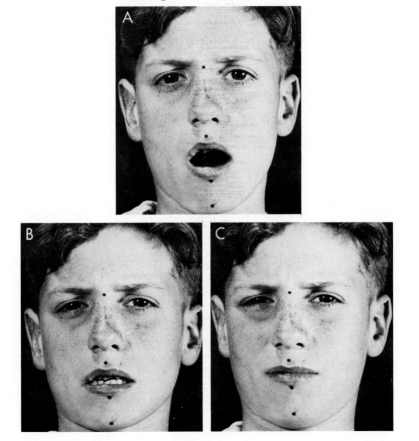

Detailed procedures for analyzing occlusal interferences and registering jaw relationships are given in Chapter XI. Since a brief functional analysis of the occlusion must be a part of the cursory examination, the following procedures are suggested:

(*a*) With the patient sitting upright and the head supported by the headrest, or supported in such a way that the Frankfurt plane is parallel to the floor, have the patient open and close his jaws slowly. Pay particular attention to the chin and mandibular incisors during the last stages of closing. Changes in the overjet relationship as the teeth come into occlusion are typically noted. The use of dots marked on the midlines of the face, or a straightedge held to the midlines, is useful in diagnosing lateral shifts of the jaws (Fig. VIII-17). The Facial Form Analysis makes use of such a functional evaluation (see Fig. VIII-10).

(*b*) Correlate the two denture midlines, asking the patient to move the mandible forward gently while you guide it so that the midlines still coincide (Fig. VIII-18). As the patient moves the jaw gently forward and backward with the midlines coincident, a quick and clear view of cuspal interferences sometimes can be noted. Often they are found in the primary cuspid region during the mixed dentition.

(*c*) Gently guide the mandible into its retruded contact position and note any cuspal interferences between the retruded contact position and the usual occlusal position.

(*d*) Place the jaw in the retruded contact position and guide the patient slightly into lateral occlusion on either side to observe occlusal impedance to lateral function (Fig. VIII-19).

(*e*) Observe carefully jaw movements during the unconscious swallow (q.v.) to ascertain whether it is completed with the teeth together or the teeth apart.

(*f*) Ascertain any abnormal movements of the jaw during speech and mastication.

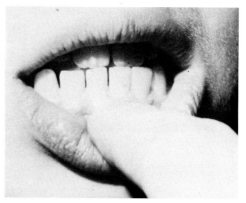

Fig. VIII-18.—Checking for occlusal interferences during protrusion.

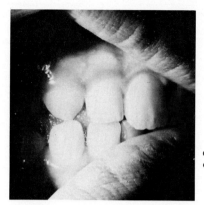

Fig. VIII-19.—Checking for occlusal interferences in lateral excursive occlusion.

(*g*) Even during this quick functional analysis of the occlusion, one may mark any interfering cusps with articulation paper, noting in the written record the teeth involved.

Step 8. COMPLETE THE PERMANENT RECORD

Three permanent records are derived from the cursory examination—the case history, record casts and radiographs. Memory cannot be trusted to recall minute details at a later date. Furthermore, subsequent problems missed in the initial examination but observed later may be clarified by referral to the original record. Many problems in dental practice are reasonably static and can be expected to remain unchanged until corrected. The signs and symptoms of malocclusion often are fleeting and ever changing; therefore, it is essential that a continuous record be kept of changes in the developing dentition.

a) *The Case History (Fig. VIII-20)*

The case history should include all of the information gathered in the cursory examination as well as the usual data concerning the patient's age, parents' names, address, family physician, school, siblings, etc. The case history may include, as well, any questions that arise and must be answered later.

Factors to be studied in detail before treatment can be begun should be mentioned. The orthodontic case history must be written out and thus resembles more a medical case history than it does the usual codified representation of teeth and cavities used in restorative dentistry. Time spent in compiling a complete orthodontic case history is time productively invested, for this record is of continuing assistance during subsequent observations of the dentition's development during treatment. No dentist treating malocclusion can afford to have an improper case history.

ORTHODONTIC CASE HISTORY

NAME _____ Nickname_____ Date_____

ADDRESS _____ PHONE_____

SEX _____ AGE____ yr. ___ mo. HEIGHT _____ WEIGHT _____ BIRTH
DATE _____

SCHOOL _____ HOBBIES _____

Siblings (names and ages) _____

Family physician (name, address, tel. no.) _____
_____

I. GENERAL INFORMATION

    A. Reason for evaluation (related by parent) _____
_____

    B. Past orthodontic treatment: No_____ Yes_____ (Explain) _____
_____

    C. History of related problems:

        1. Nasorespiratory   Yes_____ No_____
        2. Tonsillitis   Yes_____ No_____
        3. Allergy   Yes_____ No_____
        4. Others   Yes_____ No_____

    D. Percentile level for: Height _____ Weight _____

    E. Patient's attitude toward problem and orthodontics:

    F. Others in family who have had orthodontic treatment:

    G. Other comments:

II. ORTHODONTIC RECORDS

	Date	**Date**	Date	Date	Date	Date	Date	Date
A. Casts with wax bite								
B. Full-mouth x-rays								
C. Lateral cephalogram								
D. Photographs								
E. Other								

Fig. VIII-20.—Orthodontic case history. This usually is supplemented by the Mixed Dentition Analysis (Fig. XI-17), the Facial Form Analysis (Fig. VIII-10), the health questionnaire (Fig. VIII-2), treatment goals (Fig. XIV-3) and one or more of the various cephalometric analyses (Figs. XII-13, 14, 15, 19). It also may be supported by such features as the Howes analysis (Fig. XI-13) and the Bolton analysis (Fig. XI-11). (*Continued.*)

III. FACIAL FEATURES (other than Facial Form Analysis)

    A. Lips:
        1. Posture at rest: Open_____   Closed_____
        2. Upper lip: Normal_____ Hypo_____ Hypertonic_____ Incompetent_____
        3. Lower lip: Normal_____ Hypo_____ Hypertonic_____ Overextended____
        4. Mentalis action: Yes____ No____ During _____

    B. Soft tissue profile: Normal_____   Abnormal_____

    C. Breathing pattern: Nasal_____   Mouth_____

                                    Acute_____   Chronic_____

    D. Other comments:

IV. INTRA-ORAL FEATURES

    A. Gingiva:

    B. Tonsils present: Yes_____   No_____   Condition_____

    C. Adenoids present: Yes_____   No_____   Condition_____

    D. Tongue action:
        1. Extent and mobility: Normal_____   Abnormal_____
        2. Postural position: Normal_____   Abnormal_____
        3. Position during speech: Normal_____   Abnormal_____
        4. Position during mastication: Normal_____   Abnormal_____

    E. Swallowing:
        1. Unconscious: Teeth together_____   Apart_____
        2. Command: Teeth together_____   Apart_____
        3. Water: Teeth together_____   Apart_____
        4. Masticatory: Teeth together_____   Apart_____
        5. Classification:
           a. Simple tongue-thrust
           b. Complex tongue-thrust
           c. Retained infantile swallow
           d. Retained infantile posture

    F. Other habits:
        1. Describe: Digital_____
                     Bruxism_____
                     Other_____
        2. Occurrence: Active_____   Inactive_____
                     Continuous   Yes_____   No_____
                     Night only   Yes_____   No____ __
                     Tension only   Yes_____   No_____
        3. Previous attempts at correction:
           a. By parents   Yes_____   No_____
           b. By others   Yes_____   No_____

    G. Other comments:

Fig. VIII-20 (cont.).—Orthodontic case history. (*Continued.*)

V.   DENTITION and OCCLUSION   (other than M. D. A.)

A.   Supernumerary teeth

B.   Missing teeth

C.   Malformed, impacted or ectopic teeth

D.   Teeth showing delayed development

E.   Eruption sequence, apparent

Significance:

F.   Maxillary arch form: Tapering, trapezoid, ovoid, "U" type
     Mandibular arch form: Tapering, trapezoid, ovoid, "U" type

G.   Molar relationship   I   II   III   E-E   (Circle, indicate Rt, Lt)
     Cuspid relationship   I   II   III   E-E
     Overjet _____mm.
     Overbite _____mm.
     Open bite_____mm.

H.   Midlines:
     1.   Together

     2.   Upper
          Lower to right   _____mm.   _____mm.

     3.   Upper
          Lower to left   _____mm.   _____mm.

I.   Arch asymmetry

J.   Teeth mesially displaced

K.   Other comments:

Fig. VIII-20 (cont.).—Orthodontic case history. (*Continued.*)

CLINICAL RECORD

NAME _____ NUMBER _____

DATE	CLINICAL SERVICE RENDERED	NEXT TIME

Fig. VIII-20 (cont.).—Orthodontic case history, clinical record.

b) Record Casts

It is difficult to recall minute occlusal details of every patient. It is even more difficult for the parents who see their child constantly to realize the important changes that take place with growth and orthodontic treatment. For these and obvious legal reasons, a carefully prepared set of record casts is a part of the cursory examination. Procedures for taking impressions and preparing record casts are given in Chapter XVII; for their detailed analysis, see Chapter XI.

c) Radiographic Record

If the necessary radiographs are not available, their acquisition and study becomes the last step in the cursory examination. A discussion of the several radiographic projections of use in analysis of the occlusion will be found in Chapter XI. A discussion of cephalometric analysis is contained in Chapter XII.

SUGGESTED READINGS

Ackerman, J. L., and Proffit, W. R.: The characteristics of malocclusion: A modern approach to classification and diagnosis. Am. J. Orthodont. 56:443, 1969.

Jacquez, J. A.: The Diagnostic Process: Problems and Perspectives, in Jacquez, J. A. (ed.), *The Diagnostic Process* (Ann Arbor: The University of Michigan Press, 1964).

Moorrees, C. F. A., and Gron, A. M.: Principles of orthodontic diagnosis, Angle Orthodont. 36:258, 1966.

IX

Classification and Terminology of Malocclusion

> The beginning of wisdom is to call things by their right names. —CHINESE PROVERB

IT HAS BEEN SAID that the introduction of the Angle system of classification of malocclusions was the principal step in turning disorganized clinical concepts into the disciplined science of orthodontics. This may be true. But it also is true that no phase of orthodontics is less understood or more misused. Many new and simplified systems for classifying malocclusions have been introduced, and each new system soon has many modifications. The reason for this constant search for an unfailing method of categorizing cases is due not only to inadequacies in systems already presented but to their misuse as well. Someone once said that 5% of us think, 15% of us think we think and the other 80% are looking for rules so that we won't have to think. Those who strive to devise a perfect formula that will enable them to put each case into a carefully numbered pigeonhole where all will be precisely alike and treated in exactly the same fashion obviously are in the 80% group. Unfortunately, malocclusions are not so easily sorted and typed. There is a need for clinicians in the 5% group who think, because orthodontics cannot be practiced primarily by any set of rules, however cleverly devised.

A. What is a Classification System?

To classify malocclusion, one must have a concept of normal occlusion. Since normal occlusion is the composite of many factors, some of which, if measured separately, might be outside the expected normal range, the simple classification of normal or abnormal occlusion is difficult. A person with abnormally large teeth may have a normal occlusion, provided other features are sufficiently large to compensate for the large teeth. Occlusion may be best conceptualized for classification purposes as a frequency distribution with a range of features typically found in Class I, Class II and Class III. No single feature measured is a valid clue to any class because of the overlap of the class distributions for single measurements. Certain signs and symptoms tend to cluster in typical malocclusions, producing syndromes or classes whose identification and labeling are useful.

Each time that a patient is examined, he is classified subconsciously by the examiner in many different ways. We say, for example, that this patient is an 8-year-old boy who has not yet acquired his maxillary permanent central incisors. In one sentence we have classified our patient by three different standards—sex, age and time of eruption of permanent teeth. But this classification tells us nothing concerning the plan of treatment and the prognosis. In Chapter VII on Etiology, care was taken to differentiate several factors involved: (1) the cause, (2) the time it was acting, (3) the site where its effect was felt and (4) the resulting orthodontic problem. Classification systems, to be usable, must confine themselves to the last—the resulting malocclusion, as determined for a specific developmental age.

A classification system is a grouping of clinical cases, of similar appearance, for ease in handling; it is not a system of diagnosis, method for determining prognosis or a way of defining treatment.

B. Purpose of Classifying

One well may ask, then, "Why does one classify?" There are several practical reasons for so doing. Historically, certain types always have been grouped together; thus, the literature contains many articles confined, for example, to "The Treatment of Angle Class II, Division 1 Malocclusions." It is necessary, if we are to appreciate such an article, to have a clear concept of just how an Angle Class II, Division 1 case appears. All Class II, Division 1 malocclusions are not exactly alike, their etiology is not necessarily identical, their prognoses are not similar nor do they all demand precisely the same treatment; still, it is traditional to group them together. A second reason for classifying is ease of reference. It is much easier to call a case a Class III malocclusion than to go into all of the detail necessary to describe the dentocranial morphology of mandibular prognathism. The listener will have a rough idea of the problem simply from the label "Class III" even though he does not know the etiology, the prognosis or the best treatment procedure. Experience with previous cases bearing the same label facilitates understanding of problems that may be encountered in treatment; thus, classification aids comparison. There also is a reflexive or self-communicative reason for classification. When we name a malocclusion a severe Class II, we are (1) identifying problems of which we must be wary, (2) recalling past difficulties with similar cases and (3) alerting ourselves to possible strategies and appliances that may be needed in treatment.

Classification is done for traditional reasons, for ease of reference, for purposes of comparison and for ease in self-communication.

C. When to Classify

One of the most common mistakes is that of trying to label each case immediately. Do not be too hasty to categorize. The classification is not the diagnosis. It is far better first to describe that which is wrong in a complete and precise manner. If, at the end of the examination, the case falls into a certain usable group, it should then be named. If it does not fit easily into any of the classic groupings, do not worry. Do not, in any circumstance, strain to put a case in a given classification; the fit seldom is perfect. There was good reason in Chapter VIII for leaving the process of classification until the fifth step of the cursory examination. Immediate classification may prejudice later thinking. Study the malocclusion carefully; describe it in detail; then, if possible, classify it.

D. Systems of Classification

Of all the many methods of classifying malocclusions presented to the profession, only two persist and are widely used today. One of these, the Angle system,[1] is used intact, but the other, the Simon system,[3] is used in its entirety by very few clinicians. However, certain fundamental concepts contained in it have had a great influence, and for that reason it will be described briefly.

1. ANGLE SYSTEM

This system is based on the anteroposterior relationships of the jaws with each other (Fig. IX-1). Angle originally presented his classification on the theory that the maxillary first permanent molar invariably was in correct position. Subsequent cephalometric research has not substantiated this hypothesis. Emphasis on the relationship of the first permanent molars caused clinicians to ignore the facial skeleton itself and to think solely in terms of the position of the teeth. Therefore, malfunction of muscles and problems of growth of bones often were overlooked. Even today, there is a tendency in the inexperienced to center too much attention on this one tooth relationship. The first molar relationship changes during the various stages of development of the dentition (see Chapter VI). A better correlation between Angle's concepts and treatment is obtained if one uses the Angle groups to classify skeletal relationships. A Class II molar relationship may result in several different ways, each requiring a different strategy in treatment, but a Class II skeletal pattern is not misunderstood, since it dominates the occlusion and its treatment. Clinicians now use the Angle system differently than it was originally presented, for the basis of the classification has shifted from the molars to skeletal relationships.

The Angle system does not itself take into account discrepancies in a vertical or lateral plane. Although the anteroposterior relationship of the teeth may be the most important single consideration, this classification system sometimes causes the uninitiated to overlook such problems as overbite and narrowness of the arches. Despite these and other criticisms, the Angle method of classifying cases is the most practical and hence the most popular in use at present.

Fig. IX-1.—Angle classification. Facial profile and molar relationship; note how the two change together. It would be difficult, for example, to have a Class III molar relationship in a Class II profile. (*Continued.*)

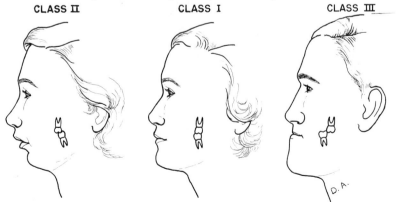

CLASS II   CLASS I   CLASS III

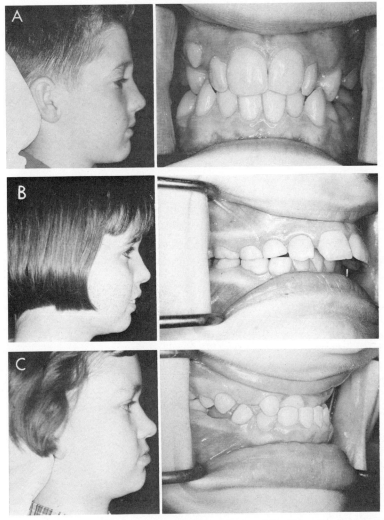

Fig. IX-1 (cont.).—Angle classification. The relationship of the soft tissue profile to the occlusion. **A,** a balanced profile with a Class I malocclusion. **B,** a retrognathic profile and the Class II malocclusion. Note how the lips reflect the overjet of the incisors. **C,** a Class III malocclusion. Here, the lip posture clearly indicates the presence of a Class III malocclusion.

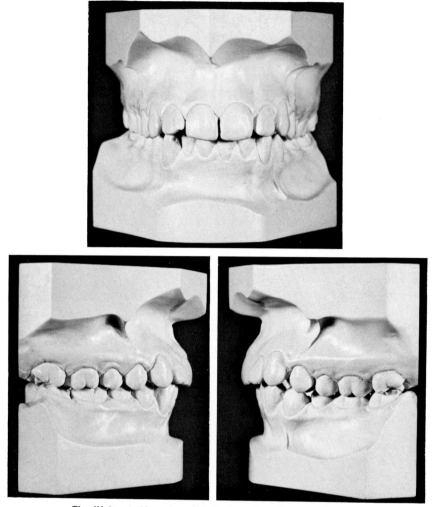

Fig. IX-2.—A Class I malocclusion. See also Figure IX-1.

a) Class I (Neutroclusion)

Those malocclusions in which there is a normal anteroposterior relationship between the maxilla and the mandible fall in this class. The triangular ridge of the mesiobuccal cusp of the maxillary first permanent molar articulates in the buccal groove of the mandibular first permanent molar. The bony base supporting the mandibular dentition is directly beneath that of the maxillary, and neither is too far anterior or posterior in relation to the cranium (Fig. IX-2).

b) Class II (Distoclusion)

Those malocclusions in which there is a "distal" relationship of mandible to maxilla make up this class. The mesial groove of the mandibular first permanent molar articulates posteriorly to the mesiobuccal cusp of the maxillary first permanent molar (Fig. IX-3).

Fig. IX-3.—A typical Class II, Division 1 malocclusion as shown in dental casts.

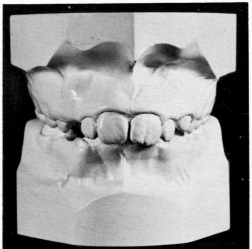

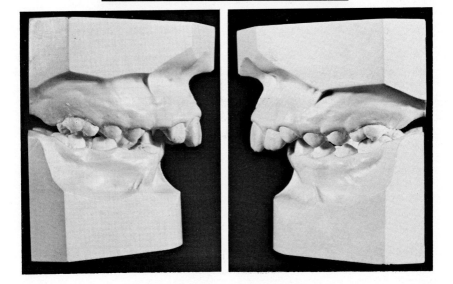

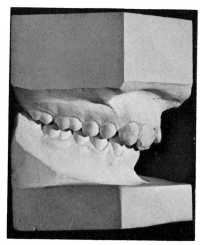

Fig. IX-4.—A typical Class II, Division 2 malocclusion. Class II, Division 2 malocclusions ordinarily do not show the basic skeletal retrognathism seen in Class II, Division 1. The maxillary central incisors seem to be tipped lingually and the lateral incisors are in labioversion. This incisal relationship is the most typical diagnostic sign for Class II, Division 2, although the lingual tipping of the central incisors is more apparent than real.

1) DIVISION 1.—Distoclusion in which the maxillary incisors are typically in extreme labioversion (Fig. IX-3).

2) DIVISION 2.—Distoclusion in which the maxillary central incisors are near normal anteroposteriorly or slightly in linguoversion, whereas the maxillary lateral incisors have tipped labially and mesially (Fig. IX-4).

3) SUBDIVISIONS.—When the distoclusion occurs on one side of the dental arch only, the unilaterality is referred to as a subdivision of its division.

c) Class III (Mesioclusion)

Those malocclusions in which there is a "mesial" relationship of mandible to maxilla make up Class III. The mesial groove of the mandibular first permanent molar articulates anteriorly to the mesiobuccal cusp of the maxillary first permanent molar (Figs. IX-1 and IX-5).

2. SIMON SYSTEM

The dental arches in the Simon system are related to three anthropologic planes based on cranial landmarks[3] (Fig. IX-6). The planes are the Frankfurt, the orbital and the midsagittal. They are used in cephalometric analyses frequently, but the only part of this system in routine current usage is some of the terminology.

a) Anteroposterior Relationships (Orbital Plane)

When the dental arch, or part of it, is more anteriorly placed than normal with respect to the orbital plane, it is said to be in *protraction.* When

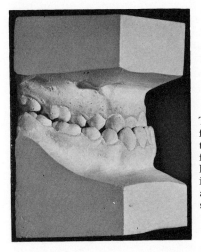

Fig. IX-5.—A Class III malocclusion. The mesiobuccal cusp of the maxillary first permanent molar occludes posteriorly to the buccal groove of the mandibular first permanent molar and the mandibular incisors occlude outside the maxillary incisors. Such an occlusal configuration almost always is the result of marked skeletal mandibular prognathism.

the arch, or part of it, is more posteriorly placed than normal with respect to the orbital plane, it is said to be in *retraction*. Simon placed much emphasis on the fact that he found the orbital plane passing through the maxillary cuspid region in a high percentage of normal occlusions. This finding was termed the Law of the Cuspid. Subsequent research by several investigators has shown that the position of the

Fig. IX-6.—The Simon system of classification of malocclusion. Tooth malpositions are related to three planes of space in the head.

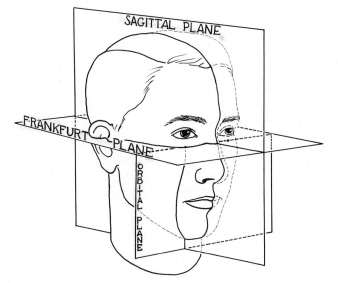

maxillary cuspid does not coincide with the orbital plane sufficiently often to have practical diagnostic value.

b) *Mediolateral Relationships (Midsagittal Plane)*

When the dental arch, or part of it, is nearer to the midsagittal plane than the normal position, it is said to be in *contraction*. When the arch, or part of it, is farther away from the midsagittal plane than the normal position, it is said to be in *distraction*.

c) *Vertical Relationships (Frankfurt Plane)*

When the dental arch, or part of it, is nearer to the Frankfurt plane than the normal position, it is said to be in *attraction*. When the dental arch, or part of it, is farther away from the Frankfurt plane than the normal position, it is said to be in *abstraction*.

Only three of these terms are in frequent use—*protraction, retraction* and *contraction*. For example, an Angle Class II case may be due to maxillary protraction, mandibular retraction or both. Similarly, a narrowed dental arch is said to be contracted. The principal contribution of the Simon system is its emphasis on the orientation of the dental arches to the facial skeleton. In addition to this, it separates carefully, by means of its terminology, problems in malpositions of teeth from those of osseous dysplasia; for example, maxillary dental protraction is differentiated from total maxillary protraction. In the former, only the teeth are anteriorly placed, whereas, in the latter, the entire maxilla and its teeth are protracted. This system probably is capable of more precision than the Angle system, and it is three-dimensional. However, in truth, it is cumbersome, confusing at times (e.g., attraction is intrusion of the maxillary teeth and extrusion of mandibular teeth) and little used in practice. Simon's concepts, however, have had a great impact on orthodontic thinking and even have altered the fashion in which the Angle system is used.

3. NAMING MALPOSITIONS OF INDIVIDUAL TEETH AND GROUPS OF TEETH

a) *Individual Teeth*

Lischer's nomenclature[2] to describe malpositions of individual teeth is in general use. It simply involves adding the suffix "-version" to a word to indicate the direction from the normal position:

a) Mesioversion—mesial to the normal position.
b) Distoversion—distal to the normal position.
c) Linguoversion—lingual to the normal position.
d) Labioversion or buccoversion—toward the lip or cheek.
e) Infraversion—away from the line of occlusion.

f) Supraversion—extended past the line of occlusion, i.e., below in the maxilla and above in the mandible.

g) Axiversion—tipped, the wrong axial inclination.

h) Torsiversion—rotated on its long axis.

i) Transversion—wrong order in the arch, transposition.

The terms are combined when a tooth assumes a malposition involving more than one direction from the normal. Thus, for example, sometimes it is said that a tooth is in mesiolabioversion.

b) *Vertical Variations of Groups of Teeth*

Deep overbite is a term applied when there is excessive vertical overlap of the incisors. Just what is excessive overlap is difficult to define, but when the soft tissue of the palate is impinged, or the health of the supporting structures is endangered, certainly that bite is excessively deep. Wide variations in depth of the bite may be seen, however, with no danger to the occlusion or health of the supporting structures.

Open bite is a term applied when there is localized absence of occlusion while the remaining teeth are in occlusion (see Fig. VIII-14, p. 292). Open bite is seen most frequently in the anterior part of the mouth, although posterior open bites are encountered also. See Chapter XV for a description of treatment of this problem.

c) *Transverse Variations of Groups of Teeth*

Crossbite is a term used to indicate an abnormal buccolingual (labiolingual) relationship of the teeth (Fig. IX-7). The most common crossbite is that seen when buccal cusps of some of the maxillary posterior teeth occlude lingually to the buccal cusps of the lower teeth. When one or more maxillary teeth are in crossbite toward the midline, it is termed *lingual crossbite*. When the lingual cusps of upper posterior teeth occlude completely buccally of the buccal cusps of the lower teeth, it is termed *buccal crossbite*.

Fig. IX-7.—Crossbite. **A,** the normal buccolingual relationship of molars. **B,** buccal crossbite. **C,** lingual crossbite. **D,** complete lingual crossbite.

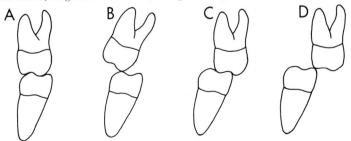

4. Etiologic Classification; Its Effect on Diagnosis

Although it is handy to be able to group cases easily, it is more important and practical to learn their origin. There is, for example, a wide diversity of malocclusions that must bear the label "Class II," yet they may have differing geneses and varying prognoses and may require diverse appliances. It will be easier to clarify this situation by a return for a moment to the etiologic concepts outlined in Chapter VII. We have seen that there are several primary tissue sites in which orthodontic problems may originate. Indeed, one may classify cases according to the tissue primarily involved, for the soundest method of precisely determining differences in similar clinical problems is to study each on the basis of the probable site of origin.

a) Osseous

This category includes problems in abnormal growth, size, shape or proportion of any of the bones of the craniofacial complex. When any bone of the face develops in a perverted, delayed, advanced or otherwise asynchronous manner, the aberration may be reflected in an orthodontic problem. Class III cases, for example, may be due to mandibular hypertrophy and Class II to mandibular inadequacy. The clinical condition may be ascribed to a genetic cause or severe malfunctions. Each facial bone has a genetically determined potential of growth that may be altered by environment. This genetic pattern of development may express itself somewhat independently of the dental area. The terms "basal bone" and "apical base" have been coined to describe the areas involved in osseous dysplasias. The remaining bone, the alveolar process, reacts largely to the needs of the dentition it supports. (NOTE: Axel Lundstrom, who introduced the term and concept of "apical base," stated that it includes an area involving the apices of the teeth. Enlow's work [see Figs. IV-10 and IV-13] supports this view, although common usage excludes the dento-alveolar region.) The alveolar process can be shaped and altered by tooth movements; the basal bone is less responsive to the forces of orthodontic appliances. Abnormal or perverted muscle contractions readily alter the conformation of the alveolar process, but it takes a greater muscular abnormality acting much longer to affect the basal bone area. Something is known concerning the effect of muscles and appliances on the alveolar process and their impact on the apical base; base relationships have been studied in detail only in recent years (see Chapter IV).

Cephalometric analysis provides the best means of studying variations of the craniofacial skeleton. It should be remembered that other parts always are affected secondarily. Malpositions of teeth in such cases are mostly the result of abnormal growth of bone, an expression or symptom of the principal fault. Orthodontic treatment may be planned to correct the fundamental osseous dysplasia or to accommodate the dentition to it. Orthodontic appliances, although mostly influencing the dento-alveolar area, also can have a profound "orthopedic" effect on basal bone as well.

Osseous dysplasia or skeletal disharmony, unfortunately, is a component of many of the malocclusions seen most frequently. Only the most naïve clinician avoids analysis of the skeletal aspects of craniofacial deformity. Correction or camouflage of skeletal disharmonies of the face is one of the primary tasks of dentists who would treat any but the most simple malocclusions. The adjective "skeletal" is applied to a high percentage of Class II problems, indicating significant osseous involvement. Most Class III malocclusions are skeletal in origin and even such apparently localized matters as deep bite or crossbite may have a skeletal basis.

b) *Muscular*

This group includes all problems in malfunction of the dentofacial musculature. Any persistent alteration in the normal synchrony of the mandibular movements or muscle contractions may result in distorted growth of the facial bones or abnormal positions of teeth. A simple lip-sucking habit may give rise to a Class II dentition and profile. Sometimes several habit patterns combine to make a complicated syndrome; for example, thumb-sucking. The sucking habit itself is a complicated neuromuscular reflex involving many muscles of the face, the temporomandibular articulation, throat, tongue and arm. Continued sucking may narrow the maxillary dental arch. This contraction of the maxillary arch gives rise to another complicated neuromuscular habit pattern, mandibular retraction. The narrowing of the maxillary arch results in tooth interference, and the mandible is then shifted posteriorly by the muscles to a position of better occlusal function. (Professor Hotz calls this "compulsive distoclusion.") A Class II molar relationship results, but each molar may be well related to its supporting bone and neither the mandible nor the maxilla be abnormal in size or conformation. In other words, the size of the bones and the positioning of the molars can be near normal and still a Class II relationship eventually obtains because the mandible is held by the muscles in a retruded position. In time, the upset of forces acting within the entire system produces the syndrome we call Class II (see Chapters IV, VI and VII).

Since such neuromuscular patterns of behavior are habits, they were once learned and hence are capable of being altered. Treatment is directed toward understanding the complete habit reflex, then removing precipitating influences or substituting other habits that are less detrimental. The prognosis usually is excellent if care is taken to learn well the entire syndrome and treatment is begun early. Neuromuscular or "functional" malocclusions always eventually bring about dental, dento-alveolar or skeletal manifestations that are not as easily reversible as the original reflex. There is near unanimity (a rare thing in orthodontics) that neuromuscular features of malocclusion should be treated as early as possible.

The role of the muscles in etiology will be found in Chapter VII, their part in dentitional and occlusal development in Chapter VI and in skeletal growth in Chapter IV. Maturation of the neuromusculature is described in Chapter V, analysis in Chapter X and treatment of the functional aspects of malocclusion in Chapter XV.

This category includes:

Functional "slides into occlusion" due to occlusal interferences.
Detrimental sucking habits, e.g., thumb, finger, lip, etc.
Abnormal patterns of mandibular closure.
Incompetent normal reflexes, e.g., lip posture.
Abnormal muscular contractions, e.g., tongue-thrusting during swallowing.

c) Dental

Dental problems involve primarily the teeth and their supporting structures. The malposition of a tooth on a bone is a totally different consideration from the growth of that bone or the muscular contractions that move bones. It is fortunate, indeed, that many clinical cases primarily involve the teeth, for they often are the easiest to intercept and retain. Care must be exercised, though, to determine whether the dental abnormality is the primary problem or whether it is secondary to aberrations in osseous growth or malfunction of muscles. Treatment is aimed at moving the teeth to their normal positions, replacing lost teeth or fitting the dentition's abnormalities to the facial skeleton and its musculature.

This category includes:

Malpositions of teeth.
Abnormal numbers of teeth.
Abnormal size of teeth.
Abnormal conformation or texture of teeth.

d) Comment

One rarely encounters a malocclusion that is solely a dental, a muscular or an osseous problem. So intimate are the interactions of growth that a change in one tissue easily affects another. Although all three tissues (bone, muscle and teeth) usually are involved in all dentofacial deformities, one is dominant—one is the primary etiologic tissue site. It is this one that largely determines the final treatment plan and prognosis, and on it we should focus our attention.

The classification has purposes other than providing a convenient tag for designating clinical problems. When thoughtfully applied, it also may help in understanding basic differences between cases that at first glance look similar.

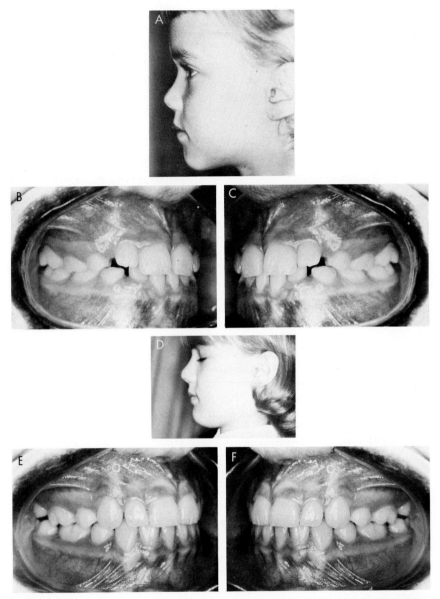

Fig. IX-8.—A Class I malocclusion. **A–C,** before treatment. **D–F,** after treatment.

E. The Class I Syndrome

Class I (neutroclusion) malocclusions are characterized by a normal molar and skeletal relationship. The skeletal profile is straight, and therefore the problem usually is dental in origin. Such problems as large teeth, open bite, deep bite, etc., are typical of Class I malocclusion. The lips and tongue are more likely to function normally than in Class II or Class III. A typical Class I malocclusion is shown in Figure IX-8. Treatment of Class I malocclusions is described in Chapter XV.

F. The Class II Syndrome

Class II (distoclusion, postnormal occlusion) is the most frequently encountered severe malocclusion syndrome. It is characterized by a mandibular dentition that is posterior to its normal relationship with the maxillary dentition. The malrelationship may be due to a basic osseous dysplasia or to forward movement of the maxillary dental arch and alveolar processes or a combination of skeletal and dental factors. The overjet is excessive in Class II, Division 1 and the bite is likely to be deep. The retrognathic profile and excessive overjet demand that the facial muscles and tongue adapt themselves by abnormal contraction patterns. Typically, there is a hyperactive mentalis muscle, which contracts strongly to elevate the orbicularis oris and effect the lip seal.

Class II, Division 2 is characterized by distoclusion, abnormal depth of bite, labioversion of the maxillary lateral incisors and more normal lip function. The Class II, Division 2 facial skeleton usually is not so dramatically retrognathic as Class II, Division 1. Figure IX-9 shows a typical Class II, Division 2 case. Figure IX-10 illustrates a typical Class II, Division 1 malocclusion.

Class II, although described here as a syndrome, is really a large grouping with many subtypes of Class II, Division 1. Some help in differentiation of the features of Class II will be found in Chapters XII and XV. See Chapter XV for the treatment of Class II malocclusion.

G. The Class III Syndrome

Class III (mesioclusion, prenormal occlusion) is characterized by mandibular prognathism, a Class III molar relationship and the mandibular incisors labially placed to the maxillary. Most frequently it is a deep-seated skeletal dysplasia, although functional Class IIIs are seen. In the adult, orthodontic treatment is aimed at camouflage of the skeletal pattern to improve aesthetics and function, but in the young child, growth may be directed to obtain a correction. Occasionally, surgery must be resorted to in order to treat well the severe Class III. Figure IX-11 illustrates a typical Class III syndrome treated in a child and

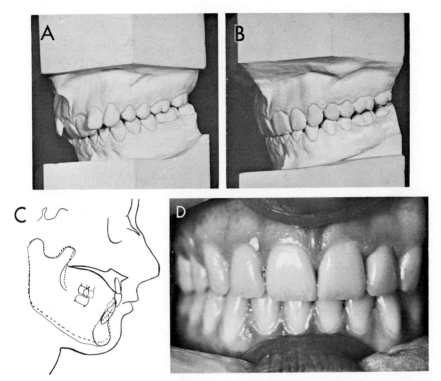

Fig. IX-9.—A typical Class II, Division 2 malocclusion treated in the permanent dentition. **A,** the casts before treatment. **B,** the casts after treatment. **C,** cephalometric tracings before treatment (*dotted lines*) and after treatment (*solid lines*). Note that the response is primarily dental and that the distal movement of the maxillary first molar also opened the bite. Further, note that the maxillary central incisors were not moved labially during treatment. **D,** intra-oral photograph after the retention period was over.

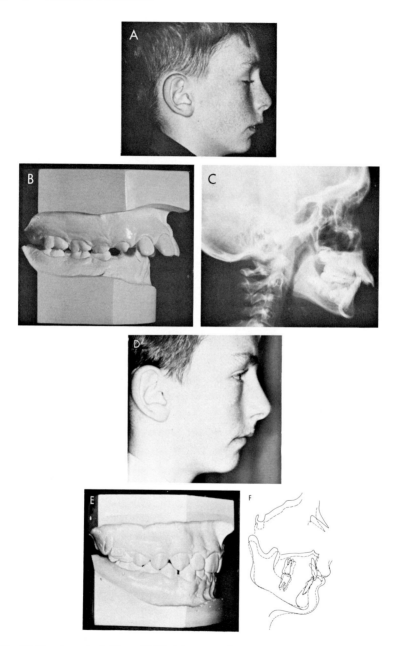

Fig. IX-10.—A typical Class II, Division 1 malocclusion. **A–C,** before treatment. Note the relationship of the lip posture to the overbite and overjet. See also how the facial skeleton, as shown in the cephalogram, determines the soft tissue profile and incisor relationship. **D–F,** the treated result. The casts were made

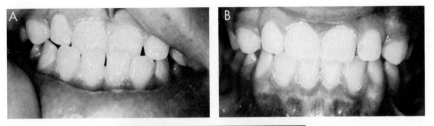

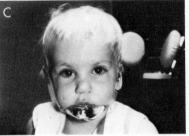

Fig. IX-11.—A Class III malocclusion treated in a young child. **A,** intra-oral photograph before treatment. **B,** intra-oral photograph a few months later. **C,** the chin cap appliance used in treatment. (Courtesy of Dr. T. M. Graber.)

during the retention period but the photograph and cephalogram are some time out of retention. Although the occlusal correction is satisfactory in this case, note the persistence of the marked skeletal retrognathism and that although the lip posture is improved and adapts nicely to the new incisor relationship, it still betrays the Class II facial skeleton. The large amount of nasal growth in this case tends to counteract some of the aesthetics achieved by the orthodontic correction.

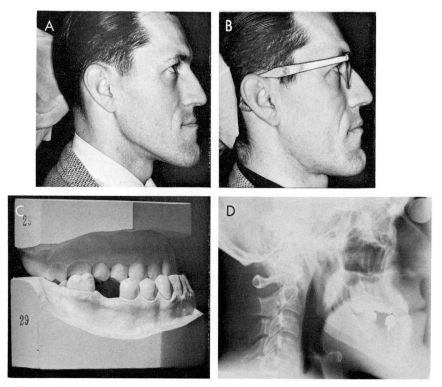

Fig. IX-12.—**A,** a typical severe Class III malocclusion due to mandibular prognathism. **B,** the profile at the end of treatment. **C,** the casts before treatment. **D,** cephalogram before treatment. **E,** intra-oral photograph before treatment. This case was corrected by combined orthodontic and surgical procedures. Note the typical incisal relationship and anterior crossbite. The latter always appears, since, as the mandible grows forward, it carries a wider part of the mandibular denture to a narrower diameter of the maxillary denture. *(Continued.)*

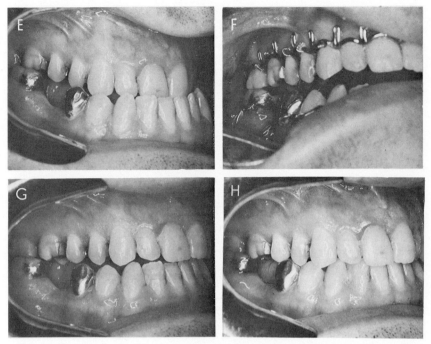

Fig. IX-12 (cont.).—F, shows the result immediately following surgery. Note the presence in the mouth of the splint for intra-oral wiring. The occlusion has not yet settled into place. **G,** after removal of the appliances and prior to occlusal equilibration. **H,** after occlusal equilibration. Compare **B** and **H** with **A, C, D** and **E.**

Figure IX-12 shows a well-treated adult case. See Chapter XV for a discussion of the possibilities of treatment of Class III.

REFERENCES

1. Angle, E. H.: *Malocclusion of the Teeth* (7th ed.; Philadelphia: S. S. White Dental Mfg. Co., 1907).
2. Lischer, B. E.: *Principles and Methods of Orthodontics* (Philadelphia: Lea & Febiger, 1912).
3. Simon, P.: *Grundzüge einer systematischen Diagnostik der Gebiss-Anomalien* (Berlin: Meusser, 1922).

X

Analysis of the Orofacial Musculature

By examining the tongue of the patient, physicians find out the diseases of the body, and philosophers the diseases of the mind. —ST. JUSTIN

A. Muscles of the lips and face

    1. Methods of examination
       a) Morphology
       b) Function
         1) Swallow
         2) Mastication
         3) Speech
    2. Differential diagnosis of lips
       a) Morphologically inadequate lips
       b) Functionally inadequate lips
       c) Functionally abnormal lips

B. Breathing

    1. Methods of examination
    2. Differential diagnosis
       a) Nasal-breathers
       b) Mouth-breathers

C. Tongue

    1. Methods of examination
       a) Posture
       b) Swallowing
       c) Mastication
       d) Speech
    2. Differential diagnosis
       a) Abnormal posture
       b) Abnormal function

D. Swallow

    1. Methods of examination

2. Differential diagnosis
  a) Normal infantile swallow
  b) Normal mature swallow
  c) Simple tongue-thrust swallow
  d) Complex tongue-thrust swallow
  e) Retained infantile swallowing behavior

E. Muscles of mastication
  1. Registering jaw relationships in the orthodontic patient
  2. Analysis of mastication

F. Speech

THE CONCEPT OF normal occlusion includes not only the relationships of the teeth to one another and the relationship of the teeth to supporting bony structures but also the relationship of the teeth to surrounding musculature and the pattern of movements of the lower jaw during function. We have a tendency to judge occlusion by the static relationship of the teeth as seen in the cephalogram or dental casts. Static malrelationships may be due to either dental factors (see Chapter XI) or skeletal features (see Chapter XII); however, what sometimes appears to be a normal relationship in the cephalogram or dental cast is functionally malrelated during muscular activities. The purpose of this chapter is to describe a series of examination procedures for analyzing the orofacial and jaw musculature.

It is a basic physiologic principle that there is a marked relationship between sensory input and motor activity. The face is a region of great and varied sensory input. Analysis of the orofacial and jaw musculature is complicated by the interrelationships among the teeth, the tongue, lips, oral mucosa, jaw muscles and pharynx. The physiologic and psychologic complications of this elaborate multisensory system are difficult to segregate and identify. As yet, no one has presented a practical clinical method of evaluating the sensory input to the mouth, although active research on lingual tactile discrimination looks hopeful.

A great diversity of motor skills is seen in the population of children. Variations in the use of the tongue, lips and jaw muscles are just as noticeable as variations in muscle skills at the ballet class or on the Little League baseball diamond. No one has yet developed a simple, orderly test of lingual, lip and jaw muscle motor abilities, although such a test is very much needed.[4] All of the diagnostic procedures listed herein would be much more meaningful if simple tests of sensory capacity and motor skill were available. What is desired is a test of the potential for better performance of the complex coordinations of speech and swallowing. In one sense, if normal hearing and opportunity to learn are assumed, speech itself is such a test and so is swallowing. Bloomer[1] has suggested diadochokinetic performance as a test of oral motor skills and potential. The child repeats each of the following sounds, first slowly to achieve perfect formation and then gradually increases the speed until he is repeating them as rapidly as he can:

1. "puh, puh, puh........."
2. "tah, tah, tah ...."
3. "kuh, kuh, kuh........."
4. "puh-tah-kuh," "puh-tah-kuh," "puh-tah-kuh........."

It is important for the examiner using diadochokinetic testing to relate performance to age.* Children whose oral movements are below the normal range for their age usually are defective speakers, often show patterns of swallowing abnormality and give evidence of dysdiadochokinesia. The child who has defective speech and/or swallowing abnormalities without dysdiadochokinesia has a better prognosis for speech therapy and retraining of the swallowing pattern.

A. Muscles of the Lips and Face

1. METHODS OF EXAMINATION[2]

a) Morphology

To a great extent, the morphologic relationships of the lips are determined by the skeletal profile (Fig. X-1). At rest, lips normally touch lightly, effecting an oral seal when the mandible is in its postural position (Fig. X-2, A). In all mouth-breathers and a few nasal-breathers, the lips will be parted at rest (Fig. X-2, C). Some quite competent lips will be found to have adapted to the malocclusion; thus, although a seal is present, it is not a lip-lip seal but a lip-tooth-lip arrangement (Fig. X-2, C). Differences in color, texture and size of lips often are related to lip malfunction. Hyperactive lips may be larger (Fig. X-2, E) and tend to be more red and moist than hypoactive or normal lips.

b) Function

1) OBSERVE THE LIP AND FACIAL MUSCLE CONTRACTIONS DURING THE VARIOUS SWALLOWS (SEE SECTION D, BELOW).

2) OBSERVE LIP FUNCTION DURING MASTICATION.—Bite-size dry breakfast food may be used to study mastication. During normal mastication, the lips are held lightly together. Strong contractions of the mentalis and circumoral muscles will be seen in teeth-apart swallowers. These same muscles also contract strongly in severe Class II malocclusions with large overjet and overbite.

3) STUDY LIP FUNCTION DURING SPEECH (SEE SECTION F, BELOW).— Most abnormal lip function during speech of children with malocclusions is an adaptation or accommodation to the tooth position, not an etiologic factor in the malpositioning of the teeth.

---

*Note: Rate norms for chronological ages have been developed. However, speed of movement is only one factor—accuracy, patterning of lingual movement and independence of lingual-mandibular action are thought to be of equal significance in distinguishing normal from abnormal action.

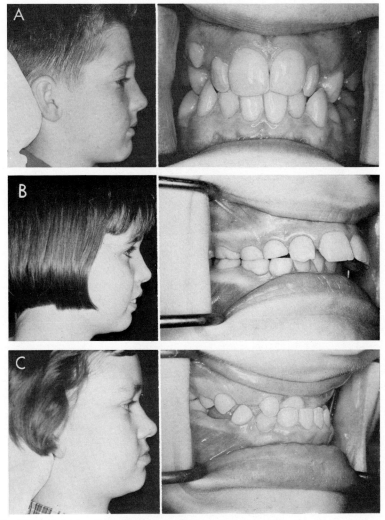

Fig. X-1.—Relationship of the soft tissue profile to occlusion. **A,** Class I malocclusion. **B,** Class II malocclusion. **C,** Class III malocclusion.

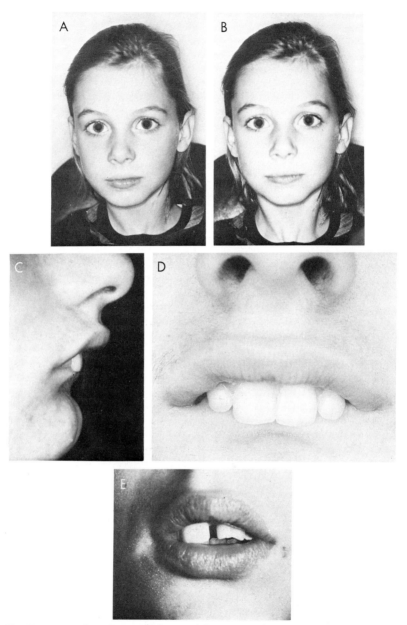

Fig. X-2.—A, relaxed normal lips. **B,** the same subject swallowing. Note that the lip posture position does not change markedly during a normal swallow. Only the contraction of the muscles in the neck betrays that a swallow is occurring. **C** and **D,** adaptation of the lips to a severe skeletal Class II malocclusion. **E,** lips parted at rest in a mouth-breather.

2. Differential Diagnosis of Lips[2]

a) Morphologically Inadequate Lips

Only on rare occasions is the upper lip morphologically short (Fig. X-3). The significance of the morphologically short upper lip to malocclusion, speech disorders and retention of orthodontically treated cases often is overstated. Lips originally diagnosed as morphologically inadequate often are found to be quite adequate because the tooth movements permit normal lip function to be restored spontaneously. Modern orthodontic technics involving bodily retraction of maxillary incisors and midface orthopedics permit many an alleged short upper lip to fall into position and function normally. Surgical intervention for supposed short upper lips is to be discouraged except in the rarest cases and then

Fig. X-3.—A and **B,** an anatomically short upper lip prior to orthodontic treatment and the malocclusion associated with it. **C** and **D,** the same patient after orthodontic therapy. Note the position of the lip posture, even though orthodontics is completed.

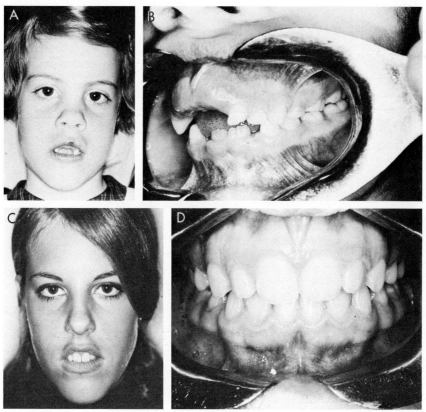

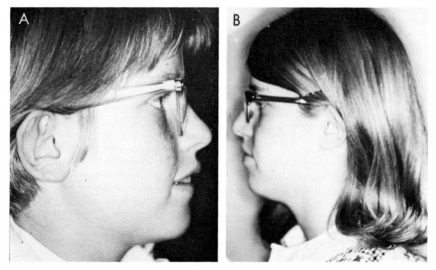

Fig. X-4.—Functionally inadequate lips, which improve with treatment. **A,** before treatment. **B,** after treatment.

undertaken only after orthodontic therapy is completed. In my experience, it has not been necessary, except for cleft lip cases.

b) Functionally Inadequate Lips

Sometimes lips are adequate in size but fail to function properly; for example, the maxillary lip in extreme Class II, Division 1 malocclusion. The hyperactive lower lip forms the oral seal with the lingual surfaces of the maxillary incisors whereas the maxillary lip scarcely functions at all (see Fig. X-2, *C*). After retraction of the incisors, spontaneous normal lip function usually occurs (Fig. X-4). If it does not, a regimen of lip exercises may be prescribed (see Chapter XVII).

c) Functionally Abnormal Lips

One of the most frequent abnormal functions of the lips and facial muscles is seen with tongue-thrust swallowing[3] (see Section D, below). The mentalis muscle frequently is hypertrophied, as is the inferior orbicularis oris muscle. When the lower lip is gently pulled away from the gingivae, the latter may be rubefacient and hypertrophied. Gingivitis in the mandibular incisor region in the absence of maxillary gingivitis is indicative of hyperactive mentalis function (Fig. X-5, *A*), whereas gingivitis in both anterior regions is seen frequently with mouth-breathing (Fig. X-5, *B*). Methods for correction of abnormal mentalis muscle and lip function will be found in Chapter XV.

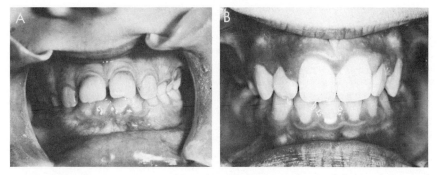

Fig. X-5.—A, gingivitis associated with hypertrophy and hyperactivity of the mentalis muscle. **B,** gingivitis associated with mouth-breathing.

Fig. X-6.—Effect of mouth-breathing on control of the alar musculature. **A** and **B,** mouth-breather inhaling and exhaling through the nose. Although he can breathe through his nose, the diameters of the external nares do not change. **C** and **D,** nasal-breather inhaling and exhaling. Note that the size and shape of the external nares change during inhalation.

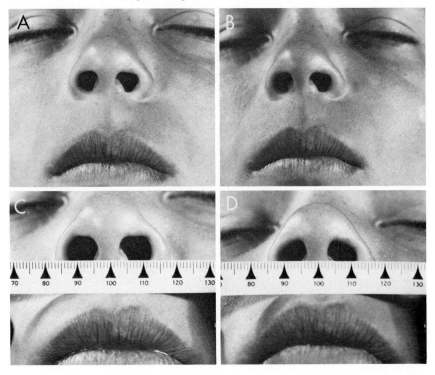

B. Breathing

1. METHODS OF EXAMINATION

1) STUDY THE PATIENT'S BREATHING UNOBSERVED.—Nasal-breathers usually hold the lips touching lightly during relaxed breathing, whereas mouth-breathers' lips must be parted.

2) ASK THE PATIENT TO TAKE A DEEP BREATH.—Most respond to such a request by inspiring through the mouth, although an occasional nasal-breather will inspire through the nose with the lips lightly closed.

3) ASK THE PATIENT TO CLOSE HIS LIPS AND TAKE A DEEP BREATH THROUGH HIS NOSE.—Nasal-breathers normally demonstrate good reflex control of the alar muscles, which control the size and shape of the external nares; therefore, they dilate the external nares on inspiration (Fig. X-6, *C* and *D*). Mouth-breathers, even though they are capable of breathing through the nose, do not change the size or shape of the external nares (Fig. X-6, *A* and *B*), and occasionally actually contract the nasal orifices while inspiring. Even nasal-breathers with temporary nasal congestion will demonstrate reflex alar contraction and dilation of the nares during voluntary inspiration. Unilateral nasal function may be diagnosed by placing a small two-surfaced steel mirror on the upper lip (Fig. X-7, *A*). The mirror will cloud with condensed moisture during breathing. A cotton butterfly (Fig. X-7, *B* and *C*) may be used also.

2. DIFFERENTIAL DIAGNOSIS

a) Nasal-Breathers

Lips touch lightly at rest, nares dilate on command inspiration.

b) Mouth-Breathers

Lips parted at rest. Nares maintain size or contract on command inspiration with lips held together.

C. Tongue

1. METHODS OF EXAMINATION

The tongue and lips are integrated and synchronized in their activity; thus, one infers tongue malfunction from observed lip and facial muscle malfunction.[2] When the lips are parted by the mouth mirror or the cheeks are withdrawn by retractors, normal tongue activity is inhibited and what is observed is accommodation to the stretching of the lips and cheeks. The paradoxic problem of the tongue examination is to examine the tongue in its normal functions without displacement of it or the lips.

1) OBSERVE THE POSTURE OF THE TONGUE WHILE THE MANDIBLE IS IN THE POSTURAL POSITION.—This may be done in a cephalogram taken

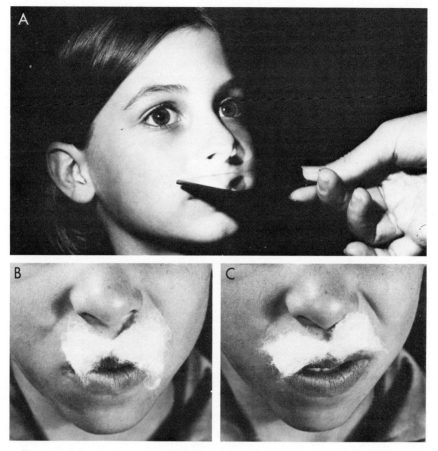

Fig. X-7.—A, use of a two-surfaced mirror to check the method of breathing. When the mirror is held in this position, if the child is a nasal-breather, the upper surface will cloud; if a mouth-breather, the lower surface will cloud. **B** and **C,** use of a cotton butterfly to diagnose nasal breathing. **B,** bilateral use of nostrils. **C,** breathing through only one nostril.

at the postural position or it may be done by gently and casually examining the tongue-lip relationship while the patient is seated in an upright position in the dental chair. During mandibular posture, the dorsum touches the palate lightly, whereas the tongue tip normally is at rest in the lingual fossae or at the cervices of the mandibular incisors (Fig. X-8, *A* and *B*). Abnormal positions found are (1) the tip atop the lower incisors, producing an open bite (Fig. X-8, *D*), or (2) a retracted or "cocked" tongue, which does not cause a malocclusion (Fig. X-8, *C*).

2) OBSERVE THE TONGUE DURING THE VARIOUS SWALLOWING PROCEDURES (SEE SECTION D, BELOW).—It is necessary to observe the tongue

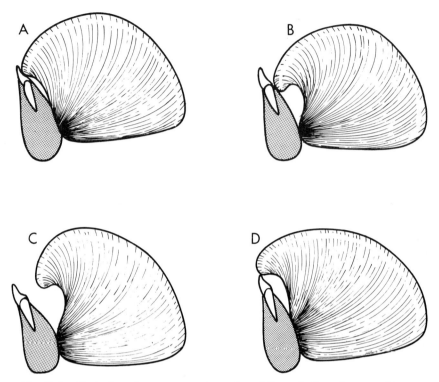

Fig. X-8.—Variations in tongue posture. **A** and **B,** variations in normal tongue posture. **C,** retracted tongue posture. **D,** the retained infantile tongue posture.

during the unconscious swallow, the command swallow of saliva, the command swallow of water and the unconscious swallow during mastication.

3) OBSERVE THE ROLE OF THE TONGUE DURING MASTICATION.—This procedure is very difficult except for the most obvious abnormalities and it is combined with the observations of swallowing during chewing.

4) OBSERVE THE ROLE OF THE TONGUE IN SPEECH (SEE SECTION F, BELOW).

2. DIFFERENTIAL DIAGNOSIS (TABLE X-1)

a) Abnormal Posture

Tongue posture has been related to skeletal morphology; for example, in severe Class III skeletons, the tongue tends to lie below the plane of occlusion (Fig. X-9, *A*) and in Class II facial skeletons with a steep mandibular plane, the tongue tends toward forward positioning (Fig.

TABLE X-1.—Differential Diagnosis of Tongue
Posture Problems

Signs and Symptoms	Posture		
	Normal (Mature)	Protracted (Infantile)	Acquired Protracted
Tongue between teeth	No	Yes	Yes
Endogenous	No	Yes	No
Pharyngeal or tonsillar inflammation	No	No	Yes
Mandibular stabilization by facial contractions	No	No	No

X-9, B). Two significant variations from the normal tongue posture can be seen: (1) the retracted or "cocked" tongue, in which the tongue tip is withdrawn from all the anterior teeth (see Fig. X-8, C), and (2) the protracted tongue posture, in which the resting tongue is between the incisors (Fig. X-8, D). The retracted tongue posture is seen in less than 10% of the children; however, it is more frequent in edentulous adults. In the latter, undoubtedly the tongue has lost some of its positional sense with the removal of the periodontal ligaments and it retracts itself in order to establish proprioceptive contact laterally with the alveolar mucosa for a better seal during the swallow. Although the retracted tongue is unsettling to mandibular artificial dentures, its significance in adolescence is not yet known. The protracted tongue posture may be a serious problem, since it usually results in an open bite.

There are two forms of the protracted tongue posture: (1) the endog-

Fig. X-9.—A, tongue posture in Class III malocclusion. The tongue is postured lower than normal. Note that the dorsum is below the incisal tip and occlusal level. **B**, typical tongue posture associated with a Class II malocclusion that has a steep mandibular plane relationship.

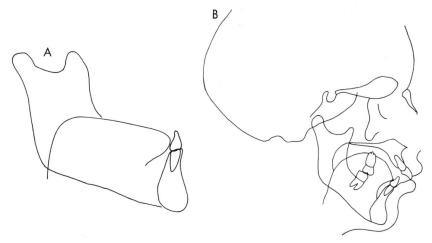

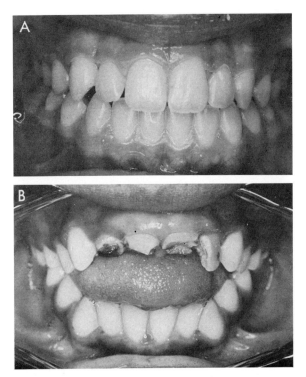

Fig. X-10.—Open bites associated with abnormal tongue posture. **A,** Class II, Division 1 malocclusion 2 years out of orthodontic retention. Note the return of a very mild open bite. This case was re-treated twice and it returned each time to this incisal relationship. Note the absence of functional occlusal stops in the entire incisor and cuspid region. **B,** a severe open bite due to abnormal tongue posture. In this instance there was no tongue-thrust on swallowing; rather, the tongue remained in this position most of the time.

enous protracted tongue posture and (2) the acquired protracted tongue posture. The endogenous protracted tongue posture is a retention of the infantile postural pattern. Some persons, for reasons not yet known, do not change their tongue posture during the arrival of the primary incisors, and the tongue tip persists between the incisors. For the great majority of patients with endogenous protracted tongue posture, the open bite is very mild and not a serious clinical problem but, on rare occasions, quite serious open bites are present (Fig. X-10). There is no known certain treatment for endogenous tongue posture problems. The acquired protracted tongue posture is a more simple matter, since it usually is a transitory result of pharyngitis or tonsillitis. It may be diagnosed by swabbing the throat with a viscous topical anesthetic and allowing the patient to swallow a tiny bit of the material. When the acutely inflamed throat regions are thus anesthetized, the adaptive protracted posture of the tongue will spontaneously correct to its more normal position. As long as the precipitating pain mechanism is present in the throat, the tongue will posture itself forward, and any repositioning of the incisors will not be stable. Therefore, it is best to refer such patients to a physician for correlative therapy. Occasionally, the nasopharyngeal condition no longer exists but the tongue reflexly remains in a forward position. Treatment of such tongue posture problems is described in Chapter XV.

To summarize, there are two problems in abnormal posture of the tongue that have clinical significance: (1) the endogenous protracted tongue posture for which the prognosis is poor, and around which, unfortunately, the occlusion must be built and (2) the acquired protracted tongue posture, which usually is easily corrected.

b) Abnormal Function

Abnormal tongue function ordinarily is seen during swallowing, mastication or speech and therefore is discussed in Sections D, E and F of this chapter. Bizarre tongue activities, e.g., tongue-sucking, may be observed rarely and are primarily psychologic, not dental, in their therapeutic needs.

D. Swallow

1. Methods of Examination[2]

For examinations of the swallow, it is imperative that the patient be seated upright in the dental chair with the vertebral column vertical to and the Frankfurt plane parallel to the floor. Try to observe, unnoticed, several unconscious swallows. Then place a small amount of tepid water beneath the tongue tip and ask the patient to swallow, noting mandibular movements. In the normal swallow, the mandible rises as the teeth are brought together during the swallow, and the lips touch lightly, showing scarcely any contractions. The facial muscles do not contract in the normal mature swallow. Next, place the hand over the temporal muscle, pressing lightly with the fingertips against the head (Fig. X-11). With the hand in this position, give the patient more water and ask for a repeat swallow. During normal swallow, the temporal muscle can be felt to contract as the mandible is elevated and the teeth are held together. During teeth-apart swallows, no contraction of the temporal muscle will be noticed. Place a tongue depressor or mouth mirror on the lower lip and ask the patient to swallow (Fig. X-12). Patients with a normal swallow can complete a command swallow of saliva while the lip is so held. Those with a teeth-apart swallow will have the swallow inhibited by depression of the lip, since strong mentalis and lip contractions are needed for mandibular stabilization in the teeth-apart swallow.

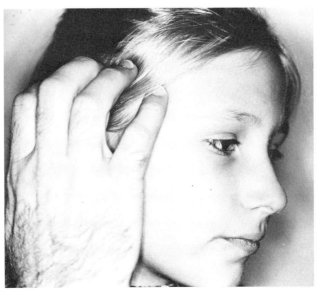

Fig. X-11.—Palpation of the temporal muscle to ascertain its activity during the swallow.

Fig. X-12.—Use of a tongue depressor to check the role of the lower lip during the swallow.

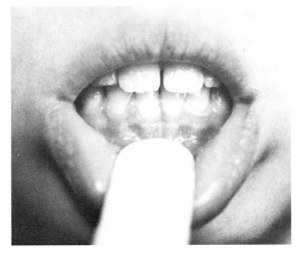

The unconscious swallow may be examined as follows: place more water in the patient's mouth, and, with the hand on the temporal muscle, ask the patient to swallow one more "last time." After the swallow is completed, turn away from the patient as if the examination were over, but retain the hand against the head. Most patients will, in a few moments, produce an unconscious clearing swallow. Unconscious swallowing behavior is not always the same as on command, particularly in those patients who have had some form of tongue-thrust therapy or to whose attention an abnormal swallow has been called.

2. Differential Diagnosis

a) Normal Infantile Swallow

The normal infantile swallow is seen only prior to the eruption of the buccal teeth in the primary dentition and, therefore, rarely is discovered in the dental examination.[3] During the normal infantile swallow, the tongue lies between the gum pads and the mandible is stabilized by strong contractions of the facial muscles.[3] The buccinator muscle is particularly strong in the infantile swallow.

b) Normal Mature Swallow

The normal mature swallow is characterized by absence of lip and cheek activity, but the mandibular elevators contract, bringing the teeth into occlusion, thus enclosing the tongue in the oral cavity.

c) Simple Tongue-Thrust Swallow

The simple tongue-thrust swallow is characterized by contractions of the lips, mentalis muscle and the mandibular elevators (Fig. X-13); therefore, the teeth are in occlusion as the tongue protrudes into the open bite. The open bite in a simple tongue-thrust is well circumscribed; that is, it has a definite beginning and ending (Fig. X-14). Patients with a simple tongue-thrust ordinarily are nasal-breathers with a history of digital sucking—the tongue-thrust maintaining an open bite previously created by thumb-sucking. If dental casts of a patient with a simple tongue-thrust are examined, they will be found to have a good occlusal fit. There is good intercuspation, even though a malocclusion may be present, because the occlusal position is continually reinforced by teeth-together swallows. Treatment of a simple tongue-thrust is described in Chapter XVII.

d) Complex Tongue-Thrust Swallow

The complex tongue-thrust swallow is defined as a tongue-thrust with a teeth-apart swallow. Therefore, these patients display contractions

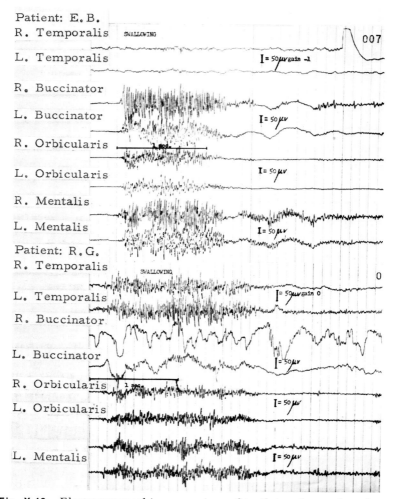

Fig. X-13.—Electromyographic comparison of teeth-together and teeth-apart swallows. The record at the bottom (R. G.) is a typical mature swallow. Note the strong contractions of the temporal muscles, which indicate that the mandible has been elevated into occlusion during the swallow. The record at the top (E. B.) is of a child of the same age. Note, however, that this child has a teeth-apart swallow, since there is little or no activity of mandibular elevators and a far greater relative activity of the facial muscles.

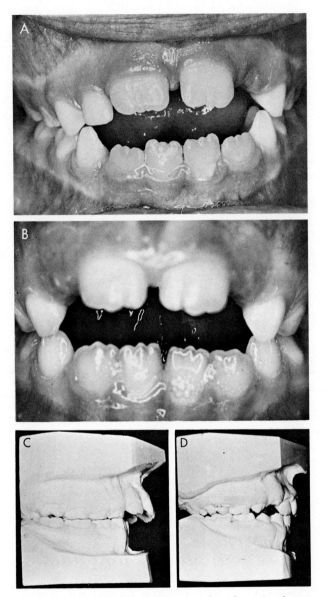

Fig. X-14.—Examples of open bites associated with a simple tongue-thrust. Note in each instance that there is a highly circumscribed open bite and good occlusal fit posteriorly even if the molar relationship is not correct. **A, B** and **C** are examples before treatment; **D** is the same subject shown in **C** but after correction of the molar relationship and retraction of the incisors. Although correction of the malocclusion is not yet complete, the open bite has been corrected spontaneously without tongue therapy.

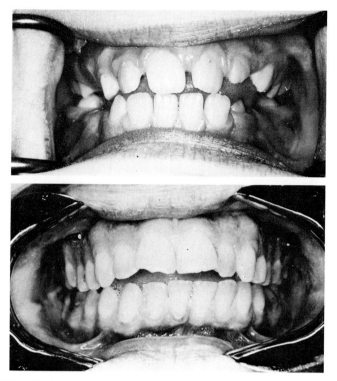

Fig. X-15.—Typical examples of open bites associated with a complex tongue-thrust. Note in each instance that the open bite is not as circumscribed as in the simple tongue-thrust and that the posterior occlusal fit is not as precise. (*Continued.*)

of the lips and facial and mentalis muscles, no contraction of the mandibular elevators (see Fig. X-13), a tongue-thrust between the teeth and a teeth-apart swallow. The open bite associated with a complex tongue-thrust usually is more diffuse and difficult to define (Fig. X-15). Indeed, on occasion, complex tongue-thrusters have no open bite at all. Examination of the dental casts reveals a poor occlusal fit and instability of intercuspation, since the intercuspal position is not reinforced during the swallow. Since swallows of water often produce teeth-apart swallows, it is important to test the patient with a dry food bolus when a complex tongue-thrust is suspected. Patients with a complex tongue-thrust usually demonstrate occlusal interferences in the retruded contact position. They also are more likely to be mouth-breathers, frequently giving a history of chronic nasorespiratory disease or allergies. Treatment of the complex tongue-thrust is described in Chapter XV.

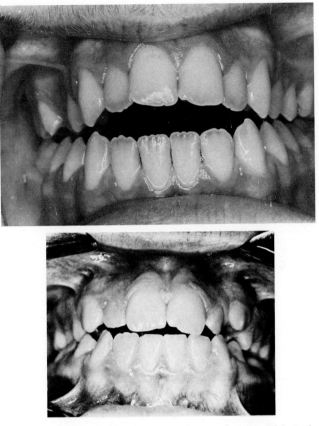

Fig. X-15 (cont.).—In the complex tongue-thrust, the mandible is dropped and the teeth are apart during the swallow; hence, the more diffuse nature of the open bite.

e) *Retained Infantile Swallowing Behavior*

Retained infantile swallowing behavior is defined as predominant persistence of the infantile swallowing reflex after the arrival of permanent teeth. Fortunately, very few people have a true retained infantile swallow. Those who do, demonstrate very strong total contractions of the lips and facial musculature, often visualized as a massive grimace. The tongue thrusts violently between the teeth in the front and on both sides. The facial and buccal musculature is powerful; particularly noticeable are contractions of the buccinator muscle. Such patients have very inexpressive faces, since the VIIth cranial nerve muscles are not being used for the delicate purposes of facial expression but rather for the massive effort of stabilizing the mandible during the

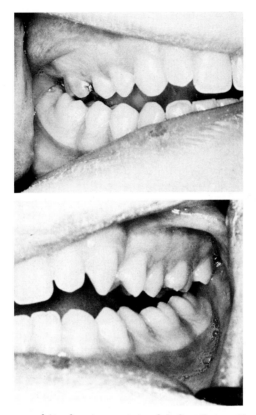

Fig. X-16.—An open bite due to a retained infantile swallow. Usually, the teeth occlude on the last molar in each quadrant. This patient was treated by a very competent orthodontist who had banded all of the patient's teeth with an edgewise mechanism. The photographs above were taken 1 month after the removal of the retainers.

TABLE X-2.—SUMMARIZING TABLE OF SYMPTOMS ASSOCIATED WITH VARIOUS TONGUE PROBLEMS

	RETAINED INFANTILE TONGUE POSTURE	SIMPLE TONGUE-THRUST SWALLOW	COMPLEX TONGUE-THRUST SWALLOW	RETAINED INFANTILE SWALLOW
Tongue-thrust on swallowing	−	+	+	+
Well-defined open bite	+	+	−	−
Good occlusal fit	+	+	−	−
"Slide into occlusion"	−	−	+	+
Teeth-together swallow	+	−	−	−
Digital sucking habit	+	−	−	−
Nasorespiratory distress	−	−	+	−

TABLE X-3.—DIFFERENTIAL DIAGNOSIS OF SWALLOWING TYPES: NORMAL AND ABNORMAL

SIGNS AND SYMPTOMS	SWALLOWING		TONGUE-THRUSTING		
	Infantile	Mature	Simple	Complex	Retained Infantile Swallowing
Tongue between teeth	Yes	No	Yes	Yes	Yes
Endogenous	Yes	No	No	No	Yes
Mandibular stabilization by facial contractions	Yes	No	No	Yes	Yes
Teeth-together swallow	No	Yes	Yes	No	No
Lip and mentalis contractions	Yes	No	Yes	Yes	Yes
Enlarged tonsils and adenoids (or history of)	No	No	No	Yes	No
Low gag reflex threshold	No	No	No	No	Yes

swallow. Patients with a retained infantile swallow have serious difficulties in mastication, since ordinarily they occlude on only one molar in each quadrant (Fig. X-16). The gag threshold is typically low. These patients may restrict themselves to a soft diet and state frankly that they do not enjoy eating. Food often is placed on the dorsum of the tongue and "mastication" occurs between the tongue tip and palate due to the inadequacy of occlusal contacts. The prognosis for conditioning of such a primitive reflex is very poor. Fortunately, true retained infantile swallowing behavior is a rare occurrence.

Table X-2 summarizes the important differentiating characteristics and symptoms of the several tongue functions, both normal and abnormal, whereas Table X-3 compares tongue-thrusting and swallowing functions.

E. Muscles of Mastication

1. REGISTERING JAW RELATIONSHIPS IN THE ORTHODONTIC PATIENT

Although registration of jaw relationships is truly an analysis of muscle function, the technical procedures for registration of jaw relationships are given in Chapter XI, Section E, since such a registration is used primarily for analysis of the occlusion.

2. ANALYSIS OF MASTICATION

Some clinicians prefer to palpate the masticatory muscles to ascertain asymmetries of size, which are symptomatic of asymmetry of function, and to identify hypertrophy of the masseter muscles. This procedure is a rather crude static analysis of muscle morphology that may be augmented by watching the patient chew bits of dry breakfast food as a functional evaluation of mastication, the masticatory musculature and the masticatory swallow. These procedures, although superficial evaluations only, are useful. Patients with common malocclusions usually do not have impaired masticatory function to the extent that might be imagined.

F. Speech*

Although the dentist is not a speech pathologist, he should be familiar with a few simple technics of speech analysis in order that children with obvious speech disorders may be referred to a speech pathologist for diagnosis or therapy. The relationship between speech and malocclusion often is overstated, since many patients with gross malocclusions have intelligible speech. Because of the remarkable adaptive characteristics of the lips and tongue, good speech can be produced through skillful control of lingual and labial movements in mouths with severe malocclusions. If abnormal tongue activity is noted during speech, there is a basic question that must be answered: "Is the abnormal tongue activity adaptive or etiologic to the malocclusion, or is it attributable to an etiology unrelated to either?" Usually it will be found to be adaptive, but

TABLE X-4.—PLACE AND MANNER OF ARTICULATORY VALVING

MANNER OF ARTICULATORY VALVING

PLACE OF ARTICULATORY VALVING	Articulatory Valve Narrowed PV-c (Glides)	Articulatory Valve Constricted PV-c (Fricatives)	(Affricates)	Articulatory Valve Closed PV-c (Stops)	PV-o (Nasals)
1. Glotto-pharyngeal		h			
2. Linguo-velar				k g̲ A	ŋ (ng)
3. Linguo-palatal	r̲ j̲(y)	ʃ(sh) ʒ̲(zh)	tʃ dz̲ (ch)(j̲)		
4. Linguo-alveolar	l̲	s z̲		t d̲	n
5. Linguo-dental		θ(th) ð̲(th)			
6. Labio-dental		f v̲			
7. Bilabial	ʍ(hw) w̲			p b̲	m̲

NOTES: 1. Palatopharyngeal valve closed and open are indicated by PV-c and PV-o, respectively.
2. The presence of voicing is indicated by underlining.
3. The English spelling equivalents of phonetic symbols are indicated in parentheses.

*Prof. Harlan H. Bloomer, Director of the Speech Clinic, The University of Michigan, helped in the writing of this section. He devised the ingenious speech tests described herein.

it may reflect an etiology that is common to both the speech defect and the neuromuscular aspects of the malocclusion. Maturational delays in development of oral motor coordinations or neural pathologies affecting oral coordinations may not be an adaptation to the malocclusion but may contribute to the malocclusion. On the other hand, environment or factors of learning may produce abnormal speech in a normally formed mouth. The existence of a disorder of speech articulation can be tested by having the patient repeat a few key sentences designed to assist in the identification of those consonants which may be defective.

The basic elements of American speech which contribute to meaning are the 25 consonants, 14 vowels and prosodic elements such as melody, stress and rhythm. Consonants and vowels are formed by a complex series of oral movements that continually modify the sounds of speech. A critical phase of articulatory movements in consonant production can be described as an "articulatory position" and the corresponding consonants can be classified in this context according to their "place of articulation." Table X-4 presents a classification of consonant phonemes according to: (1) the presence or absence of voicing, (2) the anatomic structures by which the valve is created (place), (3) the degree of valve closure required to produce the phoneme and (4) the manner of articulation (glides, fricatives, affricates, stops, nasals). Reference to such a table (and to Table X-5) can help us to understand how abnormalities of structure and maladaptive movements of the articulators may interfere with the production of satisfactory consonant phonemes. Although this table is relatively simple, some tables and charts provide elaborate and detailed information concerning the phonetic parameters of speech.

A simple test the dentist may use to evaluate the relationship between speech and malocclusion has been devised. The patient is asked to count from 1 to 10 or 1 to 20. The dentist (1) *watches* closely how the tongue and lips adapt to the structures with which they are supposed to articulate and (2) *listens* to how the consonants sound.

The word one tests	w and n
" " two tests	t
" " three tests	th and r
" " four tests	f and r
" " five tests	f and v
" " six tests	s and k
" " seven tests	s, v and n
" " eight tests	t
" " nine tests	n
" " ten tests	t and n
" " eleven tests	l, v and n
" " twelve tests	t, w, l and v
etc.	

This simple procedure provides a test of 10 consonants, 7 of which (th, r, f, v, s, l, k) are frequent offenders. It also includes 8 of the 14 vowels and diphthongs common in American speech.

The fricative consonants require very precise positioning of the speech organs and, consequently, are those sounds frequently defective. They are affected in quality by maladaptive placement of the tongue or lips or by malocclusion. Actually, the sibilants, a subgroup of the fricatives, are the ones most likely to be affected.

The proficiency of a patient to make such consonants can be tested in various ways. The mini-test of speech articulation presented in Table X-5 was devised as a simple procedure to test speech articulation by place of articulation and by manner of articulation. In this test, the subject is requested to read or to repeat after the examiner a brief series of short sentences while the examiner observes and notes whether the consonant failures or successes fall into the numbered or lettered categories around which the sentences are structured. Inasmuch as more than one instance of the articulatory category may be provided, it is suggested that the examiner listen especially for the consonants underlined as belonging to the selected category under test.

Place of articulation categorizes the consonants according to the valves that are assumed to play the predominant role in the formation of the sound, e.g., (1) labial, (2) labiodental, (3) linguodental, (4) linguoalveolar, (5) linguopalatal, (6) linguovelar and (7) glottopharyngeal (Table X-4).

Manner of articulation categorizes the consonants according to the main acoustic features by which the consonants are recognized, i.e. (a) plosive, (b) fricative, (c) affricate, (d) glides and (e) nasals (Table X-5).

The first test sentences identify consonants by *place of articulation,* that is, the position assumed by the oral articulators at a critical point in the enunciation of the consonant. Many of the 25 consonant phonemes that occur in American English occur in articulatory pairs; for

---

TABLE X-5.—MINI-TEST OF SPEECH ARTICULATION

By Place of Articulation
1. Bilabials—hw w m p b
2. Labiodentals—f v
3. Linguodentals—th th
4. Linguoalveolars—t d n l s z
5. Linguopalatals—y sh zh tsh dzh r
6. Linguovelars—k g ng
7. Glottopharyngeal—h

By Manner of Articulation
A. Plosives—p b t d k g
B. Fricatives—f v th s z sh zh h
C. Affricates—tsh dzh
D. Glides—hw w l y r
E. Nasals—m n ng

We bought my father/ two
1   1   1 2 3   4

new sun lamps.
4   4   4

You should choose a red
5   5   5   5

coat hanger.
6   7 6

Bobby pulled down two go carts.
  *   *   *   *   *   *

The thing is very full. Send his shoe measure
  *   *   *   *   *   * * *   *

to Charlie Jones.
      *   *

Why won't you let her run?
  *   *   *   *   *   *

Mary never sang.
  *   *   *

example, p and b̲, s and z̲, etc., in which the lips and tongue function in nearly identical ways to produce the sound. The audible distinction between them is created by the presence or absence of voicing. In the listing of the phonemes in the mini-test, the voiced member of each pair is underlined. In the test sentences, the articulatory position being tested is indicated by a numerical subscript that identifies the "place of articulation" group to which the consonant belongs. There are, of course, other instances of consonant occurrence, and the informed listener can easily pick them out and listen for them as the speaker repeats the sentence (for instance, the t in "taught," the z in "choose," the d in "should," etc.).

        *   *   *

The second group of sentences identifies the consonants by *manner of articulation*. Instances of voiced consonants are underlined, and each example of the consonant that illustrates the category is identified by a subscript asterisk. Whenever feasible, words have been selected in which the initial consonant is illustrative of the sound to be tested.

Inasmuch as American orthography is only partially phonetic, it would have been desirable to indicate the consonants by phonetic symbols, such as those employed in the International Phonetic Alphabet. For readers who are not phonetically trained, the consonants have been spelled to illustrate the pronunciation; for example, tsh for the ch in

Charlie, zh for the middle consonant in measure and so forth. As in the first sentences, some consonants occur in several places, but only one instance of each has been identified by the asterisk.

Some patients, by concentrating, will produce perfect speech, whereas, when speaking unobserved, they may make repeated errors. Oral sensory deficits or lack of orofacial motor skills may be common to both swallowing and speech disorders; however, the presence of abnormal tongue function during swallowing is not necessarily an indication that there will be abnormal tongue function during speech.

REFERENCES

1. Bloomer, H. H.: Speech defects in relation to orthodontics, Am. J. Orthodont. 49:920, 1963.
2. Moyers, R. E.: The Role of Musculature in Orthodontic Diagnosis and Treatment Planning, in Kraus, B. S., and Reidel, R. A. (eds.), *Vistas in Orthodontics* (Philadelphia: Lea & Febiger, 1962).
3. Moyers, R. E.: The infantile swallow, Tr. European Orthodont. Soc. 40:180, 1964.
4. Moyers, R. E.: Postnatal development of the orofacial musculature. Presented at the Ann Arbor Conference on Orofacial Development, March, 1970, A.S.H.A. Reports, no. 6, 1971.

Suggested Readings

Bloomer, H. H.: Speech defects in relation to orthodontics, Am. J. Orthodont. 49:920, 1963.
Bosma, J. F.: Deglutition: Pharyngeal stage, Physiol. Rev. 37:275, 1957.

Bosma, J. F.: *Symposium on Oral Sensation and Perception, 1964* (Springfield, Ill.: Charles C Thomas, Publisher, 1967).

Bosma, J. F.: *Symposium on Oral Sensation and Perception, 1967* (Springfield, Ill.: Charles C Thomas, Publisher, 1970).

Cleall, J. F.: Deglutition: A study of form and function, Am. J. Orthodont. 51:566, 1965.

Graber, T. M.: The three M's: Muscles, malformation, and malocclusion, Am. J. Orthodont. 49:418, 1963.

Jacobs, R. M.: Muscle equilibrium: Fact or fancy?, Angle Orthodont. 39:11, 1969.

Mathews, P. B. C.: Muscle spindles and their motor control, Physiol. Rev. 44:219, 1964.

Moyers, R. E.: The Role of Musculature in Orthodontic Diagnosis and Treatment Planning, in Kraus, B. S., and Reidel, R. A. (eds.), *Vistas in Orthodontics* (Philadelphia: Lea & Febiger, 1962).

Ricketts, R. M.: Respiratory obstruction syndrome, Am. J. Orthodont. 54:495, 1968.

Subtelny, J. D.: Examination of current philosophies associated with swallowing behavior, Am. J. Orthodont. 51:161, 1965.

Subtelny, J. D.: Malocclusions, orthodontic corrections and orofacial muscle adaptation, Angle Orthodont. 40:170, 1970.

XI

Analysis of the Dentition and Occlusion

> If we could first know where we are and whither we are tending, we could better judge what to do and how to do it.—ABRAHAM LINCOLN

A. Diagnostic data
1. Intra-oral examination
2. Dental casts
3. Radiographs
   a) Intra-oral periapical survey
   b) Bite-wing radiographs
   c) Lateral jaw projections
   d) Occlusal plane projections
   e) Panoramic radiographs
   f) Oblique cephalogram
   g) Lateral cephalogram
4. Photographs

B. Analyses of tooth development
1. Calcification
2. Eruption
   a) Predicting eruption
   b) Sequence of eruption
3. Number of teeth
4. Position of teeth
5. Anomalies

C. Size of teeth
1. Individual teeth
2. Size relationships of groups of teeth
   a) Bolton tooth ratio analysis
3. Relationships of tooth size to size of supporting structures
   a) Howes' analysis
   b) Diagnostic setup
4. Relationships of tooth size and available space during the mixed dentition (Mixed Dentition Analysis)

A. Diagnostic Data

1. INTRA-ORAL EXAMINATION

Most of the intra-oral features usually are noted in the cursory examination (see Chapter VIII). Some pertinent items in the analysis of the dentition and occlusion can be seen only intra-orally, for example, oral hygiene, gingival health, tongue size, shape and posture, dental restorations and so forth. The functional analysis of occlusal relationships is discussed separately (see Section E, below).

2. DENTAL CASTS

The record dental casts are one of the most important sources of information for the dentist doing orthodontic treatment. Technical details of impression taking, cast pouring and trimming are given in Chapter XVII. The time required for the precise construction of record casts is time well spent. A good set of dental casts should show the alignment of the teeth and the alveolar processes as far as the impression material can displace the soft tissues (Fig. XI-1). From the occlusal view, one can analyze the arch form, arch asymmetry, alignment of the teeth, palate shape, tooth size, tooth shape, rotations of teeth, etc. While holding the casts together in the usual occlusal position, the occlusal relationships can be observed as well as midline coincidence, attachment of the frena, the occlusal curve and axial inclinations of teeth.

The lingual view of occlusion can be studied only with dental casts (Fig. XI-1).

3. RADIOGRAPHS

a) *Intra-oral Periapical Survey*

The periapical survey is a necessity for any orthodontic diagnosis. From it may be learned the eruption sequence, congenital absence of

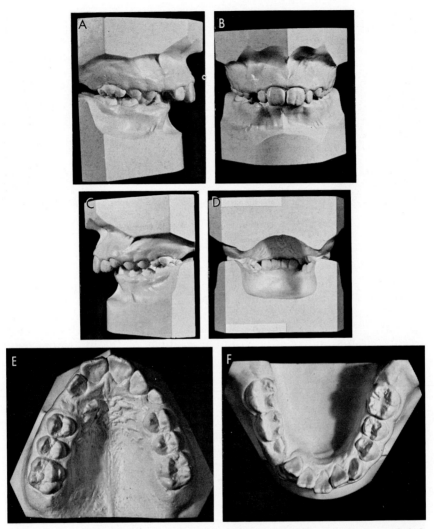

Fig. XI-1.—A good set of diagnostic dental casts. **A,** right side. **B,** front. **C,** left side. **D,** lingual view. **E,** maxillary occlusal view. **F,** mandibular occlusal view.

teeth, impactions, abnormalities, supernumerary teeth, developmental progress of teeth, etc. (Fig. XI-2).

b) Bite-wing Radiographs

Bite-wing radiographs, although essential for the detection of interproximal caries, are of little use in the orthodontic analysis.

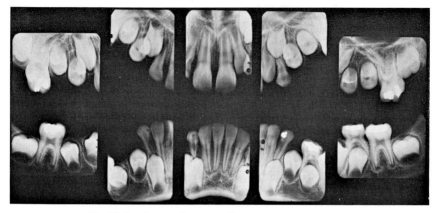

Fig. XI-2.—A complete set of periapical radiographs.

c) *Lateral Jaw Projections*

Lateral jaw projections are particularly useful during the mixed dentition, since they show the relationship of the teeth to one another and to their supporting bone better than any of the other standard radiographic projections. They also are useful for assessing the developmental status and relative eruptive positions of the individual teeth (Fig. XI-3).

Fig. XI-3.—A typical example of a well-taken lateral jaw radiograph.

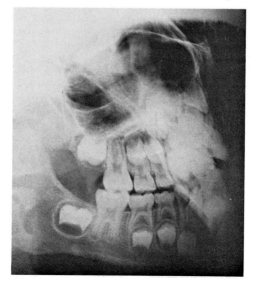

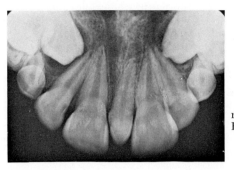

Fig. XI-4.—An occlusal plane radiograph. (Courtesy of Dr. K. A. Easlick.)

d) Occlusal Plane Projections

Occlusal plane projections are useful to locate supernumerary teeth at the midline and to ascertain accurately the position of impacted maxillary cuspids (Fig. XI-4).

e) Panoramic Radiographs

In the newly popular panoramic radiographs, one can (1) visualize, in one film, the relationships of both dentitions, both jaws and both temporomandibular joints, (2) study the relative developmental status of the teeth and progressive resorption of primary teeth and (3) ascertain

Fig. XI-5.—An example of one type of panoramic radiograph. In this form, the film must be cut and spliced. The panoramic projection, as can be seen, provides excellent views in one film of most items to be considered in analyzing a case in the mixed dentition.

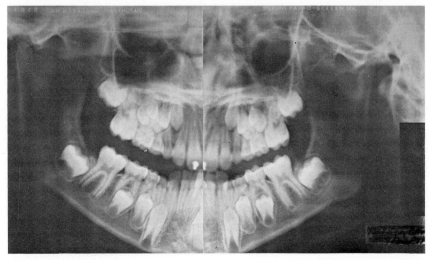

pathologic lesions. As ordinarily taken, the panoramic radiograph shows differential enlargement and therefore cannot be used for most "cephalometric measurements" (Fig. XI-5).

f) Oblique Cephalogram

The oblique cephalometric view is of particular use in analysis of the developing dentition, since it combines most of the advantages of the lateral jaw view, the intra-oral periapical survey and the panoramic radiograph, plus a standardized cephalometric registration that makes possible measurements of bone size, eruptive movements, etc. (Fig. XI-6). Cephalometric procedures are discussed in Chapter XII.

g) Lateral Cephalogram

The lateral projection is the cephalogram used most frequently for evaluation of the dentition's relationships to the osseous skeleton. See Chapter XII for a more detailed discussion of cephalometrics.

4. PHOTOGRAPHS

Standardized intra-oral and extra-oral photographs are supplemental to other diagnostic data. Parents and patients usually can interpret conditions and changes during treatment better in photographs than in casts or radiographs (Fig. XI-7). Photographs also serve to record

Fig. XI-6.—An example of an oblique cephalogram. The oblique cephalogram is a standardized cephalometric lateral jaw radiograph.

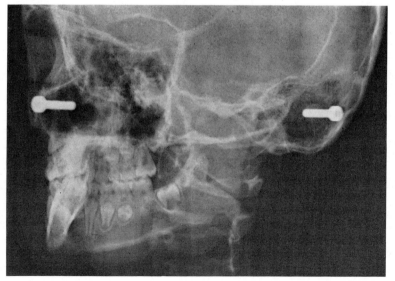

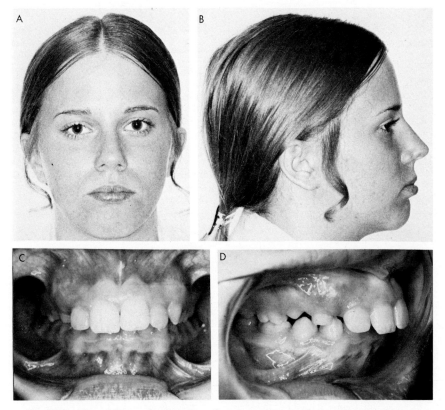

Fig. XI-7.—A and **B,** good examples of correct extra-oral photographs. (Courtesy of Dr. Michael Riolo.) **C** and **D,** good examples of intra-oral photographs.

changes in appliances used during treatment. Furthermore, some developmental anomalies actually may be visualized better in the intra-oral photograph than elsewhere; for example, mottled enamel, discoloration of enamel due to antibiotic therapy, hypoplastic enamel, amelogenesis imperfecta, etc.

B. Analyses of Tooth Development

1. CALCIFICATION

Calcification standards derived from populations of children, e.g., those by Nolla[14] (see Fig. VI-5) or those from the Center for Human Growth and Development (Table XI-1) may be used in the following ways: (a) to compare the individual patient to an appropriate population in order to determine whether his dental development is normal, advanced or retarded, (b) to compare the child to his own pattern of devel-

TABLE XI-1A.—RELATIONSHIP OF ROOT LENGTH DEVELOPMENT TO ERUPTION OF MANDIBULAR TEETH (MALES)

AGE	CANINE			FIRST PREMOLAR			SECOND PREMOLAR			FIRST MOLAR			SECOND MOLAR		
	% Age of Root Length Achieved		% Age of Eruption Achieved	% Age of Root Length Achieved		% Age of Eruption Achieved	% Age of Root Length Achieved		% Age of Eruption Achieved	% Age of Root Length Achieved		% Age of Eruption Achieved	% Age of Root Length Achieved		% Age of Eruption Achieved
	MEAN	SD		MEAN	SD		MEAN	SD		MEAN	SD		MEAN	SD	
5 yrs	3.75	5.16	0.00	0.00	0.00	0.00	0.00	0.00	0.00	26.37	8.78	0.00	0.00	0.00	0.00
6 yrs	9.38	5.36	.28	0.00	0.00	0.00	0.00	0.00	0.00	53.25	17.78	18.98	0.00	0.00	0.00
7 yrs	19.10	7.97	5.21	1.58	7.31	4.72	0.00	0.00	4.42	68.45	16.86	39.70	0.00	0.00	5.83
8 yrs	32.41	11.39	12.21	12.89	9.60	12.23	4.92	9.81	7.06	78.00	10.84	52.30	7.34	10.03	8.62
9 yrs	44.91	15.03	24.04	27.91	15.61	20.62	17.61	16.86	14.07	86.99	7.60	56.70	17.35	13.82	14.79
10 yrs	60.90	15.06	38.21	44.17	18.77	33.11	30.34	16.86	21.97	90.85	6.87	60.30	34.08	17.51	22.86
11 yrs	76.56	12.44	61.13	59.96	20.13	49.93	47.61	24.12	38.23	92.34	5.76	65.01	54.09	20.94	39.01
12 yrs	87.32	9.01	75.15	78.62	16.07	64.74	63.92	23.20	48.64	94.63	3.79	68.92	68.13	20.23	51.83
13 yrs	95.59	4.82	79.85	91.52	8.59	76.32	83.16	18.84	68.16	96.71	2.74	72.08	88.49	14.15	67.71
14 yrs	96.81	5.59	88.80	97.31	5.14	88.51	93.38	10.12	87.00	96.74	3.19	84.74	95.51	6.95	85.96
15 yrs	97.13	3.02	90.94	96.07	7.94	92.18	97.71	4.19	94.02	98.21	2.41	89.89	97.65	2.74	91.52
16 yrs	98.99	2.01	94.58	99.73	.54	95.15	100.00	0.00	95.76	95.67	6.99	97.58	99.19	1.61	98.58

Note in Tables XI-1A and *B* that active eruption does not begin until root formation starts. The greatest variability is seen during puberty; hence the impracticability of applying mean times of eruption to an individual clinical problem.

TABLE XI-1B.—RELATIONSHIP OF ROOT LENGTH DEVELOPMENT TO ERUPTION OF MANDIBULAR TEETH (FEMALES)

AGE	CANINE			FIRST PREMOLAR			SECOND PREMOLAR			FIRST MOLAR			SECOND MOLAR		
	% Age of Root Length Achieved		% Age of Eruption Achieved	% Age of Root Length Achieved		% Age of Eruption Achieved	% Age of Root Length Achieved		% Age of Eruption Achieved	% Age of Root Length Achieved		% Age of Eruption Achieved	% Age of Root Length Achieved		% Age of Eruption Achieved
	MEAN	SD		MEAN	SD		MEAN	SD		MEAN	SD		MEAN	SD	
5 yrs	8.15	5.44	0.00	0.00	0.00	0.00	0.00	0.00	0.00	35.86	14.79	10.08	0.00	0.00	0.00
6 yrs	16.64	13.30	5.12	0.00	0.00	4.66	0.00	0.00	1.57	49.30	16.54	38.98	0.00	0.00	3.78
7 yrs	27.78	12.43	10.48	8.27	7.83	7.89	1.92	10.30	3.46	69.73	9.60	64.65	4.58	9.84	8.84
8 yrs	43.95	13.83	23.79	22.19	11.13	18.49	13.56	14.32	10.11	78.73	9.71	74.80	15.28	12.41	14.75
9 yrs	62.50	13.36	45.17	37.61	15.65	32.10	25.76	18.22	18.49	87.11	7.95	78.03	31.36	19.99	21.82
10 yrs	76.44	15.21	63.43	58.71	19.92	51.96	41.04	20.94	32.54	92.54	6.07	82.91	43.18	22.19	33.98
11 yrs	89.36	10.24	80.38	74.41	17.99	69.97	63.32	25.75	53.73	95.48	4.08	85.83	65.18	22.38	56.91
12 yrs	94.55	7.31	90.50	87.40	14.34	82.84	81.63	21.90	65.95	98.32	2.33	86.69	85.09	22.46	73.85
13 yrs	98.13	4.34	96.68	96.63	7.01	97.51	92.86	14.98	86.38	97.98	2.33	95.04	91.29	14.23	91.62
14 yrs	97.26	1.91	98.73	95.41	6.71	97.46	92.19	13.02	92.43	98.86	1.22	94.96	95.45	5.18	89.32
15 yrs	99.60	.72	100.00	99.76	.36	100.00	98.06	2.74	100.00	98.00	2.86	100.00	96.69	8.10	100.00

opment, i.e., to ascertain whether there are individual teeth developing aberrant to his own general pattern and (c) to predict the time of completion of root development, diminution of pulp size or intra-oral eruption. Since Nolla's[14] and Moorrees *et al.*'s[11] stages of development are ordinal stages, it must not be assumed, for example, that the same amount of development takes place between stages 2 and 3 as takes place between stages 6 and 7. Nor is any stage necessarily exactly the same in one tooth as in another. Such ordinal stages have limited use in research in which quantification is necessary but are of help in analyzing and understanding the dentitional development of an individual child. The tabular presentation of our data (Table XI-1) makes possible a quick and useful comparison.

Before planning any orthodontic treatment in the mixed dentition, it is essential to know the developmental status of each individual tooth and the probable time each tooth will achieve future developmental stages. The use of group averages simply is not sophisticated enough for a practical clinical analysis. Research is done by the hundreds— treatment is done one by one. The purpose of dentitional evaluation is to evaluate the developmental status of each tooth in one child. Therefore, more is learned by comparing the child with himself than with a popular table of values or norms of a group to which he may not belong. Calcification of the primary teeth is discussed in Chapter VI, Section B-1 and of the permanent teeth in Chapter VI, Section D-1.

2. ERUPTION

a) Predicting Eruption

Shumaker and El Hadary[15] provide a few crude rules of thumb for predicting eruption, utilizing Nolla's stages (Fig. XI-8). Movement begins when the crown formation is complete (stage 6). The crest of the alveolar process is pierced when the root is roughly two-thirds completed (stage 8). Intra-oral emergence occurs when three-fourths of the root is formed. Occlusion is achieved when the root length is almost completed but the apex is still open (stage 9).

By referring to Table VI-4 (pp. 176 and 177), one can, in a crude way, predict the eruption of an individual tooth in the following fashion. First, compare the stage of calcification of the tooth to the mean stage of development for the appropriate chronologic age. For example, if one wishes to predict the time of emergence of a mandibular cuspid in a 6-year-old girl, he learns, by referring to Table VI-4, that on the average this tooth has reached one-third of the way between Nolla's stages 6 and 7, i.e., that the root formation has just begun. If the average 6-year-old girl has just begun eruption of the mandibular cuspid, it can be predicted that this tooth, in the average girl, will pierce the alveolar crest at age 8, when it coincidentally reaches stage 8. By comparing the individual patient's deviations from the normal pattern, crude estimates of the

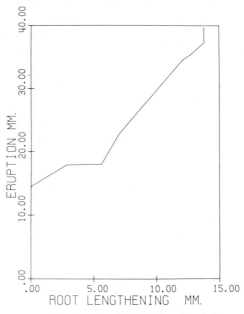

Fig. XI-8.—A computer plot showing the relationship between root lengthening and eruption. This plot is of a single mandibular cuspid. "Root lengthening" is a measure of total tooth length including crown height. "Eruption" is the distance from the lower border of the mandible. The plateau in the curve coincides with the completion of the crown. The most accelerated period occurs just after crown completion. Little, if any, eruption occurs prior to crown completion.

time of piercing the alveolar crest and reaching occlusal contact can be made. Note that these estimates are based on the time of piercing of the alveolar crest, not the gingival emergence.

b) *Sequence of Eruption*

One should always ascertain the implications to therapy of the sequence of eruption exhibited by the patient (see Chapter VI, Section D-2-e). Certain sequences tend to shorten the arch perimeter more rapidly, whereas others are useful in retaining arch perimeter. It should not be assumed that any given sequence of development will be the exact sequence of emergence in the mouth.

3. NUMBER OF TEETH

Strange as it may seem, failure to count the teeth is a common mistake. Counting must include not only the teeth seen but those developing —or not developing—within the jaws. Particular mention should be made of the determination of the congenital absence of teeth. Reference to Nolla's[14] data provides help for determination of the congenital absence of teeth. For example, if a boy of 8 years has not begun to calcify his mandibular third molar, the region should be studied regularly with radiographs, since the average boy begins calcification of mandibular third molars at age 7 (see Table VI-4A, p. 176).

4. Position of Teeth

Position of teeth must be interpreted solely in the light of the normal position for that tooth at the appropriate stage of development. For example, maxillary lateral incisors flare slightly while crowns of the erupting cuspids are changing their direction of movement toward the occlusion. As soon as the cuspid has uprighted itself and moved off the lateral incisor's root, the crown of the lateral incisor moves back into alignment in the dental arch (see Figs. VI-42 and VI-58). Thus, this slight labial position of the maxillary lateral incisors, called by Broadbent "the ugly duckling stage," is not a malposition in the mixed dentition but is a malposition in the completed permanent dentition. Simply noting malpositions of teeth is of little use; their significance to anticipated or expected tooth movements must be determined as well.

5. Anomalies

An immediate decision concerning the effects of any anomalies of development, size, shape or position of teeth on the anticipated therapy should be made. Usually, it is a mistake to postpone decisions concerning anomalies.

C. Size of Teeth

1. Individual Teeth

When considering the size of teeth, several measurements and concepts seem confusing. Indeed, the word "arch" is used to designate any or all of the dimensions shown in Figure XI-9. Some definitions may help clarify the important concepts involved.

The *basal arch* is the arch formed by the corpus mandibularis or maxillaris. Its dimensions probably are unaltered by the loss of all permanent teeth and resorption of the alveolar process. It is the arcal measurement of the apical base.

The *alveolar arch* is the arcal measurement of the alveolar process. The dimensions of the alveolar arch may not coincide with those of the basal arch if, for example, the teeth are tipped labially off the basal arch.

The *dental arch* usually is measured through the contact points of the teeth and represents a series of points where the muscle forces acting against the crowns of the teeth are balanced. When the crowns are tipped markedly off the basal bone, the dental arch and alveolar arch are not synonymous.

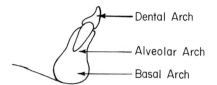

Dental Arch

Alveolar Arch

Basal Arch

Fig. XI-9.—The relationship of the three arches. The basal arch is largely determined by the configuration of the mandible itself. The alveolar arch joins the tooth to the basal arch and thus always is a compromise in size and shape between the basal arch and the dental arch. The dental arch reflects the relationship between the combined sizes of the crowns of the teeth, tongue, lip and buccal wall function, angulation of the teeth, anterior component of force, etc. When the combined mesiodistal diameters of the teeth are harmonious with the size of the basal arch and the relationship of the maxillary to the mandibular basal arch, the dental arch is synonymous with the combined sizes of the teeth.

The combined mesiodistal widths of the teeth constitute still another measurement.

Hopefully, during orthodontic treatment, all of the teeth will be so aligned that the combined widths of the teeth will be identical with the dental arch measurement and the dental arch will be so positioned over the basal bone that gross differences in the dental arch, alveolar arch and basal arch perimeters will not obscure cosmetics or complicate occlusal function and stability.

The distribution of crown sizes for the primary dentition is given in Table VI-3A and B (pp. 170 and 171) and for the permanent teeth in Table VI-5 (p. 193). For orthodontic diagnostic purposes, size of teeth is entirely a relative matter. Large teeth do not always result in a malocclusion, since the available space may be sufficiently large to include them nicely. Simple size of teeth tells little. Comparison of tooth size and available space (see Section C-4, below), determination of the effects of the size of the teeth on overbite and overjet (see Section C-2, below) and the identification of disharmonies of tooth size within the arch are, however, of great clinical import. It is not unusual to achieve a perfect Class I molar relationship during orthodontic treatment and not be able to achieve a similar cuspid interdigitation because of tooth size discrepancies in the lateral segments.

The localization of intra-arch and interarch disharmonies and their implications to treatment planning are aided by use of the Bolton Tooth Ratio Analysis (see below).

2. SIZE RELATIONSHIPS OF GROUPS OF TEETH

a) Bolton Tooth Ratio Analysis

Bolton[2, 3] studied the interarch effects of discrepancies in tooth size to devise a procedure for determining the ratio of total mandibular ver-

Over-all Ratio

$$\frac{\text{Sum mandibular 12} \_\_\_ \text{ mm.}}{\text{Sum maxillary 12} \_\_\_ \text{ mm.}} \times 100 = \text{Over-all ratio} \%$$

Mean 91.3 = 0.26
S.D. (σ) 1.91
Range 87.5 - 94.8

Maxillary 12	Mandibular 12	Maxillary 12	Mandibular 12	Maxillary 12	Mandibular 12
86	77.6	94	85.8	103	94.0
86	78.5	95	86.7	104	95.0
87	79.4	96	87.6	105	95.9
88	80.3	97	88.6	106	96.8
89	81.3	98	89.5	107	97.8
90	82.1	99	90.4	108	98.6
91	83.1	100	91.3	109	99.5
92	84.0	101	92.2	110	100.4
93	84.9	102	93.1		

Patient Analysis

If the over-all ratio exceeds 91.3 the discrepancy is in excessive mandibular arch length. In above chart locate the patient's maxillary 12 measurement and opposite it is the correct mandibular measurement. The difference **between** the actual and correct mandibular measurement is the amount of excessive mandibular arch length.

Actual mandibular 12 − Correct mandibular 12 = Excess mandibular 12

If over-all ratio is less than 91.3:

Actual maxillary 12 − Correct maxillary 12 = Excess maxillary 12

Anterior Ratio

$$\frac{\text{Sum mandibular 6} \_\_\_ \text{ mm.}}{\text{Sum maxillary 6} \_\_\_ \text{ mm.}} \times 100 = \text{Anterior ratio} \%$$

Mean 77.2 = 0.22
S.D. (σ) 1.65
Range 74.5 - 80.4

Maxillary 6	Mandibular 6	Maxillary 6	Mandibular 6	Maxillary 6	Mandibular 6
40.0	30.9	45.5	35.1	50.5	39.0
40.5	31.3	46.0	35.5	51.0	39.4
41.0	31.7	46.5	35.9	51.5	39.8
41.5	32.0	47.0	36.3	52.0	40.1
42.0	32.4	47.5	36.7	52.5	40.5
42.5	32.8	48.0	37.1	53.0	40.9
43.0	33.2	48.5	37.4	53.5	41.3
43.5	33.6	49.0	37.8	54.0	41.7
44.0	34.0	49.5	38.2	54.5	42.1
44.5	34.4	50.0	38.6	55.0	42.5
45.0	34.7				

Patient Analysis

If anterior ratio exceeds 77.2:

Actual mandibular 6 − Correct mandibular 6 = Excess mandibular 6

If anterior ratio is less than 77.2:

Actual maxillary 6 − Correct maxillary 6 = Excess maxillary 6

Fig. XI-10.—The Bolton analysis of tooth size discrepancies. The sizes of the individual teeth are measured and recorded on the form. The anterior ratio and the over-all ratio are computed separately.

sus maxillary tooth size and anterior mandibular versus maxillary tooth size. Study of these ratios helps in estimating the overbite and overjet relationships that will obtain after treatment is finished, the effects of contemplated extractions on posterior occlusion and incisor relationships and the identification of occlusal misfit produced by interarch tooth size incompatibilities. Figure XI-10 is the suggested data form for use in recording and computing both the over-all and anterior tooth ratios.

The procedure is as follows: the sum of the widths of the mandibular 12 teeth is divided by the sum of the maxillary 12 teeth and multiplied by 100. A mean ratio of 91.3, according to Bolton, will result in ideal overbite-overjet relationships as well as posterior occlusion. If the over-all ratio exceeds 91.3, the discrepancy is due to excessive mandibular tooth material. In the chart, one locates the figure corresponding to the patient's maxillary tooth size. Opposite is the desired mandibular measurement. The difference between the actual and the desired mandibular measurement is the amount of excessive mandibular tooth material when the ratio is greater than 91.3. If the ratio is less than 91.3, the difference between the actual maxillary size and the desired maxillary size is the amount of excess maxillary tooth material. A similar ratio (anterior ratio) is computed for the 6 anterior teeth (incisors and cuspids). The desired anterior ratio is 77.2, which will provide ideal overbite and overjet relationships if the angulation of the incisors is correct and if the labiolingual thickness of the incisal edges is not excessive. If the anterior ratio exceeds 77.2, there is excess mandibular tooth material; if it is less than 77.2, there is excess maxillary tooth material.

When one is contemplating the extraction of 4 premolars, it is useful, before selecting the teeth for extraction, to ascertain the effects of various extraction combinations on these ratios. Care must be taken in the use of this analysis, since Bolton's formulae do not take into account quantitatively the incisor's angulation.

3. RELATIONSHIPS OF TOOTH SIZE TO SIZE OF SUPPORTING STRUCTURES

a) Howes' Analysis

Howes[7-9] drew attention to the fact that crowding could result not only from excessive tooth size but inadequate apical bases as well. He devised an ingenious formula for determining whether the apical bases of the patient could accommodate the patient's teeth.

The procedure is as follows: Tooth material (TM) equals the sum of the mesiodistal widths of the teeth from the first permanent molar forward. Premolar diameter (PMD) is the arch width measured at the tip of the buccal cusps of the first premolars. Premolar diameter to tooth material ratio ($\frac{PMD}{TM}$) is obtained by dividing the premolar diameter by the sum of the widths of the 12 teeth. Premolar basal arch width

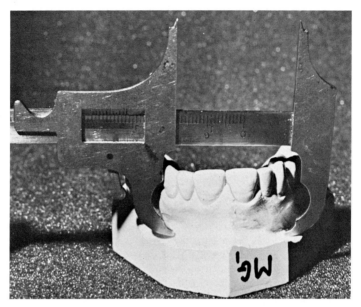

Fig. XI-11.—Measuring the canine fossa diameter.

(PMBAW) is obtained by measuring, with the bowed end of the Boley gauge, the diameter of the apical base on the dental casts at the apices of the first premolars (Fig. XI-11). The ratio of the premolar basal arch width to tooth material ($\frac{\text{PMBAW}}{\text{TM}}$) is obtained by dividing the premolar basal arch width by the sum of the width of the 12 teeth. Basal arch length (BAL) is measured at the midline (Fig. XI-12) from the estimated anterior limits of the apical base to a perpendicular that is tangent to the distal surfaces of the two first molars. The ratio of basal arch length to tooth material ($\frac{\text{BAL}}{\text{TM}}$) is obtained by dividing the arch length by the sum of the widths of the 12 teeth. Figure XI-12, *B* shows the mean values and the range of values found for both arches from a study of normal occlusion. Howes[7] believed that the premolar basal arch width (he called it the canine fossa diameter) should equal approximately 44% of the mesiodistal widths of the 12 teeth in the maxilla if it is to be sufficiently large to accommodate all the teeth. When the ratio between basal arch width and tooth material is less than 37%, Howes considers this to be a basal arch deficiency necessitating extraction of premolars. If the premolar basal width is greater than the premolar coronal arch width, expansion of the premolars may be undertaken safely. Since this method was introduced, palate splitting has come into use (see Chaps. XV and XVII). The Howes analysis is useful in planning treatment of

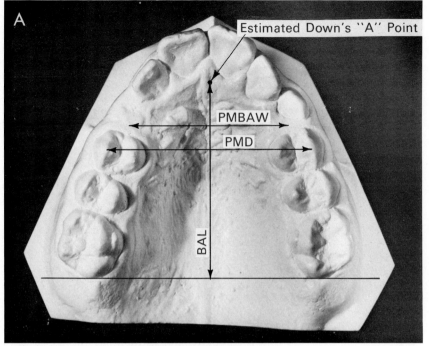

A
Estimated Down's "A" Point
PMBAW
PMD
BAL

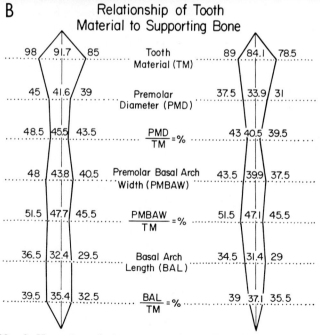

B   Relationship of Tooth
      Material to Supporting Bone

98	91.7	85	Tooth Material (TM)	89	84.1	78.5
45	41.6	39	Premolar Diameter (PMD)	37.5	33.9	31
48.5	45.5	43.5	$\dfrac{PMD}{TM}$ = %	43	40.5	39.5
48	43.8	40.5	Premolar Basal Arch Width (PMBAW)	43.5	39.9	37.5
51.5	47.7	45.5	$\dfrac{PMBAW}{TM}$ = %	51.5	47.1	45.5
36.5	32.4	29.5	Basal Arch Length (BAL)	34.5	31.4	29
39.5	35.4	32.5	$\dfrac{BAL}{TM}$ = %	39	37.1	35.5

Fig. XI-12.—A, Howes' analysis measurements. See also Figure XI-11. **B,** see text for details of use.

367

problems with suspected apical base deficiencies and deciding whether to (1) extract, (2) expand or (3) split the palate.

b) Diagnostic Setup

It is useful in difficult space management problems to ascertain, before orthodontic treatment is begun, precisely the amount and direction each tooth must be moved. Useful as the Mixed Dentition Analysis is (see Section C-4, below), it is at best a mathematical representation of the problem during the mixed dentition. A popular practical technic for visualizing space problems in three dimensions in the permanent dentition is that of cutting off the teeth from a set of casts and resetting them in more desirable positions (Fig. XI-13). This procedure is called a diagnostic or prognostic setup. The record casts are not used for this technic, since they must be saved for comparison with the diagnostic setup and with progressive record casts.

Steps in the technic are as follows:

1. Obtain an accurate wax bite (see Section E).

2. Drill a hole through the alveolar portion of the cast well below the gingival margin of the teeth.

3. Insert a fine saw blade through the hole and cut up to the crest of the gingival margin between two of the teeth. Cut laterally, well beneath the gingival margin of the teeth and come up again at the point of the gingival crest below the contact point on the opposite side of the tooth. Repeat this for all the teeth to be cut off the cast. Do not cut through the contact points. Cutting up to the gingival crest will permit gentle breaking of the plaster without damage.

Fig. XI-13.—The diagnostic setup. **A,** before, and **B,** after the teeth have been cut off and set in a corrected position.

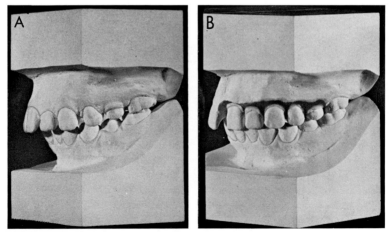

4. Align the teeth and wax them into their desired positions. It is best not to cut off all of the teeth so that the bite relationship can be kept.

A more accurate method involves taking a wax bite in the retruded contact position, mounting the casts on an adjustable articulator and finishing the diagnostic setup within the limits of the jaw relationships thus imposed (see Section E).

When extractions are contemplated as part of the orthodontic treatment, the diagnostic setup will demonstrate vividly the amount of space created by the extractions and the tooth movements necessary to close that space. It will also aid in choosing which teeth to extract.

4. RELATIONSHIPS OF TOOTH SIZE AND AVAILABLE SPACE DURING THE MIXED DENTITION (MIXED DENTITION ANALYSIS)

The purpose of the Mixed Dentition Analysis is to evaluate the amount of space available in the arch for succeeding permanent teeth and necessary occlusal adjustments. To complete an analysis of the mixed dentition, three factors must be noted: (1) the sizes of all the permanent teeth anterior to the first permanent molar, (2) the arch perimeter and (3) expected changes in the arch perimeter, which may occur with growth and development (see Chapter VI).

Many methods of Mixed Dentition Analysis have been suggested; however, all fall into two strategic categories: (1) those in which the sizes of the unerupted cuspids and premolars are estimated from measurements of the radiographic image and (2) those in which the sizes of the cuspids and premolars are derived from knowledge of the sizes of permanent teeth already erupted in the mouth. The method presented here is of the latter type. Mixed Dentition Analyses have been misused in several ways. First, they have been applied mechanically without proper regard for the biologic dynamics of a critical stage in dentitional development (see Chapter VI). Second, naïve assumptions have been made, e.g., universal 1.7 mm. late mesial shift. Third, many have presumed them to have an accuracy that is not present in any of the methods yet presented (Fig. XI-14).

The method presented here is advocated for the following reasons: (1) it has minimal systematic error and the range of such errors is known, (2) it can be done with equal reliability by the beginner and the expert— it does not presume sophisticated clinical judgment, (3) it is not time-consuming, (4) it requires no special equipment or radiographic projections, (5) although best done on dental casts, it can be done with reasonable accuracy in the mouth and (6) it may be used for both dental arches.

The genetic fields within which permanent tooth size is controlled extend to involve a number of teeth (see Chapter VI, Section E-1). Therefore, people with large teeth in one part of the mouth tend to have large teeth elsewhere. Moorrees and Reed[12] annotated the variability between combinations of teeth in the permanent dentition and concluded that

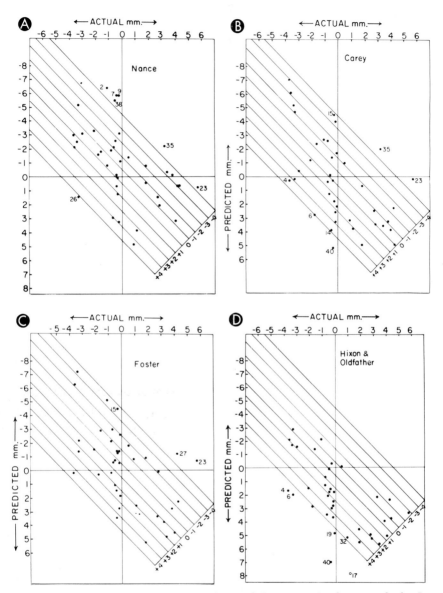

Fig. XI-14.—A comparison of several Mixed Dentition Analysis methods. In **A–F,** the charts compare the estimated spacing and crowding (vertical axis) with what actually appeared (horizontal axis) in 40 cases using six different Mixed Dentition Analysis methods. Those cases identified by number are those in which the prediction differed from the actual value by 5 mm. or more. If all the predicted values were perfect, the dots would lie in a straight line within the diagonal channel marked 0. (*Continued.*)

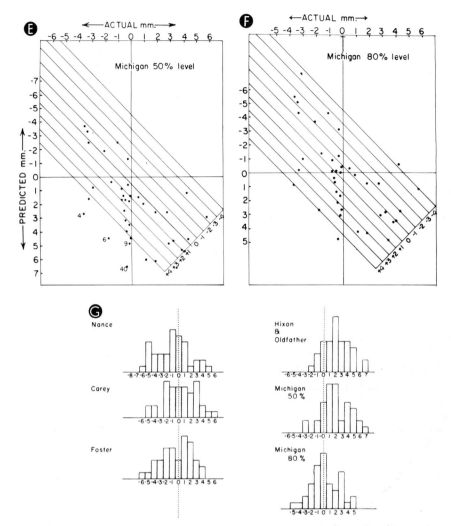

Fig. XI-14 (cont.).—Predictions that were more optimistic than actuality are in the positive channels to the left of 0. Predictions that were more pessimistic than actuality are in the channels to the right of 0. Thus, for example, Case No. 26 (Nance diagram, **A**) was predicted by that analysis to show nearly 2 mm. of spacing, whereas more than 3 mm. of crowding occurred. Therefore, the prediction is more than 4 mm. on the optimistic side. Conversely, Case No. 35 in the Nance diagram (**A**) was predicted by this Mixed Dentition Analysis to show between 2 and 3 mm. of crowding, whereas, in reality, there was 3 mm. of spacing, a prediction on the pessimistic side of about 5 mm. **G** summarizes these predictions. If all were perfect, there would be a single vertical bar in the histogram at 0. Note that some analyses, e.g., Nance, systematically make pessimistic predictions and others, e.g., Hixon and Oldfather and Michigan 50%, systematically predict optimistically.

the correlations among groups of teeth are not really very high. However, the correlation between the sizes of the mandibular incisors and the combined sizes of the cuspids and premolars in either arch is high enough to predict within rather close limits the amount of space required during space management procedures. Clauss,[4] Barber[1] and others[13] (Fig. XI-14) have found the method presented here to be superior to others tested. However, none of the Mixed Dentition Analyses are as precise as one might like, and all must be used with judgment and knowledge of development. The mandibular incisors have been chosen for measuring, since they are erupted into the mouth early in the mixed dentition, are easily measured accurately and are directly in the midst of most space management problems. The maxillary incisors are *not* used in any of the predictive procedures, since they show too much variability in size, and their correlations with other groups of teeth are too low to be of practical value. Therefore, the lower incisors are measured to predict the size of *upper* as well as lower posterior teeth.

a) Procedure in the Mandibular Arch

1. Measure with the tooth-measuring gauge (Fig. XI-15) or a pointed Boley gauge the greatest mesiodistal width of each of the 4 mandibular incisors. Record these values in the Mixed Dentition Analysis Form (Fig. XI-16).

2. Determine the amount of space needed for alignment of the incisors. Set the Boley gauge to a value equal to the sum of the widths of the left central incisor and left lateral incisor. Place one point of the gauge at the midline of the alveolar crest between the central incisors and let the other point lie along the line of the dental arch on the left side (Fig. XI-17). Mark on the tooth or the cast the precise point where the distal tip of the Boley gauge has touched. This point is where the distal surface of the lateral incisor will be when it has been aligned. Repeat this process for the right side of the arch. If the cephalometric evaluation shows the mandibular incisor to be too far labially (see Chap. XII), the Boley gauge tip is placed at the midline, but moved lingually a sufficient amount to simulate the expected uprighting of the incisors as dictated by the cephalometric evaluation.

Fig. XI-15.—A tooth-measuring gauge.

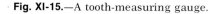

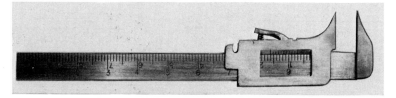

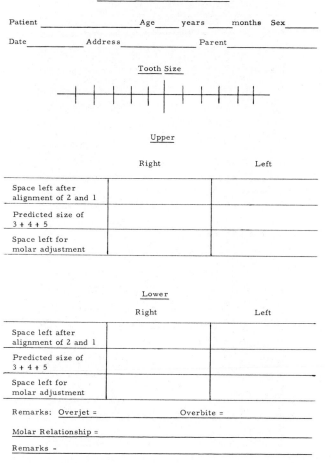

MIXED DENTITION ANALYSIS

Patient _____ Age _____ years _____ months Sex _____

Date _____ Address _____ Parent _____

Tooth Size

Upper

Right   Left

	Right	Left
Space left after alignment of 2 and 1		
Predicted size of 3 + 4 + 5		
Space left for molar adjustment		

Lower

Right   Left

	Right	Left
Space left after alignment of 2 and 1		
Predicted size of 3 + 4 + 5		
Space left for molar adjustment		

Remarks: Overjet = _____   Overbite = _____

Molar Relationship = _____

Remarks - _____

Fig. XI-16.—Chart for recording data of the Mixed Dentition Analysis. The tooth sizes are inserted in the proper positions on the chart after measurements on the casts or in the mouth. The predicted size of the cuspids and premolars is taken from the 75% level of probability in the probability chart (Fig. XI-19).

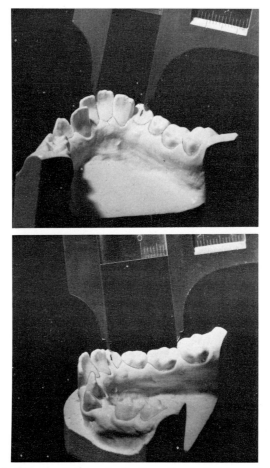

Fig. XI-17.—Marking the distance in the line of arch that is needed for the alignment of central and lateral incisors. This distance shows how much of the arch perimeter will be taken up during alignment of the mandibular incisors. It is repeated for both sides.

Fig. XI-18.—Measuring the space left in the arch after incisor alignment. After it has been ascertained how much space is needed for the incisors, it is necessary to measure the space left for cuspids and premolars and molar adjustment.

3. Compute the amount of space available after incisor alignment. To do this step, measure the distance from the point marked in the line of the arch (step 2, above) to the mesial surface of the first permanent molar (Fig. XI-18). This distance is the space available for the cuspid and 2 premolars and for any necessary molar adjustment after the incisors have been aligned. Record the data for both sides on the Mixed Dentition Analysis Form.

PROBABILITY CHART FOR PREDICTING THE SUM OF THE WIDTHS OF $\underline{345}$ FROM $\overline{21/12}$

$\overline{\Sigma 21/12}$ =	19.5	20.0	20.5	21.0	21.5	22.0	22.5	23.0	23.5	24.0	24.5	25.0
95%	21.6	21.8	22.1	22.4	22.7	22.9	23.2	23.5	23.8	24.0	24.3	24.6
85%	21.0	21.3	21.5	21.8	22.1	22.4	22.6	22.9	23.2	23.5	23.7	24.0
75%	20.6	20.9	21.2	21.5	21.8	22.0	22.3	22.6	22.9	23.1	23.4	23.7
65%	20.4	20.6	20.9	21.2	21.5	21.8	22.0	22.3	22.6	22.8	23.1	23.4
50%	20.0	20.3	20.6	20.8	21.1	21.4	21.7	21.9	22.2	22.5	22.8	23.0
35%	19.6	19.9	20.2	20.5	20.8	21.0	21.3	21.6	21.9	22.1	22.4	22.7
25%	19.4	19.7	19.9	20.2	20.5	20.8	21.0	21.3	21.6	21.9	22.1	22.4
15%	19.0	19.3	19.6	19.9	20.2	20.4	20.7	21.0	21.3	21.5	21.8	22.1
5%	18.5	18.8	19.0	19.3	19.6	19.9	20.1	20.4	20.7	21.0	21.2	21.5

PROBABILITY CHART FOR PREDICTING THE SUM OF THE WIDTHS OF $\overline{345}$ FROM $\overline{21/12}$

$\overline{\Sigma 21/12}$ =	19.5	20.0	20.5	21.0	21.5	22.0	22.5	23.0	23.5	24.0	24.5	25.0
95%	21.1	21.4	21.7	22.0	22.3	22.6	22.9	23.2	23.5	23.8	24.1	24.4
85%	20.5	20.8	21.1	21.4	21.7	22.0	22.3	22.6	22.9	23.2	23.5	23.8
75%	20.1	20.4	20.7	21.0	21.3	21.6	21.9	22.2	22.5	22.8	23.1	23.4
65%	19.8	20.1	20.4	20.7	21.0	21.3	21.6	21.9	22.2	22.5	22.8	23.1
50%	19.4	19.7	20.0	20.3	20.6	20.9	21.2	21.5	21.8	22.1	22.4	22.7
35%	19.0	19.3	19.6	19.9	20.2	20.5	20.8	21.1	21.4	21.7	22.0	22.3
25%	18.7	19.0	19.3	19.6	19.9	20.2	20.5	20.8	21.1	21.4	21.7	22.0
15%	18.4	18.7	19.0	19.3	19.6	19.8	20.1	20.4	20.7	21.0	21.3	21.6
5%	17.7	18.0	18.3	18.6	18.9	19.2	19.5	19.8	20.1	20.4	20.7	21.0

DEPARTMENT OF ORTHODONTICS   SCHOOL OF DENTISTRY   UNIVERSITY OF MICHIGAN

Fig. XI-19.—Probability charts for computing the size of unerupted cuspids and bicuspids. The top chart is for the upper arch. The bottom chart is for the lower arch. Measure and obtain the mesiodistal widths of the 4 permanent mandibular incisors and find that value in the top horizontal column. Reading downward in the appropriate vertical column, obtain the values for expected width of the cuspids and premolars corresponding to the level of probability you wish to choose. Ordinarily, the 75% level of probability is used. Note that the mandibular incisors are used for the prediction of both the mandibular and maxillary cuspid and premolar widths.

4. Predict the size of the combined widths of the mandibular cuspid and premolars. This prediction is done by use of probability charts (Fig. XI-19). Locate at the top of the mandibular chart the value that most nearly corresponds to the sum of the widths of the 4 mandibular incisors. Beneath the figure just located lies a column of figures indicating the range of values for all the cuspid and premolar sizes that will be found for incisors of the indicated size. For example, note that for incisors of 22.0 mm. combined width the summated mandibular cuspid and premolar widths range from 22.6 mm. at the 95% level of confidence down to 19.2 mm. at the 5% level. This means that of all the people in the universe whose lower incisors measure 22.0 mm., 95% will have cuspid and premolar widths totaling 22.6 mm. or less and only 5% will have cuspids and premolars whose widths total as low as 19.2 mm. No one figure can represent the precise cuspid-premolar sum for all people, since there is a range of posterior tooth widths seen even when the incisors are identical. The value at the 75% level is chosen as the estimate, since it has been found to be the most practical from a clinical standpoint. In this instance, it is 21.6 mm., which means that three times out of four the cuspid and premolars will total 21.6 mm. or less. Note also that only five times in a hundred will these teeth be more than 1 mm. greater than the estimate chosen (21.6 mm.). Theoretically, one should use the 50% level of probability, since any errors would then distribute equally both ways. However, clinically, we need more protection on the down side (crowding) than we do on the up side (spacing). Record this value in the proper blanks for right and left sides, since it is the same for both.

5. Compute the amount of space left in the arch for molar adjustment. This computation is done by subtracting the estimated cuspid and premolar size from the measured space available in the arch after alignment of the incisors. Record these values in the proper blanks on each side.

From all the values now recorded, a complete assessment of the space situation in the mandible is possible.

b) *Procedure in the Maxillary Arch*

The procedure is similar to that for the lower arch, with two exceptions: (1) a different probability chart is used for predicting the upper cuspid and premolar sum (see Fig. XI-19) and (2) allowance must be made for overjet correction when measuring the space to be occupied by the aligned incisors. Remember that *lower* incisors' widths are used to predict upper cuspid and premolar widths.

Figure XI-20 illustrates the application of the Mixed Dentition Analysis to a specific clinical problem. Note that the localization of any space shortages helps greatly in selection of the space management appliance. Discussion of the treatment of space problems is found in Chapter XV.

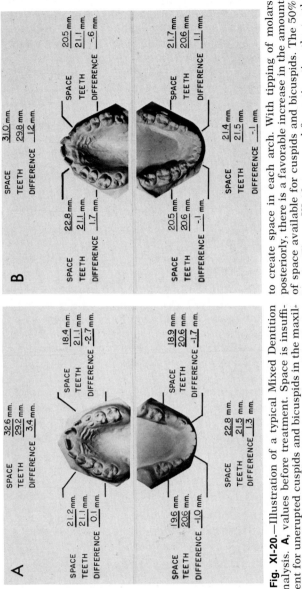

Fig. XI-20.—Illustration of a typical Mixed Dentition Analysis. **A,** values before treatment. Space is insufficient for unerupted cuspids and bicuspids in the maxillary left posterior quadrant and in both mandibular posterior quadrants. **B,** a few months later, after maxillary and mandibular acrylic appliances have been worn to create space in each arch. With tipping of molars posteriorly, there is a favorable increase in the amount of space available for cuspids and bicuspids. The 50% line in Figure XI-19 was used for estimating the teeth size in this instance.

It is good practice to study the periapical, lateral jaw or oblique cephalometric radiographs when the Mixed Dentition Analysis is done in order to note absence of permanent teeth, unusual malpositions of development or abnormalities of crown form. For example, mandibular second molars sometimes have two lingual cusps. When they are so formed, the crown is larger than might be expected from the probability chart and, therefore, a higher predictive value is used. One may, of course, measure the size of the crowns of the unerupted cuspid and premolars in periapical radiographs for supplemental information or corroboration of the Mixed Dentition Analysis estimate.

c) *Modifications*

Huckaba[10] provides a technic for Mixed Dentition Analysis that compensates nicely for radiographic enlargement of tooth images in periapical films. It is based on the assumption that the degree of magnification for a primary tooth will be the same as that for its underlying permanent successor on the same film. (1) Measure the width of the primary tooth on the x-ray film (Y') and the width of its underlying permanent successor (X') on the x-ray film. (2) Measure the primary tooth (Y) directly in the mouth or on the dental cast. The width of the unerupted permanent tooth (X) can then be calculated by simple mathematical proportion: $X:X' = Y:Y'$ or $X = \dfrac{X'\,Y}{Y'}$.

For example, if the image of the second primary molar on the x-ray film (Y') is 10.5 mm., the image of the underlying second premolar (X') is 7.4 mm., and the width of the second primary molar as measured on the cast (Y) is 10.0 mm., then $X = \dfrac{7.4 \times 10}{10.5}$ or $X = 7.0^+$ mm. This procedure is particularly useful when planning treatment for space supervision problems (see Chapter XV) in which every fraction of a millimeter must be accounted for. Inaccuracy in radiographic tooth size measurements is not the dentist's fault. It occurs because the developing teeth are not always placed exactly at right angles to the central ray; therefore, the radiographic image of the tooth, when slightly rotated or tipped, is significantly larger than the actual size of the tooth. A technic has been developed at Washington University using special vertical occlusal plane projections to obviate such distortion.[5]

A problem arises when considering the space left for molar adjustment. If this value in the chart is negative, that is, the predicted sizes of 3, 4 and 5 are greater than the space left after the alignment of the incisors, then crowding will occur in the arch without the needed forward molar adjustment. When the first permanent molars are in an end-to-end relationship (i.e., a flush terminal plane of the second primary molars), approximately 3.5 mm. of space (one-half a cusp width) is required to convert to a Class I molar relationship. This needed 3.5 mm. might be acquired in any of three ways: (1) 3.5 mm. more late mesial shift of the mandibular first permanent molar than the maxillary, (2) at least 3.5 mm. more forward growth of the mandible during this period than occurs in the maxilla or (3) some combination of dental adjustment and differential skeletal growth. Since we cannot yet predict accurately the amount of differential skeletal growth that will occur, treatment planning is based solely on dental adjustment factors. If differential skeletal growth occurs during this period, alterations in the molar relationship will be seen and the Mixed Dentition Analysis predictions must be altered accordingly. When there is a Class I molar relationship in the mixed dentition (mesial step of the second primary molars), no part of the arch perimeter need be pre-empted for molar adjustment and all the space is available for incisors, cuspids and premolars.

It has become the fashion in many Mixed Dentition Analysis procedures to assume that every child will require precisely 1.7 mm. of late mesial shift. Such fallacious reasoning is unfortunate, since it leads to errors in treatment planning. One cannot assume average mesial shift values any more than one can assume average tooth sizes. As was stated earlier, some children will require no mesial shift of the first permanent molars (Class I molar relationship), the greatest number of children will require approximately 3.5 mm. late mesial shift (end-to-end molar relationship) and some children will require as much as 7 mm. or even more molar adjustment (Class II molar relationship). The suggestion of a 1.7 mm. universal estimate was based on an erroneous derivation. Unfortunately, most children require more space. To be practical, any Mixed Dentition Analysis must be theoretically correct and technically precise; it must be a custom analysis of one child's problem. The primary purpose of the Mixed Dentition Analysis is to learn the space requirements of one mouth.

D. Arch Dimensions

1. Changes in Arch Dimensions

A discussion of the expected changes in arch dimensions during growth and development and methods of measuring arch dimensions will be found in Chapter VI. Clinically, the problem of arch dimensions is how to analyze what space is needed and which dimensions can be increased therapeutically to acquire the needed space. Figure XI-21 summarizes in a simplistic way dimensional changes in the primary and mixed dentitions that occur during growth and those that might be possible with treatment. What nature does and what we are able to do clinically often are different; for example, the mandibular arch perimeter, one of the most critical of all dimensions, usually decreases markedly at the time of exfoliation of the primary teeth and cannot easily be increased significantly by therapy in the mixed dentition. Since maxillary dimensions can be altered much more easily by treatment, it is natural for Mixed Dentition Analyses to emphasize mandibular measurements.

	PRIMARY DENTITION		MIXED DENTITION	
	GROWTH	TREATMENT	GROWTH	TREATMENT
MANDIBLE				
WIDTH	O	+	O	O
PERIMETER	O	O	− −	O
MAXILLA				
WIDTH	+	+	+	+ +
PERIMETER	O	+	O	+ +

O Same   + Mild Increase Occurs or can be Obtained
− − Decreases Greatly   + + Significant Increase Occurs or can be Obtained

Fig. XI-21.—A summary of the expected dimensional changes in the dental arches compared with the treatment possibilities. Note that the opportunities for altering the maxillary dental arch dimension are far greater than those for the mandible. Note, too, that normal growth and development results in a radical shortening of the mandibular arch perimeter unless it is stopped by treatment.

2. A WORD ABOUT INDICES

Several attempts have been made to determine what arch dimensions teeth of known size require for ideal alignment. The dimensions that are necessary for ideal alignment and those clinically achievable are not necessarily the same. There has been, in recent years, an unfortunate revival of the use of Pont's Index in an indiscriminate manner. Pont's Index of Ideal Arch Form simply suggests ideal maxillary premolar and first molar diameters according to the mesiodistal diameters of the maxillary incisors. To know desired maxillary dimensions for a case may be useful but it is more difficult to achieve the corresponding mandibular dimensions that are necessary to maintain balanced occlusal relationships. Pont's Index does not account for the relationship of the teeth to supporting bone, corresponding mandibular dimensions or the difficulties in increasing mandibular dimensions. It seems sur-

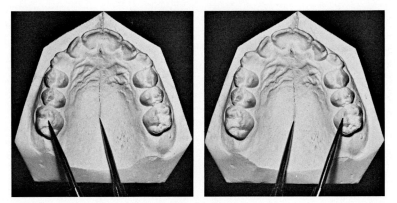

Fig. XI-22.—Method of using dividers to measure from the median raphe to estimate asymmetries of the dental arches.

prising that some today still attempt to use a crude procedure abandoned many years ago by most clinicians.

3. ASYMMETRIES OF ARCH DIMENSION AND TOOTH POSITION

Figure XI-22 shows a method to estimate asymmetries of tooth position in the arch. Figure XI-23 illustrates the use of a symmetrograph

Fig. XI-23.—Use of a symmetrograph to determine asymmetry in the dental arch.

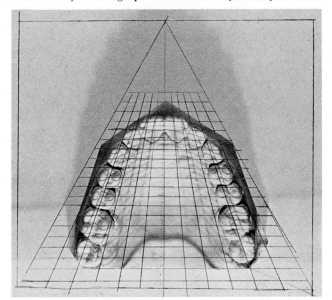

to determine asymmetry within the maxillary arch. The symmetrograph, a transparent plastic device with an inscribed grid, may be purchased or made. Place the maxillary cast on its base and carefully mark the median raphe with a series of tiny dots. It has been shown by Harvold *et al.*[6] that the median raphe is a proper representation of the skeletal midline. Orient the symmetrograph so that its midline is directly superposed over the median raphe and parallel to the occlusal surface. Total and partial arch asymmetry are quickly visualized and localized, as are drifting, tipping and rotations of individual teeth. This simple step is most useful in planning individual tooth movements and determining appliance design. A similar analysis of the mandibular dentition is likely to be a bit less precise, since the mandibular lingual frenum is not as reliable a midline structure as the median raphe. Harvold *et al.*[6] devised an ingenious system for analysis of asymmetries of teeth and arches in both casts and a method for correlating the casts and the cephalograms. The device used, however, is not generally available, and the method is a bit complicated.

E. Registration of Jaw Relationships

It is important to ask at the start which jaw position is to be registered and for what purpose. The ideal occlusal position and the retruded contact position are used for different purposes and should not be confused (see Chapter V, Section D). Neither the ideal occlusal position nor the retruded contact position is necessarily synonymous with the patient's usual occlusal position. The primary purpose of registering jaw relationships for orthodontic analysis is to determine any clinically significant differences in these three jaw positions: the usual occlusal position, the ideal occlusal position and the retruded contact position.

1. Retruded Contact Position

Every dentist has a favorite technic for recording retruded contact position. It is used in restorative and prosthetic dentistry when it is necessary to mount casts reliably on an articulator. It is used in restorative dentistry, periodontics and orthodontics as a starting position for occlusal equilibration (see Chapter XVII). It is not so precisely useful in children with malocclusion, since the immaturity of their temporomandibular joint structures often permits a more posterior retruded contact position than will be noted when the patient is older or the malocclusion corrected. Changes in the retruded contact position (centric relationship) can and do occur frequently during and after orthodontic therapy—a point often confusing to dentists working primarily with adult patients. Since most patients' jaws are reflexly prehensile when biting, I prefer the wax bite method illustrated in Figure XI-24 to the usual horseshoe method. The illustrated wax bite method has been found to be easier, since no wax touches the incisors and thus the ten-

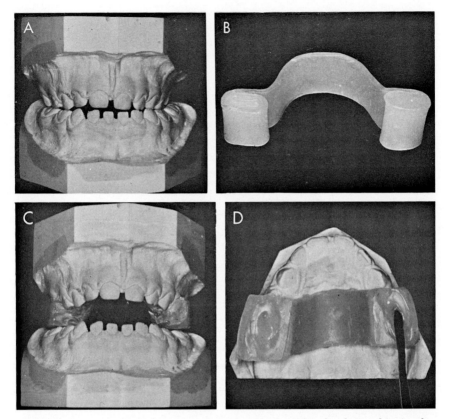

Fig. XI-24.—Procedure for registering the ideal occlusal relationship in the primary or mixed dentition. **A,** the original eccentric relationship. **B,** bite registration wax is rolled to form a scroll and adapted to the maxillary cast in the mid-palatal region. **C,** the fit in the maxillary arch. Note the vertical size of the occlusal wax pads. Ordinarily, the wax bite will stay in position by itself, but sometimes it is necessary to reinforce it with hard base plate wax. Do not use the base plate wax over the occlusal pads. **D,** softening the occlusal pads. The patient is seated upright with the Frankfurt plane parallel to the floor. The bite registration wax is introduced into the mouth and the patient is told to close his jaws gently until he just feels the wax. *(Continued.)*

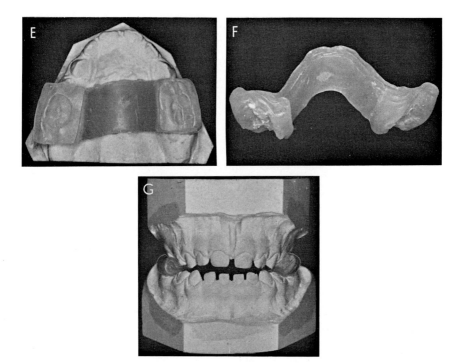

Fig. XI-24 (cont.).—E, the bite wax placed on the maxillary cast after first jaw closure. Usually, it is necessary to soften the wax about two or three times and to reintroduce it into the mouth in order to obtain the final registration. Do not let the patient bite through the wax. **F,** the final wax bite registration. **G,** the wax bite record in place on the cast. Compare with **A.** Note that the midlines now coincide. This registration is much more critical anteroposteriorly and mediolaterally than it is vertically. Therefore, it does not matter that the teeth are not in occlusion. Indeed, they must not be or the old eccentric occlusionship will be recorded instead of the ideal occlusal relationship.

dency of most people to bite protrusively is diminished. The use of a solid sheet of wax is definitely contraindicated, since the tongue is displaced, making accurate recording of the true retruded contact position much more difficult.

2. IDEAL OCCLUSAL POSITION

The ideal occlusal position is a position of muscle balance—the position of the jaws during the unconscious swallow. Unfortunately, it is rather awkward to say to the patient, "Won't you please swallow unconsciously in order that I may record your jaw relationship?" The ideal occlusal position cannot be recorded as reliably as the retruded occlusal position; hence, it does not have practical use for precise restorative and prosthetic construction technics. The ideal occlusal position is not dependent on teeth as is the usual occlusal position, nor is it a bony relationship as is the retruded contact position; rather, it is a jaw relationship determined by a primitive reflex (see Chapter V, Section D). When there is a Class II malocclusion or a functional crossbite, the retruded contact position may be of less clinical usefulness than the ideal occlusal position. The ideal occlusal position is used for equilibration procedures in the primary and mixed dentitions (see Chapter XVII). It also is used for diagnosis of all functional malocclusions.

3. STEPS IN PROCEDURE

A length of beeswax or special jaw registration wax, ½ inch wide and approximately 5 inches in length, is rolled from each end and adapted across the palate and occlusal surfaces of the posterior teeth on the maxillary cast (Fig. XI-24, *B*). The rolled portion of the wax becomes an occlusal pad into which the mandibular teeth will bite; therefore, the rolled portion should be flattened and made parallel to the occlusal plane. The wax is removed and the portion directed toward the lower teeth on either side is softened. With the patient sitting upright in the chair and the Frankfurt plane parallel to the floor, the wax is reinserted into the mouth and the patient instructed to close his jaws gently until the teeth just feel the wax. The dentist must not guide, direct or touch the patient's jaws or give directions concerning biting or retruding. The patient is simply told to close the teeth gently until he first feels wax. The wax is then removed and a hot spatula is plunged into the impression made in the wax by the lower teeth (Fig. XI-24, *D*). The wax is reinserted and the procedure repeated, usually two or three times, until the jaw has been closed far enough to record the relationship but not so far as to perforate the wax (Fig. XI-24, *E*).

The wax insulates the teeth from those of the opposite arch, enabling one to record a late stage in the balanced path of closure (Fig. XI-24, *G*). The final wax bite record thus obtained may be kept with the casts as a part of the patient's permanent records (Fig. XI-24, *F*). It also may serve to show the direction and extent of functional malocclusions and those interfering teeth that need grinding during equilibration procedures in the primary and mixed dentition (see Chap. XVII).

F. Relationships of the Teeth to Their Skeletal Support

The appraisal of the buccolingual relationships of the teeth to alveolar processes and skeletal support usually is determined from the dental casts. The relationship of the dentition to the skeletal profile is best done in the cephalometric analysis or the Facial Form Analysis (see Chapter XII). However, the relationship of the incisors to their supporting structures also must be analyzed during function (see Chapter X). It is important when using casts for analysis, e.g., the Mixed Dentition Analysis or the diagnostic setup, to keep in mind the relationships of the teeth to their supporting bases and the skeletal profile. Sophisticated diagnosticians try to relate tooth positions on diagnostic casts to their positions in the cephalogram *after* treatment and growth.

REFERENCES

1. Barber, T.: Personal communication.
2. Bolton, W. A.: Disharmony in tooth size and its relation to the analysis and treatment of malocclusion, Angle Orthodont. 28:113, 1958.
3. Bolton, W. A.: The clinical application of a tooth-size analysis, Am. J. Orthodont. 48:504, 1962.
4. Clauss, W. J.: An Evaluation of Analyses of the Mixed Dentition. Thesis, Department of Orthodontics, The University of Michigan, Ann Arbor, 1955.
5. Fabric, F. A.: Clinical undergraduate orthodontic program, Washington Univ. Dent. J. 31:2, 1964.
6. Harvold, E. P., Truque, M., and Viloria, J. O.: Establishing the Median Plane in Postero-Anterior Cephalograms, in Salzmann, J. A. (ed.), *Roentgenographic Cephalometrics* (Philadelphia: J. B. Lippincott Company, 1961).
7. Howes, A. E.: Model analysis for treatment planning, Am. J. Orthodont. 38:183, 1952.
8. Howes, A. E.: Expansion as a treatment procedure—Where does it stand today?, Am. J. Orthodont. 46:515, 1960.
9. Howes, A. E.: A polygon portrayal of coronal and basal arch dimensions in the horizontal plane, Am. J. Orthodont. 40:811, 1954.
10. Huckaba, G. W.: Arch size analysis and tooth size prediction, Dent. Clin. North America, July, 1964, p. 431.
11. Moorrees, C. F. A., Fanning, E. A., and Hunt, E. E., Jr.: Age variation of formation stages for ten permanent teeth, J. Dent. Res. 42:1490, 1963.
12. Moorrees, C. F. A., and Reed, R. B.: Correlations among crown diameters of human teeth, Arch. Oral Biol. 9:685, 1964.
13. Moyers, R. E.: Unpublished data.
14. Nolla, C. M.: The development of the permanent teeth, J. Dent. Child. 27:254, 1960.
15. Shumaker, D. B., and El Hadary, M. S.: Roentgenographic study of eruption, J.A.D.A. 61:535, 1960.

XII

Analysis of the Craniofacial Skeleton

In collaboration with

W. STUART HUNTER, D.D.S., Ph.D.

Professor of Orthodontics, Faculty of Dentistry,
University of Western Ontario

The essence of wisdom is the ability to make the right decision on the basis of inadequate evidence.—ALAN GREGG

A. Purposes of the skeletal analysis
1. Classification of facial types
2. Study of the relationships of the parts of the face
3. Identification of skeletal contributions to malocclusion
4. Prediction of facial growth

B. Facial Form Analysis

C. Cephalometrics
1. History
2. Uses
   a) Study of craniofacial growth
   b) Diagnosis of craniofacial deformity
   c) Planning orthodontic treatment
   d) Evaluation of treated cases
3. Equipment and technics
   a) Cephalometric equipment
   b) Conventions in taking cephalograms
      1) The lateral projection
      2) The posteroanterior (PA) projection
      3) Oblique cephalograms
   c) Technics of tracing cephalograms
4. Cephalometric anatomy

5. Landmarks and planes of reference
    a) Cephalometric landmarks
        Anatomic landmarks
        Derived landmarks
        Posteroanterior landmarks
    b) Cephalometric planes
6. Cephalometric analyses
    a) Analysis for diagnosis
        1) Assessment of skeletal relationships
        2) Assessment of dentitional relationships
        3) Analysis of function
            The Downs Analysis
    b) Analysis for planning treatment
        The Steiner Analysis
    c) Analysis for prediction of growth
        The Ricketts Analysis
    d) Assessment of treatment results
    e) Evaluation of growth
        1) landmarks and points
        2) Planes and axes
7. Limitations of cephalometrics
    a) Errors in taking cephalograms
    b) Enlargement and distortion
    c) Tracing errors
    d) Misuse of the method
    e) Conceptual problems
8. The future of cephalometrics

SINCE THE OCCLUSAL RELATIONSHIPS of the teeth are determined primarily by the relationship of their bony supporting bases, it is necessary for those who would analyze occlusion to analyze the craniofacial skeleton. Slight disharmonies in maxillomandibular relationships can be compensated for by variations in tooth position or inclination. However, imbalances in maxillomandibular relationships to a degree beyond which dental compensation can be made result in malocclusion. Because osseous dysplasia accounts for such a large percentage of severe malocclusions, it is imperative that the bony facial skeleton be analyzed carefully before the treatment of many malocclusions.

Craniofacial skeletal analyses are of two types—visual and radiographic. Prior to the introduction of radiographic cephalometry, it was necessary to analyze the patient's head and face solely by visual inspection or by caliper measurements. Such procedures persist today largely as an important part of the cursory examination (see Chapter VIII). Radiographic cephalometry has literally revolutionized orthodontic diagnosis and treatment. Cephalometric procedures have become so useful that they are routine in the offices of many dentists treating significant numbers of malocclusions.

A. Purposes of the Skeletal Analysis

1. Classification of Facial Types

Similarly shaped faces are grouped together for ease in communication and thinking. Such groupings according to type usually are based on the profile (see Fig. IX-1). The orthognathic, retrognathic and prognathic profiles are closely related to the Angle classes of occlusion. The profile type is determined by the relative anteroposterior position of the most anterior points in the cranial base, nasomaxillary complex and mandible. Although satisfactory occlusions can be found in a wide variety of skeletal relationships, skeletal morphology dominates tooth inclinations and occlusal relationships. Some facial types are seen more frequently in some races than in others and there is a crude relationship between somatotype and craniofacial type.

Care must be taken in the clinical application of the concept of facial typing. Whether an individual patient deviates significantly from the mean for his own ethnic, sex and age group is not important clinically; what is important clinically is whether such deviations imply impairment of function or disturbed aesthetics.

Fig. XII-1.—Form and growth diagram.

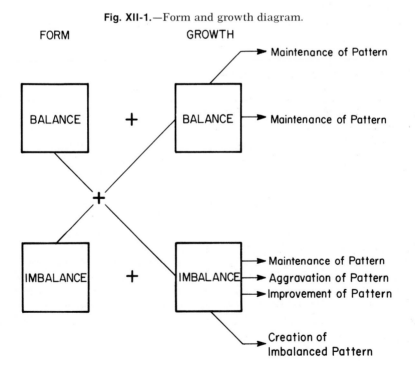

2. STUDY OF THE RELATIONSHIPS OF THE PARTS OF THE FACE

There is wide variability in the way that the facial components are put together, and the same profile type may be achieved in several varying fashions, for example, a long or protracted nasomaxillary complex, or a long or protracted cranial base, or combinations of these features. It is necessary when analyzing the facial skeleton to ascertain the relationships of the parts of the face to one another and their relative contributions to the facial type. Clinical analysis of the facial skeleton is an individualized matter; therefore, a mandible may be "long" with respect to the population but still be proportionately in balance within its own face.

3. IDENTIFICATION OF SKELETAL CONTRIBUTIONS TO MALOCCLUSION

In the craniofacial skeleton, a balanced form plus balanced growth maintains its pattern through time, but form or growth that is imbalanced likely will result in malocclusion. In Figure XII-1, the arrows represent real clinical situations. Note that treatment involves planned imbalanced growth to compensate for imbalanced form. It is essential to identify both the static skeletal contributions to malocclusion, as seen in the present form, and the anticipated dynamic contributions of growth.

4. PREDICTION OF FACIAL GROWTH

Analysis of form really is not enough to satisfy the discerning clinician, since form changes with time. For this reason, there has been an increased interest in recent years in the prediction of craniofacial growth. At this time, no reliable and generally adopted method of prediction has been presented, although a number of ingenious and promising methods are in use (see later Section, 6-c, p. 412).

B. Facial Form Analysis

The Facial Form Analysis is a procedure to provide a quick and systematic appraisal of the relationships of the various parts of the craniofacial skeleton and their contributions to occlusion. It is used as part of the cursory examination (see Chapter VIII, Section B) and when cephalograms are not available, but it is not a satisfactory substitute for cephalometric methods. The Facial Form Analysis is subjective and crude, yet useful for the purposes for which it is intended. A detailed description is given in Chapter VIII.

C. Cephalometrics

A cephalogram is a standardized radiograph of the head and face. The standardization usually is accomplished by means of a head holder or cephalostat (Fig. XII-2), which holds the subject's head in a fixed relationship to the central ray of the x-ray source so that the x-rays coincide with the transmeatal axis.

1. History

The first paper on radiographic cephalometrics probably was that by Pacini[12] in 1922, but credit for standardizing and popularizing the procedure goes to Broadbent,[2] whose classic paper in 1931 was received with excitement throughout orthodontics. At the same time, Hofrath[8] published in Germany, and Higley,[6] Margolis[10] and others were working with radiographic cephalometrics, although their initial papers came a bit later.

Fig. XII-2.—A typical cephalometric setup. At the top is the head positioner, at the lower right-hand corner is the x-ray tube. The distance between the x-ray target and the midsagittal plane of the head is exactly 5 feet. With this cephalostat, the child and the head positioner are rotated to obtain the P-A and oblique films. (Courtesy of The University of Michigan Facial Growth Study.)

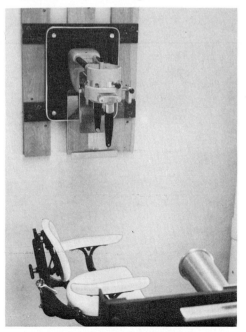

2. USES

The cephalometric technic has many uses, including the following.

a) *Study of Craniofacial Growth*

Because of the method's reliability, subjects may be examined repeatedly, permitting comparisons of the cephalograms. Serial cephalometric growth studies of both humans and animals have been a major factor in broadening our knowledge of craniofacial growth (see Chapter IV).

b) *Diagnosis of Craniofacial Deformity*

The first cephalometric studies revealed considerable variability in craniofacial form and suggested that osseous variability likely was a major contributing factor to malocclusion. Shortly thereafter, various "cephalometric analyses" were devised for identifying gross variations in the craniofacial pattern. The many cephalometric analyses subsequently introduced provide the most precise method available today for the diagnosis of craniofacial deformity, for they reveal the relationships of the various parts of the face and their contributions to the deformity.

c) *Planning Orthodontic Treatment*

Although cephalometric studies revealed that a normal occlusal relationship could obtain in a variety of skeletal forms, clinicians soon began to realize that some positions of teeth were more stable than others after treatment and that orthodontic treatment goals could be quantified by means of cephalometric geometry. Thus, cephalometric analyses evolved, permitting the orthodontist to plan, prior to treatment, the desired position for each tooth within a given patient's craniofacial skeleton.

d) *Evaluation of Treated Cases*

Cephalometric analyses of treated orthodontic cases have revealed much concerning the nature of orthodontic relapse and the stability of treated malocclusions.

3. EQUIPMENT AND TECHNICS

a) *Cephalometric Equipment*

Cephalometric equipment consists of a cephalostat or head holder, an x-ray source and a cassette holder. Head holders or cephalostats are of two types.

The Broadbent-Bolton method utilizes two x-ray sources and two film holders so that the subject need not be moved between the lateral and posteroanterior exposures. Although this method makes more precise three-dimensional studies possible, it requires two x-ray heads, more space and precludes obtaining oblique projections (see later).

The second method, originated by Higley, involves the use of one x-ray source and film holder and a cephalostat capable of rotating so that the patient may be repositioned for the various projections (see Fig. XII-2). This latter method is more versatile but there is less reliability, since the head's relationship to the cephalostat may alter slightly during repositioning. Almost all modern cephalostats, however, are of the rotating type.

The x-ray source must produce sufficiently high voltage (usually above 90 kvp) to penetrate the hard tissues well and to provide good delineation of both hard and soft structures. A small focal spot (frequently obtained by a rotating anode) results in sharper radiographic images.

The x-ray film is held within a cassette that usually also contains intensifying screens used to reduce the exposure significantly. A fixed or moving grid also may be used in conjunction with the cassette film holder to produce a sharper image. A grid resembles a Venetian blind, permitting only those rays coming directly from the source to proceed to the film. It thus absorbs the secondary radiation produced by deflections from the bones. Such secondary radiation tends to obscure the images, producing a fuzzy appearance of the bony shadows.

b) Conventions in Taking Cephalograms

1) THE LATERAL PROJECTION.—The midsagittal plane of the subject's head is placed 60 inches from the target of the x-ray tube with the left side of the subject toward the film. The central beam of the x-rays coincides with the transmeatal axis, that is, with the ear rods of the cephalostat. Under most circumstances, the distance from the midsagittal plane to the film is held constant, usually at 18 cm. However, in the Broadbent-Bolton Cephalometer, this distance is varied according to the subject and the exact distance recorded. Holding the midsagittal plane film distance constant makes compensation for enlargement easier. The head usually is placed so that the Frankfurt plane is parallel to the floor, although slight tilting of the head around the transmeatal axis does not affect the accuracy of the lateral cephalogram. The lateral projection generally is taken with the teeth together in their usual occlusal position, that is, centric occlusion (Fig. XII-3). It also may be taken with the mandible in its postural position, which may be achieved by exposing after a swallow or several repetitions of the word "Michigan" or the letter "M." If the ear rods are too large or too firmly placed in the external auditory meati, a false reading may be obtained, which is more troublesome in the lateral and oblique projections.

2) THE POSTEROANTERIOR (PA) PROJECTION.—The head is rotated 90

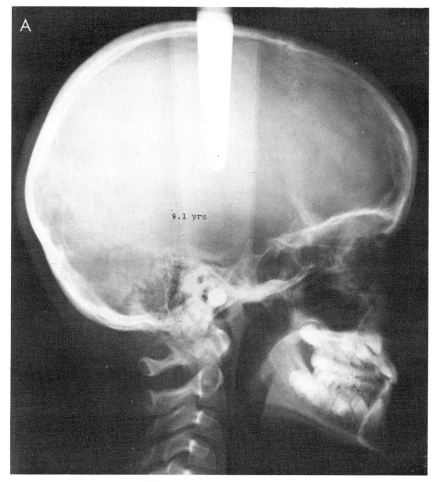

Fig. XII-3.—Typical lateral cephalogram.

degrees so that the central ray bisects the transmeatal axis (Fig. XII-4). It is very important when taking the PA cephalogram to maintain a standard horizontal relationship of the head, since, if the head is tilted, distortions occur and measurements of vertical distances are unreliable.

3) OBLIQUE CEPHALOGRAMS.—The right and left oblique cephalograms are taken at 45 degrees and 135 degrees to the lateral projection, the central ray entering behind one ramus in order to obviate superimposition of the halves of the mandible (Fig. XII-5). It is absolutely necessary that the subject be maintained on the Frankfurt plane for oblique cephalograms, since slight tipping introduces distortion and, hence, errors in measurement. The oblique cephalogram is very popular for analysis of patients in the mixed dentition.

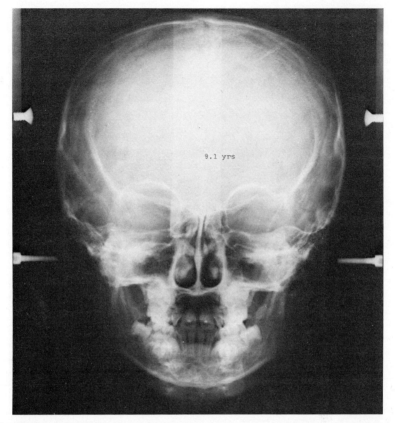

Fig. XII-4.—Posteroanterior cephalogram of the patient shown in Figure XII-3.

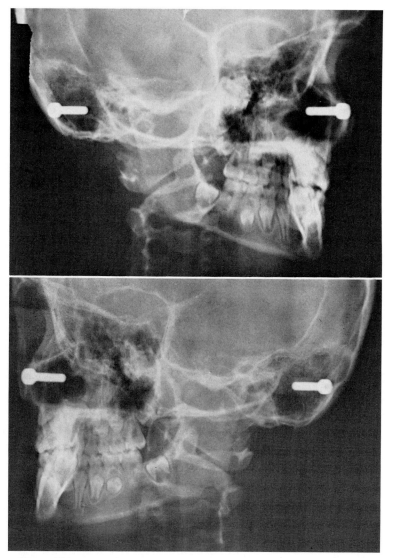

Fig. XII-5.—Oblique cephalogram of the patient shown in Figures XII-3 and XII-4.

c) Technics of Tracing Cephalograms

Most cephalometric analyses are made from tracings rather than directly from the cephalogram, permitting superpositioning of successive tracings for analysis of the effects of growth or orthodontic treatment. The cephalogram is taped to a tracing box or x-ray illuminator that has an even, well-diffused light source. Frosted acetate .003″ thick is taped to the top margin of the film, which permits lifting of the tracing from time to time for better inspection of the cephalogram. Tracings are best done in a darkened room, with all of the light box covered by black paper except that part occupied by the x-ray film. A hard pencil (4H) is used to maintain fine lines.

Tracing should be systematic. Begin with a general inspection of the cephalogram, locate and identify standard landmarks and then trace anatomic structures in a logical sequence. Finally, locate derived landmarks and planes. Although tracing cephalograms undoubtedly is an art, it must be emphasized that accurate cephalometric tracings cannot be obtained without a thorough knowledge of the underlying anatomy (see Section C-4, Cephalometric Anatomy). Although every anatomic structure will not need to be traced, all must be recognized and understood if the desired ones are to be located accurately. Usually, bilateral images are averaged, but many insist on drawing both the right and left shadows. Proper cephalometric tracings require a good cephalogram, a thorough understanding of cephalometric anatomy, meticulous care and artistic precision.

4. Cephalometric Anatomy

Figure XII-6 is a lateral cephalogram of a skull of a 9-year-old child on whom markers have been placed along the sagittal plane of the

Fig. XII-6.—Lateral cephalogram of a child's skull (see text). (From Enlow.[4])

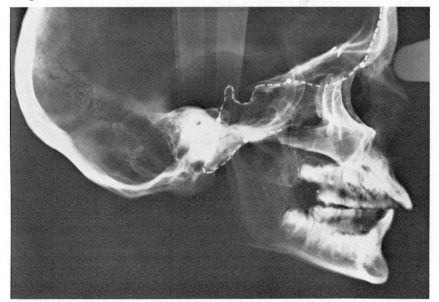

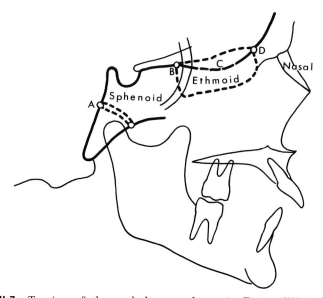

Fig. XII-7.—Tracing of the cephalogram shown in Figure XII-6. **A,** spheno-occipital synchondrosis. **B,** spheno-ethmoidal synchondrosis. **C,** cribriform plate. **D,** foramen cecum. The structures traced with dotted lines sometimes are not seen in the radiographs. (From Enlow.[4])

Fig. XII-8.—The sphenoid bone. **Left,** lateral projection: **A,** lesser wings; **B,** greater wings; **C,** pterygoid processes. **Right,** posteroanterior projection: **A,** lesser wings; **B,** greater wings; **C,** pterygoid processes; **D,** dorsum sella; **E,** the floor of the hypophyseal fossa; **F,** spheno-occipital synchondrosis. The greater wing at **G** is the floor of the middle cranial fossa and coincides with the orbital outline. (From Enlow.[4])

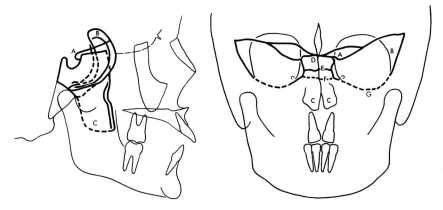

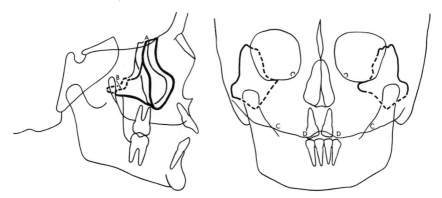

Fig. XII-9.—The zygomatic bones. **Left,** lateral projection: **A,** zygomatic frontal suture; **B,** zygomatic temporal suture. **Right,** posteroanterior projection: **C,** inferior surface of the occipital bone; **D,** occipital condyles. (From Enlow.[4])

cranial base and lead shot at the suture sites. In addition, the accessible surfaces of the zygomatic bones were covered with thin lead foil. Figure XII-7 is a tracing of the skull shown in Figure XII-6.

Sphenoid bone

Figure XII-8 shows in heavy outline those structures of the sphenoid bone seen most readily in the lateral and PA cephalogram.

Zygomatic bones

Figure XII-9 depicts the structures of the zygomatic bones ordinarily visualized in the lateral and PA cephalogram.

Fig. XII-10.—The maxillary bones. **Left,** lateral projection: **A,** frontomaxillary sutures; **B,** pterygomaxillary fissure. **Right,** posteroanterior projection: **A,** frontomaxillary sutures; **B,** palatal surface; **C,** alveolar process. (From Enlow.[4])

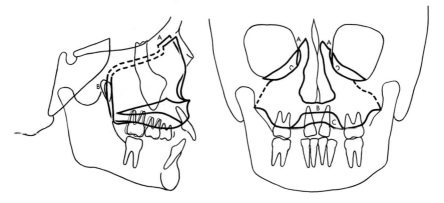

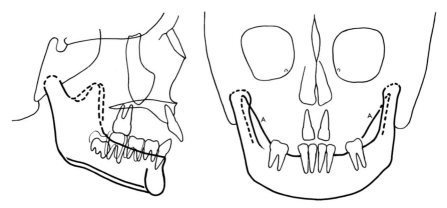

Fig. XII-11.—The mandible. **Left,** lateral projection. **Right,** posteroanterior projection showing the coronoid process, marked **A.** (From Enlow.[4])

Maxillae

Figure XII-10 shows the maxillary structures as visualized in the lateral and PA cephalogram.

Mandible

Figure XII-11 illustrates mandibular structures seen in the lateral and PA cephalogram.

5. LANDMARKS AND PLANES OF REFERENCE

a) Cephalometric Landmarks

A landmark is a point serving as a guide for measurement or the construction of planes. Ideally, a landmark should be located easily and reliably, have anatomic relevance and its behavior during growth should be consistent. Most cephalometric landmarks do not meet these specifications. Cephalometric landmarks frequently are used solely because of their ease in location or because of tradition. The landmarks listed are among those in most common use, although each individual analysis usually has certain landmarks singular to it. It should not be assumed that all landmarks are equally reliable and valid. The reliability of a landmark is affected by the quality of the cephalogram, the experience of the tracer and possible confusion with other anatomic shadows, whereas the validity of the landmark is determined largely by the way the landmark is used. Some of the most unreliable landmarks, unfortunately, are among the most popular, for example, "A" point, Orbitale, anterior nasal spine, posterior nasal spine and so forth.

Cephalometric landmarks are divided into two types: (1) anatomic and

(2) derived. Anatomic landmarks are those that represent actual anatomic structures of the skull. Derived landmarks are those that have been constructed or obtained secondarily from anatomic structures in a cephalogram. An example of the latter is the use of an intersect of two cephalometric planes as a landmark. In the following discussion, each landmark will be named, its usual cephalometric abbreviation given, its anatomic relationship defined and its location in the cephalogram explained. All references are made to Figure XII-12.

ANATOMIC LANDMARKS (Fig. XII-12, *A*)

Nasion (Na)

The junction of the frontonasal suture at the most posterior point on the curvature at the bridge of the nose.

Orbitale (Or)

The lowest point of the bony orbit. In the posteroanterior cephalogram, each may be identified; in the lateral cephalogram, the outlines of the orbital rims overlap. Usually, the lowest point on the averaged outline is used.

Anterior Nasal Spine (ANS)

The most anterior point on the maxilla at the level of the palate. Palatal plane is quite useful and precise for vertical measurements but ANS (the anterior landmark of palatal plane) is of little use for anteroposterior analyses, since the actual spine often cannot be seen and its location varies considerably according to the radiographic exposure.

Subspinale ("A" point)

The most posterior point on the curve between ANS and SPr (see below). "A" point usually is determined by a tangent to the bony curvature from Na. Superposition of cheek contours often is obfuscating. "A" point usually is found approximately 2 mm. anterior to the apices of the maxillary central incisor roots. "A" point is used only for anteroposterior measurements.

Superior Prosthion (SPr)

The most anterior inferior point on the maxillary alveolar process, usually found near the cemento-enamel junction of the maxillary central incisors. Superior Prosthion is analogous to Supradentale.

Infradentale (Id)

The most anterior superior point on the mandibular alveolar process, usually found near the cemento-enamel junction of the mandibular central incisors. Inferior Prosthion is analogous to Infradentale.

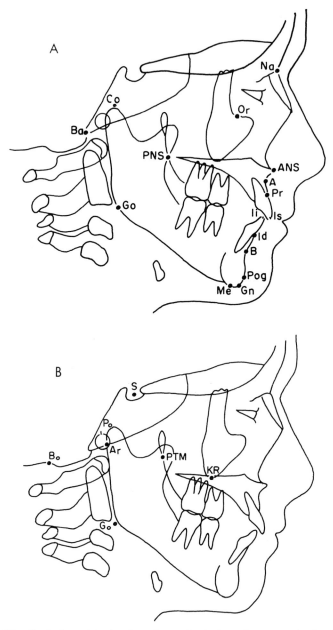

Fig. XII-12.—Cephalometric landmarks and planes. **A,** anatomic landmarks. **B,** some derived landmarks. (*Continued.*)

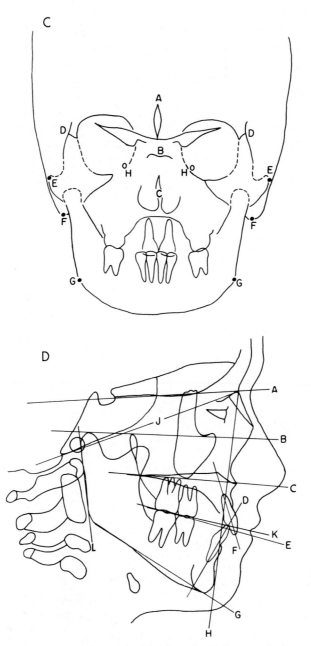

Fig. XII-12 (cont.).—C, posteroanterior landmarks. **D,** lines and planes. (See text for details and explanations.) (From Enlow.[4])

Incision Inferius (Ii)

The incisal tip of the most anterior mandibular incisor.

Incision Superius (Is)

The incisal tip of the most anterior maxillary incisor.

Supramentale ("B" point)

The most posterior point of the bony curvature of the mandible below Inferior Prosthion and above Pogonion (see below). The profile of the chin is not always concave and, in such instances, "B" point may be determined by locating a tangent to the region from Nasion. "B" point usually is found near the apical third of the roots of the mandibular incisors. The radiographic shadow often is obscured during eruption of these teeth, and referral to preceding and succeeding films is useful.

Pogonion (Pog)

The most anterior point on the contour of the chin. Pogonion usually is located by erecting a tangent perpendicular to the mandibular plane or by a tangent dropped to the chin from Nasion.

Gnathion (Gn)

The most anterior inferior point in the lateral shadow of the chin. Gnathion usually is best determined by selecting the midpoint between Pogonion and Menton on the contour of the chin.

Menton (Me)

The lowest point on the symphyseal outline of the chin. Menton usually is determined by using the mandibular plane as a tangent to the symphyseal curve.

Gonion (Go)

The most posterior inferior point at the angle of the mandible. It may be determined by inspection or derivation. The latter is done by bisecting the angle formed by the junction of the ramal and mandibular planes.

Condylion (Co)

The most posterior superior point on the condyle of the mandible. Condylion is used to measure mandibular length and ramus height.

Basion (Ba)

The most inferior posterior point in the sagittal plane on the anterior rim of the foramen magnum.

Posterior Nasal Spine (PNS)

The most posterior point on the bony hard palate in the sagittal plane. The inferior and superior surfaces of the hard palate converge; their point of meeting usually is used as Posterior Nasal Spine. As a determinant of palatal plane, PNS is reliable for vertical but not for anteropos-terior measurements.

DERIVED LANDMARKS (Fig. XII-12, *B*)

Sella (S)

The center of the hypophyseal fossa (sella turcica).
The following are bilateral landmarks. When both sides are visible, the midpoint between the two landmarks usually is used.

Articulare (Ar)

The intersection of the radiographic images of the inferior surface of cranial base and the posterior surfaces of the necks of the condyles of the mandible. Articulare is used as a substitute for Condylion when the latter is not clearly discernible.

Pterygomaxillary Fissure (PTM)

A bilateral teardrop-shaped area of radiolucency, the anterior shadow of which is the posterior surfaces of the tuberosities of the maxilla. The landmark itself is at the most anterior inferior confluences of the curvatures.

Porion (Po)

The top of the ear rods' shadow, the external auditory meati.

Key Ridge (KR)

The lowest point on the outline of the zygoma.

LANDMARKS SEEN IN THE POSTEROANTERIOR PROJECTION (Fig. XII-12, *C*)

Midline Structures

Crista galli. A vertically elongated diamond shape, to help establish the sagittal plane (*A*).
The floor of the hypophyseal fossa (*B*).
The septal structures of the nose (*C*).

Bilateral Structures

Frontozygomatic sutures. Seen as dark lines on a gray background (*D*).
Zygomatic processes. The lateral surfaces may usually be seen (*E*).
Mastoid processes (*F*). Gonial areas of the mandible (*G*).
Foramen rotunda. In medial inferior portion of orbital outlines (*H*).

b) *Cephalometric Planes* (Fig. XII-12, D)

Cephalometric planes are derived from at least two landmarks (pref-erably three or more). Such planes are used for measurements, separation of anatomic divisions, definition of anatomic structures or relating parts of the face to one another. The planes listed are those used most commonly; each analysis may have planes singular to it.

Sella-Nasion (A)

From Sella to Nasion.

Frankfurt (B)

In cephalometrics, Frankfurt plane is drawn from Porion to Orbitale.

Palatal (C)

From posterior nasal spine to anterior nasal spine.

Basion-Nasion (J)

From Basion to Nasion.

Occlusal (K, E)

There are two occlusal planes in common use:
Occlusal plane (Downs)—drawn from the midocclusal points of the first permanent molar to a point midway between the upper and lower central incisors, that is, one-half the incisal overlap or open bite (*E*).
Natural occlusal plane (or functional)—is a line averaging the points of posterior occlusal contact, usually the first permanent molar and primary molar or bicuspid region. It avoids incisor landmarks (*K*).

Mandibular (G)

Several mandibular planes are in use. The classic mandibular plane is simply a tangent to the lower borders of the mandible. The mandibular plane also may be drawn tangent to the posterior portion of the lower border of the mandible and to the symphyseal curve (Menton or Gnathion). Another method is to join Gonion and Menton.

Ramal (L)

Tangent to the posterior borders of the ramus and the condyles.

Facial (H)

Nasion to Pogonion.

6. CEPHALOMETRIC ANALYSES

Cephalometric analyses have been devised for (1) the diagnosis of abnormalities in craniofacial form or growth, (2) the planning of orthodontic treatment goals, (3) the prediction of craniofacial growth and (4) the assessment of results of orthodontic treatment. Most cephalometric analyses are static in concept; that is, the analysis concerns itself solely with the form of the subject at one time, with no attempt to determine the dynamic effects of future growth. Growth and orthodontic treatment bring about changes that make any cephalogram almost immediately out of date. There are, of course, great conceptual and technical difficulties in making quantified dynamic usage of a static two-dimensional image.

Cephalometric analyses are attempts by means of linear and geometric measurements to portray the form or growth of the face in a manner that more readily provides comparisons to known standards or idealized norms. Since the standard scores or norms used in cephalometric analyses have been derived in many different ways, it is essential to know the source and nature of the original data. In the following discussion, the basic concepts used in each of the four types of analyses will be discussed and one popular method, typical of each type, will be presented in summary.

a) Analysis for Diagnosis

Diagnostic analyses typically are divided into three sections: (1) assessment of skeletal relationships, (2) assessment of dentitional relationships and (3) analysis of function.

1) ASSESSMENT OF SKELETAL RELATIONSHIPS.—Some of the usual ways of assessing typical skeletal relationships are shown in Table XII-1.

2) ASSESSMENT OF DENTITIONAL RELATIONSHIPS.—Some method of evaluating the relationships of the dentition to the facial skeleton is included in each analysis (see Figs. XII-13–XII-15).

3) ANALYSIS OF FUNCTION.—The cephalometric technic has been used to study mandibular movements, palatal function during speech and assessment of the freeway space, but functional analysis in the cephalogram, although useful, has many limitations. The occlusal distance (freeway space) and the path of closure may be assessed by comparing lateral cephalograms taken in the postural and usual occlusal positions.

TABLE XII-1.—TYPICAL MEASUREMENTS OF
SKELETAL RELATIONSHIPS

RELATIONSHIP	TYPICAL MEASUREMENTS
Maxilla to cranium	SNA angle
	NA to FH angle
Mandible to cranium	SN-Pog angle
	Facial angle
	Mandibular plane angle
Maxilla to mandible	ANB angle
	AB angle
	Angle of convexity (Downs)
Direction of growth	"Y" axis angle
Vertical proportions	$\dfrac{\text{Upper face height}}{\text{Total face height}}$ ratio

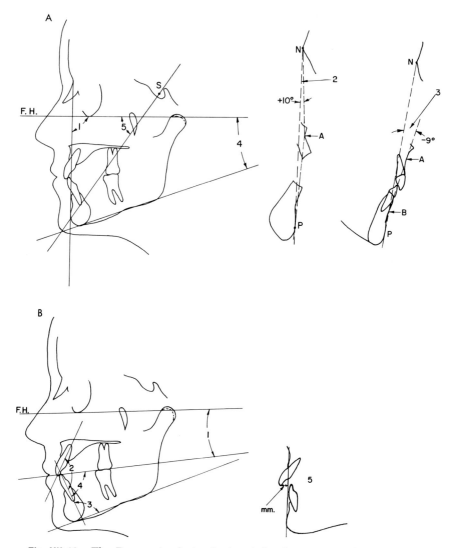

Fig. XII-13.—The Downs Analysis. **A,** the skeletal pattern. *1,* the facial angle formed by the intersection of the Frankfurt plane and a line joining Nasion and Pogonion. The inferior posterior angle is measured. It reflects mandibular protrusion or retrusion. *2,* the angle of convexity (Pogonion, Nasion, A point). If the angle PNA is formed ahead of the Nasion-Pogonion plane, the angle is read in positive degrees. If the angle is formed behind the Nasion-Pogonion plane, the angle is read in negative degrees. The angle of convexity is a measurement of maxillary prognathism. *3,* the A–B angle formed by the intersection of a line drawn through *A* and *B* points intersecting the Nasion-Pogonion line. The A–B angle is used to relate the denture bases to each other and to the skeletal profile. *4,* the Frankfurt mandibular plane angle. The relationship of the Frankfurt plane

TABLE XII-2.—Downs' Means

Skeletal	Mean	S.D.
Facial angle	88°	6°
Angle of convexity	0°	10°
A-B plane angle	−4.6°	4.5°
Mandibular plane angle	21.9°	6°
Y-axis	59°	7°

Dentition to Skeletal Pattern	Mean	S.D.
Cant of occlusal plane	9.3°	4°
$\underline{1}$ to $\bar{1}$ angle	135.4°	5.7°
$\bar{1}$ to occlusal plane	14.5°	3.5°
$+\bar{1}$ to mandibular plane	91.4°	3.8°
$\underline{1}$ to A-Pog plane	2.7 mm.	1.8 mm.

The Downs Analysis.—The first systematic cephalometric analysis was presented by Downs,[3] who selected 20 subjects between the ages of 12 and 17 years with "good occlusal relationships and good faces" and computed 9 angular measurements and 1 metric measurement that depicted the skeletal pattern and the relationship of the dentition to the skeletal pattern. Downs believed that although there was considerable variation in facial type and pattern, persons with good functional balance and aesthetics have "certain common profile characteristics." Since growing faces change in proportion as well as size, angular measurements have been used by Downs and others to depict "pattern" and minimize the effects of size increases. Figure XII-13 shows the measurements used in the Downs Analysis and Table XII-2 gives the mean and range values that Downs found for his small select group.

to a line tangential to the lower border of the mandible is a measurement of the relationship between anterior face height and posterior face height. 5, the Y axis measured as the anterior inferior angle where the Frankfurt horizontal plane is intersected by a line drawn from Sella to Gnathion. The Y axis is believed by some to be the direction of downward and forward facial growth. **B,** the relationship of the dentition to the skeletal pattern. *1,* the cant of the occlusal plane. The angle between the Frankfurt horizontal plane and the occlusal plane is measured. Downs measures the occlusal plane by bisecting the cusp height of the first molars and the incisor overbite. *2,* the interincisal angle. Lines drawn through the long axis of the maxillary and mandibular central incisors are intersected. The posterior angle is read. It is a measurement of the procumbency of the incisors. *3,* the incisor mandibular plane angle. A line representing the long axis of the mandibular incisor is intersected with the mandibular plane. The posterior superior angle is read. *4,* the mandibular incisor-occlusal plane angle. The posterior inferior angle is read and 90 degrees subtracted from it. *5,* the relationship of the maxillary incisor to the A–P line. The distance between the edge of the maxillary incisor and a line joining A point and Pogonion is measured.

b) *Analysis for Planning Treatment*

Some cephalometric analyses are designed primarily to give the clinician a clear geometric image of the individual patient and his deviations from an idealized treatment goal. In such analyses, the treatment goals admittedly are graphic and numerical representations of personal concepts and are not to be considered as population means. In clinical application, such analyses are used in three steps: First, the determination of the nature, extent and location of the dentofacial abnormality. Second, the depiction of the specified treatment goal for that particular patient. Third, the derivation of a plan of treatment.

The Steiner Analysis.—One of the most popular of the treatment-planning analyses is that devised by Steiner.[14] In addition to the skeletal measurements (Fig. XII-14), a number of dental measurements are made in the mandibular dental arch. These mandibular measurements are concerned primarily with the alignment and repositioning of teeth during treatment and the effects of such repositioning and anchorage

Fig. XII-14.—The Steiner Analysis. **A,** landmarks and average values. (*Continued.*)

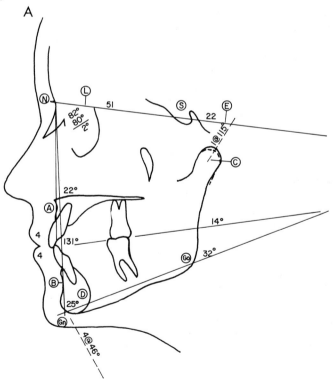

B

Name: _____ No.: _____ Age: _____ Sex: _____

CEPHALOMETRIC ANALYSIS
STEINER

		Ref. Norm.							
SNA	(angle)	82°							
SNB	(angle)	80°							
ANB	(angle)	2°							
SND	(angle)	76° or 77°							
1 to NA	(mm)	4							
1 to NA	(angle)	22°							
ī to NB	(mm)	4							
ī to NB	(angle)	25°							
Po to NB	(mm)	not established							
Po & ī to NB	(Difference)								
1 to ī	(angle)	131°							
Occl to SN	(angle)	14°							
GoGn to SN	(angle)	32°							
SL	(mm)	51							
SE	(mm)	22							
Arch length discrepancy									

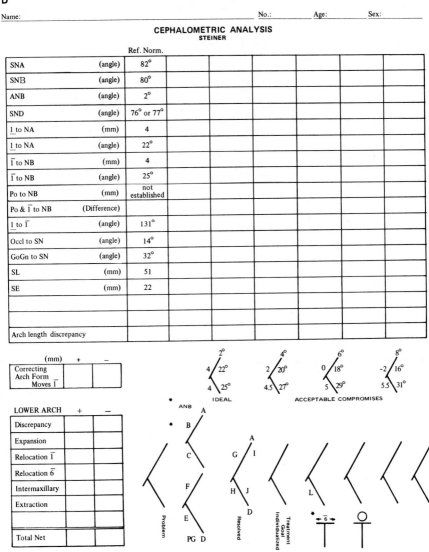

These estimates are useful as guides but they must be modified for individuals.

Fig. XII-14 (cont.).—B, the analysis sheet. For details of how to complete the bottom part of this form, see **C.** (*Continued.*)

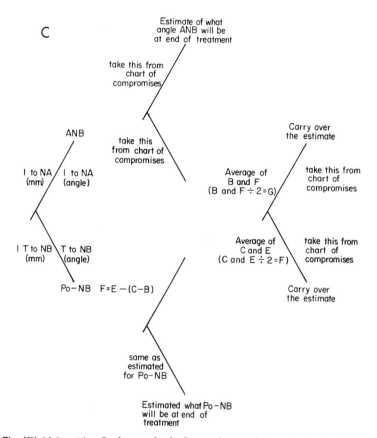

Fig. XII-14 (cont.).—C, the method of completing the analysis sheet (**B**).

loss on the arch perimeter. The dental measurements provide data on which a decision concerning extraction as a part of therapy can be made. Figure XII-14 shows the Steiner Analysis forms and indicates briefly how this analysis is done.

c) Analysis for Prediction of Growth

The problem of cephalometric analysis during orthodontic treatment is complicated by the fact that the patient will grow during treatment, thus making the original analysis obsolete, and that orthodontic treatment may affect not only the arrangement of the teeth but the directions, timing and amounts of skeletal growth as well. Accordingly, attempts have been made to make more dynamic use of the cephalometric analysis. Ricketts[13] analyzed a large number of treated cases and, on the

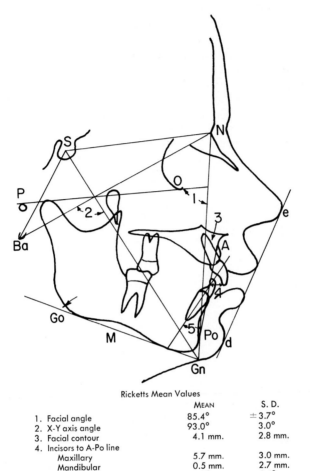

Ricketts Mean Values

	MEAN	S. D.
1. Facial angle	85.4°	± 3.7°
2. X-Y axis angle	93.0°	3.0°
3. Facial contour	4.1 mm.	2.8 mm.
4. Incisors to A-Po line		
Maxillary	5.7 mm.	3.0 mm.
Mandibular	0.5 mm.	2.7 mm.
5. Mandibular incisor to A-Po line	20.5°	6.4°

Fig. XII-15.—The Ricketts Analysis. *1*, facial angle (Downs). *2*, X–Y axis angle measured as the posterior inferior angle formed by the intersection of the Sella-Gnathion line and the Nasion-Basion line. *3*, measurement of facial contour. The distance from A point to the Nasion-Pogonion line. Each millimeter of distance is equal to about 2 degrees of convexity as measured by Downs' angle of convexity. *4*, incisor tips to the A point-Pogonion line. The A point-Pogonion line is used as a measurement of the relationship of the denture to the facial skeletal profile. *5*, the angle of the lower incisor to the A point-Pogonion plane.

basis of growth during and response to treatment, he devised an interesting method of growth prediction (see later). The Ricketts Analysis is based on the assumption that the individual patient under treatment will respond in the same manner with respect to direction and amount of growth as the mean of Ricketts' sample. It is too much to hope that this assumption will be true in every case; however, the method is very popular, since it enables the clinician to think easily of the changes in the facial pattern wrought by growth and treatment. Having more clearly defined his treatment goals, the clinician is in a better position to achieve them, and thus his skill frequently aids in making the analysis come true.

Others, for example, Johnston[9] and Balbach,[1] have attempted prediction of craniofacial growth by regression methods, whereas Hirschfeld[7] and Moyers and Hirschfeld[11] have suggested the use of time series analysis, a method of prediction based solely on values derived from the individual patient with no reference to population.

The Ricketts Analysis.—Figure XII-15 depicts the Ricketts Analysis used for growth estimation.

Fig. XII-16.—Superpositioning in the cranial base to assess the over-all effects of growth and treatment on the craniofacial pattern.

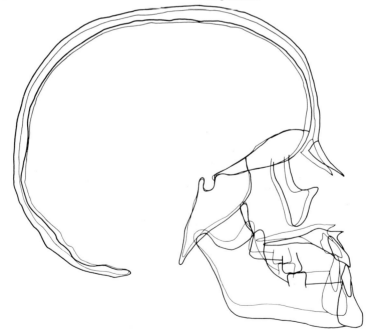

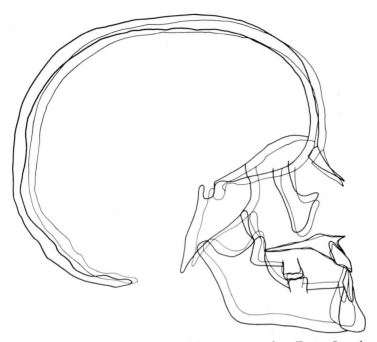

Fig. XII-17.—Superpositioning in the palate to assess the effects of tooth movements in the maxillary region.

d) Assessment of Treatment Results

The combined effects of orthodontic treatment and growth usually are appraised by superpositioning before and after tracings on some cranial base orientation (Fig. XII-16). Maxillary growth and dentitional changes during therapy may be separated by superpositioning on the palatal plane and registering at the superior portion of the palatal curvature behind the maxillary alveolar process (Fig. XII-17). Mandibular growth and dentitional changes may be separated by superpositioning on the mandibular canal and registering on the lingual aspect of the mandibular symphysis (Fig. XII-18).

e) Evaluation of Growth

Although several of the analyses described earlier have been used to study growth, the *Analysis of Growth Equivalents* (see page 422) was designed specifically for the evaluation of growth (Fig. XII-19). The landmarks and planes in this analysis were chosen specifically for their biologic significance. The analysis is based on the concept that the parts

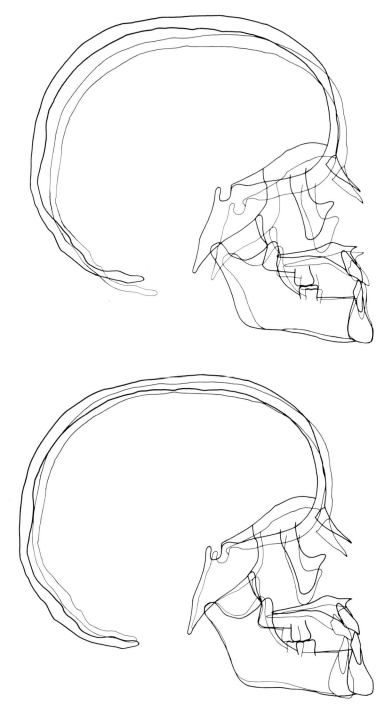

Fig. XII-18.—Superpositioning in the mandible to assess the effects of mandibular tooth movements and growth.

of the face are so interrelated that change in one region will produce "equivalent" change in corresponding areas elsewhere. The form is analyzed by comparing "equivalent" (not necessarily the anatomic) bony measurements. The effects of growth are studied by comparing growth equivalents to ascertain whether growth is aggravating, maintaining or correcting the original dysplasia (see Fig. XII-1).

Most of the traditional cephalometric landmarks and planes are not appropriate or usable in this analysis, since the procedure is based on an evaluation of *effective* dimensions between specific anatomic *equivalents* of structure. Therefore, a simple series of planes has been defined that serves to delineate these particular equivalent dimensions. In most instances, the entire dimensions of the bones are not involved, since the planes themselves are constructed in such a way that only the effective dimensions of each bone are utilized.

1) LANDMARKS AND POINTS.—The landmarks used are bilateral, but it is recommended they be averaged consistently (Fig. XII-19, *A*).

SE point (sphenoethmoidal): The intersection of the great wing of the sphenoid and the cranial floor as seen in lateral head films. The purpose is to represent the sphenoethmoidal junction, which is located slightly posterior to this intersection. The sphenoethmoidal junction separates that part of the cranial floor associated with the maxilla from the portion associated with the ramus and postmaxillary pharynx. Note that the posterior surface of the maxillary tuberosity characteristically aligns with this juncture. This anatomic feature is utilized as a key relationship for the construction of the basic horizontal and vertical planes drawn on the head film tracings.

FMS point (frontomaxillary suture): The superior-most point of the suture at its articulation with the nasal and frontal bones. The purpose is to identify a relevant point for determining the effective vertical height of the anterior nasomaxillary complex. Use the posterior corner of the suture for consistency.

Co (condylion): The most posterior-superior point on the mandibular condyle. This point is used to establish the effective horizontal and vertical dimensions of both the ramus and the cranial floor.

"A" point (subspinale): The most posterior point on the anterior shadow of the maxilla above the central incisor. "A" point is used to determine the basal length of the maxillary bony arch.

"B" point (supramentale): The most posterior point on the anterior surface of the symphyseal outline. "B" point is used to measure the basal length of the mandibular corpus exclusive of the alveolar process and mental protuberance.

SPr point (superior prosthion; supradentale): The point of contact between the alveolar margin and the two central maxillary incisors.

IPr point (inferior prosthion; infradentale): The point of contact between the alveolar process and the two central incisors of the mandible.

"X" point: The intersection of the PM vertical plane and the *neutral* occlusal axis (see below). "X" point is used to establish the over-all

effective height of the posterior nasomaxillary complex. It also is utilized to determine the direction and the extent of any occlusal rotation present.

LT point (lingual tuberosity): A point that represents, in the mandible, an equivalent of the posterior surface of the maxillary tuberosity (as identified by PTM). LT point is used to determine the horizontal dimensions of both the corpus and the ramus. It is located by determining the horizontal dimension of the ramus from its anterior to posterior margins along the *functional occlusal plane* (see below). This same dimension is then extended anteriorly from the intersection of the occlusal plane and the Ra vertical lines (dividers may be used for this purpose). The resulting point is the location of the lingual tuberosity.

Since LT cannot be visualized in head films, its location must be approximated as described above. The ramus and the corpus characteristically overlap, so that the ramus extends anteriorly for a distance well beyond the posterior limit of the corpus (the lingual tuberosity). However, the ramus is obliquely disposed, and the distance of ramus-corpus overlap is offset and approximately equaled by the distance from the posterior edge of the ramus to the Ra vertical plane (see below).

SO point (derived): The point of intersection of SO vertical and SO horizontal planes.

2) PLANES AND AXES (Fig. XII-19, *A*)

PM vertical (posterior nasomaxilla): A line drawn inferiorly from SE point along the posterior surface of the maxillary tuberosity. For serial consistency, the line is regularly passed through the inferior and posterior-most point of PTM. The PM vertical plane is used to determine the vertical dimension of the posterior nasomaxillary complex, and it also serves to delineate the effective horizontal dimensions of the maxillary body and the cranial floor posterior to it. This important plane *should be the first construction line placed on the tracing, since most of the other planes and lines are then drawn either perpendicular or parallel to it.*

UM horizontal (upper maxilla): A perpendicular to PM vertical extending anteriorly from SE point.

AM vertical (anterior nasomaxilla): A line drawn inferiorly from FMS point parallel to PM vertical. The measurement from the intersection of this line with the UM horizontal line down to the functional occlusal plane (see below) represents the effective (not over-all) height of the anterior maxilla.

SO horizontal (spheno-occipital): A perpendicular to PM vertical extending posteriorly from SE point to the intersection with SO vertical. This defines the effective horizontal dimension of the cranial base relative to its equivalent, the ramus.

SO vertical: A perpendicular from SO horizontal (parallel with PM vertical) extending inferiorly from SO point to condylion. This is the effective (not over-all) height of the cranial floor.

Ra vertical (ramus): An inferior extension of the SO vertical line from condylion down to the functional and neutral occlusal planes.

This identifies the effective (not over-all) height of the ramus relative to the vertical dimensions of the maxilla.

Neutral occlusal axis (NOA): A perpendicular from PM vertical extending anteriorly through the posterior and inferior-most maxillary molar contact point. Only a fully erupted molar is used. If the last molar, although erupted, is situated higher than the occlusal plane common to the other maxillary molars and premolars, *the next-to-last molar should be used.* The purpose of this plane is to establish the *maximum* effective height of the posterior portion of the nasomaxillary complex.

Functional occlusal plane (FOP): A line drawn anteriorly from the inferior, posterior-most maxillary-mandibular contact point (as explained above) to the maxillary-mandibular contact point of the tooth situated on the AM vertical line. The incisors are not considered in the construction of this line, and it therefore is not the occlusal plane customarily defined (Downs). It will be found that the "functional" and the "neutral" occlusal lines coincide in many faces that have balanced dimensional equivalents. If some vertical imbalance exists, however, either an upward or a downward rotation results, and the functional and neutral planes will diverge.

Maxillary and mandibular contact planes: If a vertical dimensional imbalance has produced occlusal rotation, either up or down, so that the functional plane not only diverges from the neutral occlusal axis but the maxillary contact plane also diverges from the mandibular contact plane, it is then necessary to identify them separately. A line is drawn from their posterior-most contact point(s) to the contact points (not cusp tips) of corresponding teeth that would be situated on the AM vertical line if occlusion were closed. These lines are then extended back to the Ra vertical line in order to calculate the extent of their respective divergence relative to the ramus.

D. Outline of Procedure

1) FORM ANALYSIS

The different measurements described below are shown in Figure XII-19, *B* and correspond to the blanks in the form analysis data sheet (Fig. XII-19, *C*) used in the following section so that the reader can refer from one to the other. Thus, a measurement for the value "A-1," as described below, is entered in the space designated A-1 in the form analysis data sheet.

A. Vertical

1. *Posterior maxilla (PM vertical).* Measure from SE point to "X" point.
2. *Anterior maxilla (AM vertical).* Measure from the *intersection* of the AM and UM lines inferiorly to the functional occlusal plane. If open bite occurs at the premolars, the maxillary contact line is to be used, since a functional occlusal plane here does not exist as such. This measurement represents the effective (not total) dimension of the anterior nasomaxillary complex. If any cranial floor axis rotation has occurred, it will change the dimension

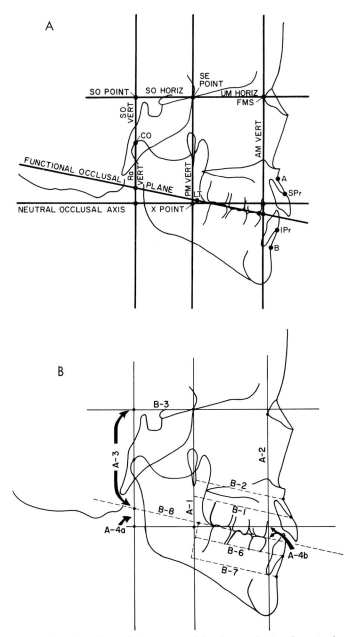

Fig. XII-19.—A, landmarks and planes used in the analysis of equivalents (see text for details and explanations). **B,** measurements used in the analysis of equivalents. The letters and numbers, e.g., *A-1,* refer to the forms used in recording the measurements (**C** and **D**). (*Continued.*)

C

Name_____ Date _____

FORM ANALYSIS

A. VERTICAL

1. Posterior Maxilla (PM Vertical) _____
2. Anterior Maxilla (AM - UM Intersection to Functional Occlusal Plane) _____
3. Composite Ramus - Cranial Floor (Ra - SO Verticals)
   a. Cranial floor (SO - vertical) if desired _____
   b. Ramus (Ra - vertical) if desired _____
4. Functional Occlusal Plane Divergence from Neutral Axis
   a. Measured at Ra vertical _____
   b. Measured at AM vertical _____
5. Mandibular - Maxillary Contact Plane Divergence from Each Other (if Premolar Open Bite Exists) _____
6. Maxillary - Mandibular Incisor Relationships _____
7. Commentary on Vertical Balance: _____

B. HORIZONTAL

1. Nasomaxilla (SPr to PM Vertical) _____
2. Nasomaxilla (A Point to PM Vertical) _____
3. Cranial Floor (SO Horizontal) _____
4. Total (1 + 3) _____
5. Total (2 + 3) _____
6. Mandibular Corpus (IPr to LT) _____
7. Mandibular Corpus (B Point to LT) _____
8. Ramus (LT to Ra Vertical) _____
9. Total (6 + 8) _____
10. Total (7 + 8) _____
11. Commentary on Horizontal Balance: _____

D

Name_____

	date	date	date

GROWTH ANALYSIS

A. VERTICAL

1. Posterior Maxilla (PM Vertical)

	age	age	age

2. Anterior Maxilla (AM - UM Intersection to Functional Occlusal Plane) ___ ___ ___
3. Composite Ramus - Cranial Floor (Ra - SO Verticals)
   a. Cranial Floor (SO Vertical) if desired ___ ___ ___
   b. Ramus (Ra vertical) if desired ___ ___ ___
4. Commentary on Vertical Incremental Balance Relative to Dimensional Balance at the Two Ages: ___ ___ ___

B. HORIZONTAL

1. Nasomaxilla (SPr to PM Vertical) ___ ___ ___
2. Nasomaxilla (A Point to PM Vertical) ___ ___ ___
3. Cranial Floor (SO Horizontal) ___ ___ ___
4. Total (1 + 3) ___ ___ ___
5. Total (2 + 3) ___ ___ ___
6. Mandibular Corpus (IPr to LT) ___ ___ ___
7. Mandibular Corpus (B Point to LT) ___ ___ ___
8. Ramus (LT to Ra Vertical) ___ ___ ___
9. Total (6 + 8) ___ ___ ___
10. Total (6 + 8) ___ ___ ___
11. Commentary on Horizontal Incremental Balance Relative to Dimensional Balance at the Two Ages: ___ ___ ___

Fig. XII-19 (cont.).—C, form analysis. **D,** growth analysis.

above the UM-AM intersection point. However, the dimension as measured below this point also incorporates any influence of rotation on this effective vertical dimension.

3. *Composite ramus-cranial floor (SO and Ra verticals).* Measure from SO point inferiorly to the intersection of the Ra vertical plane and the *functional* occlusal plane. If open bite occurs, measure to the *mandibular* contact line.

4. *Functional occlusal plane divergence.* If the functional and neutral occlusal lines do not coincide, measure the distance between them where they each intersect (a) the Ra vertical line and (b) the AM vertical line.

5. *Maxillary-mandibular contact divergence.* If open bite exists, measure from the maxillary to the mandibular contact line along the Ra vertical plane. This is the actual extent of imbalance between them relative to the ramus. The distance of either from the neutral occlusal axis indicates the extent of imbalance, relative to this ideal plane, that has produced the degree of rotation observed.

6. *Incisor relationships.* If occlusal rotation has occurred, note whether the maxillary incisor meets or bypasses the functional occlusal plane to provide a 3 or 4 mm. overlap with the mandibular incisor. If it does not, would simple lingual tipping alone be sufficient to place it in functional occlusion? Have the mandibular incisors bypassed the functional occlusal plane? Enter comments on the data sheet concerning the necessary incisor positioning.

7. Compare and evaluate the measured values for 1, 2, and 3 above. If they

match, the functional and neutral occlusal planes exactly coincide and these vertical dimensions (equivalents) are thus in balance with each other. If a dimensional imbalance exists, either an upward or (more commonly) a downward occlusal rotation has occurred. The extent of this imbalance is indicated by 4 above. If occlusal rotation has taken place in a uniform manner, open bite is not present. If a differential exists between them, however, the actual extent of maxillary-mandibular divergence is indicated by 5 above. Summarize the evaluation on the data sheet.

B. Horizontal

1. *Nasomaxilla (at SPr)*. Measure from SPr to the PM vertical line parallel to the *functional* occlusal plane (or neutral occlusal axis if they both coincide, or to the maxillary contact plane if premolar open bite exists).
2. *Nasomaxilla (at "A" point)*. Measure from "A" point to the PM vertical line parallel to the appropriate occlusal line.
3. *Cranial floor (SO horizontal)*. Measure from SO point to FMS point.
4. *Total* the values for 1 and 3 above. Record.
5. Total the values for 2 and 3 above. Record.
6. *Mandibular corpus (at IPr)*. Measure from IPr to LT point parallel to the *functional* occlusal plane (or to the neutral occlusal axis if they both coincide, or the mandibular contact line if premolar open bite occurs).
7. *Mandibular corpus (at "B" point)*. Measure from "B" point to LT point parallel to the appropriate occlusal plane. Record.
8. *Ramus*. Measure from LT point to the *Ra vertical line* along the appropriate occlusal line.
9. *Total* the values for 6 and 8 above.
10. Total the values for 7 and 8 above.
11. Compare and evaluate the measured values: 1 with 6; 2 with 7; 3 with 8; 4 with 9; and 5 with 10. If a significant dimensional imbalance occurs between any two of the *individual* equivalents, does a reciprocal imbalance occur between the others that offsets the effect of imbalance and "adjusts" their *aggregate* dimensions? If not, analyze the nature of the imbalances present to ascertain *which* equivalents mismatch. Relate this to the nature of any skeletal problems, malocclusion, overbite, etc., that occur as a consequence. Note: *maxillary length, either as an individual or as an aggregate measurement, may exceed mandibular length in an approximate 0 to 3 mm. normal range.* Within this range, dimensions may be regarded as "balanced." Summarize evaluation on the data sheet.

2) GROWTH ANALYSIS

Vertical. The increments of growth are determined by subtracting the measured values for the various dimensions at the younger age from those at the older age. The itemization on the growth data sheet (Fig. XII-19, *D*) corresponds to that on the form data sheet (Fig. XII-19, *C*).

Analyze the meaning and significance of the different growth increments relative to the status of *dimensional* balance at the ages involved. If balance of form originally occurred, did the growth increments maintain this balance? If a dimensional imbalance existed at the younger age, did the increments of growth (a) improve them, (b) sustain them without material change or (c) aggravate them?

Horizontal. Calculate the increments of growth from the previously measured values at the two age levels involved. Enter these values in the data form. Analyze and evaluate the balance of growth relative to the particular nature of the dimensions at these ages. Determine if (a) increments maintained an original balanced facial form, (b) sustained an imbalanced form, (c) improved an imbalanced form or (d) aggravated an imbalanced form. Does *aggregate balance* of the growth increments between the different sets of equivalents serve to compensate for any deficiency or excess in some individual dimension?

E. Analysis of the Effects of Treatment

A. To study the over-all effects of growth plus treatment,
  —orient on PM plane and register at SE point.
B. To separate growth from treatment in the midface region,
  —orient on PM and register at the posterior portion of
  the palatal diploë.
C. To visualize mandibular growth alone,
  —orient on condyle, registering on condylion;
  —orient on mandibular canal registering on anterior
  margin of the cortical plate forming the posterior
  portion of the symphysis.
D. To visualize mandibular rotation alone,
  —orient on PM and register at condylion.
E. To visualize the effects of mandibular growth on occlusal
  relationships,
  —orient on PM and register at the PM-NOA intersection
  ("X" point).
F. To visualize the effects of vertical growth on the occlusal
  relationships,
  —orient on NOA, holding the 2 PMs parallel, sliding the
  tracings until the "B" points are above one another. One
  now may orient on the inferior mandibular outline to study
  mandibular alveolar growth and occlusal plane changes
  or the palatal outline to study maxillary alveolar
  vertical changes.
G. To visualize changes in direction of condylar growth, i.e.,
  mandibular rotation,
  —orient on mandibular canal and symphysis as in C.
H. To visualize cranial base rotations under treatment,
  —orient on PM and register on PTM.

7. LIMITATIONS OF CEPHALOMETRICS

There are limitations inherent in cephalometrics. Even though the method is popular and useful, one may be handicapped if he is not aware of the possible sources of error.

a) *Errors in Taking Cephalograms*

Errors in this category include improper positioning of the patient, inadequate radiographic exposure, inconsistent or unrecorded mid-sagittal plane-film distance, etc. Such errors are largely controllable by proper technics.

b) *Enlargement and Distortion*

The greater the distance between the x-ray target and the film the more nearly parallel are the x-rays and the less the distortion and magnification. The closer the film is to the object being radiographed the less the enlargement. When a three-dimensional, highly irregular object such as the face is radiographed, there always will be enlargement and distortion. The cephalometric technic attempts to minimize and standardize these factors even though they are always present.

c) *Tracing Errors*

Tracing errors are due to lack of technical skill, improper cephalometric exposure or inadequate knowledge of the anatomic parts. Although tracing is as much an art as it is a science, there is no substitute for knowledge and experience.

d) *Misuse of the Method*

Perhaps the most significant limitation is simply misuse of the method. When one presumes to reduce a three-dimensional biologic entity as complicated as the human face to a two-dimensional geometric figure as simple as a triangle, and then attempts to interpret accurately all of the changes taking place during growth and treatment, the possibilities for misuse of the method are made apparent.

e) *Conceptual Problems*

Misconceptions concerning the nature of craniofacial growth are not corrected by careful cephalometric technics. Although the condyle of the mandible is growing upward and backward with an accompanying displacement of the mandible in a downward and forward direction, the gnathion often is said to be "growing downward and forward." Such loose statements may be semantic in origin or may be due to complete misconceptions concerning the nature of craniofacial growth. If the cephalometrist is to be more than a mere technician, it is necessary that he have a firm grasp of the essentials of craniofacial growth before attempting cephalometric analyses.

8. The Future of Cephalometrics

Many believe that the well of conventional static cephalometrics has run dry. Therefore, the future may bring use of the method in a more individualized and dynamic fashion. Attempts to predict precisely the amount, direction, timing and velocity of growth for the individual patient certainly are to be expected. Also, we may see the method used more exhaustively for genetic studies of craniofacial growth. The concept of form and growth equivalent measurements likely will be used in racial studies, prediction and the separation of various clinical types. Hopefully, in the future there will be less simplistic geometry and more applied biology.

REFERENCES

1. Balbach, D. R.: The cephalometric relationship between the morphology of the mandible and its future occlusal position, Angle Orthodont. 39:29, 1969.
2. Broadbent, B. H.: A new x-ray technique and its application to orthodontia, Angle Orthodont. 1:45, 1931.
3. Downs, W. B.: Variations in facial relationships: Their significance in treatment and prognosis, Am. J. Orthodont. 34:812, 1948.
4. Enlow, D. H.: *The Human Face* (New York: Hoeber Medical Division, Harper & Row, Publishers, 1968).
5. Enlow, D. H., Moyers, R. E., Hunter, W. S., and McNamara, J. A., Jr.: A procedure for the analysis of intrinsic facial form and growth. An equivalent balance concept, Am. J. Orthodont. 56(1):6, 1969.
6. Higley, L. B.: A new and scientific method of producing temporomandibular articulation radiograms, Internat. J. Orthodont. & Oral Surg. 22:983, 1936.
7. Hirschfeld, W. J.: The application of time series and exponential smoothing methods to the analysis and prediction of growth, Growth 34:129, 1970.
8. Hofrath, H.: Die Bedeutung der Röntgenfern- und Abstandsaufnahme für die Diagnostik der Kieferanomalien, Fortschr. Orthodont. 1:232, 1931.
9. Johnston, L., Jr.: A statistical evaluation of cephalometric prediction, Angle Orthodont. 38:284, 1968.
10. Margolis, H. I.: Standardized x-ray cephalographics, Am. J. Orthodont. 27:725, 1940.
11. Moyers, R. E., and Hirschfeld, W. J.: Prediction of craniofacial growth: The state of the art, Am. J. Orthodont. 60:435, 1971.
12. Pacini, A. J.: Roentgen ray anthropometry of the skull, J. Radiol. 42:230, 322 and 418, 1922.
13. Ricketts, R. M.: Cephalometric analysis and synthesis, Angle Orthodont. 31:141, 1961.
14. Steiner, C.: Cephalometrics as a Clinical Tool, in Kraus, B. S., and Riedel, R. A. (eds.), *Vistas in Orthodontics* (Philadelphia: Lea & Febiger, 1962).

XIII

Biomechanics
of Tooth Movements

> Every body continues in its state of rest, or of uniform
> motion in a right line, unless it is compelled to change that
> state by forces impressed upon it.—SIR ISAAC NEWTON,
> *Philosophiae Naturalis Principia Mathematica.* Laws of
> Motion I.

A. Essentials of theoretical mechanics (as related to tooth movements)

B. Biologic reactions to orthodontic forces

  1. Periodontal drift and physiologic tooth movements

  2. Factors in tooth movement

    a) Manner of force application

      1) Continuous forces

      2) Dissipating forces (Reitan's interrupted type)

      3) Intermittent forces

      4) Functional forces

    b) Amount of force application

    c) Duration of force application

    d) Direction of force application

      1) Tipping

      2) Translation

      3) Rotation

      4) Intrusion

      5) Extrusion

      6) Torque

    e) Occlusal function

    f) Age

  3. Tissue response

    a) Initial reaction

    b) Secondary response

    c) Root resorption

C. Design of appliances for tooth movements

  1. Methods of delivering force

  2. Selection and control of orthodontic forces

  3. Optimal orthodontic forces

A CLINICIAN'S ABILITY to perform satisfactory tooth movements depends on his understanding of (a) theoretical mechanics, (b) oral tissue response to force application and (c) clinical observations based on an accumulated knowledge of biomechanics.[1, 4] Orthodontic appliances theoretically are designed to produce a force that will elicit the optimal tissue response within the periodontal ligament and bone.[4] However, mathematical models of forces and histologic demonstrations of cellular changes must all be monitored by clinical experience, since not all the pertinent variables of tooth movement are as yet sufficiently known to permit routine control in orthodontic practice.

A. Essentials of Theoretical Mechanics (As Related to Tooth Movements)

Mechanics is the science dealing with the action of forces on the form and motion of bodies. In this instance, the bodies are the teeth, the periodontal ligaments and the bones. The forces are those delivered by orthodontic appliances or by muscle contractions against the teeth or through intercuspation of the teeth. Any orthodontic appliance is a force system storing and delivering forces against the teeth, muscles or bone and creating a reaction within the periodontal ligament and alveolar bone that permits movements of the teeth.[4] Therefore, if tooth movements are to be understood, the theoretical mechanics of the orthodontic force system must be understood.

A few definitions should be recalled.

A *force* is the action of one body on another—a push or a pull. A force has magnitude, direction and a point of application. The effect of a force on a rigid free body is independent of the point of force application on a given line of action (Fig. XIII-1).

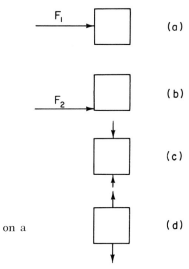

Fig. XIII-1.—The effect of force on a rigid free body.

Strain is a change in form or size of a body as it responds to an applied force[9] (Fig. XIII-2). A coil spring undergoes strain as it is stretched; a wire strains as it is bent.

Stress is the internal molecular resistance to the deforming action of external forces. Stress is equivalent, in rigid bodies, to the strength of the body.

If a force is applied to a free body on its center of mass, *translation* will occur (Fig. XIII-3). The greater the force applied to a free body the greater the translation. If a force is applied away from a center of mass, the body will move exactly the same distance it would if the force were

Fig. XIII-2 (left).—Strain. C = areas of compression; T = tension.[9]
Fig. XIII-3(right).—Translation.

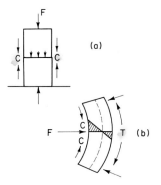

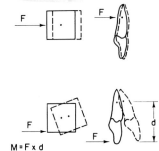

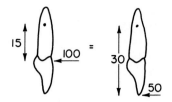

M_1 = 15mm.x 100 Gm. = M_2 = 30mm. x 50 Gm.

Fig. XIII-4.—Equivalent moments with varying forces and distances.

applied to the center of the mass, but it also will turn on an axis, developing a moment (see Fig. XIII-3).

A *moment* is the tendency of a force to cause rotation of a body around the fixed axis. Given the same free body and the same force, a moment gives the same translation as if the force were applied through the center of mass, but it also produces a rotational tendency. An equivalent moment can be produced by varying the force and the distance (Fig. XIII-4).

It is possible to rotate a body without translation by two moments that are equal, parallel, in the opposite direction and noncollinear—an arrangement of forces called a *couple*[1] (Fig. XIII-5). A couple always induces a pure rotational tendency. A force applied at different points on the body will produce different movements, but it does not make any difference where a couple is applied. A moment is one force producing a sliding vector. A couple is two forces equal, parallel, opposite and noncollinear in producing a free vector. If one desires translation, that is, bodily movement of a tooth, it could be achieved by applying force through the centroid or the center of resistance of the tooth. No appliance has yet been designed that will effect such a force application, since the centroid of most teeth is somewhere in the root. Working with a force alone at the crown of the tooth will develop a moment and tipping around the center of resistance (see Fig. XIII-3). If, however, two equal

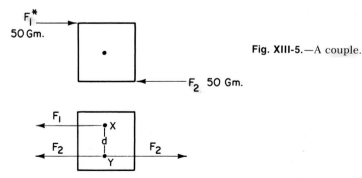

Fig. XIII-5.—A couple.

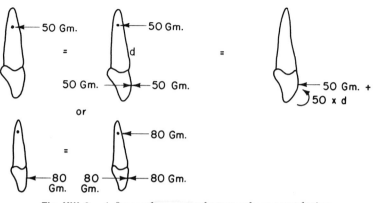

Fig. XIII-6.—A force plus a couple to produce translation.

and opposite forces (a couple) also are applied to the crown, bodily movement, i.e., translation, is achieved (Fig. XIII-6). It will be seen that any force can be replaced by a force plus a couple. Thus, translation of the tooth is achieved even though it is impossible to apply the force directly to the center of resistance (see Fig. XIII-6).

Any orthodontic appliance, when activated, delivers more than one force and, thus, is a force system. Any force system can, for analytical purposes, be reduced to either one force, one couple or one force plus one couple. Thus, it is theoretically possible to analyze any orthodontic appliance force system.[1] Forces delivered by orthodontic appliances are studied by electronic strain gauges, mechanical gauges or by mathematical calculations. If we are truly to understand an orthodontic force system for tooth movement, we must consider the magnitude of the force, its direction and the point of force application.

All of the discussion thus far has been based on assumptions that are not completely true in practice, since many of the forces are acquired from elastically deformed wires and the tooth is not a free body but is attached to bone by means of the periodontal ligament. Therefore, it is necessary to understand the biologic responses of the periodontal ligament and alveolar bone to orthodontically imposed forces.

B. Biologic Reactions to Orthodontic Forces

1. PERIODONTAL DRIFT AND PHYSIOLOGIC TOOTH MOVEMENTS

During growth of the mandible and maxilla, the teeth undergo constant changes in position that require an adjustment mechanism so that a tooth can remain attached by the periodontal ligament to the alveolar bone in a continuous and uninterrupted manner. The adjusting movements of the teeth include eruption and vertical development as well as progressive drifting, usually mesially, but also buccally, lingually or even distally, according to the tooth and the skeletal pattern. The drifting movements of teeth contribute to the progressive and continuous process of relocation of the dentition in relation to the growing, remodeling and relocating of facial bones. The periodontal ligament is provided with an intrinsic mechanism that enables it to move continuously in a manner corresponding to the various bone and tooth movements of either side. Just as the teeth and alveolar bone drift together, the periodontal ligament itself undergoes a corresponding process of

Fig. XIII-7.—Periodontal drift.

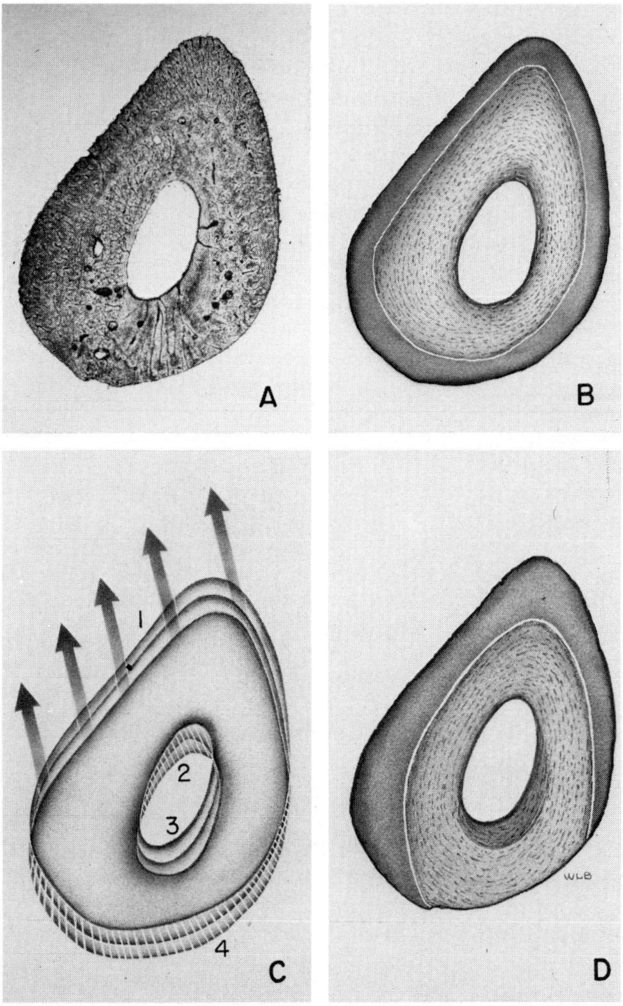

drift that permits differential movements between the root of the tooth and its surrounding alveolar wall while maintaining continuous attachment between them. This complex process involves two basic and different mechanisms of drift; one is associated with resorbing alveolar surfaces and the other with depository surfaces. The mechanisms of periodontal drift and corresponding movements of the alveolar wall are shown schematically in Figure XIII-7. This adjustment phenomenon has been studied and reported in detail by Enlow.[8]

A more general term—physiologic tooth movements—is used to describe the movements of the tooth in the alveolus during function, the changes in the tooth's position during eruption and the transitional dentition and the natural changes in tooth position that accompany occlusal and interproximal wear of the crown during adult life. Physiologic tooth movements are adjustments to normal growth and occlusal wear. Therefore, the tissue reactions that occur during physiologic tooth movements are normal and seen in every tooth. It is important to know the expected direction of physiologic tooth movements for every tooth (see Chapter VI).

All orthodontic tooth movements probably are best studied on a background of understanding of periodontal drift and physiologic tooth movements. There are two primary differences between orthodontic tooth movements and periodontal drift and physiologic tooth movements: (1) purposeful orthodontic tooth movements are brought about more rapidly and thus produce more extensive tissue changes and (2) orthodontic tooth movements often are undertaken against the normal direction of physiologic tooth movement and periodontal drift.

2. FACTORS IN TOOTH MOVEMENT

The wide variation in biologic response toward orthodontic tooth movements is due to many factors, some of which are discussed briefly below.

a) *Manner of Force Application*

The amount, duration and direction of force may be combined in various manners, according to the intent of the dentist and the appliance being used (Fig. XIII-8).

1) CONTINUOUS FORCES.—Continuous forces maintain approximately the same force magnitude over an indefinite time, for example, a coil spring.

2) DISSIPATING FORCES (REITAN'S INTERRUPTED TYPE).—Dissipating forces are continuous but demonstrate a decreasing amount of force within a short period, for example, a banded tooth ligated to an archwire. Many tooth movements effected by modern orthodontic appliances result from the dissipating type of force application. An advantage of this type of force over continuous forces is the period for recovery, reorganization and cell proliferation prior to the reapplication of force.

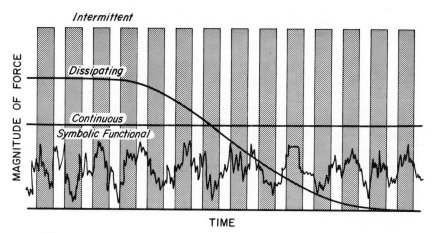

Fig. XIII-8.—Schematic presentation of manner of orthodontic force application.

3) INTERMITTENT FORCES.—Intermittent forces are associated with removable appliances. The force is active when the appliance is in the mouth and nonexistent when it is removed. Some intermittent action also is seen as the result of changes in the tooth or appliance position during mastication and speech. Fixed removable appliances, including maxillary plates with auxiliary springs and extra-oral traction appliances, are examples using intermittent tooth movements.

4) FUNCTIONAL FORCES.—Functional forces appear against the tooth only during normal oral function. Functional forces are associated with loose removable appliances. Thus, each time the patient swallows, the activator directs the force of the muscle contractions against the teeth. Functional forces are not easy to control and do not move the teeth as rapidly as dissipating or intermittent forces. It should be remembered, however, that the loose removable appliances are not designed primarily as tooth-moving appliances but rather as devices to affect the growing craniofacial skeleton.

b) Amount of Force Application

The magnitude of force determines to some extent the duration of the hyalinization[21] (see later). When excessively strong forces are applied, a longer initial hyalinization period will result as well as the formation of secondary hyalinized zones. Interruption of the heavy forces will moderate the rate of hyalinization. The amount of force that is optimal varies with the type of tooth movement; for example, if hyalinization is to be avoided during intrusion of teeth, the lightest forces must be used. A bit more force (25–30 Gm.) is useful for extrusion, and Burstone and Groves[5] have shown that 50–75 Gm. of force is satisfactory for translation of teeth. As pointed out in the discussion of manner of force application, there are two aspects of force: the amount acting at the time movements are begun and the amount acting as the teeth respond.

c) *Duration of Force Application*

Duration of force application is a factor of importance, since the periodontal ligament must have recovery periods to replenish the blood supply to the ligament and to promote cell proliferation. A heavy force of short duration may be less damaging than a light, continuous force.

d) *Direction of Force Application*

Tooth movements are named according to the direction of force application (Fig. XIII-9).

1) TIPPING.—During tipping, the crown and root are moved in opposite directions around a center of rotation within the root. Diagonally opposite areas of compression and tension are produced within the periodontal ligament. Tipping is best carried out by a light, continuous force.[21] It should be pointed out that during tipping movements, the crown of the tooth moves much more than does the root but, fortunately, that is all that is required in many instances.

2) TRANSLATION.—During translation or bodily tooth movement, the crown and root are moved in the same direction at the same time. This movement usually is brought about by a couple. At the initiation of bodily movements, a very light force is preferred. During the period of the secondary response, it has been shown that forces of 150–200 Gm. are quite satisfactory for the bodily movement of cuspids, for example, into extraction sites.

3) ROTATION.—Rotation is the movement of the tooth around its long axis. Rotation is a very complicated tooth movement, difficult to effect and difficult to retain.[21, 27] Rotations are best effected by dissipating forces with periods of stabilization between activations of the appliance.[21] Relapse of rotations is especially prominent when the tooth has been rotated rapidly with a strong, continuous force.

4) INTRUSION.—Intrusion is the movement of the tooth into the alveolus. Very light forces are used in the intrusion of teeth and, when done properly, little relapse is seen.[21] In practice, intrusion frequently is relative, that is, some teeth are intruded a little, whereas others are reciprocally *extruded* more easily.[19]

5) EXTRUSION.—Extrusion is the movement of the tooth out of the alveolus, that is, the root follows the crown. Extrusion frequently is necessary in Class II, Division 1 malocclusions with an open bite. Extrusions are best carried out using very light, continuous forces during rapid periods of alveolar growth. Heavy, intermittent forces, for example, as with strong vertical elastics, may result in relapse.[21]

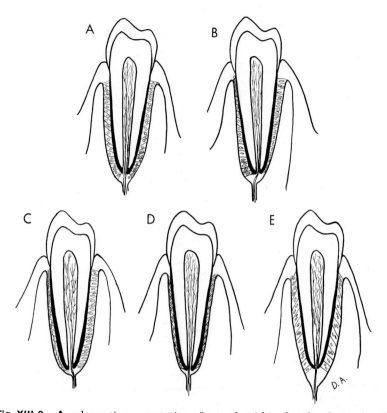

Fig. XIII-9.—**A,** schematic presentation of a tooth within the alveolar socket. The periodontal ligament is greatly enlarged. Note, however, that the tooth is situated centrally in the alveolus. **B,** as the crown is tipped, the periodontal ligament is compressed at the alveolar crest on one side and the periodontal fibers are stretched on the opposite side of the alveolar crest. Similarly, but in the opposite direction, the apex of the tooth compresses the periodontal ligament on one side and stretches the fibers on the other. **C,** translation or bodily movement of a tooth. During translation, the crown and root move in the same direction at the same time. Note that a far greater area of the periodontal ligament is compressed than when the tooth is being tipped. **D,** intrusion. During intrusion, the tooth is forced into the alveolar socket, compressing the entire periodontal ligament and thereby diminishing the periodontal circulation, thus requiring a longer recovery period than for simple tipping. **E,** extrusion.

6) TORQUE.—Torque, as used in orthodontics, is a movement of the root without movement of the crown. In other words, it is a tipping movement with the fulcrum in the bracket area, but in practice there always is some crown movement.[21] Torque may be produced by the use of rectangular wires in rectangular bracket slots or by adjuncts to a round wire. The effects of torque vary with the area of the root studied. Undermining resorption is more likely to be seen in the apical portion of the

root, where the forces are the greatest. Since the force varies along the root surface, torque usually is expressed as the amount of force at the crest of the alveolar processes. Forces of 50–60 Gm. at the alveolar crest are satisfactory for most torquing movements.[21]

e) Occlusal Function

Often, orthodontic movements are countered by the intercuspation during occlusal function, resulting in jiggling and often hypermobility. Teeth being moved may show no mobility until an occlusal interference is encountered. The use of a bite plane is helpful, but spot grinding is ill-advised, since the surface ground to relieve jiggling and mobility may be needed for occlusal stabilization in the final position.

f) Age

As a general rule, the biologic response to orthodontic forces in the adult is slower than in the child. The removal of occlusal forces is important in adult tooth movements and there is a need for light forces with longer periods of rest between adjustments.[21]

3. Tissue Response
a) Initial Reaction

It has been shown that some of the periodontal vessels are compressed a few minutes after the application of orthodontic forces.[18, 19] The pressure of the tooth only rarely results in direct resorption of the bone at the pressure site. Pathologic necrosis of bone, which was described by early workers, is not observed in studies of the effects of modern orthodontic appliances. Compression of the periodontal ligament against the wall of the alveolus usually results in the area of the compressed periodontal ligament becoming cell free, and the movement of the tooth stops until the hyalinized tissue has been removed.[21] The time necessary for undermining resorption of the bone and removal of the hyalinized tissue is roughly proportionate to the extent of the hyalinization[3, 21] (Fig. XIII-10). Thus, the initial period is longer for intrusion and translation, which occlude larger areas of periodontal circulation.[19] It is obvious, also, why an effort is made to begin such movements with very light forces to avoid the formation of excessive areas of hyalinization. The duration of the initial reaction in humans may vary from a few days to a few weeks.[21]

b) Secondary Response

Later, the periodontal space is widened and direct resorption of bone typically is seen.[19, 21] On the tension side, a proliferation of osteoblasts presages the appearance of osteoid tissue, which is followed by new

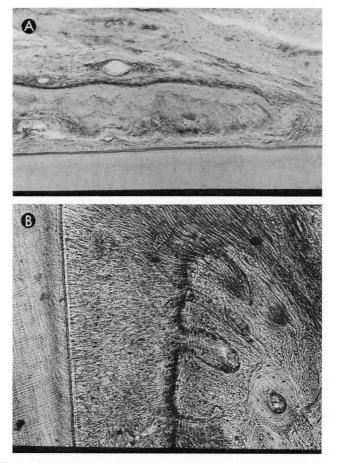

Fig. XIII-10.—A, histologic section at the pressure side of the alveolar crest under tipping force (the tooth is at the bottom). Pressure has been applied for some time, producing heavy osteoclastic activity in the bone facing the tooth. On the opposite side of the alveolar crest is a horizontal black line indicative of the heavily staining osteoblasts, which have already laid down a layer of new bone. **B,** tension side of the alveolar crest under tipping forces. The tooth at the left has been moved away from the alveolar process at the right. Note that the periodontal fibers that insert into the bone exert tension on the bone and that new bone is rapidly being laid down in the direction of the tooth movement by heavy osteoblastic activity. (From Moyers and Bauer.[19])

bundle bone. The rate and direction of new bone formation is in response to the tension exerted by the periodontal fibers (see Fig. XIII-8).

c) Root Resorption

Three types of root resorption are seen in orthodontic patients: (1) *microresorption,* which is local, superficial, confined to the cementum and routinely repaired; (2) *progressive resorption,* which involves increasing amounts of the apical end of the root; and (3) *idiopathic resorption,* in which the root resorption is not related to the orthodontic forces. Microresorption is likely to be seen to some extent on the roots of most teeth that have been moved. The cemental area heals quickly and the result may be regarded as no more than the minor scar of the orthodontic procedure. Indeed, it cannot be seen radiographically but only in the microscopic preparation. Progressive resorption of the root, on the other hand, appears first at the site of continuous and heavy apical pressure and may involve the entire apex. Since some patients have a far greater disposition to resorption than others, any teeth that must be moved great distances or for long times should be checked frequently and thoroughly by radiographs. Patients with idiopathic resorption usually show evidence of the condition before orthodontic therapy, and the orthodontic forces only aggravate the problem.

Since the first research on periodontal response to tooth movements, the problem of root resorption has been studied extensively.[21] Some of the factors that influence resorption are[18, 19]:

1. Magnitude of the force.
2. Duration of force application.
3. Direction of movement.
4. Age of the patient.

Root resorption is more likely to be seen when heavy forces are active for too long a period on small rooted teeth. Translation, torque and intrusion are the movements that are most likely to cause root resorption.

C. Design of Appliances for Tooth Movements

1. METHODS OF DELIVERING FORCE

Most orthodontic appliances derive their forces from bending of spring wire or from the torsional properties of wire. Elastics are another routine source of orthodontic forces. Screw forces are used much less frequently because they are difficult to control in the lower force range. Orthodontic forces may be applied to the tooth directly or by means of brackets or attachments. When round wires are used in brackets, ordinarily there is control in two directions only. Rigid attachments, for example, with a rectangular wire and a rectangular slot, permit control of the tooth in all three directions.

2. SELECTION AND CONTROL OF ORTHODONTIC FORCES

When designing an orthodontic appliance, a number of questions must be answered:

What is the amount of force to be used?
What is the distance the force must act?
What is the duration of time the force should act?
How will the force be dissipated during movements of the tooth?
What is the direction of force application desired?
What is the distribution of stress created within the periodontal ligament by the orthodontic force?

When an orthodontic wire is shaped to make a simple spring and the forces in that spring are measured at different deflections, it will be found that the forces increase proportionately to the distance of the deflection. This is Hooke's law, which states that the deflection is proportional to the load. Thus, in the orthodontic spring throughout the range of its normal activation, the applied force divided by the deflection produces a constant known as the load deflection rate.[4] Orthodontic springs that have a low load deflection rate deliver more constant forces, since there is less change in force with each unit change in activation. This principle underlies the theory of the "light-wire" appliances. The ideal orthodontic spring has a large range of activation (the distance through which a spring can be activated without permanent deformation) and a low load deflection rate.[4] However, to design such an ideal spring into an orthodontic appliance, we need to know several other factors, viz., the characteristics of the alloy from which the spring is made, the cross-sectional size of the wire and the length of the wire.

In clinical practice, it is desirable to apply known forces over a predetermined distance and for a specified length of time. In order to achieve these goals, it is necessary to understand how the diameter of the wire and the length of the spring affect the characteristics of the spring. The force created by deflection in a specific length of wire increases sixteen times per deflection unit when the diameter of the wire is doubled.[4, 11] Increasing the length of the spring without altering the diameter has a dramatic effect on the load in the spring, since the force that is created is reduced to one-eighth when the spring length is doubled.[4] In practice, it usually is much easier and more desirable to increase the length of a spring than to alter other variables. However, space in which to increase the spring length is an important consideration; hence, the ingenious use of helices, coils and loops (Fig. XIII-11).

Considerable variation in the force, duration of force expenditure, direction of force application and distribution of forces within the periodontal ligament is achieved by skillful use of loops and helices in the archwires.[29] Controlled tooth movements are achieved only when one has control of the moment-to-force ratio applied to the crown of the tooth. It is this ratio that determines how the tooth is going to move,

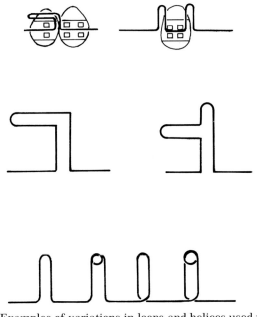

Fig. XIII-11.—Examples of variations in loops and helices used to vary the force and direction of force applied to teeth.

not the absolute force applied. Simple auxiliary springs applied to the naked crown of the tooth produce tipping, but it is uncontrolled tipping.

3. Optimal Orthodontic Forces

The optimal orthodontic force for any given tooth movement is that which initiates the maximal tissue response without pain or root resorption and maintains the health of the periodontal ligament throughout the movement of the tooth.[19, 21] The rate of tooth movement is determined by a number of other variables not discussed here, for example, the effects of occlusion and intercuspation of the teeth, the root surface area of the tooth to be moved, whether the direction of tooth movement is aided by natural tooth drift or not and so forth.

4. Concepts of Anchorage

Anchorage is the word used in orthodontics to mean resistance to displacement. Every orthodontic appliance consists of two elements— an active element and a resistance element. The active member or members of the orthodontic appliance are the parts concerned with tooth movements and thus are the elements discussed so far in this

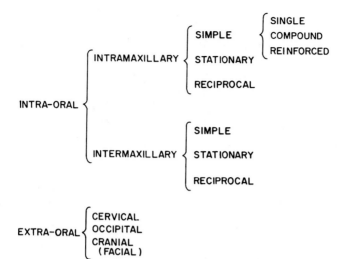

Fig. XIII-12.—Outline of various kinds of orthodontic anchorage.

chapter. The resistance elements are those that provide the resistance that makes tooth movements possible. According to Newton's Third Law there is an equal and opposite reaction to every action. Therefore, in orthodontics, all anchorage is relative and all resistance is comparative.

We may classify anchorage in a number of varying fashions (Fig. XIII-12).

a) According to the Manner of Force Application

1) SIMPLE ANCHORAGE.—Resistance to tipping, that is, the tooth is free to tip during movement.
2) STATIONARY ANCHORAGE.—Resistance to bodily movement, that is, the tooth is permitted to translate only. (The term "stationary anchorage" has always seemed to me to be one of the most ridiculous in orthodontic jargon.)
3) RECIPROCAL ANCHORAGE.—Two or more teeth moving in opposite directions and pitted against each other in the appliance. Usually, the resistance to each other is equal and opposite.

b) According to the Jaws Involved

1) INTRAMAXILLARY.—Anchorage established in the same jaw.
2) INTERMAXILLARY.—Anchorage distributed to both jaws.

c) *According to Site of Source of Anchorage*

1) INTRA-ORAL ANCHORAGE.—Anchorage established within the mouth, that is, utilizing the teeth, mucosa or other intra-oral structures.
2) EXTRA-ORAL ANCHORAGE.—Anchorage obtained outside the oral cavity.

Cervical.—Utilizing the neck for anchorage.

Occipital.—Utilizing the occipital region for anchorage.

Cranial.—Involving the cranium as a source of anchorage.

3) MUSCULAR ANCHORAGE.—Anchorage derived from action of muscles.

d) *According to the Number of Anchorage Units*

1) SINGLE OR PRIMARY ANCHORAGE.—Anchorage involving only one tooth.
2) COMPOUND ANCHORAGE.—Anchorage involving two or more teeth.
3) REINFORCED ANCHORAGE.—The addition of nondental anchorage sites, for example, mucosa, muscles, head, etc.

5. CONTROL OF ANCHORAGE

In practice, care is taken to maintain control of anchorage so that the conditions for movements of teeth are optimal in the active elements of the appliance and satisfactory for anchorage in the resistance elements. Routine precautions include (a) securing anchorage so far as possible outside the teeth themselves, for example, mucosa, muscles, cranium, etc., (b) selecting larger numbers of teeth in the resistance parts of the appliance and (c) varying the amount, direction and manner of force application between active and resistance elements. Adherence to the principles of anchorage control is an essential factor in successful orthodontics.

D. Retention, Relapse and Occlusal Stabilization

Retention is the procedure in orthodontics of maintaining a newly moved tooth in position for a long enough period to ensure maintenance of the correction.

Relapse is the term applied to the loss of correction achieved by orthodontic treatment.

Occlusal stabilization must carry the idea of homeostatic stabilization, that is, the masticatory system should be self-stabilizing after orthodontic therapy.

There have been many ideas and concepts of retention. Stability of orthodontic results has been said to be dependent on the angulation of the mandibular incisors, the relationship of the teeth to their apical bases, occlusal relationships, etc. I was part of a long-term research study of retention and relapse that produced the primary finding that there were diverse causes of relapse, but the most important were (1) failure to place the teeth in occlusion in harmony with the reflex position of the mandible during the unconscious swallow (see Chapter V) and (2) untoward intrusion of new vectors of growth after orthodontic therapy was finished.[6, 7, 12-17, 20] These findings relate primarily to occlusal corrections in toto, whereas many other studies describe the relapse of individual tooth movements. Riedel[26] has listed in interesting fashion a number of theorems that are popular explanations of the phenomena of retention of moved teeth and relapse. I shall list them and summarize the support or denial of each, but it should be noted that some of these theorems consider but one factor alone. One cannot remove the tooth from its total functioning environment, even for discussion purposes.

Theorem 1—*Teeth that have been moved tend to return to their former positions.* This certainly is not totally true for all tooth movements, but it is particularly true for rotations. The theorem is more true for incisors than for posterior teeth, which have a firmer occlusal relationship.

Theorem 2—*Elimination of the cause of malocclusion will prevent recurrence.* Most "causes" of malocclusion are not known (see Chapter VII), although the theorem is true for such obvious factors as tongue-thrusting and thumb-sucking.

Theorem 3—*Malocclusion should be overcorrected as a safety factor.* This rationale is very popular in practice, but there is little real data to support the idea.

Theorem 4—*Proper occlusion is a potent factor in holding teeth in their corrected positions.* The occlusion usually referred to is the intercuspal relationship seen in the cases (the usual occlusal position). Our own findings[13, 15, 16] indicate that the occlusal relationship obtaining during primitive reflex functions, for example, unconscious swallowing (see Chapter V), is a very important factor in stabilization of the corrected malocclusion.

Theorem 5—*Bone and adjacent tissues must be allowed time to reorganize around newly positioned teeth.* This idea is the reason for the use of retainers after active tooth movements. There is good histologic evidence that it takes some time for the adjacent tissues to return to normal after tooth movements.[21] However, this theorem presumes that mature bone provides more stability for the teeth and, further, that newly moved teeth are no longer the victims of unsettling forces. If the occlusion is not in harmony with the reflex position of the mandible during the unconscious swallow, it makes very little difference what kind of retainer is worn, for the bone is not really reorganizing as hoped for and the moment the retainers are removed, relapse will begin until the occlusion returns to harmony with the muscles.

Theorem 6—*If the lower incisors are placed upright over basal bone they are more likely to remain in good alignment.* This theorem has some value but has been overextended, since it so often avoids the implications of facial type and the mesial migration of the teeth throughout life. Further, the incisal angle that is "correct" at 12 years of age may not be "correct" for the same child at 18, after the mandible has grown disproportionately more than the midface.

Theorem 7—*Corrections carried out during periods of growth are less likely to relapse.* This theorem seems valid and logical, but there is little solid evidence to support it. Treatment during growth presumably allows the tissues involved to adjust better to the intrusions of the dentist.

Theorem 8—*The farther teeth have been moved the less is the likelihood of relapse.* This theorem is strange in logic and there is no evidence to support it.

Theorem 9—*Arch form, particularly the mandibular arch, cannot be altered permanently by appliance therapy.* The strongest support for this idea comes from the analysis of cases treated by multibanded therapy after most growth is over. Treatment during the mixed dentition with bite plates, extra-oral traction[10] or functional jaw orthopedic appliances has been shown many times to *permit* a natural widening of the mandibular arch diameters. The best evidence, though, shows that *purposeful* alteration of the bicanine diameter in the mandibular arch is hazardous to stability.[26]

The preceding theorems are those of Riedel but the commentary is mine. To the theorems might be added the following:

Theorem 10—*Many treated malocclusions require permanent retaining devices.* This rarely is true for cases treated during growth and cases treated by clinicians who hold due regard for proper goals of therapy and the dynamics of growth and occlusal function. The less the dentist knows about occlusal physiology the more cases he will be tempted to retain permanently.

Most of our treatment goals thus far have been stated in cephalometric terms, which are useful but not complete. All occlusions treated orthodontically most likely were stable before therapy. If, at the end of treatment, they are not, it may be the fault of the dentist. Eventually, all treated malocclusions must be returned from control by appliances to control by the patient's own musculature. Proper goals of treatment, careful mechanotherapy, precise occlusal equilibration (see Chapter XVII) and well-chosen retention procedures play a role in achieving occlusal homeostasis.

REFERENCES

1. Baril, C.: Biomechanics, in University of Montreal, Department of Orthodontics, manual for students.
2. Bien, S. M.: Fluid dynamic mechanisms which regulate tooth movement, Advances Oral Biol. 2:173, 1966.
3. Burstone, C. J.: The Biomechanics of Tooth Movements, in Kraus, B. S., and Riedel, R. A. (eds.), *Vistas in Orthodontics* (Philadelphia: Lea & Febiger, 1962).
4. Burstone, C. J.: Biomechanics of the Orthodontic Appliance, in Graber, T. M. (ed.), *Current Orthodontic Concepts and Techniques* (Philadelphia: W. B. Saunders Company, 1969).

5. Burstone, C. J., and Groves, M. H.: Threshold and optimum force values for maxillary anterior tooth movement, J. Dent. Res. 39:695, 1961.
6. Campisciano, V., and Shiba, S.: A Study of the Effects of Occlusal Equilibration on Orthodontic Retention, M. S. thesis, University of Michigan, Ann Arbor, 1961.
7. Eggleston, W. B., Jr., and Ekleberry, J. W.: An Electromyographic and Functional Evaluation of Treated Orthodontic Cases, M.S. thesis, University of Michigan, Ann Arbor, 1961.
8. Enlow, D. H.: *The Human Face* (New York: Hoeber Medical Division, Harper & Row, Publishers, 1968).
9. Evans, F. G.: *Stress and Strain in Bones. Their Relation to Fractures and Osteogenesis* (Springfield, Ill.: Charles C Thomas, Publisher, 1957).
10. Graber, T. M. (ed.): *Current Orthodontic Concepts and Techniques* (Philadelphia: W. B. Saunders Company, 1969).
11. Halderson, H., Johns, E. E., and Moyers, R. E.: The selection of forces for tooth movement, Am. J. Orthodont. 39:25, 1953.
12. Jacob, T.: An Electromyographic Study of Orthodontic Retention Patients before and after Occlusal Equilibration, M.S. thesis, University of Michigan, Ann Arbor, 1960.
13. Moyers, R. E.: Unpublished study.
14. Moyers, R. E.: Equilibration, band removal, and retainers. Taped slide sequence prepared for the American Association of Orthodontics, Miami, Florida, 1969.
15. Moyers, R. E.: The strategy of retention. Taped lecture, Orthodont. Digest, 1969.
16. Moyers, R. E.: Some Comments About the Nature of Orthodontic Relapse, in *Nederlanse Vereniging Voor Orthodontische Studie, Studieweek* (Leiden, Netherlands: Kluwer-Veventer Pub., 1970).
17. Moyers, R. E.: Clinical Steps Suggested for Obviating Orthodontic Relapse, in *Nederlanse Vereniging Voor Orthodontische Studie, Studieweek* (Leiden, Netherlands: Kluwer-Veventer Pub., 1970).
18. Moyers, R. E.: The periodontal membrane in orthodontics, J.A.D.A. 40:22, 1950.
19. Moyers, R. E., and Bauer, J. L.: The periodontal response to various tooth movements, Am. J. Orthodont. 36:572, 1950.
20. Moyers, R. E., and Ekleberry, J. W.: Band removal, finishing, and retainers. Taped slide sequence prepared for the American Association of Orthodontics, Miami, Florida, 1969.
21. Reitan, K.: Biomechanical Principles and Reactions, in Graber, T. M. (ed.), *Current Orthodontic Concepts and Techniques* (Philadelphia: W. B. Saunders Company, 1969).
22. Reitan, K.: Bone Formation and Resorption during Reversed Tooth Movement, in Kraus, B. S., and Riedel, R. A. (eds.), *Vistas in Orthodontics* (Philadelphia: Lea & Febiger, 1962).
23. Reitan, K.: Tissue reaction as related to the age factor, Dent. Rec. 74:271, 1954.
24. Reitan, K.: Continuous bodily tooth movement and its histological significance, Acta odont. scandinav. 6:115, 1947.
25. Reitan, K.: Effects of force, magnitude and direction of tooth movement on different alveolar bone types, Angle Orthodont. 34:244, 1964.
26. Riedel, R. A.: Retention, in Graber, T. M. (ed.), *Current Orthodontic Concepts and Techniques* (Philadelphia: W. B. Saunders Company, 1969).
27. Skillen, W., and Reitan, K.: Tissue changes following rotation of teeth in the dog, Angle Orthodont. 10:140, 1940.
28. Smith, R., and Storey, E.: The importance of force in orthodontics; the design of cuspid retraction springs, Australian D. J. 56:291, 1952.
29. Stoner, M., and Lindquist, J.: The Edgewise Appliance Today, in Graber, T. M. (ed.), *Current Orthodontic Concepts and Techniques* (Philadelphia: W. B. Saunders Company, 1969).
30. Storey, E.: Bone changes associated with tooth movement. A histological study of the effect of force for varying durations in the rabbit, guinea pig and rat, Australian D. J. 59:209, 1955.
31. Storey, E., and Smith, R.: Force in orthodontics and its relation to tooth movement, Australian D. J. 56:11, 1952.

Suggested Readings

Burstone, C. J.: Biomechanics of the Orthodontic Appliance, in Graber, T. M. (ed.), *Current Orthodontic Concepts and Techniques* (Philadelphia: W. B. Saunders Company, 1969).
Reitan, K.: Biomechanical Principles and Reactions, in Graber, T. M. (ed.), *Current Orthodontic Concepts and Techniques* (Philadelphia: W. B. Saunders Company, 1969).
Thurow, R. H.: *Atlas of Orthodontic Principles* (St. Louis: The C. V. Mosby Company, 1970).
Thurow, R. H.: *Technique and Treatment with the Edgewise Appliance* (St. Louis: The C. V. Mosby Company, 1962).

XIV

Planning Orthodontic Treatment

Always take hold of things by the smooth handle.—
THOMAS JEFFERSON

Nothing in progression can rest on its original plan.
We might as well think of rocking a grown man in the
cradle of an infant.—EDMUND BURKE

A. Selection of orthodontic cases in general practice
   1. Appraisal of the family and the patient
   2. Typifying the case
      a) Timing of treatment
      b) Skeletal pattern
      c) Available space

B. Organizing the therapy
   1. Defining goals
      a) Ideal treatment
      b) Compromise treatment
      c) Symptomatic treatment
   2. Disposition of the case
   3. Specifying the tooth movements required
   4. Selection of the appliance(s)
   5. Planning the retention

C. Treatment planning in the primary dentition
   1. Reasons for treatment
   2. Conditions that should be treated
   3. Conditions that may be treated
   4. Contraindications to treatment in the primary dentition

D. Treatment planning in the mixed dentition
   1. Reasons for treatment
   2. Conditions that should be treated
   3. Conditions that may be treated

E. Treatment planning in the permanent dentition

F. Limiting factors in orthodontic therapy
1. Factors related to the individual patient
   a) Limiting skeletal factors
   b) Limiting dental factors
   c) Limiting neuromuscular factors
2. Factors related to the individual dentist
   a) Aptitude
   b) Training
   c) Experience
   d) Attitude
   e) Adherence to poor methods
3. Factors related to the nature of orthodontics itself
   a) The nature of developmental oral biology
   b) Role of the patient in orthodontic therapy
   c) Paucity of adequate compromising alternative treatments

G. Some common mistakes

WHEN A PATIENT has a malocclusion and the parents desire orthodontic treatment for him, the dentist typically asks himself two questions: "When can I work this case into my busy schedule?" and "Which appliance shall I use?" These are not the most critical questions to be asked, but, when asked, dominate the treatment plan.

Not all patients with malocclusion need or should have treatment. Not all patients with malocclusion needing orthodontic treatment should be treated by the family dentist. This chapter is written assuming that the reader has the interest and desire to treat as many patients orthodontically as he can without compromising quality of the final result. Many dentists have a great desire to extend their orthodontic service to more patients, but enthusiasm is no substitute for ability, nor does sincerity guarantee correctness. The dentist must protect himself and his patients from well-meant but ill-planned therapy. Meticulous planning of orthodontic treatment before the case actually is accepted prevents much misunderstanding and trouble.

The purposes of this chapter are (1) to provide a procedure for typifying orthodontic treatment problems so that the dentist may test whether he knows a satisfactory treatment protocol for a particular problem and (2) to outline a plan for organizing the sequences of orthodontic treatment.

A. Selection of Orthodontic Cases in General Practice

1. APPRAISAL OF THE FAMILY AND THE PATIENT

The family dentist doing orthodontics has one great advantage over the specialist—he usually knows the patients very well and can estimate from past experience their motivation and cooperation. Even with familiar patients, though, it is wise to ask the following questions before accepting the responsibilities for orthodontic treatment:

1. Who first suggested orthodontic treatment? You? Parent? Patient? Friend?

2. Why do the patient and parents think orthodontic treatment is needed? It is always a good plan to give both the parents and the patient a chance to verbalize at this point. The mother will not say that she wants the mesial buccal cusp of the maxillary first permanent molar to occlude perfectly with the buccal groove of the mandibular first permanent molar. More likely her concern will be with cosmetics, and she must be informed of the occlusal physiology, growth, etc.

3. What is the family's idea of the expected result?

4. What does the family know about orthodontic procedures? Time necessary for treatment? Difficulties? Cost?

5. What is the patient's attitude toward orthodontics? Some patients are far more motivated for orthodontic therapy than they are for restorative dentistry.

Many orthodontic treatment plans have failed not because of a lack of diagnostic or technical skill but rather because parents and patient did not know the nature of the procedures and their patience and cooperation ran out before a satisfactory result could be achieved. One does not have the luxury of accepting for treatment only those good little boys and girls who keep appointments, brush their teeth regularly and wear their elastic faithfully. Therefore, it is necessary to identify—at the start—parental and patient attitudes in order that they may be altered, if necessary, lest they confound and complicate the plan of treatment.

2. Typifying the Case

Before starting any treatment, the family dentist must be certain that the type of case presented is amenable to treatment by some method he has already mastered. Therefore, it is necessary to typify the case in terms of treatment procedures. The Angle classification and most other diagnostic classification systems are inadequate for this purpose. The procedure suggested herein consists of answering three questions, the answers to which segregate most malocclusions into eighteen categories according to their primary characteristics (Fig. XIV-1). All of the malocclusions selected by this method for any given protocol category have the same basic and fundamental problems. They differ only in the superficial aspects of the malocclusion. This procedure is designed to keep the dentist's mind, while planning the treatment, on basic matters in order to avoid being diverted by the obvious and superficial. Treatment planning should not be directed to the ugliest aspects of the malocclusion nor to the feature that particularly worries parent or child. Successful therapy is founded on a thorough understanding of the fun-

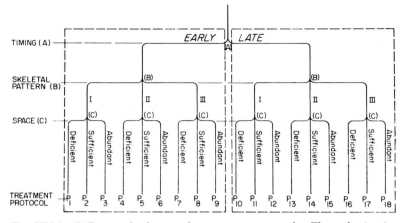

Fig. XIV-1.—Differential choice of treatment protocols. The arborization of choices based on three decisions. *A,* timing. The choice is early treatment during growth or late treatment when most of growth is over. *B,* the decision concerning skeletal profile. Three choices are available: I, a straight profile; II, a retrognathic profile and III, a profile showing mandibular prognathism. *C,* the decision concerning the available space. Three choices are available: abundant, sufficient and deficient.

damentals of the malocclusion. Superficialities treat easily if basics are understood. Figure XIV-1 is an arborization resulting from the possible answers to three questions:

1. What is the timing of treatment?
2. What is the facial skeletal pattern?
3. Is space available within the dental arch to correct the malocclusion?

As each question is asked, the most appropriate available answer is chosen and the diagram is followed to the next question. Finally, one of the eighteen protocols at the bottom of the chart is chosen. All cases within this protocol category will have similar basic features with respect to developmental age, skeletal pattern and available space.

Although this sequence is suggested for all, the more advanced clinician undoubtedly will supply more sophisticated methods of answering each query; for example, a cephalometric appraisal may be substituted for the Facial Form Analysis in order to appraise the facial skeleton.

a) Timing of Treatment (Fig. XIV-1, A)

Orthodontic treatment timing is related to dentitional growth and development. So different are the strategy and tactics for early vs. late treatment that the question of timing is asked first. Must the therapy for a case take into account facial growth or is most of the growth over, so that the therapy consists of tooth movements neither greatly aided nor hampered by growth? *Early treatment* is arbitrarily defined as treatment during the most active growth. Orthodontic treatment during very active growth sometimes capitalizes on growth and sometimes is handicapped thereby.

A method is required to assess roughly the stage of occlusal development and to estimate the time left before loss of the remaining primary teeth and the establishment of the permanent occlusion. Such a method would make it possible to determine whether there was sufficient time to complete any interceptive and guidance procedures. When the permanent occlusion is established (second molars in occlusion), a great percentage of the total growth is over and the opportunities for guidance of growth and occlusal development therefore are diminished. Furthermore, the mechanotherapy necessarily changes at this time as well; the interceptive and guidance appliances (holding arches, activators, extra-oral traction devices, etc.) give way to the multibanded precision appliances needed for careful positioning of teeth in the permanent dentition.

An arbitrary rule of thumb is applied to separate early from late treatment. This rule is based on the calcification stage of the mandibular permanent cuspid and first premolar. When they have not yet reached calcification stage $7\frac{1}{2}$ (roughly one-half the root formed), the case is considered eligible for early treatment planning (see Chapter VI, Development of the Dentition and the Occlusion, and Chapter XI, Analysis of the Dentition and Occlusion). *Late treatment* is defined as treatment begun too late to take advantage of growth or too late to be greatly complicated or confounded by growth. There still is active facial growth and dentitional development after the cuspids and premolars have reached stage $7\frac{1}{2}$, but usually there is insufficient time to complete the treatment without changing greatly the strategy and appliances. One can take advantage of growth only when growth is active and time is available to utilize it. The decision is arbitrary but has proved very satisfactory as a guideline for undergraduate students and general practitioners. The skilled orthodontist with an experienced sense of timing often can start "early" treatment at a later developmental date. *Diphasic treatment* is becoming more popular too, that is, treating the skeletal problem early when growth is active and treating the dental malalignment after the permanent teeth have erupted. The concepts of "early" and "late" treatment are working hypotheses only and offer no guarantee that unexpected growth will not disrupt a late treatment plan.

b) Skeletal Pattern (Fig. XIV-1, *B*)

In Chapter VIII, The Orthodontic Examination, and Chapter XII, Analysis of the Craniofacial Skeleton, a noncephalometric method was presented for assessing the contributions of the facial skeleton to the malocclusion. On the basis of the Facial Form Analysis or, better, a cephalometric analysis, the patient is arbitrarily assigned to one of three skeletal categories—*Class I,* essentially a well-balanced facial skeleton, *Class II,* essentially a retrognathic profile, or *Class III,* a prognathic profile. If any difficulty is encountered in choosing, for example, between Class I and Class II, it is advisable to select the more serious, that is, Class II.

c) Available Space (Fig. XIV-1, *C*)

In Chapter XI, Analysis of the Dentition and Occlusion, methods for mixed dentition analyses and dental "setups" were given. It is necessary to decide, before beginning treatment, whether there is enough space in the dental arch to provide for the alignment of all the teeth, the necessary developmental occlusal adjustments and the placement of the teeth satisfactorily over their bases. The Mixed Dentition Analysis alone cannot show how the teeth fit in the facial skeleton. Only a combined cephalometric and Mixed Dentition Analysis could be so revealing. Nevertheless, the dentist *must* make this last differentiating decision and categorize the case as having either *abundant, sufficient* or *deficient* space. By *abundant* is meant that there is more than enough space to align all of the teeth properly within the facial skeleton and enough to permit any required developmental occlusal adjustments as well. By *sufficient* is meant that there is just barely enough space to align the teeth but no arch space to aid in achieving a Class I occlusion, e.g., no space for a late mesial shift. By *deficient* is meant that there is insufficient arch perimeter in which to accommodate all of the teeth. All of these decisions are based primarily on the lower arch, since it is the more critical in matters of space.

The basic approach to treating all cases within any one protocol category is similar, for the individual malocclusions in the group will vary only in their superficial aspects. For example, all patients in protocol 13 will have most of their permanent teeth erupted, a severe skeletal Class II and inadequate space in the dental arch to align the teeth. Some may have more labioversion of the maxillary incisors than others, there will be variability in the depth of the bite and dissimilarity in a number of other superficial or localized aspects of the malocclusion. The dentist now can more easily decide whether he knows a protocol of therapy that will provide satisfactory treatment for the patient who has just been typified. All parts of Figure XIV-2 should be studied carefully, for each group illustrates the application of the method to actual cases. These cases have been chosen to show the differential utility of this simple procedure.

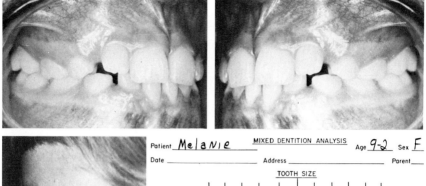

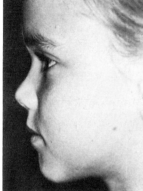

Fig. XIV-2.—See legend at foot of page 453.

Patient __Melanie__   MIXED DENTITION ANALYSIS   Age __9-2__ Sex __F__

Date _____   Address _____   Parent____

TOOTH SIZE

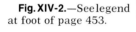

| 6.4 | 5.8 | 5.9 | 6.4 |

Upper

	Right	Left
Space left after alignment of 2 and 1	19.3	19.8
Predicted size of 3 + 4 + 5	23.4	23.4
Space left for molar adjustment	−4.1	−3.6

Lower

	Right	Left
Space left after alignment of 2 and 1	17.9	18.4
Predicted size of 3 + 4 + 5	23.1	23.1
Space left for molar adjustment	−5.2	−4.7

Remarks: Overjet = **3.9**   Overbite = **4.8 mm**

Molar relationship = **Class I , Class I**

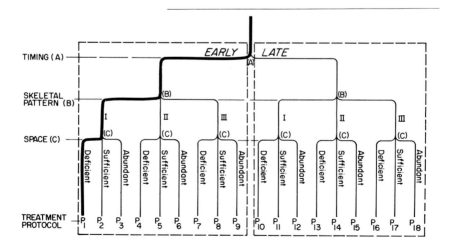

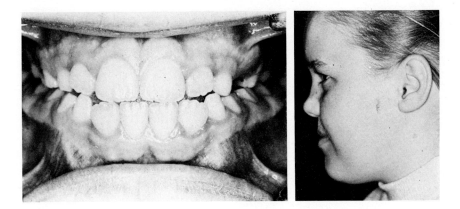

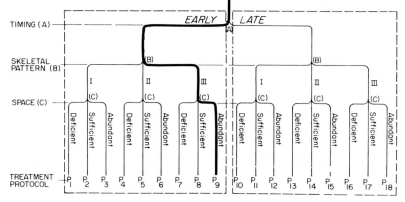

Fig. XIV-2 (cont.).—Example of arborization. (*Continued.*)

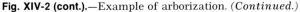

Fig. XIV-2.—Examples of arborization applied to actual cases. Look at the photos, make the three decisions as best you can and check your choices against the chart available for each patient. (*Continued.*)

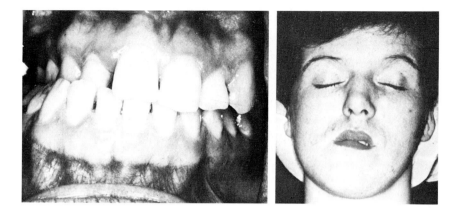

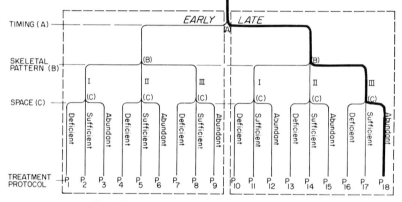

Fig. XIV-2 (cont.).—Example of arborization.

B. Organizing the Therapy

1. DEFINING GOALS

There are three kinds of orthodontic treatment goals: (1) treating to the most ideal result permitted by the case, (2) compromise treatment and (3) symptomatic treatment.

1. *Ideal treatment.* First, always define the ideal goal for the case and do not abandon that goal without clearly understanding why it is necessary to do so. The "ideal" result may be impractical or even harmful to oral health. What is ideal from an aesthetic point of view may not be ideal from the standpoint of periodontal health, occlusal function or practicality. The ideal goal in orthodontic treatment often is rejected because of a lack of needed technical skills or because such a goal seems "impractical." In orthodontics, practicality often is determined largely

by stability of result. An unstable occlusion, however nicely the teeth are aligned, may be the most impractical result. Some reasons for abandoning the ideal goal are: (1) the nature of the malocclusion does not permit an ideal result—for example, extraction of teeth is necessary; (2) you do not know how to treat to the ideal result; (3) the cost of ideal treatment may be prohibitive.

The goals listed here include concepts of health, function and cosmetics, whereas the family may be concerned solely with aesthetics. We must be very careful not to impose our own concepts and standards of aesthetics. Often a trait has been accepted without question or even cherished as a family characteristic until the dentist calls undue attention to it.

When the nature of the case does not permit ideal treatment, the only compromise treatment that can be accepted, of course, is that which most clearly approximates the ideal. When the clinician does not know how to treat to an ideal result, two alternatives are available: he may refer the patient to a specialist or he may suggest a compromise treatment plan. The latter alternative cannot be followed ethically unless the first alternative has been suggested and rejected by the patient and the nature of the compromise and its difficulties have been presented clearly and accepted by the family. When patients cannot afford the cost of ideal treatment, it is well, before suggesting a compromise treatment, to remember that no patient can afford an unstable result and that most malocclusions are stable until meddling begins. An alternative procedure under these circumstances may be not to treat at all in the hope that at a later time the ideal treatment can be achieved.

2. *Compromise treatment.* Before beginning compromise treatment, it is well to ask several questions: "What is being compromised?" "Why is compromise treatment considered?" "Who pays how big a price for the compromise?" Some malocclusions simply cannot be treated ideally, and any therapy is a compromise with perfection. On the other hand, to compromise the goal because of clinical inability to treat to the best goal may be to ask the patient to pay too big a price in oral health and raises serious questions of ethics.

Unfortunately, there are three common problems in orthodontics that do not lend themselves to compromise. The Class II malocclusion cannot be treated partially toward a Class I relationship or it will revert to the original condition. Occlusal function and the protective occlusal reflexes tend to destroy partly corrected Class II cases, for the occlusion must settle into either a Class I or a Class II relationship. The second difficult matter to compromise is that of the correction of gross tooth size-space discrepancies. If there is a discrepancy of 3 mm. in a quadrant, there is no 3-mm. tooth that can be extracted to alleviate exactly that amount of crowding. The dentist must extract a tooth that usually is about 7 mm. in width. Although the space is thus easily provided for alignment of 3 mm. of crowding, one cannot compromise the fact that 4 mm. of space

OUTLINE OF TREATMENT PLAN

Name _Charlie L._   Age _9-1_

Parent _Clyde_   Date _1-13-71_

_____ Interceptive or Guidance   _____ Compromise

_____ Comprehensive   __X__ Diphasic (i. e. Guidance)
                                                 + Comprehensive

Specified Compromises and Reasons for Accepting Same

1. _None_

2. _____

3. _____

Goals of Treatment	Strategies of Treatment
(In Order of Importance)	**(In Time Sequence)**
1. Secure a cl. I molar relationship.	I. Space supervision Conventional mandibular protocol when cuspids start to erupt (2).
2. Preserve mandibular arch perimeter and prevent late mesial shift of 6/6.	II. Extra oral traction to 6/6 soon after I (1 and 2)
3. Correct overjet and overbite.	III. Band and retract 21/12 when class I molar relationship is obtained (3).

Fig. XIV-3.—Treatment plan form. The case must be cataloged for planning purposes into one of the four classes. Do not choose two. If the case is cataloged as a compromise case, it is important at the very start to specify what the compromises are that are being accepted and the precise reason for doing so; if this is not done, the compromises may be forgotten later. The goals of treatment are specified in short, clear sentences and listed in order of importance. The strategies of treatment, that is, the methods of treatment, are listed in time sequence. Note that each item under strategies of treatment is followed by a number in parentheses. The number refers to the goals listed at the left.

closure remains to be carried out to complete the treatment, and the tooth movements necessary to effect 4 mm. of space closure are much more difficult than the tooth movements that provide 3 mm. of alignment. A third uncompromising situation is the inability of the jaw musculature to adapt to gross occlusal interferences. For example, some are tempted to extract a single mandibular incisor to relieve crowding. The incisors are then easily aligned but they usually have no antagonistic occlusal stops in the upper arch and therefore erupt toward the palate, whereas the posterior intercuspation has been altered so much that it cannot even be equilibrated into stability.

Unfortunately, there are not as many compromise methods of treatment in orthodontics as we would like and as often are available for other dental services. One of the most difficult tasks in orthodontics is that of planning sensible and practical compromise treatment. An equally difficult problem involves retreatment of cases that have worsened because of unfortunate mistakes in compromise therapy. The basic rule to remember is easy—one cannot compromise stability.

3. *Symptomatic treatment.* The treatment of symptoms of malocclusion rather than the malocclusion itself very rarely is advised and nearly always should be followed by treatment of the basic problem itself. A good example of acceptable symptomatic therapy is the retraction of maxillary incisors in extreme labioversion during the early mixed dentition in order to minimize their accidental fracture. But even the palliative retraction of maxillary incisors often is done just as easily by treating the Class II occlusal relationship simultaneously.

Figure XIV-3 shows a form I use to outline the treatment plan. Note that the goals are specified in order of importance prior to listing the steps of treatment in sequence. Figure XIV-3 illustrates a typical treatment plan completed for a mixed dentition case.

2. Disposition of the Case

Precise definition of goals makes easier the decision concerning disposition of the case. One wants to treat only those patients he can treat well to a stable result, refer those patients needing treatment that he cannot provide and keep under careful surveillance those patients for whom the best treatment must come later. There is no excuse for observing a case because of ignorance or indecision. Referrals can be made for diagnostic consultation as well as for treatment. The patient should not suffer longer or more expensive treatment because of diagnostic inabilities on the part of the family dentist, nor should a colleague have his task made more difficult by another's indecision.

3. Specifying the Tooth Movements Required

It is impossible to choose an appliance for treating a malocclusion without a clear idea of the tooth movements required for correction, i.e., the strategy to be employed. Therefore, it is necessary to specify the direction and distance each tooth is to be moved as well as its final angulation and occlusal relationship. The cephalogram or dental cast setup is very useful for visualizing the expected treatment result.

The treatment may best be broken down into stages or phases. It is imperative to write into the case history the aim of each phase and the tooth movements to be achieved during that stage of treatment. The written details of tooth movement probably are the most important single step in the treatment plan, since they help define the appliance that must be constructed and permit the dentist, before starting treatment, to test whether he knows a way to complete each necessary phase. Far too frequently a dentist attacks a malocclusion with a favorite appliance, only to learn after a few months that it is inadequate for the job. One works with greater comfort, surety and speed when he has, at the start, a precise idea of the sequence of treatment and the ordered tooth movements necessary.

The following list provides, in a very general way, the sequence of steps in the treatment of most malocclusions. It does not apply to adult malocclusions and may, of course, be varied to suit the individual problem.

a) Removal of all interferences to normal function and growth. These interferences include conditions resulting from pressure habits, those causing abnormal patterns of mandibular closure and conditions resulting from disease that are amenable to treatment.

b) Correction of disharmonies between the dentitions. These disharmonies may be either anteroposterior, e.g., maxillary dento-alveolar protraction, or lateral, e.g., maxillary contraction.

c) Fitting the dentition to the osseous base. This treatment includes such procedures as mass movements of the lateral segments distally in Class II and extractions to aid in placement of the teeth over their bases.

d) Alignment of the teeth in the dental arch. This step often is combined with steps *b* and/or *c*.

4. SELECTION OF THE APPLIANCE(S)

There is an old saying in orthodontics that it is better to make the appliance fit the patient than to make the patient fit the appliance. Often we become enamored with a particular appliance but it is very important to make sure, for a given case, that we are utilizing the most efficient mechanism for that particular malocclusion. If the goals of treatment are clearly in mind, if the stages of treatment have been defined and if the specific tooth movements required for each stage have been written down carefully, one has automatically narrowed the number of appliances that might be used for each stage of treatment.

Every appliance has limitations, yet every appliance that has stood the test of time must have some virtues. Many a case drags on and on because the dentist fails to recognize the fact that the appliance he chose is inadequate for the job. Many a malocclusion is finished with an inadequate result because the dentist did not know the best appliance for the case or refused to use other than his favorite. So varied are the malocclusions and so complex the details of their corrections that all clever clinicians are constantly adding to their repertory of appliance technics. Only the naïve and stubborn marry themselves to but one appliance, even though some appliances are much more versatile than others. Those who do so, if their standards are to remain high, must limit the patients treated, either consciously or unconsciously, to those malocclusions that respond well to that particular appliance.

5. Planning the Retention

Before a dentist proceeds to prepare a Class II cavity for an inlay, he has a clear mental image of the cavity outline, the depth of the preparation, the slope of the cavity walls, etc. Without such a mental image as a goal, he could scarcely begin. In like fashion, before a malocclusion can be corrected, the clinician must have a precise concept of how the treated result will appear. Every dentist knows perfect intercuspation of the teeth. That is not what is meant; rather, one must be aware at the very start of treatment of the detailed deviations from perfect intercuspation that can be expected in a case because of the very nature of the problem; for example, if the maxillary incisors are disproportionately wide for the mandibular incisors, the most perfect mechanotherapy cannot effect a perfect posterior occlusion and an ideal overbite and overjet relationship. Under such circumstances, one usually treats to a perfect posterior occlusion and admits that the nature of the case will require a bit more overjet than would have appeared had the tooth widths been more harmonious. Thus, the retention is planned only after a clear estimate of the probable result has been formed. It always is advisable to write into the treatment plan any expected difficulties during retention or any expected tendencies to relapse. This serves to remind one, as treatment ends, of details that were fresh in mind during the thorough study always done at the start of treatment. The details of the retention phase of treatment are given in Chapter XV.

C. Treatment Planning in the Primary Dentition

1. Reasons for Treatment

Treatment in the primary dentition is undertaken for the following reasons:

a) To remove obstacles to normal growth of the face and of the dentition.

b) To maintain or to restore normal function.

2. Conditions That Should Be Treated

Conditions that *should* be treated in the primary dentition are:
a) Anterior and posterior crossbites.
b) Cases in which primary teeth have been lost and closure of space may result.
c) Unduly retained primary incisors that are interfering with the normal eruption of the permanent incisors.
d) Malpositioned teeth that may interfere with proper function or induce faulty patterns of mandibular closure.
e) All habits that cause abnormal function or may distort growth.

3. Conditions That May Be Treated

a) Distoclusions that are positional, at least in part. Occlusal equilibration or tooth movements may remove the functional aspect, the rest of the problem being treated later.
b) Open bites due to tongue-thrusting or digital sucking habits.

4. Contraindications to Treatment in the Primary Dentition

a) When there is no assurance that the results will be sustained.
b) When a better result can be achieved with less effort at another time.

D. Treatment Planning in the Mixed Dentition

The mixed dentition period is the time of greatest opportunity for occlusal guidance and the interception of malocclusion. At this time, the dentist has his greatest orthodontic challenges and his finest opportunities.

1. Reasons for Treatment

Any case may be treated in the mixed dentition:
a) Provided that the treatment does not impede normal growth of the dentition.
b) Provided that the malocclusion cannot be treated more efficiently in the permanent dentition. Emphasis should be placed on guidance of growth, interception of a developing malocclusion and elimination of the first symptoms of what might become serious malocclusions that must be treated in the permanent dentition.

2. Conditions That Should Be Treated

Conditions that *should* be treated in the mixed dentition are:
a) Loss of primary teeth endangering the length of the arch.

b) Closure of space due to the premature loss of primary teeth; the length of the arch must be regained.

c) Malpositions of teeth that interfere with the normal development of occlusal function or cause faulty patterns of mandibular closure.

d) Supernumerary teeth that may cause malocclusion.

e) Crossbites of permanent teeth.

f) Malocclusions resulting from deleterious habits.

g) Oligodontia if closure of space is preferable to prosthesis.

h) Localized spacing between the maxillary central incisors for which orthodontic therapy is indicated.

i) Neutroclusion with extreme labioversion of the maxillary anterior teeth (maxillary dental protraction).

j) Class II (distoclusions) cases of a functional type.

k) Class II (distoclusions) cases of a dental type.

3. CONDITIONS THAT MAY BE TREATED

Conditions that *may* be treated in the mixed dentition are:

a) Class II malocclusions of a skeletal type.

b) Class II malocclusions.

c) All malocclusions accompanied by extremely large teeth. If serial extractions are to be undertaken, treatment must be instituted in the mixed dentition.

d) Gross inadequacies of the apical bases.

E. Treatment Planning in the Permanent Dentition

All malocclusions possible to correct *may* be treated in the permanent dentition of the young adult, although, as noted earlier, that is not necessarily the best time for some problems. Orthodontic therapy may be carried out for adults of older ages, although, of course, tooth movements do not occur as quickly as they do in adolescents.

F. Limiting Factors in Orthodontic Therapy

1. FACTORS RELATED TO THE INDIVIDUAL PATIENT

So much variability is seen among orthodontic patients that sophisticated diagnostic technics have been developed for identifying the individual characteristics of each patient to be treated.

a) Limiting Skeletal Factors

The most limiting skeletal factors are those of gross osseous dysplasia, wherein one or more parts of the craniofacial skeleton are in disharmony with other parts of that particular face. The clinical problem then is primarily one of disharmonies within an individual face rather than deviations in absolute size from population norms (see Chapters IV and XII).

b) Limiting Dental Factors

The primary limiting dental factors include disharmony between the total tooth size and available space in the arch perimeter, variations in the number of teeth, intra-arch tooth size disharmonies and inter-arch tooth size disharmonies. The best-planned orthodontic treatments can go awry because the number and size of teeth for the patient are not in harmony with other features.

c) Limiting Neuromuscular Factors

The most important and frequent limiting neuromuscular factors are abnormal reflex activities, including lip functions, tongue-thrusting, swallowing and functional mandibular movements adaptive to occlusal disharmonies. Less frequently seen, but more severe, neuromuscular factors include the retention of endogenous orofacial infantile neuromuscular behavior and neuromuscular behavior resulting from pathologic conditions, for example, those resulting from brain deficits. Chapters V and X should be read for an understanding of the limiting neuromuscular factors in orthodontic treatment planning.

2. FACTORS RELATED TO THE INDIVIDUAL DENTIST

Just as patients and malocclusions vary, so there is wide variation in the aptitude, training, experience, personality and attitude of dentists who treat malocclusions. These variations have a marked effect on the quality of the treated result.

a) Aptitude

Aptitude, or native ability, is clearly differentiated from training or experience. The technical aptitudes and their influence on dentistry are well known. What may be less appreciated in orthodontics are the intellectual or conceptional aptitudes. Those who would treat malocclusions must adopt a long-term view; hence, treatment must await biologic response and growth. Such a philosophic point of view comes easily to some but not to all. Successful orthodontics requires a biologic point of view on the part of the dentist—an aptitude for understanding biologic response. This aptitude is clearly differentiated from the aptitudes for technical and mechanical skills. Finally, specific diagnostic capacities are of use in orthodontics. For most malocclusions there are several satisfactory treatment plans that may be followed. The dentist who requires a clear concept of right and wrong, the identification of the one best way to treat every case, etc., will encounter difficulties in orthodontics. Such narrow views are useful in achieving technical skill; they are handicapping when developing broad diagnostic capacities in orthodontics.

b) Training

Most dentists in North America have had less undergraduate orthodontic training than for most other clinical subjects. Therefore, the general dentist desiring to broaden his abilities in orthodontics begins with a handicap of which he may not be aware. Furthermore, there are not many short courses available in orthodontics for the general practitioner and very few include the actual treatment of malocclusions. Even the well-organized graduate courses for orthodontic specialty training vary according to the desires and experience of the staff available at each dental school. Furthermore, there are even today, in both undergraduate and graduate courses, occasional evidences of parochialism in orthodontic training. The dentist who would treat malocclusions must analyze carefully the advantages and disadvantages of the training he has had and the methods available to him to strengthen and improve himself.

c) Experience

The finest graduate training program in the world is not an adequate substitute for clinical experience.

d) Attitude

Any of us may have unconscious personal biases or handicapping attitudes toward ourselves and our clinical work. If we have unjustified self-esteem or overrate the training we have had, we may be handicapped in our clinical efforts. Perhaps the most important single attitude for the clinical orthodontist is that of objective criticism of his own clinical efforts.

e) Adherence to Poor Methods

One must use the best method available, but as new discoveries and innovations are made, the best methods of one period become poorer methods in another. Good orthodontic clinicians are constantly on the lookout for improvements in treatment methods. Adherence to unfounded or poorly based methods is inexcusable, since today the dissemination of orthodontic knowledge to the profession through journals and textbooks is so thorough and widespread. There is, unfortunately, some evidence of "cultism" still remaining in orthodontics; such parochial attitudes are found less frequently in the experienced and well trained.

3. Factors Related to the Nature of Orthodontics Itself

Orthodontics is a difficult clinical practice with many limiting factors that are common to the field itself and apply to all who treat malocclusions. "The rules of the game" of orthodontics are somewhat at variance with successful principles applicable in other fields of clinical dentistry. Often the dentist is unaware that the factors by which he achieves success in restorative and prosthetic dentistry are not necessarily the same factors that guarantee success in orthodontics.

a) The Nature of Developmental Oral Biology

The nature of developmental biology is such that although there is considerable variation in morphology, the unfolding of the growth pattern and the response to orthodontic therapy, the clinician is still limited by the nature of growth itself. Growth takes place at specific sites in a specific fashion, in specific directions and occurs within a rather rigid time pattern. As yet, we are limited in our predictive abilities and our control of growth processes. These limitations include our inability to condition easily all neuromuscular reflexes, produce growth of bones at will, stabilize all occlusions exactly where we might wish them to stabilize and so forth.

b) Role of the Patient in Orthodontic Therapy

The finest orthodontic treatment plan and the most meticulously made orthodontic appliance will achieve little if parents and patient are not enthusiastically supportive of the dentist's efforts. In orthodontics, as much as in any other clinical field, the patient determines the success of treatment. Dentists who treat malocclusions must exhibit skill in child psychology, patience and understanding of interpersonal dynamics if they are to be successful.

c) Paucity of Adequate Compromising Alternative Treatments

For a discussion of the problems of compromise in orthodontic therapy, see Section B-1-b.

G. Some Common Mistakes

For several years, I analyzed and categorized the types of orthodontic problems brought to me by family dentists seeking consultation. A further analysis was made of a number of cases assigned to the undergraduate clinic that were not completed there and required more comprehensive therapy than had been envisaged. No claim is made that these findings are universally applicable, but it is interesting to note that in the many cases studied, 88% involved three types of malocclusions only.

Space problems, 46%	Severe open bites, 11%
Class II, 31%	Miscellaneous, 12%

The greatest percentage of space problems arose because an inadequate diagnosis had been made and the case thus was classified erroneously, e.g., a gross discrepancy case was treated as a space supervision case. In other instances, the clinician treating the case had mistaken ideas concerning the growth of the dental arches. It is most difficult for the inexperienced clinician to comprehend just how severe a shortage of 2–3 mm. in each quadrant really is. Other difficulties arose in the handling of discrepancy cases by extraction of teeth when the clinician treating the case did not have available the skills and technics for closing the spaces remaining after alignment was achieved.

All dentists can, of course, recognize Class II molar relationship, but even the skilled cephalometrist has difficulty in assessing the skeletal contribution to that molar relationship. It is understandable that the dentist in general practice might have problems with the Class II syndrome, since all orthodontists have problems with this difficult group of malocclusions. It would seem that the more experienced the clinician the more he respects the dominance of skeletal patterning on occlusal relationships.

The enigma of open bite is best resolved by abandoning a morphologic point of view and accepting the fact that open bites may be caused by many different factors. As soon as a thorough differential diagnosis and an understanding of the etiology of open bite is appreciated, it is quickly seen that some open bites are easy to treat and others are nearly impossible.

After teaching undergraduate dental students for a number of years, and counseling many general practitioners concerning their orthodontic problems, I have become convinced that the key to orthodontic success in general practice lies in (1) a thorough knowledge of growth and development, on which is based (2) a practical diagnostic ability. The technical skills, although important for all orthodontics, are perhaps not as difficult to master as the skills in differential diagnosis. The dentist who fails to recognize the primary role of growth and development and the overriding importance of the differential diagnosis will have continual trouble with his orthodontic treatments irrespective of his technical skills. According to our own data, the family dentist's mistakes arose nine times out of ten because of his inability to appreciate and diagnose correctly a space management problem, a Class II malocclusion or a severe open bite.

TREATMENT

Here is the beginning of Chapter XV—the portion of the volume designed for ready clinical reference.

XV

Treatment of Clinical Problems

What you should put first in all the practice of our art is how to make the patient well; and if he can be made well in many ways, one should choose the least troublesome.—
HIPPOCRATES, *On Joints*

Theories are always thin and unsubstantial; experience only is tangible.—HOSEA BALLOU

A. Number of Teeth (p. 473)

1. Missing teeth
   a) Causes
      1) Heredity
      2) Ectodermal dysplasia
      3) Localized inflammations or infections
      4) Systemic conditions
      5) Expression of evolutionary changes in the dentition
   b) Diagnosis
   c) Treatment
      1) Maxillary lateral incisors
      2) Mandibular second bicuspids
      3) Multiple absence of teeth
2. Loss of permanent teeth due to trauma, caries, etc.
   a) Treatment
      1) Maxillary central incisors
      2) Maxillary lateral incisors
      3) Maxillary cuspids
      4) Maxillary first bicuspids
      5) Maxillary second bicuspids
      6) Maxillary first permanent molars
      7) Maxillary second molars
      8) Maxillary third molars
      9) Mandibular central incisors
      10) Mandibular lateral incisors
      11) Mandibular cuspids
      12) Mandibular bicuspids
      13) Mandibular molars
   b) Multiple loss of permanent teeth

3. Supernumerary teeth
    a) Diagnosis
    b) Treatment
        1) In primary dentition
        2) Teeth with conical crowns
        3) Supplemental teeth of normal size and shape
        4) Supernumerary teeth showing variations in size and shape
    c) Discussion

B. Variations in size of teeth (p. 485)

  1. Diagnosis
  2. Large teeth
  3. Small teeth
  4. Anomalies of tooth shape
    a) Maxillary lateral incisors
    b) Mandibular second bicuspids
    c) Miscellaneous anomalies of shape

C. Problems in the mixed dentition (p. 488)

  1. Space management
    a) Introduction
    b) Maintenance of arch perimeter
        1) Caries of primary teeth
        2) Loss of individual primary teeth
        3) Multiple loss of primary teeth
    c) Regaining space in the arch perimeter
        1) Mesial drift of permanent molars
        2) Distal movement of first permanent molars
    d) Space supervision
        1) Mesial step (Class I) protocol
        2) Flush terminal plane (end-to-end) protocol
        3) Distal step (Class II) protocol
    e) Gross discrepancy problems
        1) Diagnosis
        2) General rules
        3) Treatment protocol
        4) Precautions
  2. Difficulties in eruption
    a) Alterations in sequence of eruption
        1) Premature eruption of individual teeth
        2) Delayed eruption of individual teeth
    b) Ectopic eruption of teeth
        1) Maxillary first permanent molar
        2) Maxillary cuspids
        3) Mandibular incisors
        4) Other teeth
    c) Impaction of teeth
        1) Diagnosis
        2) Mandibular third molars
        3) Maxillary cuspids
        4) Mandibular and maxillary second bicuspids
        5) Other teeth

2. General principles
   a) Anchorage
   b) Space
   c) Occlusion
   d) Retention
3. Uprighting second molars
4. Congenitally missing maxillary lateral incisors
5. Crowded mandibular incisors
6. Deep bite
7. Individual tooth movements

A. Number of Teeth

1. MISSING TEETH

By missing teeth is meant those teeth whose germ did not develop sufficiently to allow the differentiation of the dental tissues. Somewhat less than 4% of the population have one or more teeth congenitally missing. Missing teeth constitute a clinical problem seen more frequently than supernumerary teeth. The teeth most frequently found congenitally missing are mandibular second bicuspids, maxillary lateral incisors and maxillary second bicuspids, in that order (see Chapter VI, Section E-2-a). Complete absence of all teeth, called anodontia, is seen only rarely.

Oligodontia is the term used when parts of the complete dentition are missing. Oligodontia often—and incorrectly—is called "partial anodontia."

a) Causes

The principal known causes of congenital absence of teeth follow.

1) HEREDITY.—There is a familial distribution of congenital absence of teeth in many instances, and heredity as an etiologic factor of importance has been accepted quite generally by investigators (see Chapter VI).

2) ECTODERMAL DYSPLASIA.—Congenitally missing teeth are noted frequently in conjunction with other clinical manifestations of disturbances in the development of ectodermal tissue; for example, anhidrosis and absence of the hair follicles.

3) LOCALIZED INFLAMMATIONS OR INFECTIONS.

4) SYSTEMIC CONDITIONS.—Rickets, syphilis and severe intrauterine disturbances are claimed by some to lead to the destruction of developing tooth germs.

5) EXPRESSION OF EVOLUTIONARY CHANGES IN THE DENTITION.—Some authorities believe that, in the future, man will have neither third molars nor maxillary lateral incisors, just as he may already have lost fourth molars.

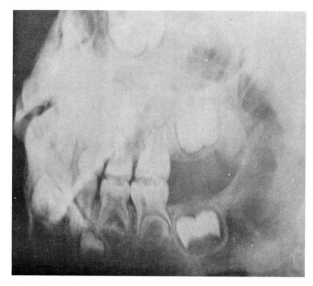

Fig. XV-1.—Tooth sac before calcification. Note that the mandibular second bicuspid tooth sac can be seen clearly even though very little calcification has started.

b) Diagnosis

The diagnosis of missing teeth is based wholly on the findings in the radiograph. The differential problem is one of distinguishing these teeth from those displaying greatly delayed calcification. In this connection, it must be remembered that the teeth show great individual variations in their patterns of development. Well-taken radiographs will show the tooth sac before calcification begins (Fig. XV-1). If, instead of a circumscribed homogeneous area in the bone, indicative of a tooth germ before calcification begins, there is trabeculation, one can assume the absence of the germ (Fig. XV-2). There can be no calcification without the germ.

Mandibular second biscuspids show the greatest variation in differentiation and calcification. Often it will seem that calcification is not to begin, and serial radiographs will suggest that the germ is dormant (Fig. XV-3). With a magnifying glass, sometimes one can detect minute signs of activity indicative of delayed or slow calcification rather than failure of the tissue to differentiate.

Ordinarily, it is possible at the age of $4\frac{1}{2}$–5 years to discern the presence or absence of all teeth but third molars in well-taken intra-oral radiographs. For this reason, it is strongly urged that a complete dental radiographic survey be taken of each patient at this age. Such a survey is one of the most important single steps in orthodontic diagnosis and the interception of malocclusion. Nothing is more embarrassing than

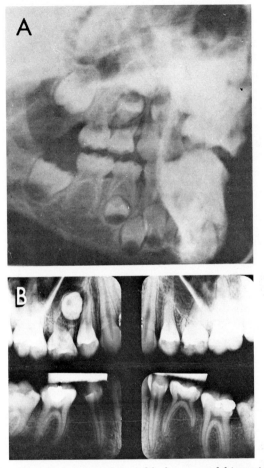

Fig. XV-2.—Congenital absence of mandibular second bicuspids. **A,** note fine trabeculae of bone of the alveolar process beneath the second primary molar. **B,** a similar situation in three of four quadrants. Even though the bicuspid is present in one quadrant, it is delayed in development, malformed and unerupted.

Fig. XV-3.—Delayed development of second bicuspids. Contrast their root development with that of the first bicuspid and cuspid.

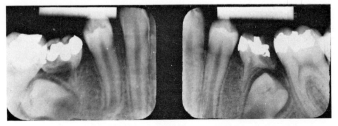

to discover the congenital absence of a tooth in a child who has been under your care for several years. If for no other reason than this problem of congenitally missing teeth, one should have on file for each young patient a complete radiographic survey at the earliest possible age.

c) Treatment

1) MAXILLARY LATERAL INCISORS.—Two courses of treatment are open to the clinician: (1) moving the cuspids mesially for use in place of lateral incisors and (2) a prosthesis.

The choice is dependent on:

Age of patient.
Conformation of cuspids.
Position of cuspids.
Suitability of central incisors and cuspids as abutments.
Desires of patient.
Depth of bite.

Moving the cuspids to serve as lateral incisors:

Advantages:

Unnecessary to prepare abutment teeth.
Less chance for maxillary third molars to become impacted.
Is permanent, not necessary to replace at a later date.

Disadvantages:

Does not work well after all permanent teeth are erupted.
Can be done only in carefully selected cases.
Takes more time than the prosthetic approach.

Follow this procedure if:

The cuspids are unerupted or only partially erupted and appear of normal size and shape.
The central incisors are of normal or slightly greater than normal mesiodistal diameter.
The maxillary molars already have drifted mesially.
There are no contraindications to orthodontic therapy.
The depth of bite permits it.

Steps in treatment:

Remove the maxillary primary cuspids, if still present, to hasten the eruption of the maxillary permanent cuspids. If possible, try to get them into place in the arch before the bicuspids. Sometimes it is helpful to remove bone overlying a cuspid to hasten and direct its eruption.

The central incisors and first permanent molars may be banded and a labial archwire placed to bring the incisors together. When the cuspids can be banded,

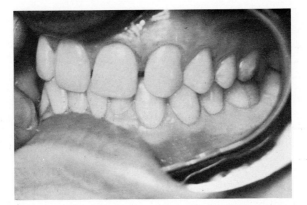

Fig. XV-4.—Treatment of congenital absence of maxillary lateral incisors without a prosthesis.

it will be easier to guide them mesially against the incisors. The archwire must not have a stop so the permanent molars and all erupting bicuspids may drift mesially.

Grind down and polish the labial surfaces of the cuspids to diminish the high curve of convexity so that they more nearly resemble lateral incisors. Grind the incisal edge until it is flat, and gently round the distal incisal angle in simulation of the lateral incisor. It also may be necessary to relieve the lingual aspects of the cuspids. This grinding and polishing should be done in several stages to avoid traumatizing the pulp.

Retain with a Hawley plate retainer.

Prognosis:

If care is taken in choosing the case, this procedure can produce satisfactory results. It is most likely to be indicated when early treatment is possible. *If there is any doubt concerning the success of this plan of treatment, do not begin it.* One must either wait until a decision can be made or use the prosthetic approach. Figure XV-4 illustrates the result in a case in which the cuspid was moved mesially in place of the lateral incisor.

Alternative procedure:

When the cuspids are erupted completely before therapy is started, they still may be moved forward but the technical demands are much greater. Maxillary cuspids are most difficult to control, since their long roots are hard to move without tipping of the crown. When treatment is to be begun this late, there should be clearly defined reasons for not following the alternative prosthetic approach. If completely erupted cuspids are to be moved mesially against the central incisors, maximal banding and complicated mechanotherapy are required in order to achieve the precise tooth movements demanded. Bodily movement of teeth and parallel positioning of roots, not simple tipping of crowns, are needed.

Prosthesis

Advantages:

Ordinarily, less movement of teeth is required.

Takes only a short time.

Can be used on all patients.

Disadvantages:

Necessary to prepare abutment teeth or construct a removable partial denture.

May have to be redone at a later date.

Aesthetic problems are difficult, i.e., matching shades, hiding gold margins, pontics, etc.

Follow this procedure if:

The cuspids are slender and pointed or otherwise ill-suited to serve as simulated lateral incisors.

The central incisors have less than normal width mesiodistally.

The maxillary molars are in complete neutroclusion (applies only if all permanent teeth are erupted).

You cannot decide which of the two plans is better. In other words, when in doubt, it is safer to plan to use bridges for lateral incisors instead of cuspids for lateral incisors.

Steps in treatment:

Preliminary orthodontic procedures.—Preliminary treatment is likely to involve moving the central incisors together and/or moving the lateral segments of the

Fig. XV-5.—Treatment of congenital absence of maxillary lateral incisors. On the patient's right side, the replacement is by a pontic. On the left side, the cuspid has been moved mesially and a pontic placed between the cuspid and the first premolar.

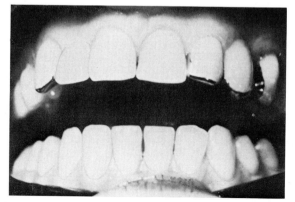

maxillary arch a slight distance distally. Do not prepare the abutment teeth until there is sufficient space for a full-size lateral incisor pontic.

Place the restoration.—Whether this is to consist of two fixed bridges or a partial denture depends on the age of the patient and individual choice.

Prognosis:

The prognosis is directly dependent on the prosthetic skill of the dentist. Figure XV-5 illustrates a case in which the right lateral incisor was replaced by a pontic and the left cuspid was moved mesially.

2) MANDIBULAR SECOND BICUSPIDS.—Again, there are two accepted procedures: (1) holding space for a restoration and (2) moving the first permanent molars forward the width of one cusp. The choice depends largely on the age of the patient and whether the mandibular second primary molar is retained. A third choice, that of keeping the second primary molar permanently in place, often is advanced. To follow this course is to guarantee to the patient a malocclusion and eventually a prosthesis, unless the primary second molar is trimmed to the width of a bicuspid. Although the crown can be cut down this much, the roots usually are still too wide and the first molar cannot move mesially as far as is desirable. The primary second molar may be pared down in this fashion, but only as a very temporary measure during the mixed dentition stage. The correct first permanent molar relationship should be established by the time of arrival of the first bicuspid and before eruption of the second molar.

Early diagnosis is the key to this problem because it greatly lessens the amount of work involved and ensures a more satisfactory result.

Moving mandibular first permanent molars:

Advantages:

Unnecessary to prepare abutment teeth.
Less chance for impacted mandibular third molars.
Is permanent; need not be redone at a later date.

Disadvantages:

Can be completed without complete banding only on rare occasions.
The buccolingual thickness of the alveolar process is not sufficient in many mouths to accommodate the first molar in a forward position when treatment is begun in the late mixed or permanent dentition. When treatment is started in the primary dentition, the first permanent molar's eruption forms a sufficient alveolar process.

Follow this procedure in:

Indicated primary and early mixed dentition cases.
Young adults who are having other orthodontic therapy. It is particularly

appropriate when there is anterior crowding and the first bicuspids must be moved distally.

Steps in treatment—if diagnosed in primary dentition

Remove the mandibular primary second molars and allow the mandibular first permanent molars to move mesially beneath the gum. This movement will take place quickly, but these teeth usually erupt before they are completely forward. In almost every instance it is necessary to band the molar and upright it.

Steps in treatment—if diagnosed in mixed dentition

After the first permanent molar has erupted, it is more difficult to move it mesially without tipping. To do so properly may require bodily movement over a considerable distance and the use of multibanded technics.

Steps in treatment—if diagnosed after eruption of mandibular second permanent molar

Unless the patient is having extensive orthodontic therapy for other reasons and the case is unusually well suited to this approach, it is advisable to place a bridge.

Prognosis:

The prognosis is favorable in all instances, but the task is much easier in the earlier dentitions. In all cases, occlusal correction will be necessary. The final result is a Class III molar relationship, but this should be of little concern.

Prosthesis:

A prosthesis is indicated for the reasons mentioned earlier or when, for any reason, it seems that mesial movement of the first molar is contraindicated. However, the bridge should not be made until eruption of the second permanent molars. During the mixed dentition, it will be necessary to extract the first and second primary molars and guide the first permanent molar into its correct relationship with the other arch.

Discussion.—In the past, I have been much too optimistic concerning the average general dentist's ability to move the first molar forward properly. In the first edition of this book, mesial movement of the first molar was recommended with enthusiasm, since I have done it satisfactorily many times. Unfortunately, there seem to be too many complications here for the unskilled. Therefore, when this seems the desired approach, study the problem carefully and approach it with caution. It is impossible to change your mind and reverse the movements.

3) MULTIPLE ABSENCE OF TEETH.—So many variations appear in the more severe types of oligodontia that it is difficult to formulate a general rule. Treatment may require a blending of orthodontic and prosthetic skills. The problem often is enhanced by small conically shaped teeth. For the most part, severe oligodontia is best handled by a specialist, at least for the orthodontic aspects of the problem.

2. Loss of Permanent Teeth Due to Trauma, Caries, etc.

The loss of fully developed, erupted permanent teeth is a major orthodontic problem. In the anterior region, trauma is the principal cause, whereas caries is largely responsible for early loss of the first permanent molars. Important to an understanding of the effects of loss of permanent teeth is a knowledge of physiologic tooth shifting after extraction. The tendency to shifting is more marked in the maxilla and the process begins more rapidly than in the mandible. It is difficult to predict reliably, however, the extent and direction of shifting in any given patient. Figure XV-6 shows in a diagrammatic fashion the usual direction of physiologic shifting after extraction of a permanent tooth.

Fig. XV-6.—The usual direction of drifting of permanent teeth in the alveolar process after extraction of a permanent tooth.

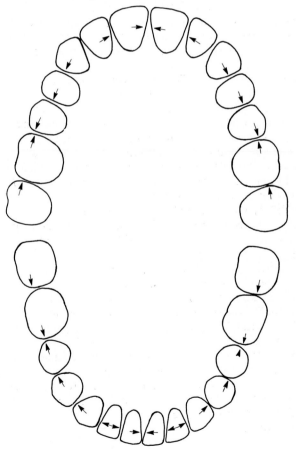

a) Treatment

1) MAXILLARY CENTRAL INCISORS.—Loss of central incisors is a common problem, particularly in boys, whose baseball bats and hockey sticks are notable etiologic agents. The opposite central incisor tends to drift across the midline and the lateral incisor and cuspid on the affected side move mesially. Spacing may occur between the lateral incisor and cuspid or distal to the cuspid. The lateral segments of the arches do not move mesially until considerable time has elapsed. An acrylic plate with acrylic pontic of a snug fit should be placed at once and worn until an age when a permanent restoration can be inserted. If drifting already has begun, treatment with an appliance is necessary to regain the lost space. The high labial archwire with auxiliary springs is a simple, efficient way to effect the necessary tooth movements, if the molar relationship is normal.

2) MAXILLARY LATERAL INCISORS.—Loss of the lateral incisor causes mesial drifting of the cuspid and distal tipping of the central incisor. The treatment is exactly the same as for the central incisor. It is possible in some cases to move the cuspid forward and use it for a lateral incisor. This procedure is described in the section on congenitally missing teeth (A-1-c-1).

3) MAXILLARY CUSPIDS.—This condition, seen rarely, gives rise to distal tipping of the central and lateral incisors with little mesial movement of the first bicuspid. The suggested course of action is to place an acrylic plate, as for the incisors, and add auxiliary springs to move the bicuspid distally and the incisors mesially. A pontic may be added for aesthetic reasons when there is sufficient space to do so.

4) MAXILLARY FIRST BICUSPIDS.—The loss of a first bicuspid without control of the rest of the occlusion is a most severe situation to handle. The incisors and cuspid drift distally and the posterior teeth tip mesially. Spacing probably will appear in the anterior segment. Only rarely can the dentist tip the remaining teeth back to near-normal positions with simple mechanics. Far more frequently multibanded mechanotherapy is required.

5) MAXILLARY SECOND BICUSPIDS.—The same general considerations apply for the second as for the first bicuspids.

6) MAXILLARY FIRST PERMANENT MOLARS.—Special consideration must be given to these molars because they often are lost early in life due to caries. If the first molar is lost before the eruption of the second bicuspid, the latter may drift into the space left by the first molar. When first molars are lost, a dipping in the line of occlusion occurs due to the change in the axial inclination of the remaining posterior teeth. There also is a concomitant closure of the bite. The result of the loss of one or more first molars at any age invariably produces a difficult clinical task. Immediate steps should be taken to control and direct the drifting of the remaining teeth.

Treatment is best carried out with an appliance involving banding of all the teeth.

The extraction of four first molars as a prophylactic measure is not to be recommended.

7) MAXILLARY SECOND MOLARS.—Loss of these teeth gives rise to mesial drifting of the third molars. The best policy is to leave this condition alone, since, in time, the third molar often comes into an acceptable occlusal relationship.

8) MAXILLARY THIRD MOLARS.—No shifting of the other teeth occurs with the loss of a third molar, which has little orthodontic significance.

9) MANDIBULAR CENTRAL INCISORS.—These are treated as are the central incisors in the maxilla (Section A-2-a-1), except that an appliance consisting of banded teeth and a labial archwire is more suited to the regaining of lost space.

10) MANDIBULAR LATERAL INCISORS.—Treatment is the same as for the mandibular central incisors.

11) MANDIBULAR CUSPIDS.—Treatment is the same as for the maxillary cuspids.

12) MANDIBULAR BICUSPIDS.—Basically, this is the same problem as with the maxillary bicuspids. However, the mandibular molars do not drift mesially as rapidly as do the molars in the maxilla.

13) MANDIBULAR MOLARS.—Treatment is the same as for the maxillary molars.

b) Multiple Loss of Permanent Teeth

When more than one tooth is lost, the same principles are kept in mind as were noted for the loss of individual teeth. In children, the etiologic factor is most likely to be an accident; in adults, caries. When the teeth are lost simultaneously, as in the case of trauma, there is little drifting of the remaining teeth. In adults who have lost their teeth gradually, the migration of the remaining teeth enhances the occlusal problem. No simple rules can be stated, but do not overlook the possibilities of improving the occlusion with orthodontic treatment before inserting a prosthesis.

3. SUPERNUMERARY TEETH

Supernumerary teeth are encountered less frequently than congenitally missing teeth. They occur more often in the maxilla, particularly in the premaxillary region, than in the mandible. The principal causative factors are said to be (1) heredity, (2) epithelial remnants and (3) gross aberrations in development, such as the supernumeraries seen with cleft palate. They often are classified according to type:

1. Teeth with conical crowns, Black's "enamel droplets." These usually are

found at the maxillary midline, either singly or in clusters. Often they erupt ectopically, even into the nasal floor.

2. Teeth of normal form and size that are supplemental to those of the regular dentition.

3. Teeth showing variation in size and cuspal form. These may be larger or smaller than normal or the occlusal surface may be deeply pitted. They are recognized by their anatomy, however, and usually are found near their "proper" place in the dental arch.

a) Diagnosis

The diagnosis is based on the radiograph and careful measurement of the teeth in question. Occlusal view radiographs are especially helpful in locating and diagnosing supernumerary teeth (see Fig. XI-4).

b) Treatment

1) IN PRIMARY DENTITION.—Supernumeraries are encountered only rarely in the primary dentition. When seen, they usually are well-formed supplemental teeth. A good rule to follow is to leave them in place unless they are causing some form of malocclusion or malfunction, for example, a functional crossbite due to tooth interference.

2) TEETH WITH CONICAL CROWNS.—These teeth only rarely can have functional use in the mouth. The treatment decision is based on ascertaining whether they may be direct causes of some form of malocclusion. Often they are so placed that the normal teeth must change their course of eruption. If such is the case, remove the supernumerary teeth, taking care not to harm the follicles of the other teeth. If the supernumerary teeth can do no harm, they may be left in position until a later time. They follow no set pattern of eruption, so they must be observed at regular intervals. Always they must be removed eventually.

3) SUPPLEMENTAL TEETH OF NORMAL SIZE AND SHAPE.—Maxillary lateral incisors are the teeth seen most frequently in this category, although maxillary central incisors are observed as well. Rarely is the size of the crowns of the supernumerary teeth exactly that of the normal teeth. If the problem is unilateral, measure all three teeth; that is, the two normal teeth and the supernumerary tooth. The mesiodistal diameter of two of the teeth will be found to be the same. The odd-sized tooth is the accessory member. Do not remove a tooth until the root formation, crown size and position have been studied. To extract the wrong tooth may cause disharmony and shifting of the midline of the dental arch. There are uncommon instances in which the supernumerary tooth is of good formation and in better position to remain in the arch than the normal tooth.

4) SUPERNUMERARY TEETH SHOWING VARIATIONS IN SIZE AND SHAPE.—Such teeth should be removed as soon as it is possible to do so without damaging the follicles of nearby normal teeth.

c) *Discussion*

Early diagnosis and careful observation will enable the operator to decide on the timing in these cases. Timing is important, since the supernumerary tooth seldom is a major orthodontic problem if it is studied early in the dentition's development. To neglect the condition is to create a more severe clinical task. Treatment with appliances may be required for alignment after the removal of the supernumerary tooth, but many of these cases are self-corrective.

B. Variations in Size of Teeth

Variation is a rule of nature, and teeth are no exception. The prosthodontist always has carefully chosen the exact size and shape of teeth to provide perfect alignment for a given dental arch. In contrast, orthodontists for years wrote and practiced as if all teeth were the same size and the size of the basal bone could be altered at will. The orthodontist, obviously, cannot choose the size of teeth with which he would deal. Further, he now knows that orthodontic therapy can bring about changes in the alveolar process only, the apical base remaining largely unaltered. A box of a given size can hold only so many marbles; the rest must spill out. A similar condition often is seen in orthodontic practice, when malalignment and jumbling of the teeth frequently is an expression of a disharmony between the size of teeth and the dimensions of the basal arch (Fig. XV-7).

The introduction of cephalometrics has provided a considerable amount of knowledge concerning the variations in the pattern of growth and dimensions of the facial skeleton. As yet, it is impossible to make a set of measurements of the facial bones and decide exactly how much

Fig. XV-7.—Dental casts of two mouths with teeth exactly the same size. Since the incisors are markedly crowded in the cast at the left and aligned in the cast at the right, the difference must be due to the size of the osseous bases.

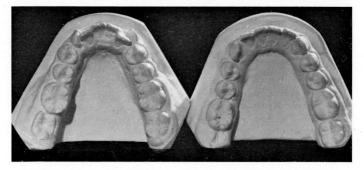

tooth substance would provide an ideal occlusion—or if this is necessarily desirable. Knowledge concerning variation in size of teeth, however, is available and is of great assistance in diagnosis. Since there is such variation in size of teeth from one individual to another, it is advantageous to learn, in each instance, the dimensions of the structures with which one must work. Table VI-5 (p. 193) gives the mean mesiodistal widths of the permanent teeth and some indication of their range in size. Certain correlations exist among the various measurements. There is, in fact, a rather high correlation, for biologic data, among all the widths of teeth except the four teeth developing within the premaxilla. This correlation makes it possible to measure certain of the first teeth to erupt and to predict, with some reliability, the size of the teeth not yet erupted. This procedure is explained in Chapter VIII, The Orthodontic Examination. Although it is impossible to ascertain the precise dimension of the osseous facial skeleton without elaborate cephalometric procedures, certain facts concerning the growth of the face can be utilized routinely (Chapters IV and XII). The determination of whether teeth will fit into a given arch is one of the most difficult of all orthodontic diagnostic decisions. But to try to make it without even knowing the size of the teeth is to handicap oneself unnecessarily.

1. Diagnosis

Diagnosis is carried out by use of the tooth-measuring gauge shown in Figure VIII-3 (p. 279). A Boley gauge may be used instead, although its larger size makes it less handy in the mouth. Always record the measurements of the teeth as part of the written examination record. Great help also will be obtained from the diagnostic procedures described in Chapter XI.

2. Large Teeth

The term "large teeth" is relative, for teeth that are large for one dental arch may not be large for another (see Fig. XV-7). The problem of teeth that are too large for their arch (or is it an arch too small for the teeth?) is discussed later under Space Management (Section C-1). In reading the section on space management, pay particular heed to the sections on space supervision (C-1-d) and gross discrepancy problems (C-1-e).

3. Small Teeth

Always measure the teeth to make sure that the problem is truly one of small teeth. Small teeth usually result in a generalized diastematic condition, whereas with the various sucking or tongue habits the space problem is more localized.

a) Treatment

Orthodontic therapy often is contraindicated in case of extremely small teeth because the tongue and lips often return the teeth to their original positions after the treatment is completed. Many times the case is best left alone unless the aesthetics are unusually poor; in this circumstance, a series of jacket crowns sometimes may be used. In some instances, the arch may be consolidated and bridgework placed.

4. ANOMALIES OF TOOTH SHAPE

Developmental anomalies showing alteration in coronal conformation are seen in all of the permanent teeth. The teeth affected most frequently are (1) third molars, (2) maxillary lateral incisors and (3) mandibular second bicuspids. Only the last two present practical clinical problems.

a) Maxillary Lateral Incisors

The term "peg lateral" is applied when only the middle lobe calcifies. Treatment is determined by two factors: (1) the age at which the condition is discovered and (2) the size and position of the malformed crown and its root.

If the lateral incisor's crown and root are such that the placement of a jacket crown is ill-advised, the tooth must be extracted. If the condition has been noted before eruption of the cuspids, proceed as in the case of congenitally missing lateral incisors. When the condition is noted after eruption of cuspids, one is more likely to resort to a bridge to replace the lateral incisor.

If the "peg lateral" incisor has a strong root and sufficient crown for the preparation of a satisfactory jacket crown, this type of prosthesis is favored. At the first observation of a "peg lateral" incisor, care must be taken to preserve sufficient space in the arch to insert a jacket crown of proper mesiodistal width. A high labial section on an acrylic plate often is of use in opening space for the jacket crown or for centering the tooth in the space between the central incisor and the cuspid. Banding several anterior teeth and the first molars, however, will permit the use of a labial archwire to open spaces with coil springs. It also makes possible accurate placement of each tooth in its best possible position and provides better root angulation.

b) Mandibular Second Bicuspids

This tooth frequently is seen with two lingual cusps. The tooth is thus wider mesiodistally; otherwise, the extra cusp is of little concern. When such a tooth is seen in the radiograph before its eruption, take steps to ensure that a bit more space is available in the arch than the Mixed

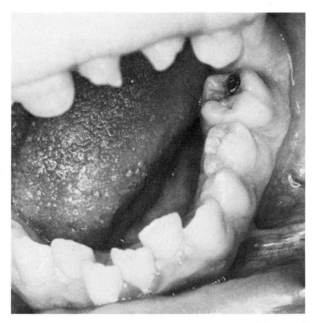

Fig. XV-8.—Abnormally shaped mandibular second bicuspids.

Dentition Analysis predicts. Bizarre ovoid or "egg-shaped" crowns (Fig. XV-8) also are observed; these are extremely difficult to place in a satisfactory intercuspation.

c) Miscellaneous Anomalies of Shape

Many other anomalies of coronal shape may be observed affecting any of the teeth. Each anomaly presents a separate problem requiring singular treatment. Among the anomalies that may create orthodontic problems are: claw form incisors, giant and pygmy forms, dilacerations, odontomas, taurodontia, gemination (twinning), fused teeth, Hutchinson's incisors, dens in dente, hypoplastic teeth and cone-shaped teeth. Certain developmental defects in the texture of dental tissues, for example, amelogenesis imperfecta, result in altered coronal conformation due to excessive wearing down of the teeth.

C. Problems in the Mixed Dentition

1. SPACE MANAGEMENT

a) Introduction

Space management is a general term that includes four subdivisions: space maintenance, space regaining, space supervision and gross dis-

TABLE XV-1.—Symptoms and Space Management Categories

Signs and Symptoms	Maintenance	Regaining	Supervision	Discrepancy
1. Early loss of primary teeth	Yes	Yes	No	No
2. Loss of space in arch	No	Yes	No	No
3. Favorable Mixed Dentition Analysis	Yes	Yes	?	No
4. Active therapy	No	Yes	Yes	No
5. Complete banding of teeth	No	No	?	Yes
6. Good prognosis	Yes	Yes	?	*

*Very dependent on the experience and skill of the dentist.

crepancies. All problems in space management will fall in one of the four categories. The differential diagnosis among them is determined primarily by the Mixed Dentition Analysis (see Chapter XI). Table XV-1 compares the distribution of symptoms associated with space management problems of the four subtypes. The effects of molar relationship on arch perimeter changes during the mixed dentition are discussed under space supervision, since the problem is more critical in that category. However, its significance should not be forgotten when treating other space problems.

b) Maintenance of Arch Perimeter

Space maintenance is undertaken only when the following conditions obtain: (1) loss of one or more primary teeth, (2) no loss of arch length and (3) favorable mixed dentition prediction. Before undertaking any space management therapy, one should understand thoroughly Chapter VI, Development of the Dentition and the Occlusion, and the Mixed Dentition Analysis (Chapter XI, Analysis of the Dentition and Occlusion).

The problem of maintenance of arch perimeter is not peculiar to the mixed dentition, for the arch perimeter is likely to shorten at any time following the loss of either a primary or a permanent tooth (see Section A-2). However, certain difficulties in the mixed dentition are so singular as to require separate technics and hence separate discussion. Here, the explanation will be confined to problems of maintenance of the perimeter of the arch appearing in a normally developing dentition that has suffered from caries or unwanted loss of teeth.

It is necessary to separate these cases carefully from (1) space regaining (see Section C-1-c) and (2) space supervision (see Section C-1-d).

1) Caries of primary teeth.—The most frequent cause of arch perimeter loss in the mixed dentition is caries of the primary molars. A carious lesion on the distal surface of the second primary molar, in particular, allows the first permanent molar to tip mesially. The first step in maintaining arch perimeters is to preserve intact the size of the

primary molar crowns. The most important preventive orthodontic appliance is a properly placed restoration in a primary molar.

2) LOSS OF INDIVIDUAL PRIMARY TEETH.—Much attention has been given to the necessity for placing space-maintainers when a primary tooth has been lost. Too often, however, the effect of the tooth loss on the total arch length has been neglected. A space-maintainer to hold space after the loss of a single tooth is placed only if the following conditions obtain: (1) the permanent successor is present and developing normally, (2) the arch length has not shortened, (3) the space from which the tooth has been lost has not diminished, (4) the molar or cuspid interdigitation has been unaffected by the loss and (5) there is a favorable Mixed Dentition Analysis prediction. There is no reason to insert a space-maintainer if the permanent successor is absent, nor should one maintain 4 mm. of space for a tooth known to be 7 mm. in width. The type of space-maintainer to be used depends on the site of the loss and the operator's preference.

Primary incisors.—These teeth may be lost prematurely due to trauma, although multiple loss due to caries is, of course, seen. In most circumstances, space-maintainers are not necessary; however, this certainly is not a rigid rule. Before the permanent teeth have developed sufficiently to maintain the dimensions of the arch, the loss of a primary incisor can result in a rapid space closure (see Fig. VII-19, p. 263). In every case of premature loss of primary incisors, make a record cast and occlusal plane radiographs for diagnosis and serial study. In children in whom space loss is likely to occur, place a band with a loop of wire soldered to it to touch the tooth on the other side of the edentulous space. Leave this in place until the eruption of the permanent incisor. Space-maintainers for primary incisors rarely are needed if the primary tooth has been lost after age 4 years.

Primary cuspids.—Although the primary cuspids may be prematurely removed because of caries, the eruption of large permanent incisors is a more frequent cause of their unwanted loss. Not infrequently, a large lateral incisor will erupt lingually to the central incisors in the mandible. This is its normal eruptive position, but because of its large size there is no room for it in the arch. The combination of eruptive force and tongue pressure forces the lateral incisor against the primary cuspid's root, causing resorption. Resorption of the primary cuspid's root most likely is in the mandible, particularly if the cuspids cannot move labially and distally into the primate space. Following the loss of primary cuspids, the *mandibular arch* perimeter is likely to be shortened from the front, since the lips may tip the permanent incisors lingually, increasing the overjet and apparently increasing the overbite. As a result, the erupting mandibular permanent cuspids may move anteriorly across the roots of the lateral incisors, finally emerging in a position of labioversion. If other posterior teeth also move anteriorly, it is difficult to correct the cuspids' malposition. Such cuspid malposition

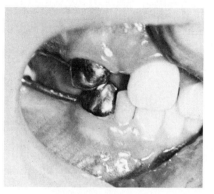

Fig. XV-9.—The misuse of space-maintainers. Fixed cast space-maintainers have prevented the natural movements of the primary cuspids during the eruption of the permanent lateral incisors.

is best averted by prevention of lingual tipping of the incisors with a well-adapted lingual archwire.

Do not tip the mandibular incisors labially with any appliance at this time unless you are very carefully uprighting them from a position of linguoversion. In the *maxillary arch,* the problem is similar, but the variation in the sequence of eruption enhances the chances for the permanent cuspid to move labially. There also seems to be a better chance for the arch to be shortened posteriorly, but there also is a better chance for distal movement of the first permanent molar to provide room in the arch for better placement of cuspids and premolars.

First primary molars.—In most cases, the loss of this tooth is not as serious as the loss of the second primary molar. The severity of the problem is dependent on the sequence of eruption of the succeeding teeth, the molar intercuspation and the age of the patient. Arch perimeter loss is most likely to occur when the first primary molar is lost before the eruption of the first permanent molar. It may occur when the permanent molars' cusps are shallow or there is an end-to-end molar relationship combined with an unfavorable eruption sequence. Many types of space-maintainers have been designed to hold space in this region. Some of those suggested are so complicated as to be ridiculous and impractical. Do not insert an appliance that locks the primary cuspid and second molar together. As the primary cuspid is exfoliated, it must have the chance to move labially and a bit distally (Fig. XV-9). After loss of a first primary molar, one may insert a removable plate or a lingual archwire if other space problems are expected in that arch. If the perimeter is not threatened, a single unit space-maintainer, for example, a preformed stainless steel crown on the second primary molar with a loop engaging the cuspid, may be placed.

Second primary molars.—The most rapid losses in the perimeter of

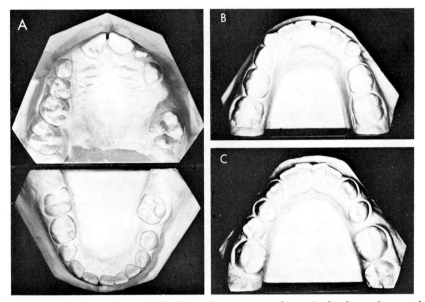

Fig. XV-10.—The effect of the loss of primary molars. **A,** the loss of second primary molars. In both arches, the first permanent molar has a strong tendency to drift mesially and rotate on its long axis. In the mandibular arch, it may tip lingually also. **B** and **C,** the effects of the loss of first primary molars. In order for this amount of space to be lost, the first primary molars must be lost very early, i.e., before the eruption of the first permanent molar.

the arch usually are due to a mesial tipping of the first permanent molar after removal of the second primary molar (Fig. XV-10). When this tooth is lost, always maintain space until the arrival of the second bicuspid. If the first permanent molar has erupted, the appliance may consist of a preformed stainless steel crown form or a band on the first primary molar carrying a wire loop to engage the first permanent molar. The first permanent molar may be banded and the strut placed mesially to engage the distal surface of the first primary molar (see Fig. XVII-30, p. 664). Overlays or crown forms for the first permanent molar are contraindicated, since they prevent the tooth from erupting to its full height. If the first permanent molar has not yet erupted, the free-end acrylic block type of maintainer shown in Figure XVII-51 (p. 694) may be used.

3) MULTIPLE LOSS OF PRIMARY TEETH.—Usually, when several primary teeth are lost, the arch perimeter is shortened and thus *maintenance* of the arch is not indicated. Sometimes it will be necessary to extract more than one primary tooth at the same appointment. If such is the plan, it usually is best to construct the appliance before the extractions and insert it the very day the teeth are removed. A lingual archwire or multiple acrylic space-maintainer will serve well. It is not

necessary to cast elaborate frameworks and meticulously carve occlusal patterns for "primary partial dentures." A block of acrylic to provide a smooth occluding surface, maintain the vertical height and prevent extrusion of the opposite teeth is all that is necessary. Many of these appliances will not even require clasps. Indeed, the occlusal carvings or acrylic tooth pontics may interfere with the normal exfoliation of primary teeth and natural-drifting permanent teeth. The mixed dentition is a dynamic, rapidly changing entity ill-suited to the application of the static prosthetic approach so successful in aged adults. Appliances used with the mixed dentition must neither inhibit nor divert the growth changes taking place. The design of any appliance is dependent on the individual situation. Several suggestions will be found in Chapter XVII.

c) Regaining Space in the Arch Perimeter

Space regaining, as used in this section, means that all of the following conditions obtain: (1) one or more primary teeth have been lost, (2) some space in the arch also has been lost to mesial drift of the first permanent molar and (3) the Mixed Dentition Analysis shows that if one could recapture what was once there, there would be adequate room for all the teeth and the normal mixed dentition adjustments. Regaining what was once there is entirely different from creating that which was never there.

Loss of arch perimeter usually is due to caries or premature loss of primary teeth. Such cases must be differentiated carefully from those in which the tooth size-osseous base relationship is so poor that there is insufficient space for the permanent teeth. The discussion at this point is centered on the cases that once had sufficient length of the arch perimeter but, due to environmental reasons, that length is now shortened. The arch becomes shortened by mesial movement of the first permanent molars or by lingual tipping of the incisors. Correction should be where the loss has occurred. Note the molar relationship, cuspid interdigitation and overjet, since they provide the key to the site of the shortening.

After locating where the arch has shortened, determine, by means of the analysis given in Chapter XI, the exact amount of space that must be regained and the most logical tooth movements to recover that space. Usually, distal movement of first permanent molars is required. But before moving first permanent molars distally it is necessary to understand the nature of the mesial movements that caused the shortening of the arch perimeter.

1) MESIAL DRIFT OF PERMANENT MOLARS.—Mesial drift of the first permanent molars involves three separate kinds of tooth movements, viz., mesial crown tipping, rotation and translation. There are distinct differences in the mode of mesial movement between the upper and lower first molars, differences caused by variations in the crown shape, number of roots and occlusal relationships. Furthermore, the time of

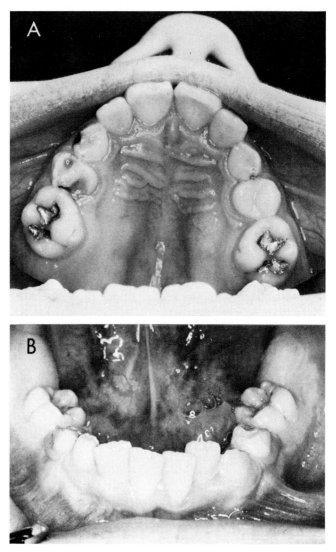

Fig. XV-11.—A, the effects of early loss of primary molars. Note that the maxillary first molars have rotated, tipped and translated mesially. **B,** the lower arch in the same mouth. In the mandibular arch, the first permanent molars, in addition to translating and rotating as they tip mesially, also have tipped lingually. The lingual tipping of the mandibular molars during mesial drifting often is due to the effects of occlusion.

loss of the primary second molar's crown is a determining factor in the type of movement seen. Maxillary first permanent molars quickly tip mesially with the loss of crown substance of the maxillary second primary molars (see Fig. XV-10). Mesial tipping causes the distobuccal cusp to become more prominent occlusally. Due to the large lingual root of the maxillary first permanent molar, rotation of the crown also is seen with mesial tipping, and the distobuccal cusp becomes more prominent buccally as well. When the second primary molar is lost prior to the eruption of the first permanent molar, translation of the first permanent molar during its eruption also may be seen. Mandibular first permanent molars display mesial tipping, crown rotation and translation as well but they also are more likely to show lingual tipping during mesial movement. The lingual tipping is caused by the absence of a lingual root and the fact that occlusal function occurs buccally to the center of mass of the lower molar, a condition aggravated as the first molar drifts mesially. Figure XV-11 illustrates clearly the differences in mesial drifting of maxillary and mandibular first permanent molars.

2) DISTAL MOVEMENT OF FIRST PERMANENT MOLARS.—The basic tooth movement necessary in space regaining is distal movement of first permanent molars, which must recapitulate in reverse the movements that occurred as the tooth drifted mesially. Therefore, the selection of the space-regaining appliance is dependent on whether tipping, rotation, translation or combinations of these movements is required. Some common mistakes in choosing space-regaining appliances should be noted: (1) Often, too complicated an appliance is chosen when a simple appliance would let the tooth fall back more easily into the position from whence it came. (2) A firm purchase on the tooth often is used but it is not necessary except for translation. Actually, tipping and rotation usually occur more readily with finger springs rather than a banded appliance. (3) Failure to achieve all of the necessary movements. It should be noted that surprising amounts of arch perimeter space often are created just by distal tipping and rotation of the first molar. Therefore, tipping and rotation should be achieved prior to attempting translation. Although this sequence may necessitate the use of two space-regaining appliances, it often will save months of treatment time and frequently permits the use of simpler appliances.

A wide variety of space-regaining appliances are available (see Chapter XVII). No more complicated appliance should be used than is required to achieve the necessary space. Table XV-2 suggests which appliances may be indicated for varying amounts of space loss in either arch. Do not overextend the space-regaining appliance. Simple finger springs cannot move molars bodily nor can they lengthen an arch perimeter past its original dimensions and retain a permanent result. Space-regaining appliances are intended to be used solely for recovering space that once was there. Space regaining is not space creating.

The timing of space regaining is important, since the position and

TABLE XV-2.—Space-Regainers for Extensive
Loss of Length of Arch

Amount to be Regained	Mandible	Maxilla
0–2 mm.	Helical spring, loop lingual, split saddle	Split saddle, helical spring
2–4 mm.	"Slingshot," split saddle	Split saddle, sliding yoke
More than 4 mm.		Extra-oral force

stage of development of the second permanent molar often is a limiting factor. When the simpler space-regaining appliances cannot complete the task, one may resort to extra-oral traction, but before using extra-oral traction, the case should be reassessed completely to make certain that the original diagnosis still obtains.

When the loss of perimeter length is so extensive as to be beyond the scope of the simpler appliances, or when there is insufficient time to recover the space before the eruption of the bicuspids and second permanent molars, a far more difficult clinical situation obtains and comprehensive multibanded appliance therapy usually is indicated.

Chapter XVII describes the construction and adjustment of several popular space-regaining appliances. It should be noted that these appliances also are useful when constructing bridges to replace lost first permanent molars, since they may be used for the uprighting and distal movement of second molars prior to their preparations as abutments. Figure XV-11 illustrates typical cases where space regaining was needed.

d) Space Supervision

Space supervision is the term applied when it is doubtful, according to the Mixed Dentition Analysis, whether there will be room for all the teeth. The prognosis for space supervision is always questionable and never good, whereas it always is good for regaining and maintenance. Space supervision cases are those that in your judgment will have a better chance of getting through the mixed dentition with your help than they will without it. Each is a calculated risk; therefore, space supervision is not to be undertaken without patient cooperation and parental understanding. Successfully treated, such cases are among the most comforting victories in interceptive orthodontics; but when fought through and lost, they provide us with our most disheartening moments, since, if extractions of permanent teeth ultimately are necessary, large amounts of space closure will be required. Misdiagnosed space supervision cases that require extractions of permanent teeth are more difficult to treat than gross discrepancy cases because (1) more space closure is needed and (2) the patient's cooperation often ceases after the planned interceptive procedure has failed. Do not oversell

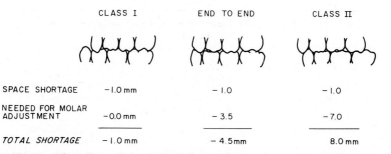

	CLASS I	END TO END	CLASS II
SPACE SHORTAGE	−1.0 mm	− 1.0	− 1.0
NEEDED FOR MOLAR ADJUSTMENT	−0.0 mm	− 3.5	− 7.0
TOTAL SHORTAGE	− 1.0 mm	− 4.5 mm	8.0 mm

Fig. XV-12.—The effect of the molar relationship on the available space. Three hypothetical situations are shown in which it is predicted that there will be a shortage of 1 mm. on each side in the mandible. Where there is a Class I molar relationship, the only problem is the 1-mm. shortage. However, where there is an end-to-end molar relationship, one must account for half a cusp's width (approximately 3.5 mm.) in addition. Where there is a Class II molar relationship, one must allow for the 1-mm. shortage plus the width of an entire cusp (approximately 7 mm.). Naturally, under such circumstances, both the end-to-end and the Class II molar relationship are treated by Class II mechanics, i.e., moving the maxillary dentition distally while preserving the mandibular dentition intact. Further, such cases are poor candidates for intermaxillary elastics, since the elastic traction tends to shorten the mandibular arch length while moving the maxillary molars distally.

space supervision to the parents. Select space supervision cases with great care and maintain careful records, since help from a colleague may be required later. Success is greatly dependent on the clinician's knowledge of the details of mixed dentition development.

Because of the critical effect of molar relationship on utilization of available space (Fig. XV-12), three space supervision protocols are needed. However, several basic principles obtain in all three: (1) space supervision is not begun until the mandibular cuspid and first premolar are in developmental stage 7; (2) primary teeth are extracted serially to provide an eruption sequence of cuspid, first premolar and second premolar in the mandible and first premolar, cuspid and second premolar in the maxilla; (3) an effort is made to keep the mandibular teeth erupting well ahead of the maxillary; (4) a late mesial shift of the mandibular first permanent molar *must not occur.*

1) Mesial step (Class I) protocol (Table XV-3).—This protocol is used when the first permanent molar has already achieved a Class I molar relationship at the time of instituting space supervision (Fig. XV-13, *A*). The first step, the removal of the mandibular primary cuspids, is begun when the mandibular permanent cuspid is at developmental stage 6 or 7 (Fig. XV-13, *C*). The purpose of the first step is to provide space in the arch for the alignment of the mandibular incisors and to induce the mandibular cuspid to erupt before the first bicuspid. One of the most important single steps in space supervision is the correct

TABLE XV-3.—SPACE SUPERVISION PROTOCOL FOR MESIAL STEP
OR CLASS I CASES

STEPS	PURPOSES	TIMING
1. Removal of $\overline{\text{C}}$	1. (a) Align incisors (b) Erupt $\overline{3}$ before $\overline{4}$	1. $\overline{3}$ is stage 6+ or 7
2. Removal of $\overline{\text{D}}$, slicing of $\overline{\text{E}}$	2. (a) Allow $\overline{3}$ to erupt distally (b) Hasten eruption of $\overline{4}$	2. When $\overline{3}$ can no longer erupt normally
3. Archwire and extraction of $\overline{\text{E}}$	3. (a) Prevent mesial drift of $\overline{6}$ (b) Erupt $\overline{5}$ before $\overline{7}$	3. When $\overline{4}$'s eruption is halted by $\overline{\text{E}}$

Fig. XV-13.—See legend on facing page.

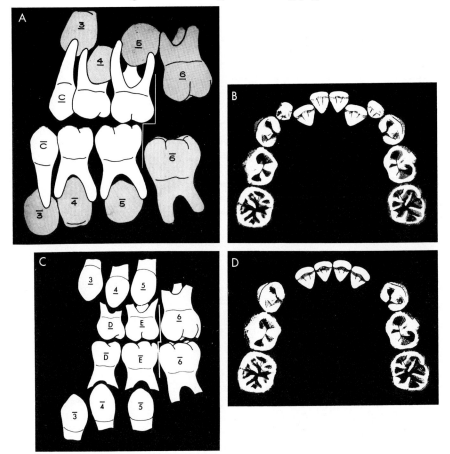

placement of the mandibular permanent cuspid after alignment of the incisors. Several months after the primary cuspids have been removed, it will be found by palpation that the permanent cuspid can no longer erupt normally without moving into labioversion. It is now time for the second step—the removal of the primary first molar and the slicing of the mesial surface of the second primary molar. The purpose of the second step is to allow the cuspid to erupt distally into the line of arch and to hasten the eruption of the first bicuspid at this time. After the cuspids have arrived in the arch there usually is insufficient space for the eruption of the first premolar, since it becomes halted at the mesial

Fig. XV-13.—Space supervision protocol for Class I or mesial step cases. **A,** the mesial step. **B,** typical crowding in the mandibular arch. Note that the primate space is closed. **C,** the first step—removal of mandibular primary cuspids. **D,** the effects on incisor alignment of the removal of primary cuspids. **E,** the second step—removal of the first primary molar and slicing of the mesial surface of the second primary molar. **F,** the effects of removing the first primary molar and slicing the second primary molar. Note, too, that the mesial surface of the second primary molar may be shaped by a small finishing stone to facilitate the eruption of the first bicuspid. **G,** the third step—placement of a lingual archwire and removal of the second primary molars. **H,** the results of the third step.

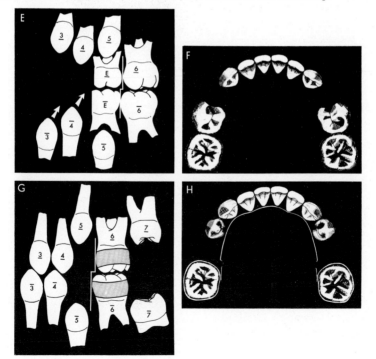

A

Patient R̲i̲c̲h̲a̲r̲d̲ ̲S̲.̲ ̲_____ MIXED DENTITION ANALYSIS Age 9̲ ̲-̲ ̲4̲ Sex M̲_____

Date _____ Address _____ Parent _____

TOOTH SIZE

| | | | | 6.0 | 5.5 | 5.6 | 5.9 | | | |
'Upper

	Right	Left
Space left after alignment of 2 and 1	23.7	23.1
Predicted size of 3 + 4 + 5	22.6	22.6
Space left for molar adjustment	+ 1.1	+ .5

Lower

	Right	Left
Space left after alignment of 2 and 1	20.8	21.5
Predicted size of 3 + 4 + 5	22.2	22.2
Space left for molar adjustment	− 1.4	− .7

Remarks: Overjet = 3.2 mm.   Overbite = 4.1 mm.

Molar relationship = Class I, Class I   cuspid relationship I - I

Fig. XV-14.—Space supervision with a Class I molar relationship. **A,** the Mixed Dentition Analysis for the case. (*Continued.*)

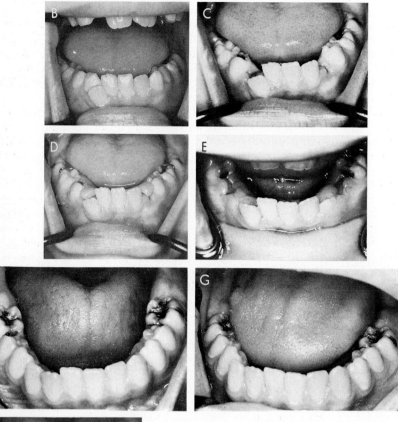

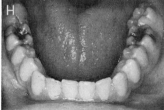

Fig. XV-14 (cont.).—B, at the start of treatment. **C,** at the time of extraction of the mandibular primary cuspids. **D,** a removable acrylic arch-holding appliance was inserted immediately after extraction of the primary cuspid, since the patient had a hyperactive mentalis muscle, which might have collapsed the incisors lingually. Ordinarily, it is better practice to place a lingual archwire in such cases. **E,** 9 months later, at the time of extraction of the first primary molars. **F,** after the loss of the second primary molars. Note the spontaneous improvement in the incisor region, although the contact is not correct between the right lateral incisor and the cuspid. This photo was taken 2 years after the start of treatment. **G,** 1 year later than **F. H,** 1 year later than **G,** or 4 years after the start of space supervision procedures. Compare this photo with **A.** It is doubtful if such a result would have occurred spontaneously by chance alone. Only the intervention and careful supervision of the loss of the primary teeth and the eruption of the permanent teeth could have guided such a result.

surface of the second primary molar. At this time, a holding lingual archwire is inserted and the mandibular second primary molars are extracted. The purposes of this third step are to prevent the mesial drift of the first permanent molar and to cause the second premolar to erupt before the second permanent molar. All of the steps in space supervision are shown in sequence in Table XV-3. Figure XV-13, *A–H* depicts diagrammatically the various steps in the mesial step protocol and Figure XV-14 illustrates a case treated in this manner.

2) FLUSH TERMINAL PLANE (END-TO-END) PROTOCOL (Table XV-4).— The protocol for space supervision with a flush terminal plane (end-to-end) relationship is quite similar to that for a mesial step—with one exception. Since the molars are not yet in a Class I relationship and a late mesial shift cannot be allowed to occur, it is necessary to achieve a Class I molar relationship by guidance of the eruption of the maxillary first permanent molar. Figure XV-15 diagrams how the distal tipping of a maxillary molar during the transitional dentition helps achieve a Class I molar relationship without a late mesial shift in the mandible. A maxillary Hawley-type appliance or Sved plate with helical springs may be used (Fig. XV-17, *C*). The Sved plate frees the occlusion, which aids in the distal tipping of the maxillary first permanent molar, helps flatten the mandibular occlusal plane and removes any occlusal interferences. Study Figure XV-16 carefully, for the details of each step of treatment are depicted in the diagrams. Figure XV-17 illustrates a case treated by this protocol.

3) DISTAL STEP (CLASS II) PROTOCOL.—In the preceding space supervision protocols it has been assumed that the problem is seen in a balanced or nearly balanced facial skeleton. A space supervision problem combined with a distal step is a much more serious matter and the space problem is quite secondary to the skeletal pattern producing the distal step. Many other problems are encountered in addition to that of the

---

TABLE XV-4.—SPACE SUPERVISION PROTOCOL FOR FLUSH TERMINAL PLANE OR END-TO-END CASES

STEPS	PURPOSES	TIMING
1. Max.—appliance. Mand.—remove $\overline{\text{C}}$	1. (a) Tip $\underline{6}$ distally (b) Align incisors (c) Erupt $\underline{3}$ before $\overline{4}$	1. $\overline{3}$ is stage 6+ or 7
2. Remove $\overline{\text{D}}$, slice $\overline{\text{E}}$	2. (a) Allow $\overline{3}$ to erupt distally (b) Hasten eruption of $\overline{4}$	2. When $\overline{3}$ can no longer erupt normally
3. Mandibular lingual archwire, extract $\overline{\text{E}}$	3. (a) Prevent mesial drift of $\overline{6}$ (b) Erupt $\overline{5}$ before $\overline{7}$	3. When $\overline{4}$'s eruption is halted by $\overline{\text{E}}$

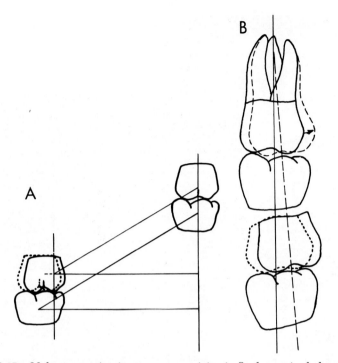

Fig. XV-15.—Molar correction in space supervision in flush terminal plane cases. **A,** the maxillary molar is restrained during the downward and forward growth of the maxilla. Thus, it comes to occupy a relatively different occlusal relationship with the mandibular first permanent molar. **B,** the maxillary first molar is tipped distally a slight amount, thus changing the axial inclination of the tooth during subsequent vertical development. The tooth is *not* moved distally in a translatory fashion; rather, its angle of vertical development is changed so that it comes to occupy a relatively different occlusal relationship with the mandibular first molar after some time has passed.

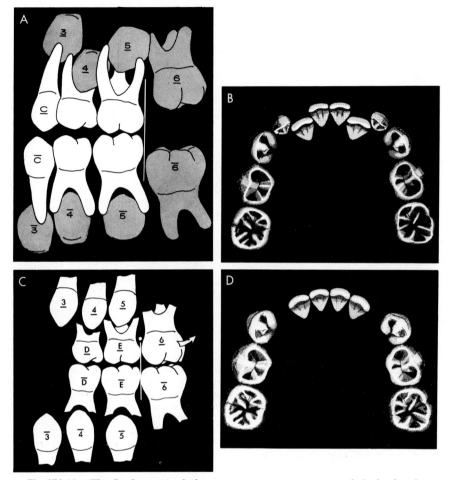

Fig. XV-16.—The flush terminal plane space supervision protocol. **A,** the developing flush terminal plane. **B,** the typical incisal configuration at the start of treatment. **C,** the first step—removal of the mandibular primary cuspids and tipping of the maxillary first molar distally. **D,** the results in the mandibular arch of the first step. (*Continued.*)

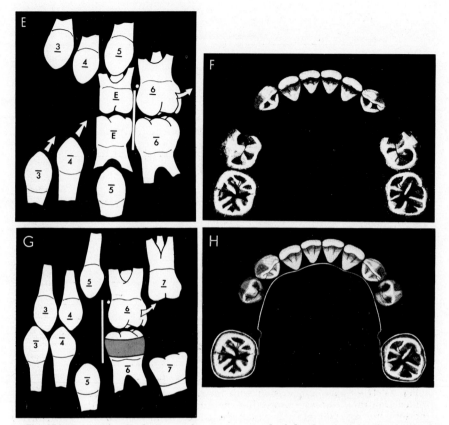

Fig. XV-16 (cont.).—E, the second step—removal of the first primary molar and slicing of the mesial surface of the second primary molar. Note that by this time there is some improvement in the first permanent molar relationship. **F,** the results in the mandibular denture of removal of the first primary molar and slicing and contouring of the second primary molar. **G,** the third step—placing the lingual archwire and removal of the second primary mandibular molars. By this time, the first permanent molars often have a Class I molar relationship. **H,** the results of the third step while awaiting the eruption of the second bicuspid.

A

Patient **Tom K.**   MIXED DENTITION ANALYSIS   Age **11-4**   Sex **M**

Date _____   Address _____   Parent _____

TOOTH SIZE

			6.1	5.7	5.6	6.1			

Upper

	Right	Left
Space left after alignment of 2 and 1	22.3	21.9
Predicted size of 3 + 4 + 5	22.9	22.9
Space left for molar adjustment	−0.6	−1.0

Lower

	Right	Left
Space left after alignment of 2 and 1	21.5	22.0
Predicted size of 3 + 4 + 5	22.5	22.5
Space left for molar adjustment	−1.0	−.5

Remarks: Overjet = **3.5 mm.**   Overbite = **4.2 mm.**

Molar relationship = *Class II, left side almost Class I. When midlines are together molar relationship is end-to-end on both sides.*

Fig. XV-17.—Space supervision with an end-to-end molar relationship. **A,** the Mixed Dentition Analysis. Note that there is scarcely enough room to align the incisors and no available space is predicted for molar adjustment. (*Continued.*)

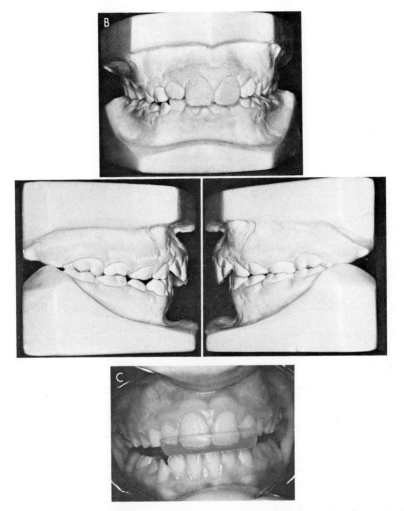

Fig. XV-17 (cont.).—B, the casts at the start of treatment. Note that the patient's right side showed a Class II molar relationship whereas on the left the molars tend toward Class I. Since the midlines do not coincide, it usually is found in such cases of unilateral molar relationship in the mixed dentition that they have an end-to-end molar relationship when a wax bite is taken. **C,** the Sved plate was used to tip the maxillary molars distally during typical serial extractions of the primary teeth in the mandible. (*Continued.*)

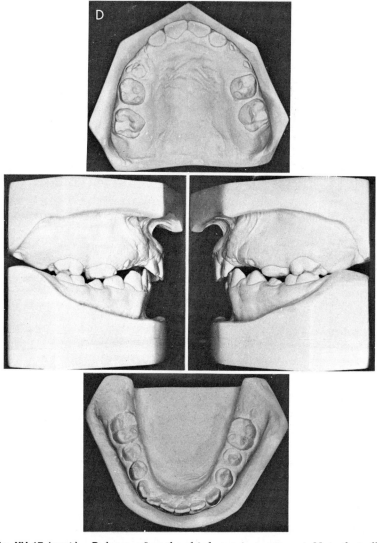

Fig. XV-17 (cont.).—D, later, after the third step in treatment. Note that all the mandibular teeth have erupted well ahead of the maxillary, as was planned. Now both molar relationships tend toward Class I. Further, there is just barely enough room to align all the mandibular teeth, so none of the molar correction has been achieved by a late mesial shift. (*Continued.*)

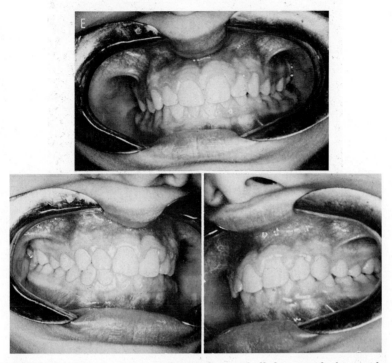

Fig. XV-17 (cont.).—E, after complete eruption of all the cuspids, bicuspids and molars.

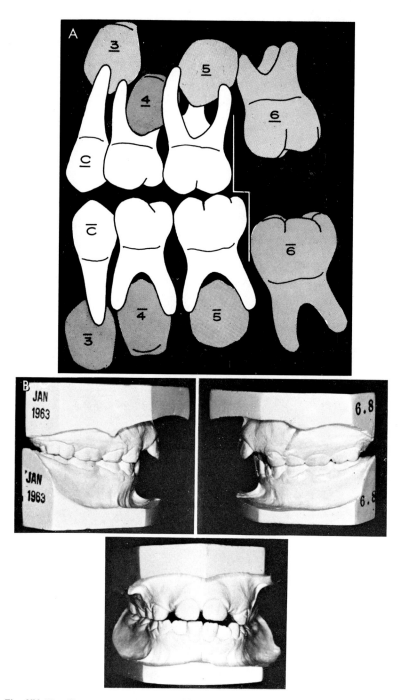

Fig. XV-18.—Space supervision in Class II. **A,** the developing distal step. **B,** the casts at the start of treatment. (*Continued.*)

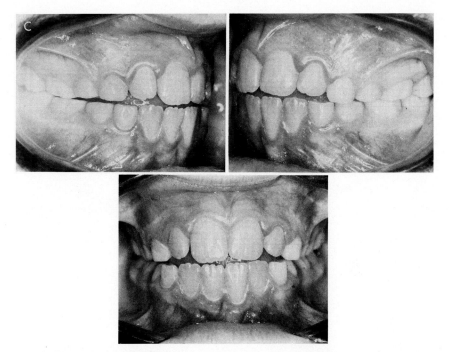

Fig. XV-18 (cont.).—C, after 1 year of treatment. An activator appliance was used to hold the mandibular arch perimeter, aid in correcting the open bite and to optimize mandibular growth. Note that a Class I molar relationship has been achieved and the space situation is better, although the open bit is not yet corrected completely. (*Continued.*)

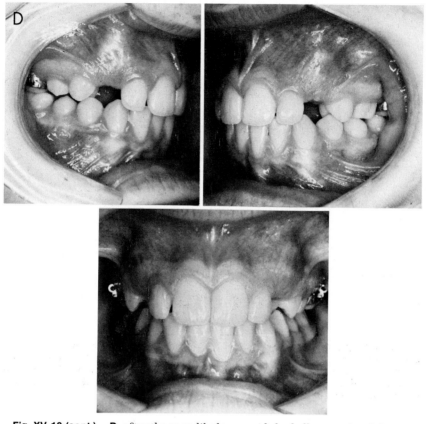

Fig. XV-18 (cont.).—D, after the mandibular cuspids had all erupted and the open bite closed successfully. The case was changed to extra-oral traction lest the Activator jeopardize the integrity of the mandibular arch perimeter. The extra-oral traction served to restrain the Class II growth of the midface and to hold the maxillary arch perimeter during the eruption of the cuspids. Note in **D¹** that the maxillary second bicuspid has been sliced to allow the first bicuspid to drop into occlusion. (*Continued.*)

space situation. The Class II malocclusion must be treated and the teeth must be positioned to camouflage the Class II facial skeleton. Furthermore, there usually are vertical occlusal problems to be corrected and abnormal tongue and lip contractions are seen frequently as well.

Distal step space supervision is begun at the time indicated in the flush terminal plane and mesial step protocols. However, more frequently in distal step space supervision, the mixed dentition therapy is followed by a period of banded appliance therapy to finish the alignment of the permanent teeth. Figure XV-18 illustrates the treatment of a distal step space supervision case.

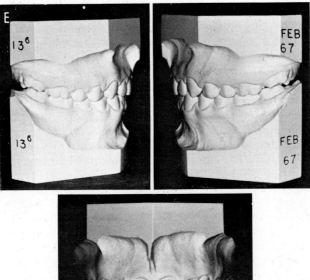

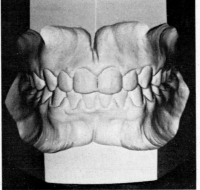

Fig. XV-18 (cont.).—E, the cases after the eruption of the second permanent molars and after the retention period was over.

e) Gross Discrepancy Problems

Gross discrepancy problems are those in which there is a great and significant difference between the sizes of all the permanent teeth and the space available for them within the alveolar arch perimeter. Gross discrepancy problems ordinarily cannot be diagnosed until the early mixed dentition, since no important correlation has been shown to exist between the size of the primary teeth and those of the permanent dentition. Table XV-1 establishes clearly how different gross discrepancy problems are from those of space maintenance and space regaining. The difference between space supervision cases and gross discrepancy problems is largely one of strategy. In space supervision, the goal is to squeeze all the permanent teeth into what obviously is minimal space. In the gross discrepancy problem, it is accepted at the start that insufficient space is available and therefore extraction of permanent teeth is necessary.

1) DIAGNOSIS.—A most meticulous Mixed Dentition Analysis is necessary (see Chapter XI); however, it must be remembered that the skeletal pattern has a significant effect on the alignment of teeth within the dental arch. The discussion herein assumes a balanced facial skeleton. A Mixed Dentition Analysis provides insufficient evidence on which to base a Class II malocclusion treatment plan. One must also study the facial skeleton to determine how the orthodontic treatment will correct or camouflage the skeletal dysplasia and to quantify what effects the comprehensive orthodontic therapy will have on the available space. Tooth movements undertaken to overcome a Class II skeletal dysplasia ordinarily shorten the arch perimeter significantly.

In the adult dentition, the space diagnosis may best be done by a diagnostic setup (see Chapter XI).

2) GENERAL RULES.—No one undertakes the extraction of permanent teeth casually. No dentist should extract permanent teeth as a part of orthodontic therapy unless he has the technical skills to correct all the sequelae of the extractions. Extraction itself provides space, some of which may be absorbed by spontaneous alignment of crowded teeth, but any remaining space is not likely to close spontaneously. Therefore, most cases in which permanent teeth are extracted require comprehensive multibanded appliance therapy to close the spaces remaining, parallel the roots, establish the occlusal plane and correct the intercuspation.

It may be useful to have a few general rules to provide insurance against involvement in unwanted complications. The following were suggested by Eisner.[2] The more a case deviates from them the more comprehensive is the mechanotherapy required to complete the case. When a case satisfies the requirements of all the rules, it may be treated by the protocol that follows with a reasonable chance for success and a minimum chance of trouble.

Rule No. 1: There must be a class I molar relationship bilaterally.

Rule No. 2: The facial skeleton must be balanced anteroposteriorly, vertically and mediolaterally.

Rule No. 3: The discrepancy must be at least 5 mm. in all four quadrants.

Rule No. 4: The denture midlines must coincide.

Rule No. 5: There must be neither an open bite nor a deep bite.

Only a few discrepancy cases will meet all the requirements of these rules, and the more a case deviates from them the more difficult it will be to treat.

3) TREATMENT PROTOCOL.—These procedures involve the planned sequential removal of primary and permanent teeth to alleviate the major dental aspects of the malocclusion seen in gross discrepancy problems. The case may be started when the mandibular first bicuspid has at least a portion of its root forming (Fig. XV-19, *A*). The first active step in treatment is the removal of the mandibular first primary molar,

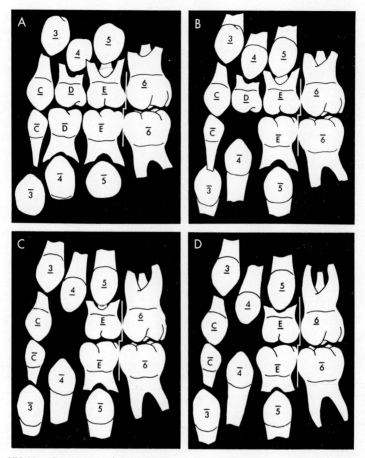

Fig. XV-19.—One protocol for serial extraction of primary and permanent teeth in gross discrepancy cases. **A,** at the start of treatment. Note the Class I molar relationship and the beginning of root development of the cuspid and the first bicuspid. **B,** the first step—removal of the lower first primary molar. **C,** the second step—removal of the upper first primary molar. **D,** the results of steps 1 and 2. Note that the first bicuspid erupts quickly, ahead of the cuspid. As it does so, its root develops and the alveolar process is completely formed in the region. This alveolar development provides bone into which the cuspids may naturally move distally. (*Continued.*)

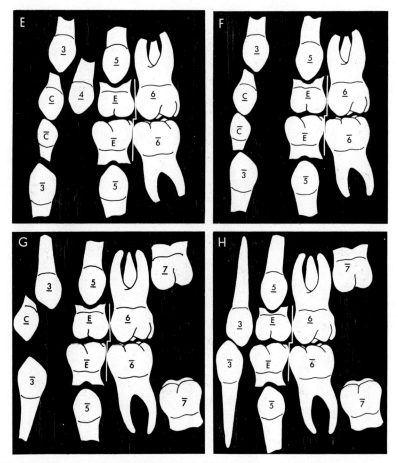

Fig. XV-19 (cont.).—E, the third step—removal of the mandibular first bicuspid. This tooth is removed *after* it has erupted into the mouth, delaying the extraction until intra-oral eruption permits the formation of normal alveolar height in the region. **F,** the fourth step—removal of the maxillary first bicuspid. **G,** the results of steps 3 and 4. The permanent cuspids now move distally into the extraction site readily, since there is sufficient bone for them. As they erupt and drift distally, they often upright themselves, although it is always necessary to band them in order to close the spaces and make the roots perpendicular. **H,** schematic presentation of the results of the serial extraction procedures. Hopefully, the case will look like this at the time of band placement.

which is completed when approximately one-third of the root of the mandibular first bicuspid has formed (Fig. XV-19, *B*). As soon as the mandibular first bicuspids are seen erupting into the extraction site, the maxillary first primary molar may be removed (Fig. XV-19, *C*). Delaying the extraction of the maxillary first primary molar guarantees the earlier arrival of the mandibular first bicuspid, allowing the mandibular arch to progress ahead of the upper (Fig. XV-19, *D*). When the mandibular first bicuspid has erupted to its approximate clinical crown height, it may be extracted. It is not advisable to extract the bicuspid earlier, since the eruption of the bicuspid forms alveolar bone in the area into which the cuspid eventually will move. To enucleate the first bicuspid is to delay the natural distal drifting of the cuspid, since the alveolar process will resorb and new alveolar bone will not appear until the cuspid is in position to erupt. Paradoxically, waiting for the eruption of the first bicuspid before it is extracted actually hastens the treatment (Fig. XV-19, *E*). In similar fashion, when the maxillary first bicuspid has erupted to full height, it may be extracted (Fig. XV-19, *F*). The results of the preceding steps are shown in Figure XV-19, *G*. Usually, the incisors align spontaneously and the cuspid eruption is delayed slightly but, as the cuspid erupts, its root often is in a surprisingly good vertical position (Fig. XV-20). Indeed, one of the primary reasons for treatment of gross discrepancy problems in the mixed dentition is to ease difficulties in cuspid positioning. The amount of space closure that will be required after the incisors and cuspids are in position is, of course, determined by the extent of the original discrepancy.

Only rarely does one encounter a case in which the discrepancy in each quadrant is exactly the same as the width of the tooth extracted in that quadrant. Some natural spontaneous space closure can be obtained by slicing the proximal surfaces of the second primary molars, but only small amounts of spontaneous closure ordinarily occur without tipping of the teeth, loss of parallelism of the roots and loss of vertical dimension. Hence, there is a need for precise control of the teeth during the finishing stages of treatment of a gross discrepancy problem. Figure XV-21 illustrates a clinical case treated by the protocol just described.

Fig. XV-20.—Oblique cephalograms showing the excellent vertical position of cuspids that can be achieved by careful timing of serial extraction procedures.

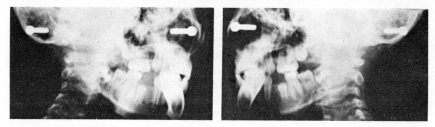

A

Patient __Me|a Ni e__   MIXED DENTITION ANALYSIS   Age __9-2__ Sex __F__

Date _____   Address _____   Parent _____

TOOTH SIZE

| | | | | | 6.4 | 5.8 | 5.9 | 6.4 | | | | |

Upper

	Right	Left
Space left after alignment of 2 and 1	19. 3	19. 8
Predicted size of 3 + 4 + 5	23. 4	23. 4
Space left for molar adjustment	—4. 1	— 3. 6

Lower

	Right	Left
Space left after alignment of 2 and 1	17. 9	18. 4
Predicted size of 3 + 4 + 5	23. 1	23. 1
Space left for molar adjustment	— 5. 2	— 4. 7

Remarks: Overjet = **3. 9**   Overbite = **4. 8 mm**

Molar relationship = **Class I, Class I**

Fig. XV-21.—A gross discrepancy case treated in the mixed dentition. **A,** the Mixed Dentition Analysis. (*Continued.*)

Many protocols for planned extractions of primary and permanent teeth as a guidance therapy have been reported in the literature (see Suggested Readings). Although many sophisticated variations of the extraction sequence have been suggested, that presented here is one of the most common and most frequently used. Other sequences involve serial removal of combinations of first and second premolars, all second premolars or a lower premolar and upper second permanent molar, according to the demands of the case. Such sophisticated procedures are beyond the scope of this book. They are mentioned lest the reader think that this difficult problem can be met in all instances by the simplistic approach presented. On the other hand, the rules given and the protocols described are sound, useful and well tested in clinical practice.

4) PRECAUTIONS.—It must be borne in mind that discrepancy cases are really the only ones in orthodontics in which extraction plays a routine therapeutic role. When the diagnosis suggests removal of teeth, extraction alone does not solve all the problems of treatment at once. It provides space in the arch, but extraction cases nearly always require difficult movements of teeth and precision appliancing to complete a

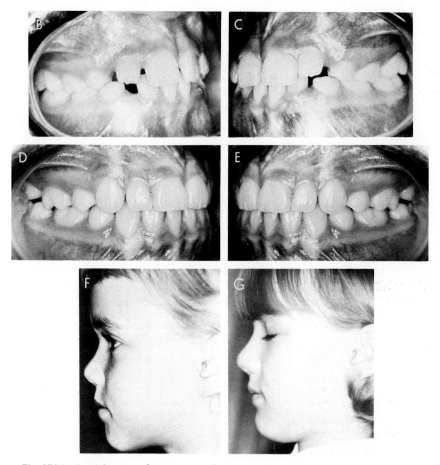

Fig. XV-21 (cont.).—**B** and **C,** intra-oral views at the start of treatment. **D** and **E,** intra-oral photographs after the removal of bands. **F,** the facial profile at the start of treatment. **G,** the profile at the end of treatment.

perfect result. Unfortunately, one can remove only a whole tooth in each quadrant and far too often the clinician removes approximately 7 mm. of space to permit alignment, which absorbs only a fraction of the space created. Perhaps it is better clinical judgment never to extract unless an appreciable percentage of the bicuspid's width is needed for alignment in each quadrant.

Many cases tempt one to extract asymmetrically and thus try to absorb the space provided on both sides of the arch. It is a sound policy to avoid extraction or to extract bilaterally except in the presence of malocclusions that are distinctly unilateral.

The dentist who has mastered the manipulation of a precision multibanded appliance has distinct advantages when treating extraction cases, for he can, by his technical skills, more satisfactorily close the spaces and consolidate the arch without creating traumatic occlusion and possible periodontal problems. The dentist who has only removable appliances in his armamentarium usually is not permitted this clinical position and must necessarily adopt a far more conservative attitude toward the extraction of the permanent teeth.

There is, in my opinion, entirely too much loose writing on the subject of extractions. Such cases should not be undertaken unless the dentist is prepared to give each case the study and careful attention it demands. There are not as many places for compromise in orthodontic therapy as we might desire. Unfortunately, the gross discrepancy problem is one of those uncompromising situations. There is simply no easy compromise with the problem of large teeth. One either leaves them in place or treats the problem comprehensively. Any other course of action is likely to leave the mouth in worse shape than it was at the start. The gross discrepancy problem is a common one in practice and there is no one safe practical approach that universally guarantees easy success in treatment. Early diagnosis enables the dentist to treat the case, if he chooses, at the optimum time and also permits him to refer those cases he chooses not to treat to a specialist without jeopardizing the chances for success. It is good policy never to begin the treatment of a gross discrepancy case unless you are prepared to follow it through to the final result. To do otherwise may handicap the colleague to whom the case is referred.

2. DIFFICULTIES IN ERUPTION

a) Alterations in Sequence of Eruption

Certain variations in the order of eruption of the teeth have been shown to be symptomatic of certain malocclusions (see Chapters VI and VII). It also is true that the normal sequence of eruption provides the best chance for maintaining arch length intact. Class II cases often show upper molars erupting ahead of the corresponding lower molars. A serious problem occurs in difficult space management situations (see Section C-1) when the second permanent molar erupts ahead of any cuspids or bicuspids. If noted early, a lingual holding arch will prevent premature shortening of the arch perimeter. If noted only after causing a loss of arch perimeter, extra-oral traction may be necessary if it is important to recover the lost perimeter.

1) PREMATURE ERUPTION OF INDIVIDUAL TEETH.—Permanent teeth may erupt unusually early if the primary predecessor has lost a considerable amount of bone from around its roots. Periapical lesions may result in early loss of the primary tooth, extensive bone resorption and increased circulation in the region. All of these conditions hasten the arrival of the permanent tooth (Fig. XV-22).

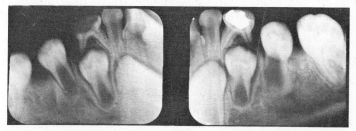

Fig. XV-22.—Premature eruption of second bicuspids due to the early loss of second primary molars. These second primary molars were lost during root development of the bicuspids. Had they been lost prior to the start of root development, the eruption of the second bicuspids might have been delayed.

When a tooth arrives so early as to have insufficient root length to maintain itself in position, instruct the patient to avoid, temporarily, tough, chewy foods and take steps to stabilize the tooth. Bands, if used, should be made with great care lest the tooth be inadvertently extracted. Small pellets of tooth-filling acrylic resin may be squeezed into the embrasures and allowed to flow over the marginal ridges. If this is done, on hardening, it will brace the tooth against stresses that might dislodge it. For obvious reasons of possible soft tissue damage, this splinting cannot be left in position very long. Check the growth of the root by serial radiographs and remove the plastic as soon as possible.

2) DELAYED ERUPTION OF INDIVIDUAL TEETH.—Individual teeth may be delayed in eruption because of retarded development, obstructions to occlusalward movement or premature loss of the primary predecessor. The mandibular second bicuspid is likely to develop in a manner disharmonious with adjacent teeth, and thus its eruptive development must be watched carefully (see Chapter XI). Retained root fragments are the most frequent obstructive impediment to eruption. When a primary tooth is removed prior to the initiation of root formation of the permanent successor, and hence the start of its eruption, bone may reform atop the permanent tooth before eruptive movements can begin and thus eruption actually is delayed by the premature loss of the primary tooth. The critical point is the amount of root formation of the permanent tooth at the time of loss of its predecessor. Such cases in delayed eruption must, of course, be differentiated from ankylosed permanent teeth.

b) Ectopic-Eruption of Teeth

The word "ectopia" and its adjective "ectopic" are among the most misused terms in dentistry. Ectopia means out of the normal position, misplaced. It means this and nothing more. Wrong therapy sometimes is advocated simply because the incorrect use of the word leads to incorrect ideas concerning treatment. Any tooth may be in ectopia during eruption, although some are more frequently so than others. Those teeth whose ectopic eruption most often is a clinical problem will be dealt with here.

1) MAXILLARY FIRST PERMANENT MOLAR

Causes:

The following, in combination, usually account for the abnormality.[6]

a) The teeth in ectopia are significantly larger than normal.

b) The maxillary first permanent molar erupting ectopically often does so at an abnormal angle to the occlusal plane. This indicates that the tooth germ probably was abnormally placed.

c) The maxillary length is normal in these cases, but tuberosity growth may lag significantly.

d) The morphology of the distal surface of the maxillary second primary molar and of the mesial surface of the maxillary first permanent molar is ideally suited for locking of the latter tooth during its eruption. The difference between the shape of these two teeth and the corresponding teeth in the mandible may be one reason why far fewer ectopic eruptions of the first molar are seen in the lower arch.

e) The size of the primary second molar is not as significant as the size of the first permanent molar, although in individual cases primary molar size may be a contributing factor.

In the typical case, the erupting maxillary first permanent molar is tipped mesially to engage closely the distal surface of the tooth and crown of the primary second molar. The permanent molar then becomes caught at the cervix of the primary tooth. Destruction of the primary tooth's crown may proceed unless the permanent tooth becomes freed (Fig. XV-23, *A*). Ectopia of the maxillary first permanent molar frequently is bilateral. When it is unilateral, excessive mesiodistal width of the tooth is not likely to be as important an etiologic factor as the misplacement of the developing tooth germ.

Treatment:

Separating wire procedure:

a) The first consideration is preservation of the length of the arch. As the permanent tooth erupts ectopically, it can greatly shorten the amount of space into which the cuspid and bicuspids must erupt. The fate of the second primary molar crown is not as important as the fate of the space that the crown occupies.

b) *Do not slice the distal surface of the second primary molar.* Such slicing will allow the first permanent molar to erupt, but it will be tipped and farther out of position. Malocclusion will always result, for there will be insufficient room for the cuspid and bicuspids.

c) Insert brass separating wire between the second primary and the first permanent molar as the first step in treatment. Tighten the wire every few days, forcing the permanent tooth distally. Later, you may have to use a doubled separating wire. When the permanent molar is freed, it will erupt to normal position. Re-

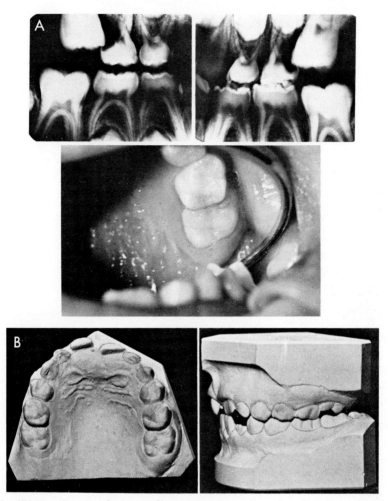

Fig. XV-23.—A case of ectopically erupting maxillary first permanent molars. This case is a bit atypical, since ectopic eruption of maxillary first permanent molars often is an indication of a shortage of space in the arch. **A,** note the undermining of the distal surface of the second primary molars, the tipped position of the maxillary first permanent molars and the Class II relationship of the permanent molars. **B,** *left,* occlusal view of the maxillary cast. *Right,* side view to show the tipping of the maxillary first molar and an anterior crossbite that corrected spontaneously. (*Continued.*)

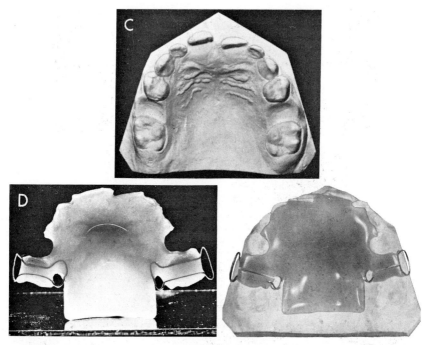

Fig. XV-23 (cont.).—**C,** results of carving the second primary molars off the *work* casts and to reproduce the mesial anatomy of the first permanent molars. **D,** *left,* the completed space-regainer, which has been made on the prepared cast shown in **C.** *Right,* the same appliance after the saddle areas have been sliced to permit activation. (*Continued.*)

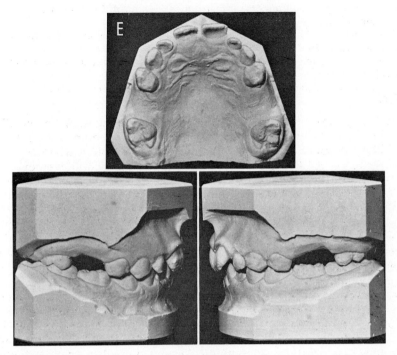

Fig. XV-23 (cont.).—E, the treatment result. The appliance now can be worn as a space-maintainer simply by filling the cracks with self-curing acrylic resin. Note the spontaneous correction of the incisor crossbite.

member that a second primary molar that has been damaged, as it usually is in this situation, is more likely to be lost early. Therefore, there is still a chance for the arch length to shorten.

If the separating wire procedure fails to dislodge the permanent molar or if you are unable to insert a separating wire, follow these steps (Fig. XV-23, *A–E* shows the steps in treatment of a typical case by this method):

Alternative procedure:

On the maxillary work cast remove the second primary molar, carving the plaster to simulate the mesial surface of the first permanent molar (Fig. XV-23, *C*).

Construct on the prepared cast an acrylic appliance of the split-saddle type. Allow the plastic to fit into the carved-away portion of the cast so that it may snugly meet the mesial surface of the first permanent molar as that tooth is freed (Fig. XV-23, *D*).

Extract both maxillary second primary molars and insert the appliance after having split it with a separating disk. The appliance must be placed immediately following the extractions, just as one would insert an immediate denture.

At subsequent appointments, adjust the springs until the desired amount of regaining is obtained (Fig. XV-23, *E*).

When the regaining is completed, fill the crack in the appliance with quick-curing acrylic resin.

The plate now may be worn as a space-maintainer until the cuspid and bicuspids are in place.

Details of construction and adjustment of this appliance are given in Chapter XVII.

2) MAXILLARY CUSPIDS.—Maxillary cuspids may develop ectopically, in which event they usually become impacted (see Section C-2-c below). Maxillary cuspids also are forced into ectopic eruption when there is insufficient space in the arch (see Section C-1, Space Management).

3) MANDIBULAR INCISORS.—Only rarely are the mandibular incisors in ectopic eruption, although the lateral incisor frequently is thought to be. When an incisor in the lower arch is or seems to be in ectopia, the condition is most likely to be caused by the prolonged retention of a primary predecessor or excessively large permanent teeth. Mandibular lateral incisors normally erupt lingually to their final position. However, they soon are moved into the line of arch by the tongue unless there is insufficient room for them.

4) OTHER TEETH.—Any tooth may erupt in ectopia, the treatment varying greatly with the tooth and the direction of its misplacement. Ectopic eruption of the mandibular first permanent molars may be seen. Maxillary permanent cuspids that erupt ectopically may result in impaction palatally; mandibular second premolars may be forced to erupt lingually because of lack of arch space. Indeed, almost any tooth may be seen to erupt ectopically due to local causes. The most serious ectopias, however, are those in which the tooth germ itself seems to form ectopically.

When planning treatment, always keep in mind three objectives: (1) placement of the tooth in its normal position, (2) retention of a favorable sequence of eruption and (3) maintenance of arch perimeter.

c) *Impaction of Teeth*

By definition, impactions are teeth that are so closely lodged in the alveolar bone as to be unable to erupt. Common usage has applied the term to any tooth that remains within its alveolus and does not erupt.

Although there are hereditary patterns leading to impacted teeth, the etiologic factors of most concern are malposed tooth germs, prolonged retention of primary teeth, localized pathologic lesions and shortening of the length of the arch.

Any tooth can be impacted, but the teeth involved most frequently are the mandibular third molar, maxillary cuspid, maxillary third molar, mandibular and maxillary second bicuspids and maxillary central incisor, in that order. The cause varies greatly with the tooth. Thus, mandibular third molar impactions may be due largely to evolution, whereas

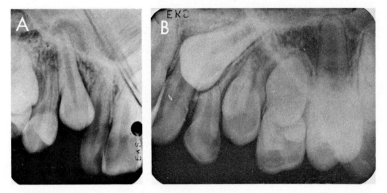

Fig. XV-24.—A, a maxillary cuspid impacted but not ectopic. **B,** a maxillary cuspid both impacted and ectopic.

those of the mandibular second bicuspids usually are due to space closure.

1) DIAGNOSIS.—The condition is diagnosed most frequently and easily when a tooth is long delayed in eruption, yet every effort should be made to make a diagnosis at an early date. For this purpose, radiographs are invaluable.

Impacted teeth may or may not be in ectopia (Fig. XV-24). Maxillary cuspids, for example, frequently are; mandibular second bicuspids are only seldom. It is important to observe in each case whether the impacted tooth is also misplaced.

2) MANDIBULAR THIRD MOLARS.—Although this tooth often is indicted as the cause of anterior crowding, one should remember that it cannot exert any effect until about 15–16 years of age. Most problems in crowding appear before this time. See Chapter IV for a discussion of current views on the role of mandibular third molars in incisor alignment.

3) MAXILLARY CUSPIDS.—This tooth may be simply impacted, as sometimes happens when the primary cuspid fails to resorb, or it may be impacted ectopically.

Treatment:

When the case is a simple impaction, follow these steps:

Measure the space available for the tooth. If insufficient, space must be gained as the first step in treatment. The size of the impacted tooth may be learned by measuring the cuspid on the opposite side of the maxillary arch or estimated by using the average width when the other teeth are average in size.

Uncover the impacted tooth. Remove the primary tooth, if present, and carefully expose the crown of the permanent cuspid. The tendency is to uncover the cuspid crown insufficiently. Excise a circular piece of palatal mucosa and with a surgical bur remove the bone surrounding the crown. Form a loop of .014″ steel

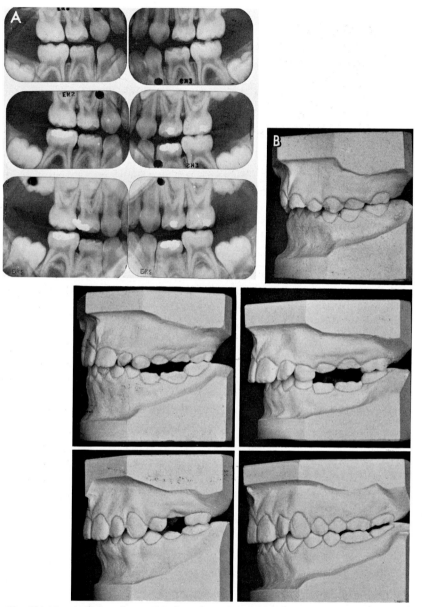

Fig. XV-25.—Ankylosed mandibular primary molars. **A,** serial intra-oral radiographs. Note the progressive loss of occlusal height in the mandibular second molar region. All the other teeth grow vertically, but the ankylosed second primary molar cannot. **B,** serial casts of a patient with 8 ankylosed primary molars. In the top illustration there is no evidence of ankylosis. No appliance therapy was used, only the carefully timed removal of the primary molars to coincide with the rapidly developing eruptive period of their successor teeth.

ligature wire, slip it around the cervix of the cuspid and allow the free ends of the ligature to extend outside the incision. The flap is sutured and the ligature wire gently wrapped around the neck of the lateral incisor or first bicuspid.

After healing, the steel ligature wire lariat is used to apply traction to the impacted tooth. The lariat may be tied to a light labial archwire or an auxiliary spring from a lingual archwire.

After the cuspid is brought into the mouth cavity, it is aligned by conventional methods of multibanded appliancing. The cuspid should be retained with the banded appliance for some time.

Occasionally, the oral surgeon can gently move the impacted tooth to a better position and stabilize it with surgical cement (e.g., Wonderpack). Several months of treatment time may be saved when this surgical repositioning is possible.

Retain with an acrylic Hawley plate.

4) MANDIBULAR AND MAXILLARY SECOND BICUSPIDS.—The impaction of these teeth is largely a matter of loss of arch perimeter. They will erupt spontaneously only if the molars are moved distally before the root length of the bicuspids is too advanced. After their roots are formed, they will no longer erupt spontaneously and traction must be applied.

5) OTHER TEETH.—When other teeth are impacted, the following principles should be held in mind when planning treatment: remove interferences to eruption before root formation is completed, hold sufficient space in the arch and bring appliance forces to bear in a gentle manner.

d) Ankylosed Primary Molars

Occasionally, a primary molar fails to maintain itself at the level of occlusion (Fig. XV-25). This condition has been erroneously called "submergence." Great variations are seen, and although many are of no practical significance, it is not unusual to see a primary molar buried beneath the cervix of adjacent teeth and partially covered by soft tissue.

Some investigators believe that "submerged" teeth are all ankylosed to the alveolar process, whereas others hold that only some are ankylosed. Nevertheless, treatment is planned as if all such primary molars were ankylosed.

Treatment:

Three possibilities must be avoided: (1) loss of the length of the arch, (2) extrusion of teeth in the opposite arch and (3) interference with the eruption of succeeding permanent teeth. When a primary molar becomes ankylosed, there is a localized arrest of eruption and alveolar growth. Adjacent teeth may proceed to greater occlusal heights. At times, first permanent molars tip mesially over the crowns of ankylosed second primary molars. Judicious use of space-maintainers and regainers is advisable. Never permit the presence of an ankylosed tooth to jeopardize the length of the arch. Should the opposite teeth begin to extrude, two courses of action are open: (1) placement of a stainless steel primary crown form on the ankylosed tooth to restore its occlusal height until it must be extracted or (2) removal of the ankylosed tooth and placement of a space-maintainer that will engage the opposing tooth. Some ankylosed primary molars cause no harm

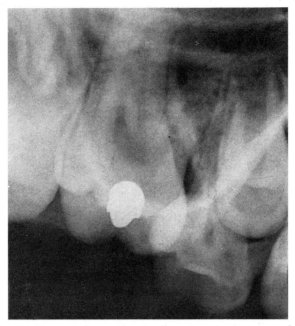

Fig. XV-26.—Ankylosis of a maxillary first permanent molar.

except interference with the eruption of their successors. All such primary molars may be left in place until the proper time for the eruption of the teeth beneath them. Indeed, with careful supervision, they often serve as excellent maintainers of the length of the arch. Figure XV-25, *B* shows an interesting series of casts of a case with all primary molars ankylosed. Each ankylosed primary molar was extracted on a schedule permitting a normal sequence of eruption.

e) Ankylosed Permanent Teeth

Although any permanent tooth may become ankylosed, first permanent molars are the most likely to do so. Two courses of action are available: (1) loosening and repositioning the tooth with forceps and (2) extraction. In the case of anterior teeth, extraction should be done only after loosening and repositioning has failed. On the other hand, in the case of first molars, extraction often is more conservative if timed correctly. Figure XV-26 illustrates a case in which the maxillary first molar was extracted and the second naturally assumed a more mesial position. If attempted later, more extensive orthodontic procedures are needed.

D. Lateral Relationships of Dental Arches

Failure of the two dental arches to occlude normally in lateral relationship may be due to localized problems of tooth position or alveolar

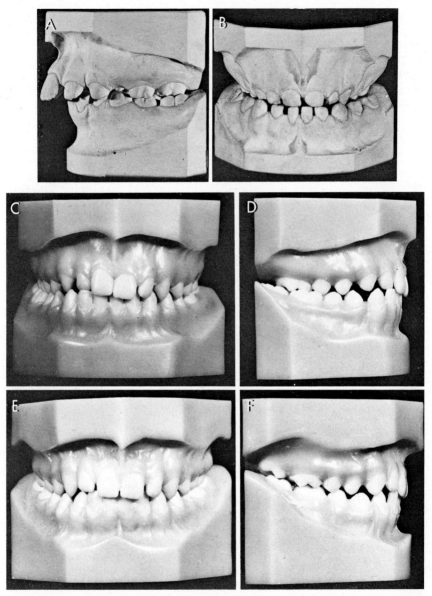

Fig. XV-27.—Dental crossbites. **A,** single-tooth crossbite. **B,** crossbite of several teeth. **C–F,** a case involving treatment of anterior and posterior crossbites of dental origin with a removable acrylic appliance and auxiliary springs. (Courtesy of the Department of Orthodontics, Faculty of Dentistry, University of Toronto.) This case was treated by an undergraduate student.

growth, or to gross disharmony between maxilla and mandible. This condition is known as crossbite. It may involve one or more teeth, usually in the lateral segments, and it may be unilateral or bilateral (Fig. XV-27). Regardless of the cause or the severity of the malocclusion, some adjustment must take place in the neuromuscular control of the mandible to provide satisfactory function. In Chapter VII, emphasis was placed on the primary etiologic site. It is important to remember that crossbites may originate in the dentition, the craniofacial skeleton or the temporomandibular musculature.

1. DIFFERENTIAL DIAGNOSIS

The principal concern of the examiner is to localize precisely where the aberration lies. Is it confined to the maxilla? Mandible? Or both? Does it involve only the alveolar process or is it a gross discrepancy in the "fit" of one jaw to the other? Is it unilateral malpositioning of teeth or bilateral contraction of the entire dental arch? It is important, too, to discern the origin of the problem, that is, the tissue first involved. Crossbites may be classified on an etiologic basis as dental, muscular or osseous.

a) Dental

This condition involves only the localized tipping of a tooth or teeth (see Fig. XV 27) and does not affect the size or shape of the basal bone. Muscular adjustments must always be made to provide an adequate accommodative occlusion. The midlines will coincide when the jaws are apart and diverge as the teeth come into occlusion. Some of the teeth in crossbite will not be centered buccolingually in the alveolar process. The most important single diagnostic point will be asymmetry of the dento-alveolar arch (see Chapter XI).

b) Muscular

"Muscular crossbite" involves functional adjustment to tooth interferences. It is similar to the dental type except that the teeth are not tipped within the alveolar process. In other words, muscular adjustment is involved more than malpositioning of teeth (Fig. XV-28). A functional analysis of the occlusal relationship is important and provides both the differential diagnosis and identification of interfering teeth (see Chapters XI and XVII). There is no clear-cut differentiation between the dental and muscular types except, perhaps, the treatment. In one (dental), teeth must be moved; in the other (muscular), the adjustments often can be gained by occlusal equilibration, which permits changes in the muscular reflexes governing mandibular positioning (see Chapter XVII, Section H). The pure muscular type is seen most often in young children. Both dental and muscular types require occlusal and muscular adjustments to complete their correction. Although many

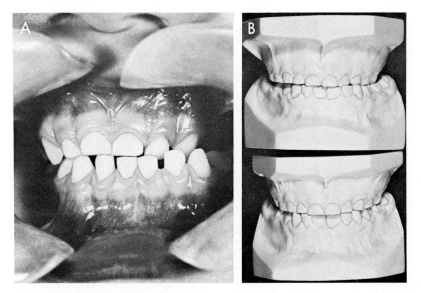

Fig. XV-28.—A functional or muscular type of crossbite of the primary dentition. **A,** intra-oral view. **B,** the casts before occlusal equilibration (*above*) and after occlusal equilibration (*below*).

muscular crossbites correct solely with occlusal equilibration, this is not sufficient for some. For these, the Porter lingual archwire (see Fig. XVII-28) is indicated. Figure XV-29 illustrates a case of functional crossbite treated by a combination of Porter archwire and equilibration. Treatment procedures include occlusal equilibration (see Chapter XVII), functional analysis of occlusion (see Chapter XI) and use of a Porter lingual archwire or a similarly acting appliance (see Chapter XVII).

c) *Osseous*

Aberrations in bony growth may give rise to crossbites in two ways: (1) asymmetric growth of the maxilla or mandible and (2) lack of agreement in the widths of the maxilla and mandible.

Asymmetric growth of the maxilla or mandible may be due to inherited growth patterns or trauma that impedes the normal growth on the affected side. Crossbites due to asymmetric bony growth are most difficult to treat. The teeth are moved to provide the best possible occlusion in the circumstances.

Lack of harmony between the maxillary and mandibular widths usually is due to a bilaterally contracted maxilla. In such cases, the muscles shift the mandible to one side to acquire sufficient occlusal contact for mastication (Fig. XV-30).

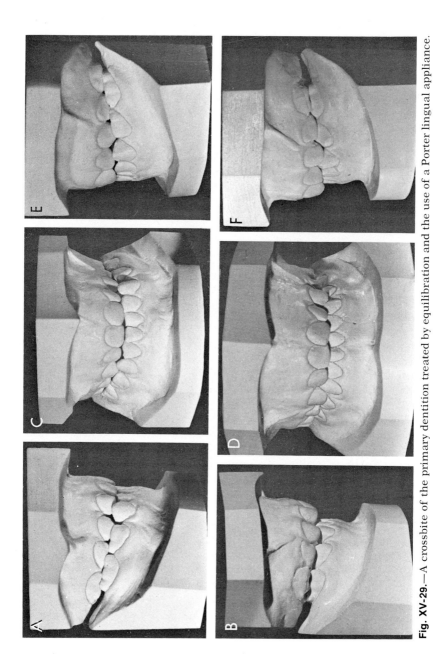

Fig. XV-29.—A crossbite of the primary dentition treated by equilibration and the use of a Porter lingual appliance.

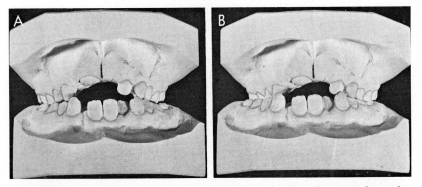

Fig. XV-30.—Maxillary dental arch contraction producing a functional crossbite. **A,** the cast placed so that the midlines are together, thus demonstrating that the contraction is bilateral. **B,** the usual occlusal position, which seems to portray a unilateral crossbite.

A more severe condition is that in which the mandibular denture occludes completely within the maxillary arch (Fig. XV-31). When this mediolateral problem is combined with a skeletal Class II malocclusion, it produces one of the most severe of all malocclusions (Fig. XV-32). In mandibular hypertrophy and prognathism, the mandible is excessively wide for the maxilla as well as unduly long; therefore, a mediolateral occlusal problem exists in addition to the Class III malocclusion.

Study carefully the closure pattern of the mandible, noting at which

Fig. XV-31.—Osseous disharmony between the mandible and the maxilla producing a typical bilateral skeletal-type crossbite. Often in such cases the mandibular teeth occlude completely inside the maxillary teeth.

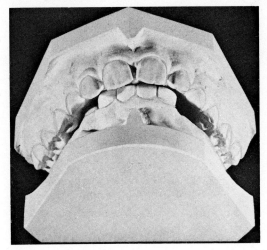

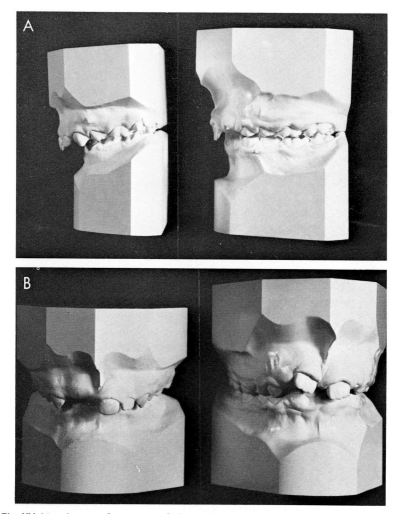

Fig. XV-32.—A case of severe mediolateral osseous dysplasia in conjunction with mandibular insufficiency. This boy was first seen for neuromuscular analysis when he was 2 years of age. He could eat nothing but pappy baby food and had not learned to chew. The results of the first phase of therapy, done by means of an activator, are shown in **A–C** (*left before; right after*). Note that although there is now bilateral occlusal function, a severe Class II relationship remains. At this time, he could chew adequately. (*Continued.*)

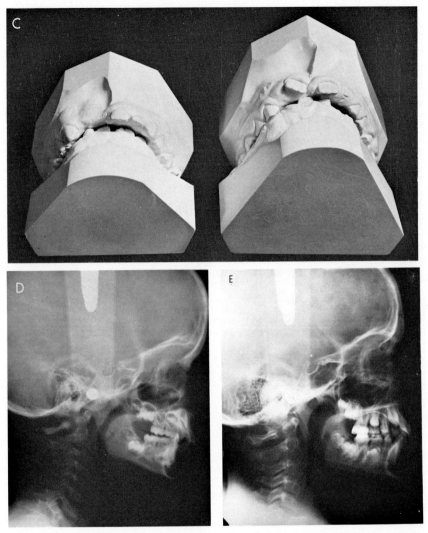

Fig. XV-32 (cont.).—D is the original lateral cephalogram. **E,** cephalogram at age 9 years, after first stage of orthodontic therapy (activator).

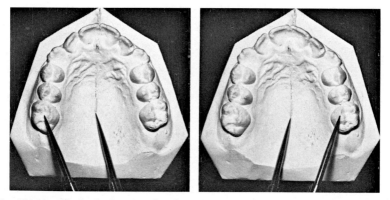

Fig. XV-33.—Method of using dividers to measure from the medium raphe to estimate asymmetries of the dental arch.

stage of closure lateral deviations occur. When the lateral shifting occurs late in closure, it usually is due to a tooth interference.

If the deviation of the midlines of the lower and upper face increases throughout opening, the primary fault is likely to be unilateral bony growth. In cases of bilaterally symmetric dental arches in each jaw with one arch grossly wider than the other, the patient may demonstrate several different closure paths and several occlusal relationships.

Place the mandible so that the midlines of the upper and lower face coincide. Many patients who show a crossbite on one side only will thus exhibit bilateral dental arch contractions (see Fig. XV-30). One also may use a set of dividers on the dental cast for more precise localization of the asymmetrically placed teeth (Fig. XV-33). A symmetrograph is essential for analysis of crossbite (see Chapter XI, Section D-3).

2. TREATMENT

a) Dental Crossbite (Individual Teeth)

1) CASE ANALYSIS.—*a*) Rarely is one tooth alone tipped. In most cases, its antagonist in the opposite arch is out of position also. Thus, the maxillary first molar may be tipped lingually, whereas the mandibular first molar is tipped slightly buccally. In such cases, usually both teeth must be moved.

b) Always measure the amount of space into which the tooth is to be moved. Many individually malposed teeth are wider than the space for them in the arch. If such is the case, that space must be increased before the crossbite can be corrected.

2) APPLIANCE.—*a*) Simple through-the-bite elastics (Fig. XV-34) are effective for molars in crossbite when both teeth are out of position and there is adequate space for them.

b) If the problem is largely a matter of tipping a single tooth rather

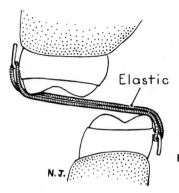

Fig. XV-34.—Through-the-bite elastics.

than reciprocal tipping of two teeth, an acrylic plate with auxiliary spring will serve well.

c) Lingual archwires with recurved auxiliary springs also are satisfactory, particularly if patient cooperation is lacking.

b) Dento-Alveolar Contraction

In this category, crossbites involve several posterior teeth (see Fig. XV-30).

1) Case analysis.—It is important to learn how much of the condition is due to actual dento-alveolar contraction and how much to muscular adaptive positioning of the mandible. The more it is a matter of the mandible adopting a new position of closure for more efficient functioning, the better the prognosis.

a) If the midlines are together when the patient occludes in his accustomed position, there usually is very little muscular adaptation and the case is purely one of narrowing of the maxillary alveolar arch.

b) If the midlines are not together when the patient occludes in his accustomed position, some functional adaptation probably has taken place.

2) Appliance.—After locating any tooth interferences when the midlines coincide, remove by grinding those interferences involving primary teeth (Chapter XVII, Section H). In such cases, the cuspids are likely to be the offenders. Do not hesitate to grind contacting inclined planes on these teeth so that, as they meet, the mandible will tend to return to its normal position (see Fig. XV-28, *B*). When the entire primary dentition is present, sometimes one can correct minor problems by occlusal adjustment alone.

Bilateral contraction of the maxillary arch

For this condition, the Porter lingual archwire is ideally suited (see Fig. XVII-28). Do not expect this appliance to widen greatly the osseous base; it can only move the teeth to a better position within their bony support.

Unilateral contraction of the maxillary arch

A lingual archwire with an auxiliary spring on one side often is the easiest appliance in these cases (see Fig. XVII-29). Note that true unilateral contraction seldom is seen; this is fortunate, for it is more difficult to treat than when reciprocal action may be used. Gross unilateral maxillary development problems are difficult; the procedures mentioned are for minor deviations only.

Mandibular dento-alveolar contraction

Unilateral contraction in the mandible is rare. Bilateral narrowing caused by lingual tipping of teeth is best handled by a lingual archwire with auxiliary springs (see Figs. XVII-28 and XVII-29).

c) Gross Disharmony between Osseous Bases

1) CASE ANALYSIS.—Most frequently, the mandibular teeth, when the midlines coincide, fail to occlude properly with any of the maxillary teeth (see Fig. XV-31). Masticatory efficiency is low, since the patient must shift the mandible completely to one side or the other for chewing. Thus, in young children, a definite fixed occlusal relationship does not exist. Figure XV-35 is an example of such a problem.

2) APPLIANCE.—These difficult cases are best treated while growth potential remains; therefore, the two appliances used most frequently are functional jaw orthopedics and palate-splitting devices. Figure XV-32 illustrates a case of marked mandibular insufficiency treated with a conventional activator because a Class II correction also was required. Improvement resulted, since the better anteroposterior relationship

Fig. XV-35.—Serial casts illustrating treatment of skeletal-type crossbite. Note the complete inclusion of the mandibular teeth within the maxillary dental arch at the start of treatment.

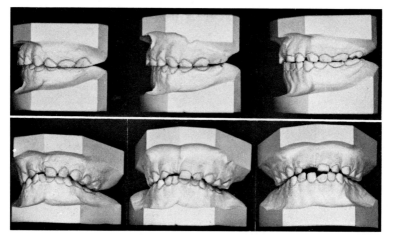

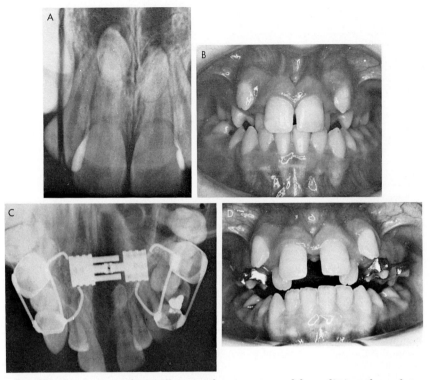

Fig. XV-36.—A case of maxillary inadequacy treated by splitting the palate. **A,** periapical radiograph at the start of treatment. Note the two supernumerary teeth. **B,** intra-oral photograph at the start of treatment. Note the bilateral crossbite and the malposed cuspids. **C,** radiograph a short time later, after the palate has been split. **D,** same time as **C.** The appliance used in this case is shown in Figure XVII-31. (*Continued.*)

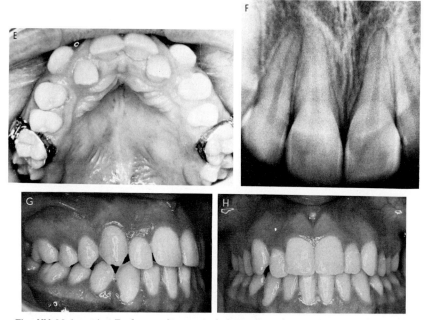

Fig. XV-36 (cont.).—E, the appliance is left in place but inactive as the median palatine suture fills with bone and the teeth drift toward the midline. **F,** radiograph at the midline at the end of treatment and after the removal of the supernumerary teeth. **G** and **H,** after the removal of the banded appliance and at the end of the retention period. (Courtesy of Dr. Robert Aldrich.)

also aided the mediolateral problem and the vertical development of the alveolar processes was altered.

In recent years, there has been a revival of the use of palate-splitting appliances for treatment of gross mediolateral osseous dysplasia resulting from an inadequate maxillary apical base. The results are swift and dramatic when the planning is correct. Figure XV-36 illustrates the use of a palate-splitting device in an appropriate case.

E. Anteroposterior Relationships of Teeth and Arches

1. Class II (Distoclusion, Postnormal Occlusion)

Class II is a common severe malocclusion. When combined with serious space management problems, it becomes a most difficult malocclusion to treat well. The term Class II is used in only the general sense, for the only thing the many varieties of Class II have in common is the molar relationship. Unfortunately, there is no standard method of identifying and segregating the types of Class II malocclusion (except for Angle's Divisions 1 and 2). In Class II, secondary features of the malocclusion, that is, those aspects other than the Class II molar relationship and the anteroposterior skeletal dysplasia, often are very important to the treatment plan. Vertical skeletal dysplasia, the muscle pattern and the arch space available for alignment of the teeth are frequent complicating factors in Class II malocclusion. It may be useful to reread or recall the facts on skeletal growth in Chapter IV, classification of malocclusion in Chapter IX, analysis of the dentition and occlusion in Chapter XI and analysis of the craniofacial skeleton in Chapter XII.

A vast literature on the diagnosis and treatment of Class II malocclusions exists throughout the world's dental journals. There are many strategies of treatment, numerous appliances and differences of opinion concerning this malocclusion class. The following pages constitute only a brief outline and are not intended in any way to suggest that all Class II malocclusions should be treated routinely in general practice. Since this malocclusion probably is the most common of the severe malocclusions, every dentist must have a correct understanding and perspective of the problem irrespective of whether he refers them all for treatment or selects the simpler types for treatment himself.

a) *Differential Diagnosis*

1) SKELETAL FEATURES.—A cephalometric analysis is a necessity when diagnosing and planning treatment of Class II malocclusions (Fig. XV-37) (see Chapter XII). Typically, the variant skeletal characteristics are found in one or more of the following regions: (a) maxillomandibular relationship. The profile is typically retrognathic or convex due to mandibular retrognathism, midface protrusion or both; (b) the cranial base. Increased length in the anterior cranial base will contribute to any midface protrusion, whereas increased obtusity of the cranial base angle or lengthening of the posterior cranial base will tend to position the temporomandibular articulation more retrusively; (c) vertical dysplasia. The anterior upper face height often is greater than normal and may be disharmonious with the posterior upper face height; (d) the occlusal plane may be steeply placed, a reflection of the vertical skeletal dysplasia.

2) DENTAL FEATURES.—The dental aspects of Class II largely are an adaptive reflection of the skeletal and muscular pattern, although they may exist alone sufficiently exaggerated to produce a Class II molar relationship in a balanced facial skeleton, i.e., facial convexity less than +5 mm. ("A" point ahead of Na-Po plane). The dental features may be studied in the cephalogram (see Chapter XII), the dental casts (see Chapter XI) or in the patient himself.

(a) *Incisors.*—The upper and lower incisors may be tipped labially off their bases (Fig. XV-38). This labioversion of incisors is particularly

A

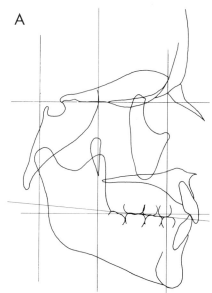

Fig. XV-37.—Comparison of a balanced facial pattern (**A**) with four different Class II problems (**B-E**). (*Continued.*)

evident when the posterior face height is less than the anterior face height. When the anterior and posterior vertical heights are balanced and the midface is normal, the maxillary incisors are likely to be more normally inclined or nearly vertical. Excessive overjet is a common feature of Class II malocclusion (except Class II, Division 2) and excessive depth of bite is a common finding. The gross deviations in incisor relationships often result in the loss of functional incisal stops, thus permitting the mandibular incisors to erupt past the posterior occlusal plane and often allowing the maxillary incisors to overerupt as well.

(*b*) *Molars.*—Mesial displacement of maxillary molars is a common finding in Class II (see Fig. XV-38). These teeth tip mesially and rotate as well as translate during the mesial drifting and thus contribute to an increase in the depth of bite. The more the maxillary posterior teeth have drifted mesially the easier it may be to correct the overbite relationship by derotating, distal tipping and distal placement of the molars. Study the maxillary cast carefully in order to identify any such mesial positioning of maxillary lateral teeth.

(*c*) *Cuspids.*—The angulation of cuspids in Class II is an important factor in diagnosis. Correlate the angulation of the maxillary cuspid with any possible mesial drifting of the molars and the angulation of the cuspids in both arches with the space analysis.

(*d*) *Occlusal plane.*—The occlusal plane posteriorly is a reflection of the vertical skeletal features of the Class II, whereas anteriorly it also betrays the role of the tongue and lip in aggravating the incisal features of the malocclusion.

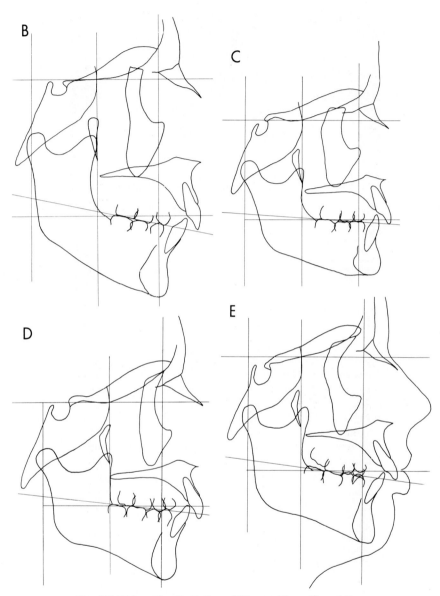

Fig. XV-37 (cont.).—B–E, four different Class II problems.

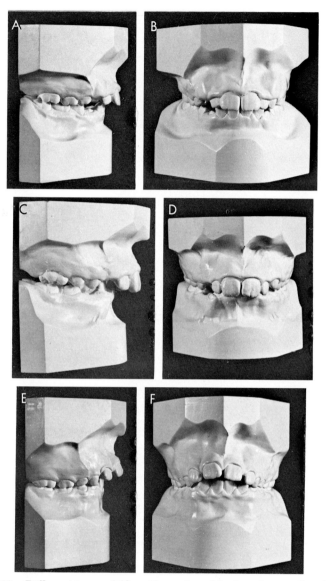

Fig. XV-38.—Different types of Class II, as viewed in dental casts. See also many other illustrations in Chapters VI, IX, XI, XVII, etc. **A–B,** a moderately severe skeletally involved Class II. **C** and **D,** a Class II complicated by large teeth. **E** and **F,** a mild skeletal Class II aggravated by a thumb-sucking habit. Casts are useful for observing details of occlusion and tooth position but how inadequate for understanding the skeletal involvement or muscular contributions.

(*e*) *Arch form.*—In Class II, the maxillary arch is more likely to be narrow and elongated and thus disharmonious with the mandibular arch form (see Fig. XV-38). The incisors' elongation and the possibility for positioning the incisors over the basal bone are key prognostic factors in appraising arch form.

3) NEUROMUSCULAR FEATURES.—The neuromuscular features seen at diagnosis often seem to be largely adaptive to the skeleton and tooth positions typical of Class II malocclusion (Fig. XV-39). But one must not quickly discount the possible etiologic role of the neuromusculature in producing the malocclusion. If muscle factors have been present from the start, their removal is essential for stability of the treated re-

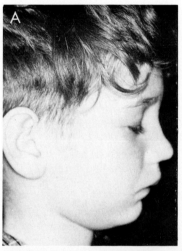

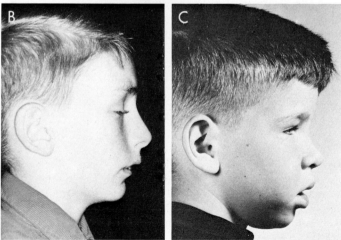

Fig. XV-39.—Variation in the profiles and soft tissue balance in Class II cases. Note the placid lips in **C**. (**C** courtesy of Dr. Arthur Storey.)

sult. The lip positions imposed by the facial skeleton cause increased labioversion of the maxillary incisors and often lingual tipping of the mandibular incisors. In other instances, both upper and lower incisors are tipped off their bases, since the lips and tongue must effect an anterior seal during swallowing and in the production of certain speech sounds. Their efforts to do so in the presence of a skeletal dysplasia often result in some aggravation of the incisal relationships.

A functional mandibular retraction is a common feature of Class II in the primary dentition and Class II, Division 2 in the mixed dentition stage. A functional retraction of the mandible is seen only occasionally in Class II, Division 1 in the mixed dentition and very rarely in the completed permanent dentition. Other common neuromuscular factors often found with Class II are mouth-breathing and tongue-thrusting. Study carefully Chapter V, Maturation of the Orofacial Musculature, and Chapter X, Analysis of the Orofacial Musculature, to understand and identify the neuromuscular features of Class II.

b) *Rationale of Class II Therapy*

1) SKELETAL FEATURES.—(a) *In the primary dentition.*—Treatment of the skeletal features of Class II in the primary dentition aims at restraining midface growth and promoting, as much as possible, mandibular growth in order to achieve a more balanced facial skeleton before eruption of the permanent teeth. These strategies seem sound but they are done routinely on children so young by only a few clinicians.

(b) *In the mixed dentition.*—Treatment of the skeletal features of Class II in the mixed dentition is routine in orthodontics. Such therapy aims at bringing about orthopedic results in the midface to minimize the anteroposterior dysplasia or attempts are made to encourage the mandible to achieve its ultimate growth potential (Fig. XV-40). Planned differential vertical growth of the alveolar processes during eruption of the teeth levels the occlusal plane and corrects some of the vertical dysplasia. Since there are distinct sexual differences in the onset of the pubescent growth spurt and in the cessation of craniofacial growth, the rationale for Class II therapy varies with the sex, that is, girls should be treated earlier and results may be achieved sooner. Obversely, the tendency for males' craniofacial growth to continue past the second decade of life is a complicating factor in retention.

(c) *In the permanent dentition.*—Camouflage of the disharmonious facial skeleton is the primary aim when treating the skeletal features of Class II in the permanent dentition (Fig. XV-41). Since the best possibilities of skeletal growth have largely been lost by this time, the clinician must resort mainly to tooth movements to mask the skeletal dysplasia. Extractions of teeth and subsequent tooth movements into the space thus made available achieve the same purpose. Treatment of Class II in the permanent dentition takes into account the dynamics

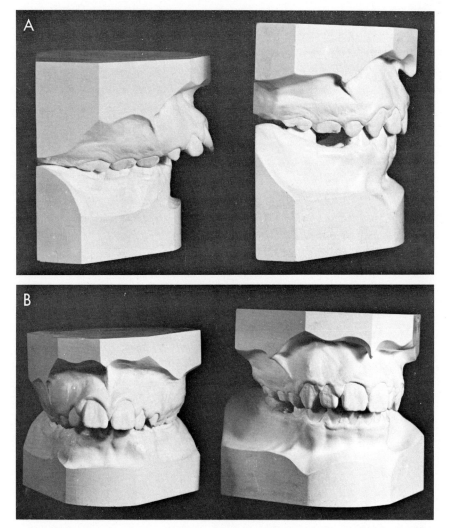

Fig. XV-40.—Treated Class II case in the mixed dentition. **A–B,** casts before and after treatment. (*Continued.*)

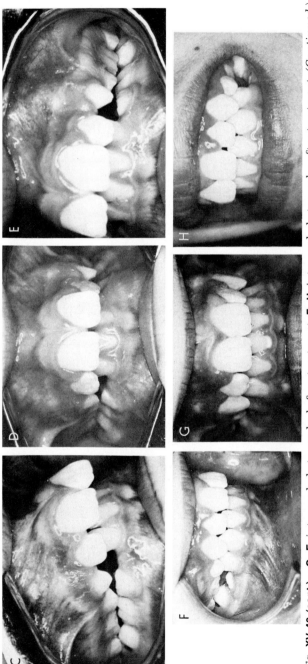
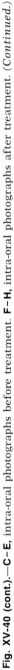

Fig. XV-40 (cont.).—**C–E,** intra-oral photographs before treatment. **F–H,** intra-oral photographs after treatment. (*Continued.*)

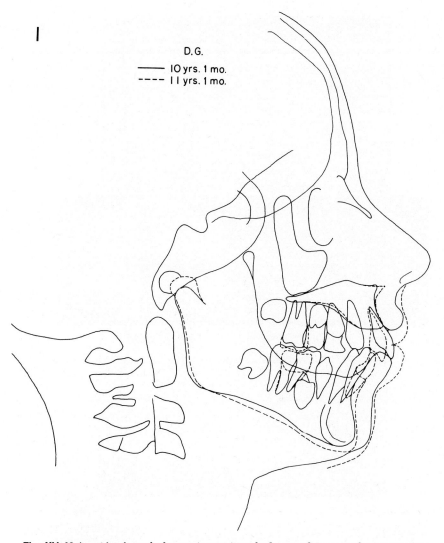

Fig. XV-40 (cont.).—I, cephalometric tracings before and 1 year after treatment with an activator. Banded appliances had not yet been placed. Note the amount of mandibular growth.

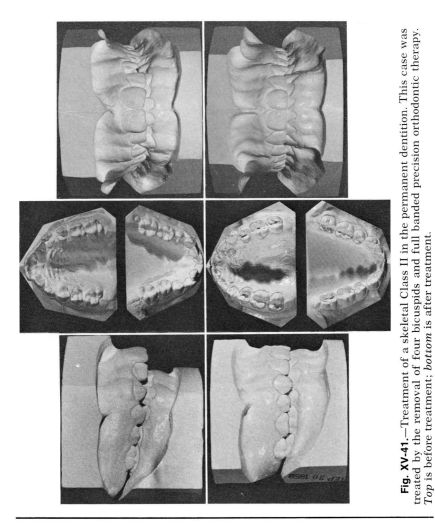

Fig. XV-41.—Treatment of a skeletal Class II in the permanent dentition. This case was treated by the removal of four bicuspids and full banded precision orthodontic therapy. *Top* is before treatment; *bottom* is after treatment.

of growth much less than when similar cases are treated in the mixed dentition.

2) TREATING THE DENTAL FEATURES.—(*a*) *In the primary dentition.*— If Class II treatment is undertaken in the primary dentition, harmonizing of the maxillary and mandibular arch forms is a primary aim. In addition, attempts are made to place the incisors well over their supporting basal bone and to create functional incisal stops and thus minimize the overbite and overjet when the permanent teeth erupt. Such therapy also aids in the maintenance of the primary dentition's flat occlusal plane into the mixed dentition. There are many problems in patient cooperation and few appliances that are usable in the primary

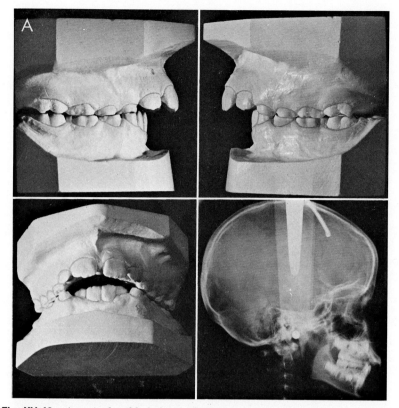

Fig. XV-42.—A typical mild skeletal Class II malocclusion treated in the mixed dentition with extra-oral traction. **A,** at the start of treatment. Note the overbite and the slight open bite associated with an active tongue-thrust habit. (*Continued.*)

dentition. Therefore, treatment of the dental features of the Class II in the primary dentition is not practiced routinely.

(*b*) *In the mixed dentition.*—The aim of treating the dental features of Class II in the mixed dentition is to produce normal molar and incisal relationships and thus establish normal occlusal function prior to the eruption of the cuspids, premolars and second permanent molars (Fig. XV-42). If this aim is achieved, the dental development of the remaining teeth produces good occlusal function and a flat occlusal plane well related to the profile. The distinct sexual differences in the eruption of teeth and the growth of the craniofacial skeleton alter the treatment strategy. Similarly, there are variations in the amount of space available in the mandible for alignment of the teeth. Therefore, the exact protocols for treatment of the dental features of Class II in the mixed dentition vary greatly but they all include the following three points:

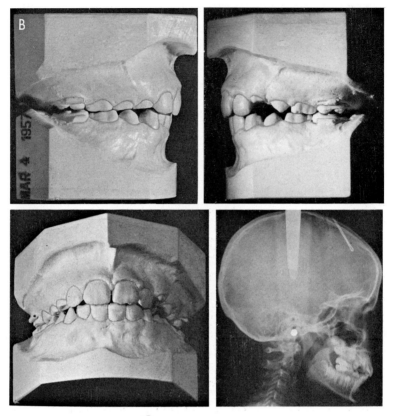

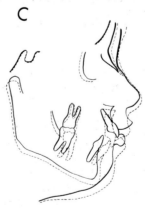

Fig. XV-42 (cont.)—B, the results at the end of 1 year of extra-oral traction to the maxillary dentition while space supervision procedures were carried out in the mandible. **C,** composite cephalometric tracings registered on the cranial base. (*Continued.*)

D

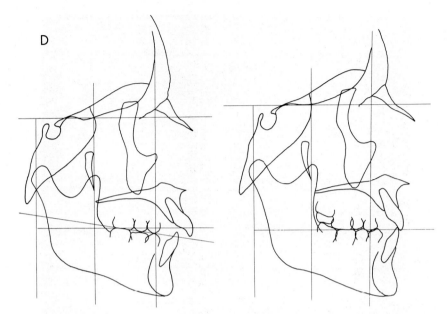

Fig. XV-42 (cont.).—D, cephalometric tracings of another case showing primarily a dental response, i.e., distal movement of maxillary teeth. (*Continued.*)

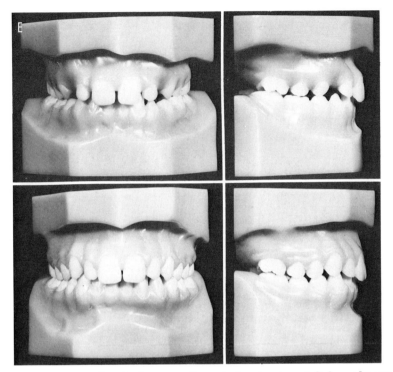

Fig. XV-42 (cont.).—E, a similar case. *Above,* before treatment. *Below,* after treatment. This case was treated by an undergraduate student. Note the good relationship of the apical bases. (Courtesy of the Department of Orthodontics, Faculty of Dentistry, University of Toronto.) (*Continued.*)

(1) distal rotation, tipping and movement of the maxillary molars to correct the Class II molar relationship, a procedure that opens the bite and lengthens the maxillary arch perimeter; (2) restraint of the maxillary dentition while the midface grows forward, thus changing the relative position of the maxillary dentition to its base; and (3) retraction and intrusion of maxillary incisors to reduce the dento-alveolar protrusion, produce normal incisor function and improve lip and tongue movements.

(c) *In the permanent dentition.*—Since skeletal growth is largely over by the time of the eruption of the permanent second molars, treatment of dental features of Class II at this time is mostly a matter of camouflaging the skeletal pattern by tooth movements. In order to acquire the space for such camouflaging tooth movements, it often is necessary to extract teeth in severe Class II malocclusions in the permanent dentition.

3) TREATING THE NEUROMUSCULAR FEATURES.—(a) *In the primary*

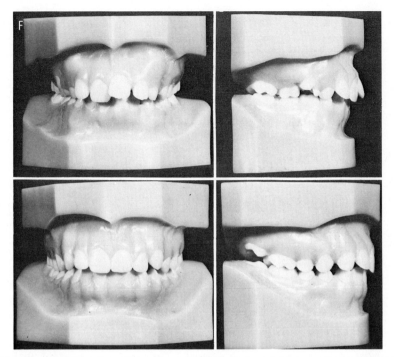

Fig. XV-42 (cont.).—F, a case with some Class II dental features that was treated solely by guidance of eruption and control of the arch perimeter. *Above,* before treatment. *Below,* after treatment. This case was treated by an undergraduate student using a labiolingual appliance. (Courtesy of the Department of Orthodontics, Faculty of Dentistry, University of Toronto.)

dentition.—Treatment of the neuromuscular aspects of Class II in the primary dentition is undertaken to promote a normal neuromuscular environment that will aid function and growth and not aggravate or distort the unfolding skeletal pattern (Fig. XV-43). Such therapy often consists of control of deleterious habits and treatment of the skeletal and dental features in order that normal neuromuscular function can obtain. In a few cases, the neuromuscular pattern is the dominant Class II theme observed in the primary dentition.

(b) *In the mixed dentition.*—The aims for treating the neuromuscular features of Class II in the mixed dentition are similar to the aims in the primary dentition. However, the molars and incisors must be corrected, since a Class II muscle pattern already controls them (see Fig. XV-43). In Class II malocclusions without severe skeletal features, correction of the dental symptoms alone often restores near-normal function of the muscles. In other cases, primarily those with a severe skeletal pattern, it is harder to achieve adaptation and conditioning of

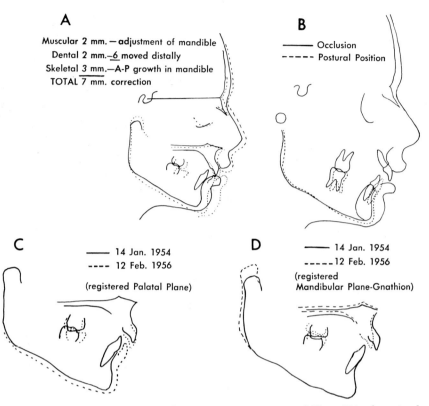

A

Muscular 2 mm. — adjustment of mandible
Dental 2 mm.—6 moved distally
Skeletal 3 mm.—A-P growth in mandible
TOTAL 7 mm. correction

B

——— Occlusion
– – – – Postural Position

C

——— 14 Jan. 1954
– – – – 12 Feb. 1956

(registered Palatal Plane)

D

——— 14 Jan. 1954
– – – – – 12 Feb. 1956

(registered
Mandibular Plane-Gnathion)

Fig. XV-43.—A, the more typical response to treatment of Class II in the mixed dentition. Here, the result is a combination of skeletal, dental and neuromuscular factors. In this case, teeth were removed, bones grew and neuromuscular reflexes adapted. **B,** the same patient, showing the slight functional mandibular retraction on closure at the start of treatment. **C,** tracings before and after treatment registered on the palatal plane to show the amount of distal movement in the upper molars and movement of the maxillary incisors. **D,** tracings registered on gnathion to show the amount of mandibular growth that took place during treatment.

the muscles, and myotherapy must be instituted in conjunction with mechanotherapy and continue throughout the retention period.

(c) *In the permanent dentition.*—When treatment of Class II malocclusion is postponed until the permanent dentition, conditioning of the neuromuscular features is more difficult and one must hope for spontaneous neuromuscular adaptation, since those reflexes that are not easily conditioned at this age often require permanent splinting-type retention devices. The two most important neuromuscular features to be treated in the permanent dentition are tongue-thrusting and eccentric occlusal reflexes caused by occlusal disharmonies (see Chapter XVII).

c) *Planning the Treatment*

Most general practitioners treat few Class II malocclusions, although all Class II malocclusions are first seen by them. Therefore, this brief outline of Class II treatment is provided for general background and an understanding of the principles involved. It will aid the dentist in (a) the recognition and grouping of cases according to their significant differences, (b) referral at the most opportune time, (c) explanations to the parents and patients and (d) cooperation with the colleague treating the case. Those dentists who treat Class II will appreciate the sketchiness of this discussion. It makes no pretense of depth or detail and is intended only as a brief—but correct—orientation on standard clinical practice for the correction of Class II malocclusion. It is not intended as a manual of practice, but rather as an orderly introduction to the various concepts and strategies employed in treatment of Class II.

1) TYPES OF CLASS II.—Figure XV-44. *A* and *B* show schematic, symbolic representations of some common types of Class II. They are intended to provide a visual image of some of the primary variations on this difficult theme. Each of the types may be complicated by vertical skeletal dysplasia (Fig. XV-44, *C*), the neuromuscular pattern, the space requirements and the vertical dento-alveolar development. Very few malocclusions will fit a single type of pattern completely in all details.

2) TREATMENT STRATEGIES FOR TYPE "A".—Malocclusions of type "A" display anteroposterior and vertical skeletal balance; therefore, the malocclusion is due to aggravation of the dental symptoms of Class II. These malocclusions may be seen with a normal overbite, with an open bite or with a deep bite. During treatment, the maxillary dentition is retracted and held while craniofacial growth goes on. The maxillary incisors may need to be retracted and may need intrusion and root torquing to correct the depth of bite. Type "A" Class II malocclusions, often called dental Class IIs, frequently are treated in the mixed dentition. The prognosis usually is good. Class II, Division 2 (Angle) is a typical example of this type (Fig. XV-44, *D*).

3) TREATMENT STRATEGIES FOR TYPE "B".—Type "B" Class II maloc-

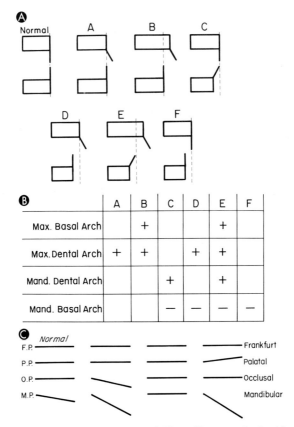

Fig. XV-44.—Schematic presentation of Class II types. **A,** the blocks represent the maxillary and mandibular bone and the perpendicular vertical lines depict the normal overbite and overjet. **B,** differential diagnosis of six Class II types: + = protruded feature; − = retruded feature. **C,** a schematic presentation of vertical dysplasia accompanying Class II. (*Continued.*)

clusions are characterized by a good mandibular base that is well positioned with respect to the anterior cranial base; the primary problem is midface protrusion, both skeletal and dento-alveolar (Fig. XV-44, *E*). There may be no vertical skeletal dysplasia. The marked facial convexity shows the "A" point more than 5 mm. ahead of the facial plane, the SNA angle higher than normal and the midface disproportionately long for the lower face. Type "B" Class II malocclusions are among the most common encountered in practice. They may be complicated by the space requirements in the mandible, vertical skeletal dysplasia or excessive vertical alveolar growth in the incisor region. They usually are treated in the mixed dentition with extra-oral force to the max-

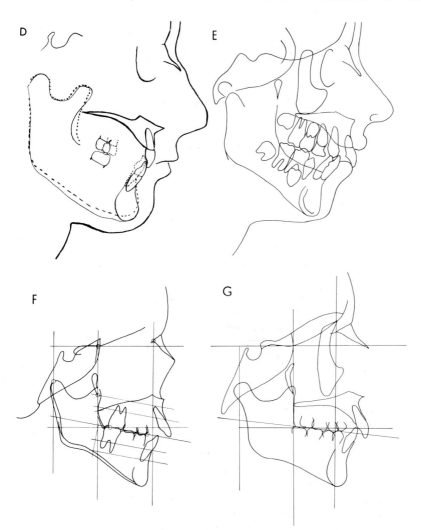

Fig. XV-44 (cont.).—D, type "A" before and after cephalometric tracings; **E,** type "B"; **F,** type "C"; **G,** type "D." (*Continued.*)

illary dentition to retract and inhibit dento-alveolar forward growth and produce orthopedic changes in the midface. The direction of the extra-oral traction is determined primarily by the vertical needs of the case. These problems are much more difficult when treatment is begun after the dentition is completed and most growth is over, since the utilization of differential growth, both anteroposteriorly and horizontally, is the prime ingredient in effecting a correction. Retention sometimes is difficult because of small residual skeletal growth during the second and third decades of life, so the extra-oral traction may be used as a retaining appliance as well. Much clinical research has been reported in the literature on the treatment of this type of Class II malocclusion in the mixed dentition (see Suggested Readings), and the treatment strategies and tactics are highly developed and used routinely in modern orthodontic practice.

4) TREATMENT STRATEGIES FOR TYPE "C".—The primary problem in type "C" Class II malocclusion is mandibular insufficiency (Fig. XV-44, *F*). This type usually has a steep occlusal plane and a steep Frankfurt mandibular plane angle. A short ramus is seen frequently; thus, the posterior vertical face height is disharmonious with the anterior face height. The vertical dysplasia is a key factor in the prognosis. The skeletal features make it necessary for the mandibular incisors to tip forward off their base, whereas the maxillary incisor angle frequently is more normal. The facial and tongue musculature is more likely to be normal in the type "C" Class II malocclusion than in the type "B," for, in the latter, it is necessary for the mandibular lips to seal between the incisors during swallowing. Type "C" Class II malocclusions are deceptively difficult to treat. Midface orthopedics may flatten the facial profile too much or cause the mandible to rotate downward and backward, whereas functional jaw orthopedics challenges the integrity of the mandibular dentition, which is already tipped off its base. Analysis of the space needs in type "C" Class II malocclusion must be done with great care, since the demands of the skeletal profile and its correction usually alter the eventual amount of space available in the mandibular arch. Modern orthodontists tend more and more to treat these malocclusions by diphasic therapy; that is, the facial skeleton is treated in the mixed dentition period and alignment of the teeth is carried out subsequently. It frequently is necessary to extract in order to provide space for the necessary alignment.

5) TREATMENT STRATEGIES FOR TYPE "D".—Type "D" Class II malocclusions are primarily a problem of mandibular insufficiency with a normal midface (Fig. XV-44, *G*). Paradoxically, there often is a good mandibular denture well placed over its basal bone. The maxillary incisors are found tipped labially and held in this position by a hyperactive mandibular lip. A tongue-thrust may be present as well. Indeed, the mandibular lip and tongue-thrust help provide a better lower arch, since they prevent labioversion and minimize overeruption of the mandibular incisors. Type "D" Class II malocclusions must be carefully discriminated from type "B," in which the midface is long, and type "C," in which the mandibular denture is off its base. Treatment aims are to offer every opportunity for mandibular growth while restraining, if possible, maxillary anterior growth. The maxillary dentition may need to be retracted and the maxillary incisors must be tipped lingually and aligned. If there has been a loss of incisal stops, it may be necessary to level the occlusal curve. Type "D" cases treat very well in the mixed dentition and usually respond positively to functional jaw orthopedic

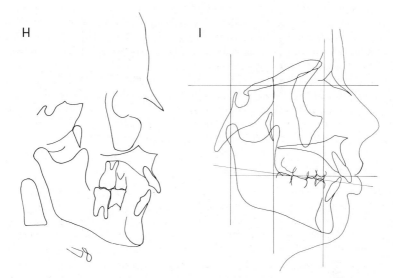

Fig. XV-44 (cont.).—H, type "E"; **I,** type "F." (See text for details.)

appliances of the activator type, if started early enough. Indeed, these are the classic activator cases. On the other hand, activators may be contraindicated if there is a borderline discrepancy problem in the lower arch. Class "C" cases are harder to treat at a later age, when skeletal growth is mostly completed.

6) TREATMENT STRATEGIES FOR TYPE "E".—Type "E" combines the worst skeletal and dental features of Class II, i.e., maxillary skeletal protrusion and dento-alveolar protraction with an insufficient mandible and labioversion of the mandibular incisors (Fig. XV-44, *H*). When these features are combined with a vertical skeletal dysplasia, as they usually are, there is constituted one of the most difficult malocclusions to treat well and retain. Space analysis is difficult, since it must be seen in light of the profile corrections necessary, corrections that invariably shorten the arch perimeter. Therefore, extractions are required more frequently than in any other Class II type. In recent times, it has become popular to treat type "E" malocclusions by diphasic treatment. Extra-oral traction, functional jaw orthopedics, or both, are employed in the mixed dentition to correct the skeletal pattern. Later, a period of multibanded appliance therapy is necessary to align the teeth and place them well over the bases and in harmony with the profile. Type "E" Class II malocclusions challenge the skills and abilities of the most experienced orthodontists.

7) TREATMENT STRATEGIES FOR TYPE "F".—Type "F" Class II malocclusions are characterized by a normal midface, mandibular insufficiency and a squarish gonial angle (Fig. XV-44, *I*). The occlusal plane

frequently is level, yet the skeletal vertical dysplasia is the key factor in the prognosis, for there always is a deep bite. The maxilla may appear normal anteroposteriorly and the maxillary dentition may be placed. It is important to check carefully the upper anterior face height, for it may be excessive. The lower dental arch usually is well placed over the mandibular base. The dental problem seen largely reflects the tooth size-space available situation except for the excessive overbite. Type "F" malocclusions frequently are treated in two phases, utilizing a flat acrylic bite plane or functional jaw orthopedics in the early mixed dentition and a later period of comprehensive appliance therapy.

2. CLASS III—MESIOCLUSION

Three rather distinct types of malocclusion often are confused, all of which at first glance may appear to be true mesioclusions. They may be separated most easily by ascertaining the primary etiologic site. The true Angle Class III, or mesioclusion, is a matter of skeletal dysplasia involving mandibular hypertrophy or, less often, marked shortening of the cranial base or maxilla. The pseudo-, or apparent, Class III involves a positional relationship brought about by early interference with the muscular reflex of mandibular closure. The pseudo- Class III is a functional mandibular protraction. The third condition, simple linguoversion of one or more maxillary anterior teeth, is caused by an abnormal axial inclination of maxillary incisors. It will be noted that the first condition is an abnormal *osseous* growth pattern, the second an acquired *muscular* reflex pattern of mandibular closure and the third a problem in *dental* positioning. In all three conditions, the maxillary anterior teeth are back of the mandibular, but only the first two show the mandibular molars ahead of their normal position. Simple linguoversion of maxillary anterior teeth is a Class I (neutroclusion) problem with an anterior crossbite. It is discussed under the heading of Anterior Crossbites, Simple (p. 574). The other two are discussed here together for ease in the differential diagnosis.

a) Differential Diagnosis

The differentiation of true and pseudo-mesioclusion requires a precise examination of the patient for the following items.

1) PROFILE.—Study the profile carefully for evidence of mandibular prognathism as seen in the soft tissues and facial musculature. Have the patient move from the postural position to occlusal contact position and note if this movement alters the profile. Lateral cephalograms are particularly helpful. These radiographs should be taken in both the occlusal contact and the postural relationship. A study of the osseous facial skeleton in such films usually can provide the complete diagnosis. In their absence, a thorough Facial Form Analysis is required (see Chapters VIII and XII).

(*a*) *True mesioclusion.*—The strong dominance of the mandible shows through the covering of soft tissue and the prognathism is seen in the profile at all times (see Fig. IX-1, *B*).

(*b*) *Pseudo-mesioclusion.*—When the lips are closed, the soft tissues may hide some of the apparent prognathism seen when the teeth alone are viewed. The profile improves as the mandible drops from occlusal contact relationship to the postural position.

2) MANDIBULAR ANGLE.—(*a*) *True mesioclusion.*—The mandibular angle invariably is obtuse, with the usual range from 130 to 140 degrees.

(*b*) *Pseudo-mesioclusion.*—The mandibular angle is more nearly a right angle, with the average near 120 degrees.

3) MANDIBULAR INCISAL ANGLE.—Study the axial inclination of the mandibular incisors to the mandibular plane.

(*a*) *True mesioclusion.*—The incisors usually are bunched and in linguoversion.

(*b*) *Pseudo-mesioclusion.*—The incisors are vertical or may be in slight labioversion when there is a pronounced anterior crossbite.

4) MANDIBULAR CLOSURE PATTERN.—(*a*) *True mesioclusion.*—These cases are more likely to have an even pattern of closure, describing a smooth arc, anteroposteriorly.

(*b*) *Pseudo-mesioclusion.*—The chin point moves forward sharply just before contact of the teeth. This can be confirmed by gently placing the fingertips over the temporomandibular joint during the closure action.

5) MOLAR RELATIONSHIP.—Note the relative positions of the first molars both in occlusion and in the postural position.

(*a*) *True mesioclusion.*—A distinct Class III relationship persists in both positions.

(*b*) *Pseudo-mesioclusion.*—Neutroclusion may be present in both positions, or there may be shift from a Class I to a Class III relationship as the mandible closes.

Manually move the mandible posteriorly to ascertain if it is possible to assume a more normal relationship with the maxilla. One also should use articulation paper as the patient attempts to close in neutroclusion. The location of the points of contact and interference on the occlusal surfaces as the teeth intermesh often is highly diagnostic. Read carefully the section on crossbites (Section D-2-a), for pseudo-mesioclusions are in reality anterior crossbites involving several teeth plus a forward positioning of the mandible.

b) Treatment

1) PSEUDO-MESIOCLUSION

(*a*) *Primary dentition.*—After all aspects of the case have been considered, treatment may proceed.

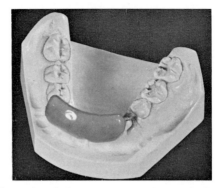

Fig. XV-45.—Acrylic inclined plane extension of incisal edges of the mandibular incisors, used for treatment of individual crossbites of anterior teeth.

Steps in treatment

In the early primary dentition, the case usually can be treated by equilibration alone (see Chapter XVII) or by the placement of an acrylic inclined plane on the mandibular incisors (Fig. XV-45). This acts as an extension of the incisal edge to contact the lingual surfaces of the maxillary anterior teeth. On closing, the mandible is forced to be retruded where it belongs. If the maxillary anterior teeth are tipped lingually, they will be moved labially into a more nearly correct position. The bevel of the appliance should be ground very carefully so that all teeth contact it evenly; the load is thus well distributed and no trauma is introduced. It may be cemented into position with a rather stiff mix of zinc oxide and eugenol. It is removed by slicing the acrylic with a carborundum disk. Do not worry about the large posterior open bite seen when the appliance is first inserted; it soon closes. Periodic observations may show that occlusal grinding is necessary to keep the load evenly distributed and to avoid the introduction of new closure patterns. Prescribe a semisolid diet for the period of treatment, usually only about a week. If marked improvement is not seen in this time, the case should be reassessed, for the original diagnosis probably was erroneous.

(b) Mixed dentition.—It should be remembered that the continual thrusting forward of the mandible and the locking of the teeth in pseudo-mesioclusion can only result in eventual perversion of the growth pattern of the facial skeleton. Thus, the older the patient the more difficult and lengthy the treatment procedure. In the mixed dentition, make doubly sure of the diagnosis before proceeding. An appliance similar to that used in the primary dentition may be satisfactory, although great variation in appliance design is necessary according to the number of teeth present. Lateral deviations on closure are more likely to be observed, owing to the greater cusp height of the permanent teeth.

Steps in treatment

Locate and remove all tooth interferences. This may involve grinding of primary teeth or use of an appliance to move interfering permanent teeth. It is un-

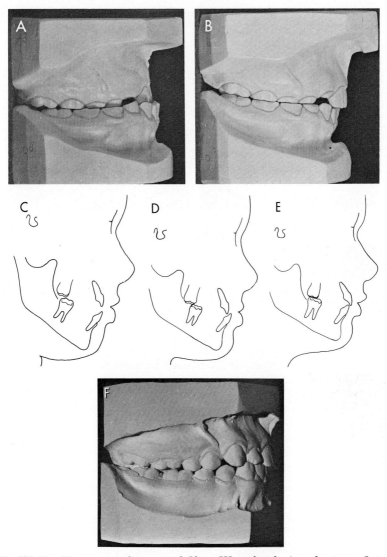

Fig. XV-46.—Neuromuscular type of Class III malocclusion. **A,** at age 8, treatment was by occlusal equilibration alone. **B,** the harmonious result obtained in a few days. **C,** the patient's postural position at the start of treatment. **D,** the patient's usual occlusal position, showing the functional mandibular protraction. **E,** the improved occlusal position obtained after occlusal equilibration. **F,** 9 years after the occlusal equilibration. No other orthodontic therapy was undertaken. Obviously, this patient has a mild skeletal Class III problem, but the occlusal equilibration at the right time prevented the case from becoming more complicated.

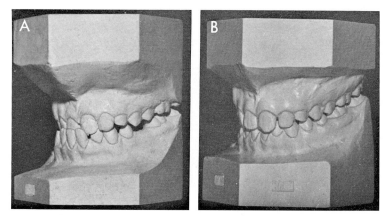

Fig. XV-47.—A, neuromuscular Class III malocclusion at the start of treatment. **B,** after treatment. The patient was 13 years of age at the start of treatment.

wise to grind permanent teeth in the mixed dentition period for this purpose, since the areas removed may be needed later for occlusal stability after the teeth's positions have been altered by growth.

Treatment is more difficult in the mixed dentition than in the primary, the prognosis is less favorable and the results are not so dramatic. Nonetheless, if the case is one of pure pseudo-mesioclusion, the results usually are satisfactory. Figure XV-46 shows a case of this kind treated successfully when the patient was 8 years of age.

(c) *Permanent dentition.*—A pseudo-mesioclusion is seen less frequently in the permanent dentition, since the continual malfunction produces aberrations of such magnitude in the facial growth pattern and positions of the teeth as to cloud the original deviation. In other

Fig. XV-48.—Comparison of the tracings of two mandibles superposed on the condyles. Note the linguoversion of the mandibular incisors in the Class III mandible and the extreme obtusity of the Class III mandible's gonial angle.

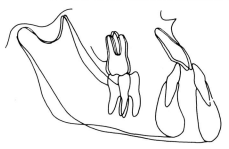

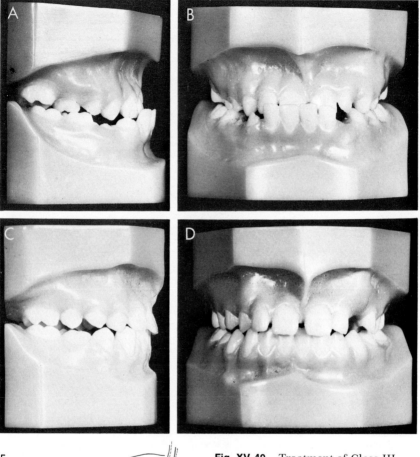

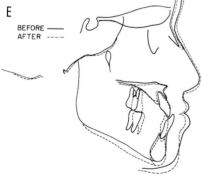

Fig. XV-49.—Treatment of Class III malocclusion. **A** and **B,** before treatment. **C** and **D,** after treatment. This case was treated with a Monobloc (Activator) appliance. (Courtesy of Dr. Ross O. Fisk, Department of Orthodontics, Faculty of Dentistry, University of Toronto.) **E,** cephalometric tracings of a Class III case before and after treatment. Note the dental adjustments made possible by the downward displacement of the mandibular growth. NOTE: this is *not* the same case shown in **A–D.**

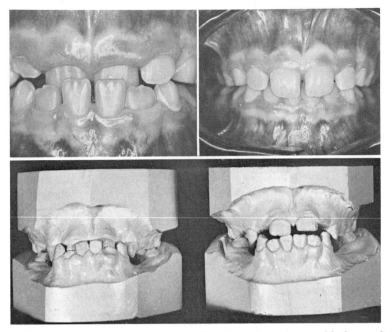

Fig. XV-50.—Above, an anterior crossbite treated with mandibular inclined plane. *Left,* before therapy. *Right,* after therapy. (Courtesy of Dr. John Mortell.) *Below,* a skeletal Class III on which a similar treatment was attempted. Note the difference in the response to treatment.

words, what originally was largely a muscular problem has now become a matter of bone growth as well. Treatment is more difficult, requires more time and the results are neither so dramatic nor so satisfactory. The same order of treatment as for the mixed dentition should be followed, but the tooth alignments take much longer and a full banded technic usually is needed. Figure XV-47 illustrates a case treated when the patient was 13 years of age.

2) TRUE MESIOCLUSION.—The term is a misnomer, since it leads one to focus attention on the molar relationship when the primary problem is truly one of osseous dysplasia (Fig. XV-48). The mandible is simply too large for the upper face and cranium with which it is associated. The etiologic factor usually is heredity, but it also is seen with certain endocrine disorders, for example, acromegaly. True mesioclusions also are due to a maxilla or cranial base that is short anteroposteriorly. In such cases, the mandibular angle is likely to be nearer normal and the mandible presents a normal appearance.

Treatment is concerned with providing a "satisfactory" functioning occlusion and attempting to hide or cover up the obvious aesthetic defects. True mesioclusion becomes progressively worse when left untreated, since the bony growth pattern is the determining factor. Some prefer to begin treatment at the earliest opportunity and attempt to retard or direct the vector of mandibular growth over a long period.

Significant advances have been made in the early treatment of Class III by Woodside and Graber. By skillful use of extra-oral traction, gross orthopedic changes are wrought as well as alterations in the vectors of mandibular growth (Fig. XV-49). Others simply leave the situation alone until young adult life and then try to create an occlusion that will hide the osseous growth defects. In extreme cases, combined surgery and orthodontics is the only recourse. In such instances, preoperative orthodontics is done; the mandible is shortened surgically, followed by another period of orthodontics for alignment of the teeth (see Fig. XV-67). True mesioclusions are among the most difficult problems the orthodontist encounters. Only in most unusual circumstances would the nonspecialist be advised to undertake their treatment. He must, however, be able to make the differential diagnosis in order to spare himself the embarrassment of mistaking a true mesioclusion for a simple pseudo-mesioclusion, and vice versa. The great difference in the prognosis of the two types makes it imperative that every dentist be able to distinguish between them clearly. Figure XV-50 shows two Class III cases treated with an inclined plane appliance, as if they both were pseudo-mesioclusions. The great difference in response is due to the fact that one was a true mesioclusion or osseous dysplasia and the other was an anterior crossbite. Continual failure of a pseudo-mesioclusion to respond to treatment can only mean a faulty original diagnosis.

3. Labioversion of Maxillary Incisors with Class I Molar Relationship

This condition seems similar to a dental type Class II, Division 1 malocclusion, since the anterior teeth of the maxilla have been brought mesially. The maxillary posterior teeth, however, have resisted the forward drifting tendencies. There usually is a good facial skeletal pattern, for if the pattern had been poor it would more likely have resulted in a Class II molar relationship. Many times the cause is a tongue-thrust and/or a thumb-sucking or finger-sucking habit. The condition may be accompanied by an open bite, particularly if the habit is still active. It also is found with a deep overbite due to the overeruption of the mandibular incisors. When the maxillary incisors were pulled forward, the lower teeth lost their antagonists and nothing prevented them from continuing upward. The result is a deep overbite and an enhanced curve of Spee. Even though the overbite may not be as severe as sometimes is seen in Class II, Division 1, this is not a condition to be taken lightly. If the overbite is severe, difficulty may be encountered in retracting the maxillary incisors unless the occlusal plane can be made level. The following discussion is centered on cases without a marked curve of Spee, for they are less difficult to correct.

Cases of this type with a marked curve of Spee and an impinging overbite are much more severe than those to be discussed and usually must be treated by a multibanded appliance to level the occlusal plane and torque and retract the incisors. Such tooth movements shorten the arch perimeter, further complicating the case.

a) Diagnosis

The diagnosis is made by ascertaining a true Class I molar relationship. This condition must be carefully differentiated from a Class II, Division 1, in which the lower teeth have drifted forward, causing anterior crowding and yet maintaining a Class I molar relationship. The lower arch ordinarily is well aligned, although there may be some increase from normal in the curve of Spee. It is most important to check carefully for the presence of an active tongue-thrust or thumb-sucking or finger-sucking habit. When they are found, the first step in treatment is correction of the habit.

b) Treatment

1) EARLY MIXED DENTITION.—A useful appliance is the hollow bite plane (Sidlow plate) shown in Figure XVII-50. This has the advantage of allowing the easy retraction of the maxillary anterior teeth while removing all tooth interferences and aiding in the flattening of the curve of the occlusal plane. The plate will maintain the length of the maxillary arch and prevent any change in the molar relationship. Another appliance that may be used is the oral shield (see Fig. XVII-59). The oral shield helps correct abnormal lip and sucking habits while utilizing lip force to move the maxillary anterior teeth lingually. This shield is not indicated for treatment of any kind of distoclusion. Figure XV-51 illustrates a treated case of labioversion of the maxillary anterior teeth.

An overt attempt is made to upset the sequence of eruption and cause the maxillary cuspids to erupt earlier than they would have otherwise. This procedure takes the cuspid pressure off the root of the lateral incisor, permitting it to be moved more easily. By removing the primary cuspid and primary first molar, the permanent cuspid and first bicuspid will begin to erupt sooner. It also may be helpful to remove some bone overlying the erupting permanent cuspid's crown. As the cuspid and first bicuspid erupt, it also is necessary to slice off the mesial bulge of the second primary molar. Thus, it is possible to supervise the loss of the primary teeth and control safely the eruption of the cuspid and bicuspids, for the Sidlow plate will prevent any forward drifting of the first permanent molar. Banding of incisors and first molars in each arch can effect an efficient correction of these problems. The lower

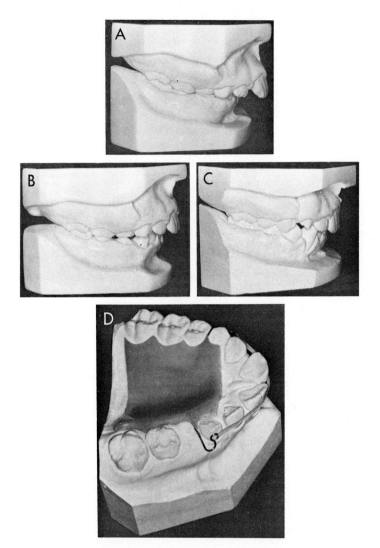

Fig. XV-51.—Treatment of labioversion in a Class I malocclusion by means of an oral shield. **A,** at the start of treatment. **B,** after 3 months. **C,** after 6 months. Note recession of the gingival tissue around the neck of the mandibular cuspid as the incisor relationship improved. The shield should have been remade so that traumatic occlusion was not introduced. The shield itself provided the trauma that produced the periodontal lesion. **D,** a modification of the maxillary acrylic palate appliance, which also may be used for such problems.

archwire is used for leveling and idealizing the arch form, whereas the maxillary archwire intrudes and retracts the incisors.

2) LATE MIXED DENTITION.—Treatment has the same objectives and strategy as in the early mixed dentition but is more difficult, since there is less time to guide the erupting teeth, and maintenance of molar relationships is more difficult.

3) PERMANENT DENTITION.—Treatment must proceed on the principles outlined for the mixed dentition.

Note carefully the interdigitation of teeth in the lateral segment. If it is normal from the cuspid back to and including the second molar, proceed as for the mixed dentition. If the lateral interdigitation is not normal, the case is likely to be a very mild Class II, Division 1 of a dental type, requiring a slight amount of distal movement of the molars.

The correction and control of deleterious oral habits is an important part of treatment at any age. If the condition is accompanied by an anterior open bite, this bite usually will be self-correcting when the habit is controlled and the rest of the treatment is begun.

The Hawley retainer with a flat bite plane is useful in these cases. When there is a residual hyperactive mentalis muscle, the modified oral shield shown in Figure XVII-72 is an efficient retainer.

4. ANTERIOR CROSSBITES, SIMPLE

Simple anterior crossbites are dental-type malocclusions due to abnormal axial inclinations of maxillary anterior teeth. These malocclusions must be clearly differentiated from the mesioclusions, which they may seem to resemble. The anterior crossbite has many other names, e.g., "in-locked" incisors and "scissors bite."

Fig. XV-52.—Crossbite of a maxillary incisor. In this instance, there was not sufficient space for the lateral incisor and it was necessary to move all of the teeth in the right lateral segment posteriorly until the crossbite could be corrected. (Courtesy of Dr. Aaron Posen.) *Left* is before and *right* is after treatment.

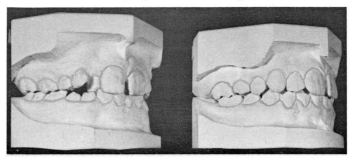

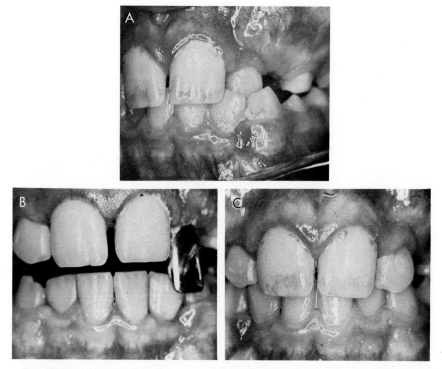

Fig. XV-53.—Lingual crossbite of a lateral incisor. Here there was sufficient space for the lateral incisor in the line of arch. **A,** before treatment. **B,** after the insertion of a stainless steel crown form, which was made unduly long in order to engage the lower teeth. Sometimes the stainless steel crown forms can be placed backward on the tooth in crossbite in order to tip them labially more effectively. **C,** 1 week later. Note the gingival hypertrophy due to the failure to maintain good oral hygiene.

a) Diagnosis

The molar relationship should be noted carefully in resting position and occlusion. If a Class II or Class III malocclusion is seen at either position, the problem is not one of simple anterior crossbite. The latter malocclusion is a matter of lingually tipped maxillary anterior teeth without serious disruption of the molar relationship. Anterior crossbites may involve one (Fig. XV-52) or more (see Fig. XV-55) teeth.

b) Treatment

1) SINGLE TOOTH.—A single anterior tooth in crossbite may be brought into alignment easily, provided there is space in the arch for it. If there

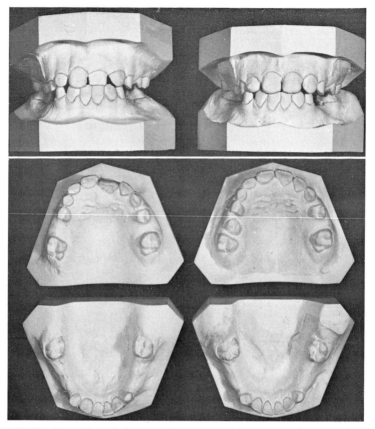

Fig. XV-54.—Crossbite of the maxillary central incisor combined with a problem in arch length. The case was treated by combining the mandibular inclined plane appliance with a regainer to upright the mandibular molars. Simultaneously, a regaining appliance was placed in the maxilla. *Left* is before treatment and *right* is after.

is not, space must be created before tipping the offending tooth labially (see Fig. XV-52). When there is sufficient space, the tooth may be brought directly into line (Fig. XV-53).

An acrylic inclined plane, as shown in Figure XV-45, also is effective. It must be adjusted carefully and not left in place unduly long. Figure XV-54 illustrates an anterior crossbite treated with an inclined plane. An auxiliary spring attached to a lingual archwire may be used or several adjacent teeth banded and the locked tooth brought to a light labial archwire by means of ligatures.

2) SEVERAL TEETH.—This condition requires the observance of the same fundamentals mentioned for a single tooth in crossbite. Lingual archwires with auxiliary springs are effective, labial archwires and

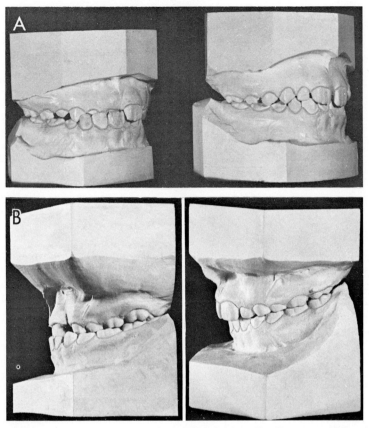

Fig. XV-55.—A, dental-type crossbite of several teeth. (Courtesy of Dr. Aaron Posen.) **B,** crossbite of several teeth. This anterior crossbite looked like a skeletal Class III but the ready response to treatment disproves that diagnosis. **A** and **B,** *left* is before treatment; *right* is after treatment.

banded anterior teeth are excellent and the inclined plane appliance may be used also. Figure XV-55 illustrates the successful treatment of one such case.

5. BIMAXILLARY PROTRUSIONS

a) Bimaxillary Prognathism

Bimaxillary prognathism is a skeletal problem in which both maxilla and mandible have a relationship more forward than normal with respect to the cranium and cranial base (Fig. XV-56). Bimaxillary prognathism is a characteristic of several races, for example, the Negroid. The

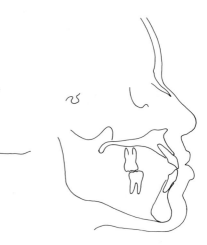

Fig. XV-56.—Cephalometric tracing of a patient with bimaxillary prognathism.

prognathic tendencies of the maxilla do not increase much after the age of 12 years. The mandible, however, continues to grow until the mid-twenties. The apparently abnormal inclinations of the teeth seen in bimaxillary prognathism are secondary to the growth of the bones, the teeth having accommodated their positions to the pattern of facial growth.

The diagnosis of bimaxillary prognathism is difficult, and it is even more difficult to predict the patient's future growth and the final relationship of the jaws. In the cephalogram, both the maxilla and the mandible are forward with respect to the anterior cranial base, that is, both the SNA and the SNB angles are large. In true bimaxillary prognathism, the axial inclinations of the teeth are nearer normal than in bimaxillary dental protrusion (see below), which makes the treatment of bimaxillary prognathism by extraction of teeth more difficult. Since bimaxillary prognathism is a problem in the basic growth pattern of the bony skeleton, interception is not a satisfactory strategy. Treatment in the young adult must be approached with caution, since the appliance procedures are difficult and the results not always fully satisfactory. A common mistake is made when the basic skeletal pattern is not recognized and attempts are made to impose too "flat" a profile by orthodontic therapy. One must take care not to confuse bimaxillary prognathism with bimaxillary dental protrusion. A definitive cephalometric analysis is required.

b) Bimaxillary Dental Protrusion

Bimaxillary dental protrusion is a condition in which procumbency of both dentitions on the bony bases is seen (Fig. XV-57). There may be strong genetic factors, as in bimaxillary prognathism, but bimax-

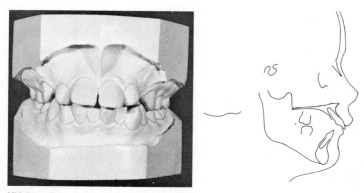

Fig. XV-57.—Bimaxillary dental protrusion. In this instance, only the teeth are protrusive. Compare the cephalometric tracing in this illustration with that in Figure XV-56.

illary dental protrusion also can arise from mesial drifting of the teeth in both arches. The condition also is seen when larger than normal teeth are found in conjunction with normal or smaller than normal osseous bases. As stated above, bimaxillary dental protrusion must be carefully differentiated from bimaxillary prognathism.

F. Vertical Relationships of Teeth and Dental Arches

1. OPEN BITE

An open bite is the result of vertical development that is insufficient to permit a tooth or teeth to meet their antagonists in the opposite arch. The result is localized absence of occlusion (Fig. XV-58). During the normal course of eruption, it is expected that the teeth and their surrounding alveolar bone will develop until the occlusal antagonist of the opposite arch is met. An interference with the normal course of

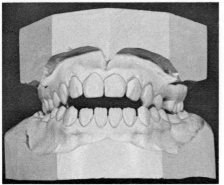

Fig. XV-58.—Anterior open bite.

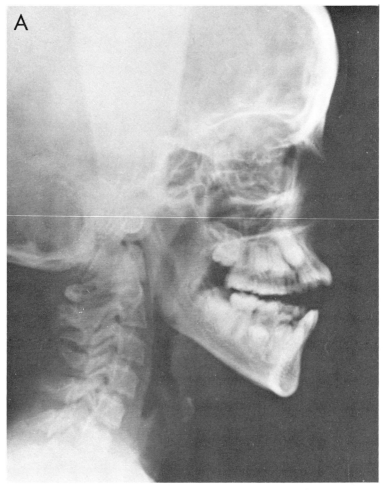

Fig. XV-59.—Gross skeletal dysplasia resulting in an open bite. Surgery early in life was undertaken to correct a bifid nose (see Fig. IV-23, *F*), which caused a further impedance to normal growth of the nasomaxillary complex. Note the upward slope of the palate (**A**). (*Continued.*)

eruption and alveolar development may result in an open bite. The causes of open bite generally may be grouped under three headings: (1) disturbances in the eruption of the teeth and alveolar growth, for example, ankylosed primary molars, (2) mechanical interference with eruption and alveolar growth, for example, a finger-sucking habit, and (3) gross osseous dysplasia. The last group is composed of but a small percentage of the total open bite cases, yet are extremely difficult to treat (Fig. XV-59).

There are two current definitions of open bite (Fig. XV-60). Through-

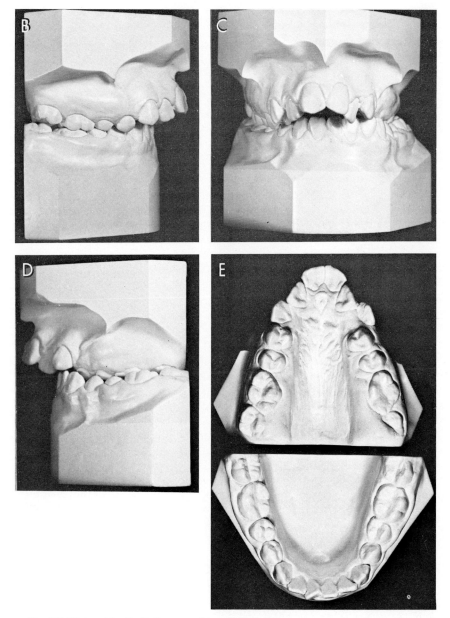

Fig. XV-59 (cont.)—B–D, the crossbite. **E,** the disharmony in the dimensions of the dental arches.

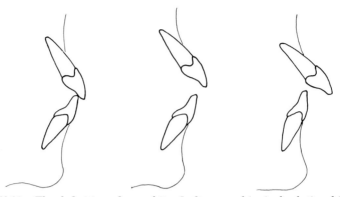

Fig. XV-60.—The definition of open bite. *Left,* normal incisal relationship. *Center,* an open bite without vertical overlap of the incisors. *Right,* an open bite with vertical overlap of the incisors. This type of open bite often is not diagnosed.

out this book, the term "open bite" means the lack of a functional antagonistic tooth.

a) Anterior Open Bite

Open bites in the anterior portion of the dental arches may be combined with labioversion of the maxillary anterior teeth. When studying anterior open bites before treatment, take great care to note the relationship of the osseous bases to the dentition. Preoccupation with the open bite may lead to erroneous diagnosis of a more basic skeletal problem.

1) DELETERIOUS HABITS AS CAUSE.—By far the majority of anterior open bites are caused by finger-, thumb-, tongue- and other sucking habits. If, during eruption, the teeth repeatedly encounter a finger, thumb or tongue placed between them, eruption is impeded and an open bite results. Always suspect a habit of some sort when an open bite first is diagnosed. In young children, it is most likely to be a thumb or finger that is sucked at night or a tongue-thrust on swallowing. Adults may suck a pipe or a pencil, with a similar result. Treatment consists, first, of controlling the habit. This alone may be sufficient and the teeth may continue to erupt to normal position. Because of the many problems unique to habit control, they are discussed under a separate heading (see Chapter XVII, section G). Retention, after treatment, of any malocclusion due to a sucking habit is almost impossible unless the habit is overcome completely and normal lip and tongue activity and function are restored.

2) GROSS OSSEOUS DYSPLASIA IN ETIOLOGY.—Micrognathia, mandibular hypertrophy and other severe disorders of the craniofacial skeleton may give rise to anterior open bites. In such instances, the open bite

is a rather minor manifestation of a gross bony discrepancy (see Fig. XV-59).

b) Posterior Open Bite

Open bites in the posterior regions of the mouth may be due to habits such as lateral thrusting of the tongue during swallowing. More frequently, the cause is related to the development of the alveolar process and eruption of the teeth. In adults, the posterior open bite may be more serious than one in the anterior part of the mouth. The older the patient the more severe the problem becomes because there is less chance for alveolar growth to correct it.

1) TONGUE-THRUSTING AS CAUSE.—Only rarely is tongue-thrusting a primary etiologic agent in posterior open bites. More frequently, the open bite is formed and afterward the tongue maintains it to effect a seal during swallowing. Treatment of posterior open bites due to tongue-thrusting is similar to that used for anterior open bites, although the design of the appliance must be altered according to the region of the open bite (see Chapter XVII).

2) ANKYLOSED PRIMARY TEETH AND OTHER CAUSES.—A localized arrest of eruption and alveolar development may occur during the mixed dentition stage. The syndrome bears many names and there is no unanimity of opinion as to the etiology. The problem is discussed under the heading Ankylosed Primary Molars (see section C-2-d).

Later in life, when a posterior open bite is observed, unless a habit can be indicted, there may be an ankylosis of the permanent teeth. Ankylosed teeth cannot be moved because the periodontal membrane is not intact. Many times, the diagnosis is difficult; certainly radiographs give only limited help. However, if a tooth does not move when orthodontic traction is placed against it, it most certainly is ankylosed, and restorative procedures must be utilized to provide occlusal function. The occlusal plane height must be established in the area of the open bite.

2. EXCESSIVE OVERBITE

Excessive overbite is a combination of skeletal, dental and neuromuscular features that causes an undue amount of vertical overlap in the incisor region. Closed bite (excessive overbite due to loss of posterior teeth) is presented separately following this discussion.

Excessive overbite may be seen with many different types of malocclusion, although it is observed most commonly in Class I and Class II. A divergence of opinion seems to exist as to what constitutes the normal range of overbite. Surely there are age variations, and the permissible amount of overbite may vary, too, with the type of facial skeleton. The overbite should not be considered excessive unless masticatory functioning is impeded, there is a functional retraction of the mandible (see Chapters X and XI), abnormal wear of teeth is induced or the integrity of certain teeth may be jeopardized in the future. Overbite must be related to the health of the soft and supporting structures, temporomandibular function and the effects of that function on growth just as carefully as to occlusion.

Cast analysis alone is insufficient, for the amount of freeway space is a critical factor in prognosis (see Chapters X and XI). When there is a larger than normal distance between the postural and the usual occlusal position, greater opportunities for treatment exist. Often, in deep bite cases, the occlusal vertical dimension is not in harmony with the neuromusculature, just as the occlusal anteroposterior position may not harmonize well with the muscle pattern.

a) Etiology

Popovich,[5] in an excellent study, found that the factors contributing to excessive overbite varied with the type of occlusion. Thus, in the ideal occlusion, the amount of overbite was determined largely by dental factors. In the Class I malocclusion with a deep overbite (more than 4 mm.) also, the overbite seemed to be controlled by dental factors, for example, length of the incisors, elevation of the maxillary first molars and the angle between the long axes of the central incisors. In Class II cases, however, skeletal features, particularly diminished lower face height and shortened ramus height, were combined with the dental factors mentioned above.

b) Diagnosis

The determination of the causative factors in a given case is perhaps the most important step in diagnosis of excessive overbite. Too frequently, excessive overbite is visualized as a separate entity. Such an approach will handicap greatly the planning of treatment. It is far better to view the overbite as a troublesome part of the total malocclusion. The more the overbite is attributable to skeletal features the more difficult the task of overcoming it. It should be noted that the dental factors are grouped easily into two distinct categories: tooth size, e.g., the length of the central incisor, and tooth position, e.g., mesial drifting of the maxillary first molar. When the overbite is caused by malpositions of teeth, it is handled much more easily than when it is due to the length of teeth. When neuromuscular factors are present, an opportunity for guiding vertical alveolar development exists. Study the freeway space carefully. Measure the interocclusal distance in the cephalogram and the direction of movement from posture to the usual occlusal position. A flat maxillary bite plane may be worn for a short time prior to the diagnostic measures. The bite plane serves to reduce the occlusal sensory input to the muscles. They become more relaxed and the interocclusal distance can be measured more validly.

An effort has been made to relate various sizes of teeth to their optimal overbite. Popovich's study shows us why we cannot predict, by tooth measurements alone, the amount of overbite a given patient will have after treatment; the problem usually is a combined dental and skeletal one. Certain cephalometric analyses of vertical dimension seem to offer much promise. In fact, cephalometric analysis seems almost indispensable in the very severe overbite problem, although the vertical analyses are not as sophisticated as those used for anteroposterior assessment (see Chapter XII).

Diagnosis thus consists of identifying the possible dental contributions, the skeletal factors and the neuromuscular attributes. Treatment depends on which features are present and the age of the patient.

c) *Planning the Treatment*

1) IN THE PRIMARY DENTITION.—On the rare occasions when an excessive overbite is seen in the primary dentition, it is most likely to have a skeletal basis. Matthews[4] has reported excellent results using simple maxillary bite planes during this early period. The activator also may be used to direct differential alveolar growth to effect a correction and reduce the interocclusal distance.

2) IN THE MIXED DENTITION.—*With Class I molar relationship.*—If the overbite seems excessive in the mixed dentition when there is a Class I molar relationship, it usually is due to one or more of the following related factors:

    1. Length of the crowns of the central incisors.

    2. Elevation of the maxillary first molars (i.e., the anatomic crown of the molar has not erupted to its full clinical crown height).

    3. Failure to recognize a normal stage of development. The overbite is greater just after eruption of the permanent incisors and decreases with eruption of the posterior teeth.

None of these factors requires heroic orthodontic treatment, although the first molars often can be aided in their eruption to full height by the wearing of an acrylic appliance with a flat bite plane or a monobloc. Such an appliance may help, too, if the curve of Spee is excessive. These appliances may be used at this age if one is certain of the cause of the excessive overbite and there is sufficient freeway space for their use.

With Class II molar relationship.—In the presence of a Class II molar relationship, the excessive overjet makes it easy for the teeth and alveolar processes in the front portion of the arch to overdevelop vertically. When the maxillary teeth and their alveolar process have no antagonists, the vertical alveolar development is excessive and the upper face height increases as the teeth descend. At the same time, the mandibular teeth erupt well lingually to their usual position of contact with the maxillary teeth and may even impinge on the soft tissue of the palate. The curve of Spee is thus enhanced considerably. Treatment is not directed to the overbite but to the total Class II problem.

The deep bite is but one aspect of a complete syndrome. There is rather general agreement that the more severe depth of bite problems can be brought to a better stable result by treating during growth rather than later. The presence of functional features and a large freeway space improve the prognosis (see Section E).

3) IN THE PERMANENT DENTITION.—When growth is completed, the treatments previously described are of little value. The flat bite plate may be used as a diagnostic appliance but it should not be left in the mouth, even though it may give some aesthetic improvement and relief from temporomandibular joint symptoms. It is far better to provide occlusal rehabilitation and any necessary periodontal therapy. Treatment of deep bite in the permanent dentition seldom is provided by orthodontic therapy alone. More often, the orthodontics is combined with periodontal and restorative or prosthetic services.

3. CLOSED BITE

Closed bite is an increased overbite due to loss of posterior teeth. The freeway space is excessive, the path of mandibular closure irregular and the condition frequently is accompanied by temporomandibular joint pain or dysfunction. Closed bite is a clinical problem of middle and old age that usually is best resolved by prosthetic procedures. Orthodontic appliances are used for two purposes only: (1) for alignment of teeth to assist in retention of the prosthesis planned and (2) for determining the ideal occlusal position. An acrylic plate with a flat anterior bite plane frees cuspal interferences, permitting the muscles that control mandibular position to hold the bone in its ideal occlusal position.

G. Spacing of Teeth

1. LOCALIZED SPACING

a) Etiology

Localized spacing may be due to many reasons other than variations of normal spacing. Treatment is highly individualized, but a knowledge of the general principles of etiology and diagnosis is very helpful.

Problems in localized spacing, that is, excessive spacing at one or a very few contact points between the teeth, usually are attributable to (1) missing teeth, (2) undue retention of primary teeth or (3) a deleterious sucking habit. One specific problem, that of spacing between the maxillary central incisors, is seen so frequently as to merit detailed discussion later.

1) ABSENT TEETH.—*Congenitally missing teeth.*—These may cause localized spacing, but the problem may not be seen in just one spot because adjacent teeth often drift into the space. (See Section A-1, Missing Teeth, for a discussion of this problem.)

Unerupted teeth.—Sometimes a tooth is impacted or remains un-

TABLE XV-5.—Percentage of Cases Showing Various Types
of Midline Spacing Problems

Supernumerary teeth at the midline (3)	3.7%
Congenitally missing lateral incisors (9)	11.0%
Unusually small teeth (2)	2.4%
Enlarged or malposed labium frenum (20)	24.4%
Spacing a part of normal growth (19)	23.2%
Imperfect fusion at midline of premaxilla (27)	32.9%
Combination of imperfect fusion and congenitally missing lateral incisors (2)	2.4%
Total (82)	100.0%

erupted. The spacing problem is then localized, and the plan of treatment is determined by the chances of bringing the tooth into its normal relationship. (See section C-2-c, Impaction of Teeth.)

Premature loss of permanent teeth.—This matter is discussed in section A-2, Loss of Permanent Teeth Due to Trauma, Caries, etc.

2) Undue retention of primary teeth.—Belated loss of primary teeth may force the erupting permanent teeth to unnatural positions. Later, when the primary tooth is exfoliated, a space results. This sequence of events is seen most frequently in the cuspid region. Obviously, the easiest and most practical treatment is removal of the primary tooth before it has deflected the permanent tooth.

3) Sucking habits.—These may cause a localized spacing of the teeth. One should read the following sections to understand this problem: XV-E-3, XV-F-1 and XVII-G.

b) Spacing between Maxillary Central Incisors

One of the malocclusions of most concern to patients is diastema between the maxillary central incisors. Excessive spacing in such a prominent place in the dentition is unsightly, although it does little to reduce masticatory efficiency. Treatment is solely for cosmetic and psychologic effects.

The data in Table XV-5 suggest that too much emphasis has been placed on the labium frenum and too little on structures and development at the midline. It also is of interest that in this series of patients nearly one fourth were developing normally.

1) Examination and differential diagnosis.—Since there are several possible causes of the condition, each requiring different forms of therapy, a careful examination is the only means of arriving at a correct diagnosis.

Steps in examination

a) Definitely decide whether the spacing is localized between the central incisors or whether generalized diastemata are present.

b) Measure the teeth and compare their sizes with the averages given in Table VI-5, page 193.

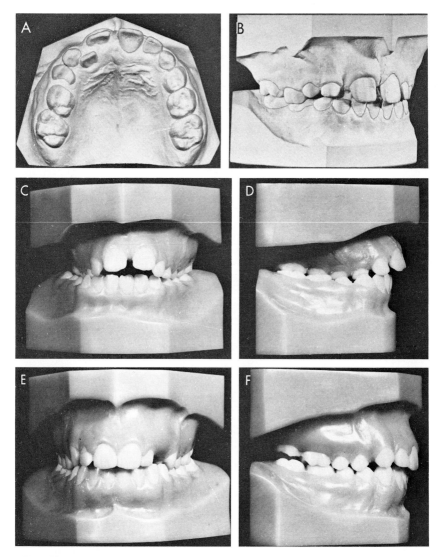

Fig. XV-61.—Crossbite problems. **A** and **B,** an interesting problem in which crossbite of the maxillary lateral incisor was combined with or caused by a supernumerary tooth at the midline. After removal of the supernumerary tooth, the incisor was moved more easily into the line of arch. **C–F,** an open bite combined with a crossbite. **C** and **D,** before treatment. **E** and **F,** after treatment. This case was treated by an undergraduate student using a maxillary lingual archwire. Often the same lingual appliance can be used to correct the crossbite, deter an oral habit and retain the treated occlusion. (**C–F** courtesy of the Department of Orthodontics, Faculty of Dentistry, University of Toronto.)

c) Lift the upper lip and while it is displaced look for blanching of the soft tissue lingual to and between the central incisors. The absence of blanching is *not* diagnostic; the presence of blanching points to a malposed labium frenum.

d) Determine, if possible, whether the space is increasing.

e) Secure periapical radiograms of the region, including both lateral incisors. Clarity in the alveolar regions is more important than interproximal details of the exposed crowns. It is essential that the central ray be directed perpendicular to the alveolar septum between the central incisors (see Figs. XV-62–XV-66). There is considerable variation in the midline structures, but there also are several abnormalities of interest that may be seen clearly only in the radiograph.

2) SUPERNUMERARY TEETH AT THE MIDLINE.—The diagnosis of this condition is based solely on radiographic studies unless the supernumerary tooth has erupted. A supernumerary tooth is the only condition likely to cause an increase in the space between the maxillary central incisors. This is discussed in Section A-3, Supernumerary Teeth. Treatment involves removal of such extra teeth as soon as diagnosed without endangering the adjacent teeth. Early removal permits the eruptive force of the incisors to close the space at the midline. Figure XV-61 illustrates the need for radiographs. The problem shown seems to be a simple matter of a lateral incisor in crossbite. Actually, a supernumerary tooth was causing the spacing at the midline and holding the lateral incisor in malposition.

3) CONGENITALLY MISSING LATERAL INCISORS.—Treatment of this

Fig. XV-62 (left).—Midline spacing in the maxilla due to congenital absence of lateral incisors.

Fig. XV-63 (right).—Spade-shaped interosseous tip between the maxillary central incisors, usually associated with an enlarged maxillary labial frenum.

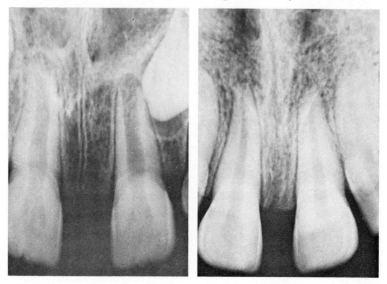

condition is discussed in Section A-1, Missing Teeth. Figure XV-62 illustrates a typical midline diastema due to congenital absence of lateral incisors.

4) ENLARGED OR MALPOSED LABIUM FRENUM

Diagnosis

The enlarged or malposed labium frenum occasionally may be diagnosed by observation alone or by lifting the lip, as described earlier. However, it is impossible to detect all enlarged or malposed frena in this manner. The final diagnosis must be based on the radiograph. The normal osseous septum between the maxillary central incisors is V-shaped and bisected by the intermaxillary suture, which sometimes is not visible in the radiograph (see Fig. XV-66). When the labium frenum inserts on the palatal side of the septum, the fibers of the frenum run across the bone, rounding it over so that the septum is spade shaped (Fig. XV-63). On occasion, a shallow trough is seen. Even when the fibers insert so deeply as not to cause blanching when the lip is displaced, the condition is diagnosed easily in the radiograph.

Treatment

Treatment consists of bringing the incisors together and excising the frenum. The incisors may be banded, a short wire ligated into the brackets and the teeth pulled together by ligatures or light elastics. In no circumstance use free elastics around the necks of unbanded teeth for this movement. It is much too easy for the patient to let one of the elastics slip up the neck of a tooth, destroying the supporting structures and endangering the tooth itself. After the central incisors have come into juxtaposition, excise the frenum and replace the orthodontic appliance while healing is taking place. The scar tissue formed will serve to help in retention. Obversely, if excision is undertaken before orthodontic movement, the teeth must be moved through the newly formed scar tissue. Although some prefer to remove the frenum by cautery, any of the several technics involving excision by scalpel are to be preferred because there is better control and less scar tissue is formed. A ligature is used to prevent reattachment of the frenum. Sometimes the orthodontic force itself will cause pressure atrophy of the frenum fibers, making excision of the frenum unnecessary.

5) IMPERFECT FUSION AT THE MIDLINE.

—The midline is a common site of development faults, such as epithelial rests and inclusion cysts. The condition illustrated in Figures XV-64 and XV-65 may be related to imperfect fusion at the midline, for histologic study of the tissue included within such osseous bifurcations has shown connective and epithelial tissue. A wide variety of forms will be observed, all of which must be differentiated from the normal suture. A distinctly W-shaped osseous septum may be associated with this condition, as well as a circumscribed irregular ovoid area (see Fig. XV-65). The separation of the osseous septum may be shallow or continue well into the alveolar process.

Treatment

This is exactly as for a malposed or enlarged labium frenum, except that the included tissue, rather than the frenum, must be excised. The excision must be

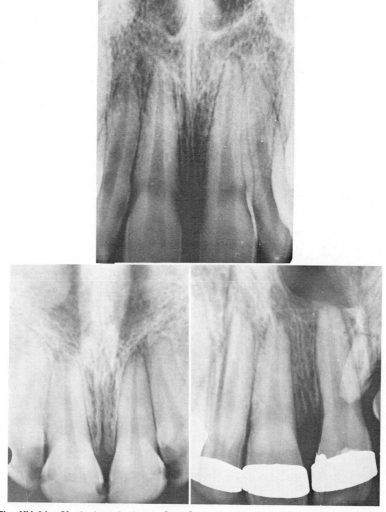

Fig. XV-64.—Variations in imperfect fusion at the midline in the maxilla. The suture can be seen clearly above the bifurcation in the interosseous tip. At the split tip will be found invaginated epithelial and periosteal tissue.

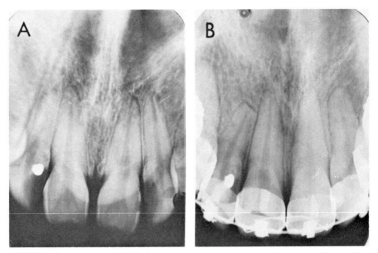

Fig. XV-65.—Imperfect midline in the dental septum. **A,** note the split of the septum or the W-shaped osseous tip between the central incisors. **B,** after treatment. The orthodontic appliance brought the teeth together. The invaginated tissue was removed surgically and the appliance used as a retainer during healing. Mere clipping of the labial frenum will not correct this problem.

Fig. XV-66.—Spacing between maxillary central incisors closing normally, with eruption of the lateral incisors.

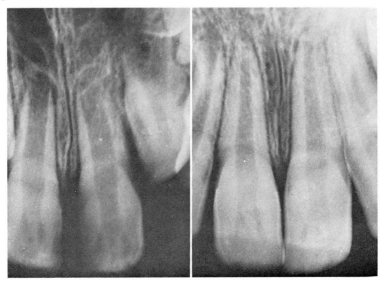

carried out thoroughly or regeneration will occur, forcing the teeth apart again. One satisfactory method is to lift a V-shaped mucosal flap directly over the septum between the central incisors The flap should flare well laterally so that later it will lie easily in place. After the alveolar bone is exposed, a surgical fissure or tapered fissure bur may be inserted gently into the cleft in the bone. With the motor turning at a slow speed, the bur will remove the included tissue and will freshen the edges of the bone as well. After excision, allow the flap to fall into place, suturing if necessary. The orthodontic appliance, which has brought the teeth together, must be replaced during healing (see Fig. XV-65). Occasionally, fibers of the frenum will insert into the suture. The same procedure may be used for their excision.

6) SPACING AS PART OF NORMAL GROWTH.—The central incisors erupt with a space between them (see Fig. VI-38). This space is diminished when the lateral incisors erupt and finally is closed by the wedging of the erupting cuspids. In the absence of abnormal midline structures or gross variations in tooth size, it can be assumed that the midline space will close naturally (Fig. XV-66).

2. GENERALIZED SPACING

a) Diagnosis

Several etiologic factors of varying frequency are involved in generalized spacing of the teeth. It is important to ascertain the presence of true generalized spacing. More frequently, a localized spacing problem is encountered.

1) SMALL TEETH.—If the teeth are unusually small for the size of the alveolar arch that includes them, generalized spacing may result. If the teeth, when measured, are very small and there are no other apparent causative factors, the smallness of the teeth alone may be at fault. Such a condition is rare and probably should not be treated orthodontically. The best treatment is by means of jacket crowns or consolidation of the arch and the placement of bridges. Whether such a heroic measure as a series of jacket crowns is to be undertaken is an individual matter, dependent on the wishes of the patient and on the cosmetic problem. Most problems of spacing due to small teeth might best be left alone.

2) LARGE TONGUE.—Another rather rare cause of generalized spacing is an unduly large tongue. Diagnosis is best made by careful examination of the tongue extended as well as in situ. The lateral edges of the tongue, when it is too large for the alveolar arch, usually display scalloping at the sites where the tongue rests against the lingual surfaces of the mandibular teeth. Treatment is contraindicated unless gross malocclusion is present, in which case a wedge of tissue is excised from the tongue. This rather heroic approach is not advocated unless a debilitating malocclusion is present.

3) SUCKING HABITS.—Sucking habits may cause rather generalized spacing of the teeth, although they are more likely to cause a localized

spacing of the maxillary anterior teeth. See Chapter VII for a discussion of digital sucking and Chapter XVII for suggested therapy in thumb-sucking and tongue-thrusting.

H. Gross Facial Deformities

Although a wide variety of gross facial deformities may be encountered, only two are seen frequently enough to merit discussion in this book—mandibular prognathism and cleft lip and palate. Ordinarily, none of the gross facial deformities are the therapeutic responsibility of the family dentist.

1. Mandibular Prognathism

This term is applied when the mandible is proportionately too large for the rest of the face and head. The condition may be due to mandibular hypertrophy, midface deficiency or combinations of the two. The condition is discussed in Section E-2, Class III—Mesioclusion. Figure XV-67 shows a case of mandibular prognathism treated with combined surgery and orthodontics.

2. Cleft Lip and Palate

Much progress has been made in cleft lip and palate therapy. One of the most important new concepts is that of positioning the segments of the maxilla by means of appliances and tension bandages prior to lip surgery. This orthodontic treatment of the young infant provides a more normal relationship of parts prior to lip surgery. The lip surgery then has a beneficial stabilizing effect, aiding more normal growth, until palate surgery can be done. Not all children are favorable candidates for this early orthodontic method.

In a similar fashion, not all cleft lip and palate children need the same schedule of surgery. Two general views of the timing of surgery are held:

a) The lip is operated on the first few weeks after birth and the palatal surgery is postponed until the age of 4–6 years. The rationale for this approach is supported by the idea that it is better to allow the face to grow along as nearly a normal path as possible for as long a time as possible. The surgery inevitably must have some effects on the growth of the facial region; therefore, postpone those effects as long as possible. Such a course of action may make the surgeon's task more difficult but the facial region will grow more normally than it would have following surgery. Orthodontic and prosthetic corrections follow, to aid the speech therapist in his important work.

b) The other school of thought wishes the surgery done at the time the surgeon can do the best job. This usually means that the lip is operated on at about the second month or a bit earlier and the palate at 18–24

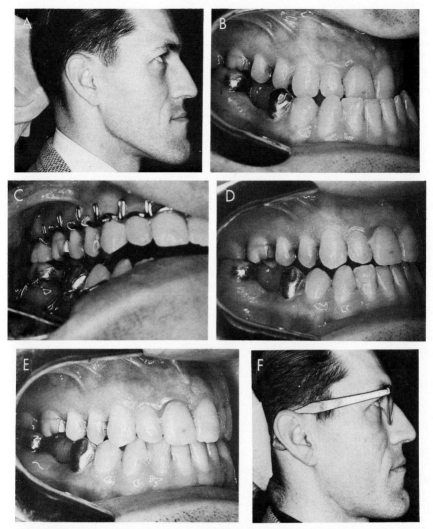

Fig. XV-67.—An extreme case of mandibular prognathism corrected by combined orthodontic and surgical procedures. **A** and **B,** the case prior to treatment. **C,** immediately following surgery. **D,** after removal of the splint appliances and prior to occlusal equilibration. **E,** after occlusal equilibration. **F,** profile at the end of treatment.

months. Studies have shown that the surgical correction of cleft palate interferes with the growth largely in the maxillary alveolar region and that proper orthodontic correction often can overcome the effects of the surgery on the growth pattern. Orthodontic correction of cleft palate should involve expansion of the lateral halves of the maxilla itself rather than the mere moving of teeth.

The needs of the child determine which surgical procedures are to be undertaken and their schedule. However, different attitudes prevail concerning the advantages and disadvantages of early surgery. Orthodontists practicing in areas in which traumatic early surgery has been seen for many years tend to want any surgery postponed. Those who have not seen the bizarre disfiguring effects of improper surgery are more comfortable with earlier intervention. So varied are the problems that no single approach serves all children well.

Excellent research shedding light on this important and difficult problem is being carried out at several cleft palate centers. The decision must be individualized for each child. The speech therapist, pedodontist,

Fig. XV-68.—A, a unilateral cleft palate prior to orthodontic treatment. **B,** the Friel lingual archwire in place. **C,** the result of maxillary expansion with the Friel lingual archwire. **D,** after positioning of the teeth with a standard orthodontic appliance, the case is now ready for a prosthesis.

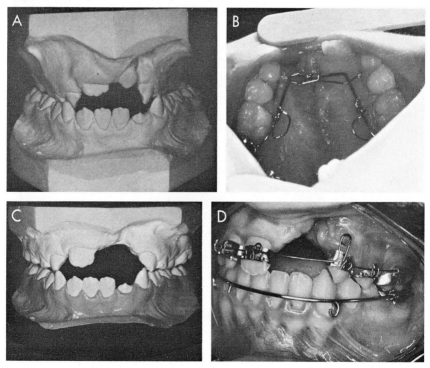

surgeon, orthodontist and prosthodontist are all involved, as may be the psychologist. However, the speech therapist and the orthodontist will spend the most time in corrective work if the decision is in error or it was impossible to achieve an ideal surgical correction.

If a child with cleft palate is brought to a family dentist, he should be referred immediately to the closest cleft palate treatment center for consultation. The team approach is the best for these children. Fortunately, cleft palate centers, where all the interested clinicians are working together, are becoming increasingly popular and widespread. Figure XV-68 shows a cleft palate malocclusion and the result of orthodontic therapy.

I. Orthodontic Aids in Crown and Bridge and Periodontal Therapy

Orthodontics for the adult patient usually involves compromise, for several reasons: (1) all growth of the craniofacial bones has ceased, (2) the tissue response is slower than in the child, (3) adult patients are less tolerant of the appliances and (4) many adult patients simply are not as cooperative as young children. It should be clearly borne in mind that some aspects of treatment can be compromised and others simply cannot. Although aesthetics is of chief importance in many adult orthodontic problems, the stability of the occlusion can never be compromised for aesthetics—or for any other reason. Many times, the biggest compromise that must be made is that of accepting the fact that the basic malocclusion itself is not to be corrected but that minor tooth movements are to be carried out for aesthetic purposes. Indeed, this field often is spoken of as "minor tooth movements" to differentiate it from comprehensive orthodontics.

1. SELECTION OF CASES

The procedures outlined in this section are best carried out when there is a normal relationship of the mandibular to the maxillary teeth and when the majority of the teeth in the arch occlude well. The technics are for localized tooth movements in adult patients as a part of periodontic treatment or as a prelude to prosthetic restorations. The following conditions should be met if successful therapy is to result:

a) The patient must want the therapy and be willing to cooperate throughout treatment.

b) It must be possible to eliminate the cause of the malposition or a prosthesis must serve as a permanent splint to maintain the teeth in new positions.

c) Sufficient anchorage must be obtainable to carry out the desired tooth movements.

d) There must be space in the arch to carry out the desired tooth movements, or that space must be readily obtainable.

e) It must be possible to free the occlusion while the tooth movements are being carried out.

f) It must be possible to retain the finished result.

2. GENERAL PRINCIPLES

a) Anchorage

The best sources of anchorage for minor tooth movements in the adult usually are the intercuspation of the teeth and/or removable acrylic appliances covering the alveolar and palatal mucosa. In my opinion, there is entirely too much "rubber band orthodontics" being done. When one joins naked teeth in the mouth with elastic bands alone without supportive anchorage, all the teeth involved may tip. Plan the anchorage control at the start of treatment. It is extremely difficult to recover lost anchorage in adult periodontic patients.

b) Space

There must be space in the line of arch to carry out the planned tooth movements. Should there be any question concerning the amount of space, a diagnostic setup will show the problem clearly. In instances of mild crowding of the mandibular incisors, some stripping of the interproximal surfaces can be carried out. This is best done by using thin linen abrasive strips. The interproximal surfaces are then treated with topical fluoride solution. Only a fraction of a millimeter can be gained from each proximal surface of a tooth, since the average enamel thickness at the contact point is approximately ½ mm. When the space is not available in the arch, and sufficient space cannot be created by stripping, extractions are the only other recourse.

A strong word of caution must be given against the promiscuous use of atypical extraction procedures. The extraction of any permanent tooth usually requires the bodily movement of adjacent teeth, which can be carried out best with a multibanded appliance. Further, it is difficult to extract in one quadrant only and achieve a balanced occlusion (see Fig. XV-74). I have seen many patients with acute temporomandibular symptoms due to the extraction of one tooth and the subsequent closing of the space created. Under these circumstances, a large slide into occlusion always occurs, resulting in trauma to teeth or the temporomandibular articulation. Such traumatic occlusion often cannot be equilibrated. The only alternative is to carry out further extractions and bring back to the occlusion the balance that was there before the original extraction. One frequently is tempted to extract a single mandibular incisor when there is gross crowding. It is imperative, when so tempted, to do a diagnostic setup. Unless the space is exactly closed by the extraction of one tooth at the midline and there still remain incisal stops between all of the lower anteriors and the maxillary anteriors, one would be well advised not to extract a single tooth. Far too frequently, the mandibular incisors are carried lingually to achieve alignment and thus no longer have maxillary antagonists. The result is overextrusion of the mandibular anteriors and impingement of the soft tissue of the palate. There are a few rare instances in which this is the therapy of choice. All such cases are clearly shown by the diagnostic setup.

c) *Occlusion*

Not only is it important to be able to remove occlusal interferences during minor tooth movement, but there must remain no interference at the end of treatment. The interference during tooth movements may be removed by the insertion of a maxillary Hawley appliance with a flat bite plane. As soon as the desired tooth movement is achieved, equilibration should be carried out to stabilize the corrected result.

d) *Retention*

No minor tooth movements should be carried out in the adult mouth unless it can be ascertained at the start that the result will be stabilized. The best retainer is the equilibrated functioning occlusion. However, in mouths suffering severe bone loss of the alveolar process, other retention may be necessary. Bridges serve as permanent splints, and in advanced periodontal disease the possibility of fixed splinting should not be forgotten.

3. UPRIGHTING SECOND MOLARS

Perhaps the most common use of orthodontics to aid crown and bridge work is the uprighting of a second molar preparatory to placing a bridge supplanting a lost first permanent molar. The appliances are the same ones that are used as space-regainers in the mixed dentition. An auxiliary spring may be used to tip the third molar distally first, or the third molar in some instances can be extracted safely prior to the uprighting of the second molar. In the lower arch, the "slingshot" appliance or the "figure 8" appliance is most applicable. After the second molar has been uprighted, the appliance may be deactivated and worn as a space-maintainer during the construction of the bridge. Inasmuch as the second molar is going to be cut down when preparing the abutment, it should not be allowed to interfere grossly with the occlusion during the tooth movements. Obviously, the bridge is the retainer.

4. CONGENITALLY MISSING MAXILLARY LATERAL INCISORS

This problem is discussed at some length in Section A-1, Missing Teeth. Also see Figures XV-70 and XV-71.

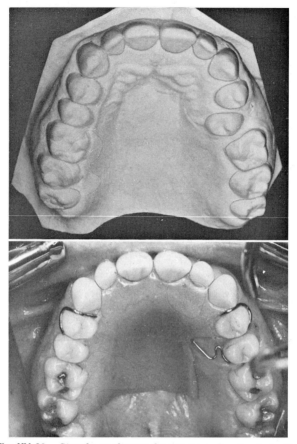

Fig. XV-69.—Simple appliance for tipping of a single tooth.

5. Crowded Mandibular Incisors

Before attempting the treatment of a case with crowded incisors as a complicating factor in periodontal disease, read Section 2-b, above. These remarks on space are most pertinent. When there is alveolar bone loss around the mandibular incisors, it is a very simple matter to tip them into alignment, provided there is space in the line of the arch. However, the retention of such a case may be nigh impossible without splinting of some sort. The tooth movements may be carried out with a removable acrylic appliance with auxiliary springs, or wire loops may be embedded into the acrylic and elastics hooked from these loops to the crowns of the teeth to tip them into position. A mandibular Hawley appliance is useful for tipping the crowns lingually if that is all that is

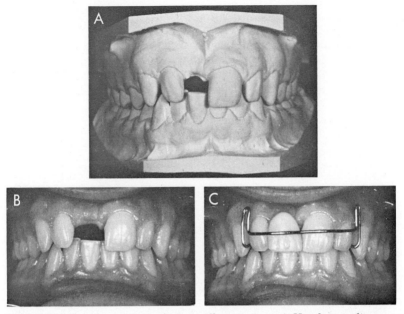

Fig. XV-70.—Accidental loss of a maxillary incisor. A Hawley appliance was used to align the teeth simply, open the bite a bit, and modified as a retainer and temporary prosthesis.

required. Satisfactory results can be obtained for many patients by a combination of minor tooth movements, some judicious stripping and careful grinding of the incisal edges.

6. DEEP BITE

Read carefully Section F, Vertical Relationships of Teeth and Dental Arches. One must differentiate carefully between a deep bite and a closed bite. In my opinion, the skeletally involved deep bite is among the most difficult of all malocclusions to treat. When seen in the adult, the most pertinent question to be asked is "Is the deep bite contributing to the patient's problem?" Many patients with deep bite have no periodontal disease and have healthy functioning masticatory systems. It is well to leave these alone. If, however, a true deep bite is complicating the reconstructive or periodontic problem, then, in most instances, multibanded therapy is indicated.

On the other hand, the closed bite often can be treated quite easily in conjunction with reconstructive and periodontic work. Removable acrylic appliances may be inserted to upright the posterior teeth and thus achieve some improvement in the loss of vertical dimension. A flat bite plane on the maxillary appliance can help to ascertain the most

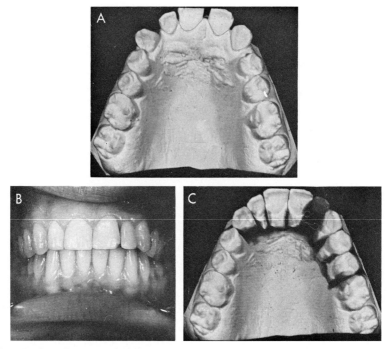

Fig. XV-71.—Congenital absence of one maxillary lateral incisor. **A,** the original condition. **B,** use of a diagnostic setup to determine whether there is sufficient room in the arch and how much each tooth must be moved during treatment. **C,** the final bridge in place. (Courtesy of Dr. Robert Aldrich.)

Fig. XV-72.—**A,** this patient had an anterior crossbite that was traumatic enough to cause the loss of maxillary incisors. A mandibular acrylic inclined plane was first inserted at the tip of the maxillary central incisors labially. **B,** the result of the first step in treatment. **C,** a maxillary acrylic palate with a high labial anterior section added, to which auxiliary springs have been attached for the positioning of the maxillary central incisors and cuspids. A bite plane has been added also. **D,** after the tooth movements were achieved with the appliance shown in **C.** A Hawley retainer with bite plane is now being worn as a temporary prosthesis. Note that some of the necessary restorative work posteriorly has been completed by this time. **E–G,** the final result. (This case was treated by an undergraduate student at The University of Michigan with the cooperation of the Departments of Orthodontics, Periodontics and Crown and Bridge Prosthesis.)

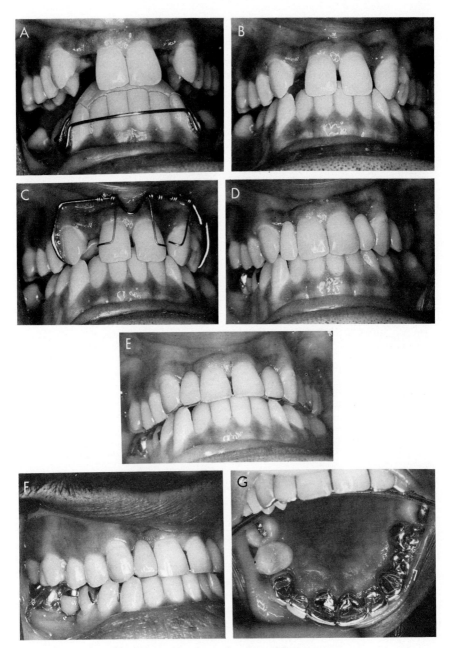

Fig. XV-72.—See legend at foot of facing page.

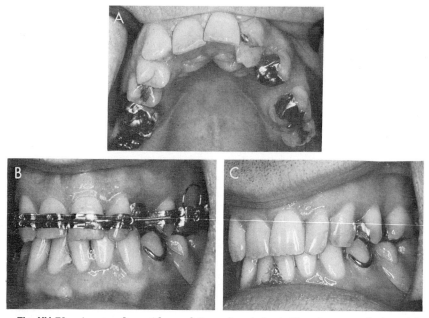

Fig. XV-73.—A case of cuspid crossbite and periodontal involvement. **A,** the original condition. There was a very deep periodontal pocket on the distal of the maxillary left first bicuspid. Note the wear facet on the inlay of this tooth. At this time there was some doubt concerning the prognosis for the first bicuspid. **B,** the maxillary orthodontic appliance. The first bicuspid was moved distally and the cuspid was banded and pulled to the line of arch. All posterior spacing was closed with this appliance. Meanwhile, the periodontal therapy on the bicuspid had been successful and the inlay with the occlusal interference had been ground down to a harmonious relationship. **C,** the finished result. Note that the first molar has been brought mesially to this new occlusal relationship, obviating the necessity for a fixed bridge in this quadrant. (This case was treated by an undergraduate student.)

likely vertical dimension to which the reconstruction can be built. Finally, the orthodontic appliance can serve as a temporary partial denture while the castings are being inserted.

A word of caution must be inserted concerning some of the "treatments" advocated for the correction of deep bite. I have been called in consultation involving several patients who had had their bite opened with removable castings or onlays on the posterior teeth. When the bite is raised beyond the original occlusal plane of the patient, the muscles intrude the posterior teeth. Indeed, one patient was seen whose mandibular posterior teeth had been intruded so that the crowns were below the gingival margin. Needless to say, such ill-conceived procedures are exceedingly destructive to the masticatory system and, in some instances, it is almost impossible to restore the mouth to health and freedom from pain. There is a great difference between restoring the patient's vertical dimension and opening the bite to heights it never knew.

7. INDIVIDUAL TOOTH MOVEMENTS

a) The incisors can be moved labially or lingually quite easily with the removable acrylic appliances described in Chapter XVII. In the maxillary arch, the high labial section is useful (see Fig. XV-72). In the posterior region, through-the-bite elastics may be used if an upper and lower tooth are in localized crossbite. Other individual tooth movements in a buccolingual way are carried out easily by inserting auxiliary springs into the acrylic (see Fig. XV-69). In both the anterior and posterior region, very light elastics may be used to move the teeth lingually. Hooks or eyelets may be inserted easily into the acrylic for the attachment of the elastics. Nylon-covered elastic thread may be tied from

Fig. XV-74.—A and **B,** the occlusion of a patient after orthodontic therapy involving unilateral atypical bicuspid extractions. The result was not stable and the multilated occlusion was deteriorating rapidly. **C** and **D,** the result of orthodontic retreatment and crown and bridge therapy. Note that in order to achieve a balanced occlusion it was necessary to reopen space in the lower right quadrant and place a bridge to replace one of the two bicuspids that, unfortunately, had been removed from there. Atypical unilateral bicuspid extractions rarely result in stable occlusions. (Courtesy of Dr. Robert Aldrich.)

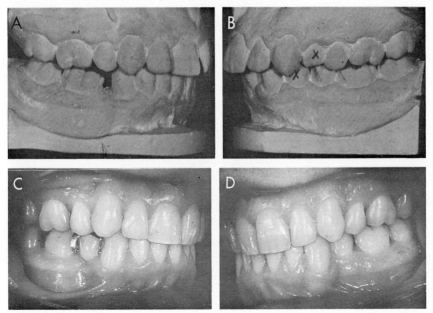

the teeth to a hook in a plate or may join two bands. It is best not to encircle the naked necks of teeth for reciprocal movement.

b) Mesiodistal tipping movements can be carried out rather easily in most instances with removable acrylic plates and attached auxiliary springs. However, when large numbers of teeth must be moved mesiodistally, this method is of little use. Furthermore, a tooth that is in its correct position mesiodistally, and is not tipped, must be moved bodily to a new position. Bodily movements of teeth ordinarily are not carried out with removable appliances. Nylon-covered elastic thread may be used for simple mesiodistal movements of teeth. Stainless steel ligatures can be used to tie two or more teeth together to augment the anchorage, the elastic ligature thread then being tied to a hook on one of the "anchored" teeth and encircled around the tooth to be moved. The simplest example of this usage is that at the midline between the maxillary central incisors. Before undertaking the treatment of any spacings among the teeth, however, read carefully Section G, Spacing of Teeth.

c) Intrusions and extrusions are very difficult to carry out with removable appliances in adult patients. Fortunately, many times an extruded tooth can be made more aesthetic by simple trimming of the crown. If generalized intrusion and extrusion must be carried out, it is best done with multibanded appliances.

The cases presented illustrate how orthodontic appliances may be used to aid in crown and bridge and periodontic therapy. No attempt has been made to demonstrate all the possibilities; rather, typical applications were chosen.

REFERENCES

1. Björk, A.: Some biological aspects of prognathism and occlusion of teeth, Orthodont. Scandinav. 9:1, 1950.
2. Eisner, D.: Comments before a conference on undergraduate orthodontic education, Ann Arbor, Michigan, 1965.
3. Jarvis, A.: The Role of Dental Caries in Space Closure in the Mixed Dentition, M.S. thesis, School of Graduate Studies, University of Toronto, 1952.
4. Matthews, J. R.: Maxillary bite plane application in Class I deciduous occlusion, Am. J. Orthodont. 45:721, 1959.
5. Popovich, F.: Cephalometric evaluation of vertical overbite in young adults, J. Canad. D. A. 21:209, 1955.
6. Pulver, F.: The etiology and prevalence of ectopic eruption of the maxillary first permanent molar, J. Dent. Child. 35:138, 1968.

SUGGESTED READINGS

NUMBER OF TEETH

Corpron, R. E.: The treatment of problems presented by congenitally missing teeth, J. New Jersey D. Soc. 31:23, 1960.
Mossmann, W. H.: Problems of supernumerary and congenitally missing teeth, J.A.D.A. 66:69, 1963.
Sabes, W. R., and Bartholdi, W. L.: Congenital partial anodontia of permanent dentition: A study of 157 cases, J. Dent. Child. 29:211, 1962.
Weber, F. N.: Supernumerary teeth, Dent. Clin. North America p. 509, July, 1964.

VARIATIONS IN SIZE OF TEETH

Lundstrom, A.: Variations of tooth size in the etiology of malocclusion, Am. J. Orthodont. 41:872, 1955.

PROBLEMS IN THE MIXED DENTITION

1. *Space Management*

SPACE MAINTENANCE

Bowden, B. D.: A clinical assessment of mixed dentition crowding, Australian D. J. 14:90, 1969.
Graber, T. M.: *Orthodontics: Principles and Practice* (2d ed.; Philadelphia: W. B. Saunders Company, 1966), pp. 649–664.
Hinrichsen, C. F. L.: Space maintenance in pedodontics, Australian D. J. 7:451, 1962.
Nance, H. N.: The limitations of orthodontic diagnosis and treatment. I and II. Am. J. Orthodont. 33:177; 253, 1947.
Proffit, W. R., and Bennett, J. C.: Space maintenance, serial extraction, and the general practitioner, J.A.D.A. 74:411, 1967.
Ryan, K. J.: Understanding and use of space maintenance procedures, J. Dent. Child. 31:22, 1964.
Zwemer, T. J.: Ten rules of the mixed dentition, J. Dent. Child. 35:298, 1968.

SPACE REGAINING

Graber, T. M.: *Orthodontics: Principles and Practice* (2d ed.; Philadelphia: W. B. Saunders Company, 1966), pp. 838–849.
Moyers, R. E.: Space regaining, Dentistry for the 70's Visu-Cassette Program, Health Information Systems, New York, 1971.
Sassouni, V.: *Orthodontics in Dental Practice* (St. Louis: The C. V. Mosby Company, 1971), Chap. 20, pp. 407–428.

SPACE SUPERVISION

Brown, W. E.: The supervision of arch length during the period of the mixed dentition, J. New Jersey D. Soc. 31:10, 1960.
Hotz, R.: Guidance of eruption versus serial extraction, Am. J. Orthodont. 58:1, 1970.
Moyers, R. E.: Space supervision: Class I Protocol, Dentistry for the 70's Visu-Cassette Program, Health Information Systems, New York, 1971.
Weber, F. N.: Corrective measures during the mixed dentition, Am. J. Orthodont. 43:639, 1957.

GROSS DISCREPANCIES (SERIAL EXTRACTION)

Dewel, B. F.: Serial extraction: Its limitations and contraindications in orthodontic treatment, Am. J. Orthodont. 53:904, 1967.
Heath, J.: The dangers and pitfalls of serial extraction, Tr. European Orthodont. Soc. p. 60, 1961.
Hotz, R.: Active supervision of the eruption of the teeth by extraction, Tr. European Orthodont. Soc. p. 34, 1947–1948.
Kjellgren, B.: Serial extraction as a corrective procedure in dental orthopedic therapy, Tr. European Orthodont. Soc., p. 134, 1947–1948.
Mayne, W. R.: Serial Extraction, in Graber, T. M. (ed.), *Current Orthodontic Concepts and Techniques* (Philadelphia: W. B. Saunders Company, 1969), Chap. 4, pp. 179–274.
Moyers, R. E.: Serial extraction in gross discrepancy cases, Dentistry for the 70's Visu-Cassette Program, Health Information Systems, New York, 1972.
Tweed, C. H., Jr.: Pre-Orthodontic Guidance Procedure: Classification of Facial Growth Trends: Treatment Timing, in Kraus, B., and Riedel, R. (eds.), *Vistas in Orthodontics* (Philadelphia: Lea & Febiger, 1962), p. 359.
Tweed, C. H., Jr.: *Clinical Orthodontics* (St. Louis: The C. V. Mosby Company, 1966), Vols. I and II.

2. *Difficulties in Eruption (Ectopic, Impacted, Ankylosed, Early, Delayed)*

Biederman, W.: The ankylosed tooth, Dent. Clin. North America, p. 493, July, 1964.
Cheyne, V. O., and Wessels, K. E.: Impaction of permanent first molars with resorption and space loss in region of deciduous second molar, J.A.D.A. 35:774, 1947.
Clark, Da Costa: The management of impacted canines: Free physiologic eruption, J.A.D.A. 82:836, 1971.

Dixon, D. A.: Observations on submerging deciduous molars, Dent. Pract. 13:303, 1963.

Moss, J. P.: The transplantation of maxillary canines, J. Clin. Orthodont. 4:77, 1970.

Pulver, F.: The etiology and prevalence of ectopic eruption of the maxillary first permanent molar, J. Dent. Child. 35:138, 1968.

Salzmann, J. A.: Effect on occlusion of uncontrolled extraction of first permanent molars: Prevention and treatment, J.A.D.A. 40:14, 1944.

LATERAL RELATIONSHIPS OF DENTAL ARCHES

Cheney, E. A.: Indications and methods for the interception of functional crossbites and inlockings, Dent. Clin. North America, p. 385, July, 1959.

Cheney, E. A.: Dentofacial asymmetries and their clinical significance, Am. J. Orthodont. 47:814, 1961.

Graber, T. M.: *Orthodontics: Principles and Practice* (2d ed.; Philadelphia: W. B. Saunders Company, 1966), pp. 821–827.

Haas, A. J.: Rapid expansion of the maxillary dental arch and nasal cavity by opening the midpalatal suture, Angle Orthodont. 31:73, 1961.

Haas, A. J.: The treatment of maxillary deficiency by opening the midpalatal suture, Angle Orthodont. 35:200, 1965.

Isaacson, R. J., Wood, J. L., and Ingram, A. H.: Forces produced by rapid maxillary expansion. I. Design of force measuring system, Angle Orthodont. 34:256, 1964.

Matthews, J. R.: Maxillary bite plane application in Class I deciduous occlusion, Am. J. Orthodont. 45:721, 1959.

Sassouni, V.: *Orthodontics in Dental Practice* (St. Louis: The C. V. Mosby Company, 1971), Chap. 24, pp. 496–500.

Wood, A. W. S.: Anterior and posterior crossbites, J. Dent. Child. 29:280, 1962.

ANTEROPOSTERIOR RELATIONSHIPS OF TEETH AND ARCHES

1. *Class II*

Coben, S. E.: Growth and Class II treatment, Am. J. Orthodont. 52:5, 1966.

Freunthaller, P.: Cephalometric observations in Class II, Div. 1 malocclusions treated with the activator, Angle Orthodont. 37:18, 1967.

Graber, T. M.: Extraoral force—Facts and fallacies, Am. J. Orthodont. 41:490, 1955.

Graber, T. M., Chung, D. D. B., and Aoba, J. T.: Dentofacial orthopedics versus orthodontics, J.A.D.A. 75:1145, 1967.

Graber, T. M. (ed.): *Current Orthodontic Concepts and Techniques* (Philadelphia: W. B. Saunders Company, 1969), Chap. 10, pp. 919–988.

Grossmann, W., and Moss, J. P.: Role of functional jaw orthopedics in orthodontics, Dent. Pract. 14:405, 1964.

Grossmann, W., and Moss, J. P.: Removable appliance therapy: Part I. Passive removable appliances, J. Pract. Orthodont. 2:28, 1968.

Harvold, E. P., and Vargervik, K.: Morphogenetic response to activator treatment, Am. J. Orthodont. 60:478, 1971.

King, E. W.: Looking back—The lessons of fifteen years of mixed dentition treatment, Am. J. Orthodont. 54:733, 1968.

King, E. W.: Treatment timing and planning in Class II, Division I malocclusions, Angle Orthodont. 50:4, 1964.

Marschner, J. F., and Harris, J. E.: Mandibular growth and Class II treatment, Angle Orthodont. 36:89, 1966.

Merrifield, L. L., and Cross, J. J.: Directional forces, Am. J. Orthodont. 57:435, 1970.

Neumann, B.: Removable Appliances, in Graber, T. M. (ed.), *Current Orthodontic Concepts and Techniques* (Philadelphia: W. B. Saunders Company, 1969), Chap. 10, pp. 817–874.

Poulton, D. R.: Three-year survey of Class II malocclusions with and without headgear therapy, Angle Orthodont. 34:181, 1964.

Poulton, D. R.: Influence of extraoral traction, Am. J. Orthodont. 53:8, 1967.

Wieslander, L.: The effect of orthodontic treatment on the concurrent development of the cranio-facial complex, Am. J. Orthodont. 49:15, 1963.

2. *Class III*

Graber, T. M. (ed.): *Current Orthodontic Concepts and Techniques* (Philadelphia: W. B. Saunders Company, 1969), pp. 927–947.

Hitchcock, H. P.: Recognition of Class III malocclusions and treatment of Class I, type 3 malocclusions, Dent. Clin. North America, p. 399, July, 1968.
Mills, J. R. E.: Assessment of Class III malocclusion, Dent. Pract. 16:452, 1966.
Sassouni, V.: *Orthodontics in Dental Practice* (St. Louis: The C. V. Mosby Company, 1971), pp. 382–389.

3. *Labioversion*

Hirschfeld, L., and Geiger, A.: *Minor Tooth Movement in General Practice* (2d ed.; St. Louis: The C. V. Mosby Company, 1966).

4. *Anterior Crossbites*

Bodenhorn, R. S., and Bodenhorn, J. A.: Etiology and treatment of anterior crossbite, Dent. Pract. 20:52, 1969.
Sassouni, V.: *Orthodontics in Dental Practice* (St. Louis: The C. V. Mosby Company, 1971), pp. 429–467.
Wood, A. W. S.: Anterior and posterior crossbites, J. Dent. Child. 29:280, 1962.

VERTICAL RELATIONSHIPS OF TEETH AND DENTAL ARCHES

1. *Open Bite*

Moyers, R. E.: The Role of Musculature in Orthodontic Diagnosis and Treatment Planning, in Kraus, B., and Riedel, R. (eds.), *Vistas in Orthodontics* (Philadelphia: Lea & Febiger, 1962), p. 309.
Moyers, R. E.: Abnormal tongue function, Dentistry for the 70's Visu-Cassette Program, Health Information Systems, New York, 1971.
Neff, C. W., and Kydd, W. L.: Open bite: Physiology and occlusion, Angle Orthodont. 36:351, 1966.
Schudy, F. F.: Vertical growth versus anteroposterior growth as related to function and treatment, Angle Orthodont. 34:75, 1964.
Subtelny, J. D., and Sakuda, M.: Open bite: Diagnosis and treatment, Am. J. Orthodont. 50:337, 1964.

2. *Excessive Overbite*

Graber, T. M.: Overbite: The dentist's challenge, J.A.D.A. 79:1135, 1969.
Sassouni, V.: Facial Types and Malocclusions, in *Orthodontics in Dental Practice* (St. Louis: The C. V. Mosby Company, 1971), pp. 121–144.

SPACING OF TEETH

Gardiner, J. H.: Midline spaces, Dent. Pract. 17:287, 1967.
Moyers, R. E.: Spacing between the maxillary incisors, Alpha Omegan 46:80, 1952.
Savin, C., Sekiguchi, T., and Savara, B. S.: Clinical method for prediction of closure of the central diastema, J. Dent. Child. 36:415, 1969.

GROSS FACIAL DEFORMITIES

1. *Mandibular Prognathism*

Proffit, W. R., and White, R. P.: Treatment of severe malocclusions by correlated orthodontic surgical procedures, Angle Orthodont. 40:1, 1970.
Robinson, M., and Doughtery, H. L.: Prognathism questions in the surgical-orthodontic team, Am. J. Orthodont. 47:531, 1961.

2. *Cleft Lip and Palate*

Grabb, W., and Rosenstein, S. W. (eds.): *Cleft Lip and Palate* (Boston: Little, Brown & Company, 1970).
Graber, T. M.: The congenital cleft palate deformity, J.A.D.A. 48:375, 1954.
Hotz, R.: *Early Treatment of Cleft Lip and Palate* (Bern: Hans Huber, 1964).
Olin, W. H.: *Cleft Lip and Palate Rehabilitation* (Springfield, Ill: Charles C Thomas, Publisher, 1960).

3. *Miscellaneous*

Pruzansky, S.: *Congenital Anomalies of the Face and Associated Structures* (Springfield, Ill.: Charles C Thomas, Publisher, 1961).

ORTHODONTIC AIDS IN CROWN AND BRIDGE AND PERIODONTAL THERAPY

Hirschfeld, L., and Geiger, A.: *Minor Tooth Movement in General Practice* (2d ed.; St. Louis: The C. V. Mosby Company, 1966).
Ramfjord, S. P., and Ash, M. M.: *Occlusion* (2d ed.; Philadelphia: W. B. Saunders Company, 1971), pp. 313–344.

XVI

Role of Orthodontics in the Profession of Dentistry

> Specialized knowledge will do a man no harm if he also has common sense, but if he lacks this, it can only make him more dangerous to his patients.—OLIVER WENDELL HOLMES

> The necessary but too rapid subdivision into specialisms and growing competition in every branch have, it would seem, been good for the technique but bad for the soul of medicine.—JOHN A. RYLE, in *Fears May Be Liars*

A. What is the need for orthodontic services?

  1. Epidemiology of malocclusion
  2. Future estimates

B. Who supplies orthodontic services?

  1. The orthodontist
    a) Training in North America
    b) Services rendered
  2. The pedodontist
  3. The general practitioner
    a) Undergraduate orthodontic training
    b) Orthodontic responsibilities of the general practitioner
    c) The changing nature of general practice

C. Problems in better serving the need

  1. Increasing the supply of services
    a) Orthodontist
    b) Pedodontists
    c) General practitioners
  2. Decreasing the need for orthodontic treatment
    a) Prevention of malocclusion
    b) Interception of malocclusion
    c) The problem of increasing demands

A. What is the Need for Orthodontic Services?

1. EPIDEMIOLOGY OF MALOCCLUSION

Only in very recent years have proper epidemiologic studies of malocclusion been provided. The difficulties are many, since malocclusion is not a discrete variable but rather is a loosely defined summation of genetic variation and the effects of extrinsic and intrinsic factors on the growth of the face and teeth. Furthermore, the basis for an epidemiologic definition of malocclusion might be very different from the reasons that prompt a parent to take a child to the dentist for treatment. It is easy to quantitate the malalignment of teeth; it is difficult to quantitate the real or imagined effects of an unaesthetic face on a sensitive developing personality. Grainger[3] and Summers[4] have developed sophisticated methods of epidemiologic studies of malocclusion. They view malocclusion as a series of syndromes scored on a scale of intensity. At what place on the scale the malocclusion becomes a clinical problem is a matter of opinion, but the method provides quantitation whatever the opinion. Further problems in understanding the need for orthodontic services are encountered if we compare the incidence and prevalence of malocclusion in a population with the demands for treatment. Fisk[2] has shown that parents seek treatment for their children in ways not necessarily related to the way the dentist views a malocclusion. For example, dentists are asked to treat certain malocclusions much earlier in girls than in boys. The number and type of malocclusions for which treatment is asked varies with the socioeconomic status of the parents and whether they themselves have a malocclusion. Further complications in understanding the true epidemiologic proportions of malocclusion are encountered if we contrast those malocclusions that require treatment for real and pressing reasons of oral or mental health with those for which treatment is sought solely for cosmetic reasons. Truly, the dental epidemiologist has an exceedingly difficult task.

Estimates of malocclusion in North American populations have varied from 20% to 100%. There are approximately 40,000,000 children in the United States between the ages of 4 and 18. Assuming that 10% of these children have severe disfiguring or handicapping malocclusion,

4,000,000 clinical problems result. The most conservative estimates assume that approximately 25-40% of the children would benefit from some degree of orthodontic treatment. Both of these estimates are at best crude and coarse. It is even more difficult to estimate the number of children being treated orthodontically in the United States, but it is likely only a small fraction of the total with measurable malocclusions.

2. FUTURE ESTIMATES

The need for orthodontic services will increase markedly for two reasons: (1) the number of children of orthodontic age likely will increase and (2) the desire by parents to have their children treated seems to be increasing with each passing year.

B. Who Supplies Orthodontic Services?

1. THE ORTHODONTIST

a) Training in North America

Most orthodontists beginning practice in North America now have completed graduate training in an approved program averaging 21-24 months. However, some programs are as brief as 18 months and some as long as 36. Approximately 300 graduate orthodontic students complete their training and enter practice each year. The ratio of orthodontists to general practicing dentists and orthodontists to the population shows considerable variability, there being greater density of orthodontists in urban areas, in areas of the highest socioeconomic level and in those states with dental schools.

b) Services Rendered

In the past, orthodontists have treated most of the malocclusions. In recent years, however, the number of pedodontists and general practitioners treating malocclusions has increased greatly, resulting in a concentration in orthodontic practice of the more severe and difficult malocclusions.

2. THE PEDODONTIST

Although there are approximately 600 pedodontists in the United States today, their training varies considerably more than that of other specialties, for example, oral surgery and orthodontics. In particular, there is some variability in the amount of training in growth and development and orthodontic therapy. Furthermore, a far smaller percentage of pedodontists have actual formal training in these subjects than do orthodontists, although the American Board of Pedodontists tests candidates for certification on growth and development and orthodontic procedures. In practice, the pedodontist is called on increasingly to treat malocclusion, for example, to supervise the developing occlusion or to correct deleterious oral habits as well as to detect incipient severe malocclusion for referral to the orthodontist. It seems that the orthodontic training received by the typical pedodontic graduate today has not kept pace with the public's demands for orthodontic services and the changing nature of pedodontic practice.

3. THE GENERAL PRACTITIONER

a) Undergraduate Orthodontic Training

Although significant advances have been made in recent years in the number of dental graduates coming to the profession, until recently little real progress had been made in undergraduate orthodontic programs. It is worth while to note some of the reasons for the inadequacy of much undergraduate orthodontic training. Orthodontics began as a specialty; other specialties have begun in general practice. The concept has been held in dentistry that the dental graduate should be able to treat capably the majority of the patients coming to his practice. Certainly our training today permits the average dentist to treat well the great majority of problems he encounters in operative dentistry, prosthetics and crown and bridge, and a significant number of the problems he encounters in periodontics, endodontics, oral surgery and pedodontics. Indeed, the graduates of some dental schools are trained to handle a very high percentage of all the cases in these clinical fields. In contrast, it is a rare dental graduate who believes that he can treat well any malocclusion at all. There are two primary reasons: (1) the historical attitude that orthodontics is a specialty practice alone and (2) the greater number of hours of instruction needed to advance the undergraduate student to the same level of competency in orthodontics as is achieved in the other fields. Most orthodontic educators estimate that it would require at least 1,500 hours of instruction to train undergraduate dental students to handle well the majority of malocclusions encountered in practice. This seems to be more time than is necessary to train a student to a level of clinical proficiency required in other fields in dentistry.

b) Orthodontic Responsibilities of the General Practitioner

Whether the family dentist has been trained in orthodontics or not, he has, by reason of his license, orthodontic responsibilities, the most important of which is to diagnose the malocclusion as early as possible and to inform the patient or the patient's parents of its implications and the possibilities for correction. It might be assumed that a family dentist need not treat any malocclusions if he so chooses, but it is difficult to see how he can avoid responsibility for diagnosis and detection of malocclusion even with little interest in orthodontic treatment. Unfortunately, undergraduate orthodontic education in the past often has been so inadequate as to leave the dentist unaware of his relative incapabilities in this field, with the result that dentists untrained in orthodontics often have naïvely rendered inadequate service to their patients.

c) The Changing Nature of General Practice

Communal fluoridation of water systems and the modern practice of dentistry have greatly altered the nature of services rendered by the family dentist. A generation ago, the majority of the family dentist's time was spent in restorative dentistry, prosthetics and surgery. With the preservation of the crowns of the teeth as a result of fluoridation, dramatic changes in dental practice have occurred. Fewer fillings are required, fewer teeth are lost to caries and more time is available for treatment of periodontal disease, interception of malocclusion, guidance of the developing dentition and other preventive services.

C. Problems in Better Serving the Need

1. INCREASING THE SUPPLY OF SERVICES

a) Orthodontists

1) INCREASING THE NUMBER BEING TRAINED.—The number of orthodontists being graduated each year in the United States has nearly doubled in the past 15 years.

2) INCREASING THE NUMBER OF CASES EACH ORTHODONTIST CAN TREAT.—The number of cases treated by each orthodontist has increased because of more frequent use of auxiliary help and laboratories, availability of prefabricated appliances, improved methods of mechanotherapy and better timing of treatments with developmental events.

b) Pedodontists

Pedodontics is one of the fastest-growing specialties in dentistry. Furthermore, there is beginning to be an improvement in the orthodontic training pedodontic graduate students are receiving. It seems reasonable to hope that pedodontists soon will expand greatly the scope of their orthodontic services.

c) General Practitioners

An increasing number of general practitioners are being graduated each year and there is evidence that the undergraduate training in orthodontics is improving. The Council on Education of the American Association of Orthodontists has worked hard the past few years to help undergraduate teachers of orthodontics improve their courses. It is difficult, however, to increase the number of hours devoted to orthodontics in the undergraduate curriculum of some dental schools. Postgraduate training in orthodontics for the general practitioner often has been advocated as a method of compensating for the lack of undergraduate orthodontic training. I do not believe this to be a completely satisfactory method. Most short courses in orthodontics for the general practitioner are of but a few days' duration and thus are no substitute for 4 years of intensive and integrated training in growth and development, diagnosis and treatment planning and the actual treatment of patients under supervision. The number of malocclusions treated *well* by general practitioners is not likely to increase significantly until undergraduate orthodontic training is improved, even though the number of general dentists treating malocclusions has increased in spectacular fashion.

Several new organizations to promote orthodontics in general practice have been started in the United States in recent years. They sponsor short courses and provide other opportunities for learning. In addition, there are an increasing number of short courses offered by the universities. A fundamental problem remains that cannot be solved by any short course or organization, viz., the matter of supervised clinical training. Good clinical orthodontic training for the nonspecialist must be obtained in undergraduate dental school or in prolonged postgraduate courses that include actual treatment of patients. The latter type of postgraduate course is not now available for many students.

2. Decreasing the Need for Orthodontic Treatment

a) Prevention of Malocclusion

The phrase prevention of malocclusion has a lovely sound but the unfortunate truth is that only a very small percentage of malocclusions truly can be prevented. Restoration of the primary teeth and the actual prevention of deleterious oral habits are the most obvious examples and these are preventable only if a normal dentition is developing within a normal craniofacial skeleton.

b) Interception of Malocclusion

It is a mistake to confuse preventive and interceptive orthodontics. Although few malocclusions actually can be prevented, serial studies at the famous Burlington Orthodontic Research Centre have documented the fact that approximately 26% of all malocclusions can be intercepted if proper procedures are undertaken at the proper time.[1] Interception, that is, skillful guidance of dental development, offers the opportunity to minimize or obliterate actual or potential abnormalities. Examples are correction of deleterious oral habits, planned serial extractions of the primary teeth, preservation of the arch perimeter during the mixed dentition, elimination of occlusal interferences causing functional crossbites and so forth.

c) *The Problem of Increasing Demands*

As our affluent society becomes more affluent, more people demand treatment of malocclusions. Furthermore, each passing year makes evident the fruits of past educational campaigns in preventive dentistry, for the public is far better educated to the problems of malocclusion than it was a generation ago. Although steps may be taken to decrease the need for orthodontic treatment of a corrective and serious nature by prevention and interception, such steps are likely to be more than countered by the increased demand for orthodontic services.

D. Administration of Orthodontic Problems in General Practice

Each dentist in general practice, whether he likes it or not, has orthodontic responsibilities. He need not treat any given patient but he must diagnose all to the best of his ability. Furthermore, he is obligated to advise the patient concerning a malocclusion and its possible treatment. The average dentist in North America has had as little training and experience in orthodontics as in any field in dentistry, but his patients do not know this. They assume that their dentist will advise them as well in orthodontics as he does in operative dentistry and prosthetics. Some men actually rationalize and deny their orthodontic responsibilities with "I didn't have a decent undergraduate orthodontic course" or "I have a fine, well-trained orthodontist who handles my cases, and he doesn't like me to fiddle with malocclusions." Every orthodontic problem is seen first in the general, not the specialty, practice. It will escape diagnosis unless the family dentist calls attention to it. The original diagnosis always is made by the family dentist. Furthermore, the orthodontist cannot treat cases he has not seen. The situation poses an unusual problem for the general practitioner, since the most difficult diagnostic problems in orthodontics may be his. There is good reason why a greater portion of this book is devoted to understanding the problem of malocclusion than to comprehensive treatment procedures.

1. RELATIONSHIPS WITH THE PATIENT

a) *Establishing Cooperation*

Many articles have been written emphasizing the importance of the first visit to the dentist's office. Since confidence of the patient is a key factor in any procedure involving pain, such articles serve a purpose. When the dentist embarks on a new orthodontic treatment, a different situation presents itself, and one should not transfer his ideas of operative dental procedures to the orthodontic patient. There is no rush; orthodontic corrections take time—time that casually may be utilized to gain the patient's confidence. No pain is involved, and knowledge of this fact is reassuring to the patient. Most children are well aware that orthodontic therapy will help them. The relationship with orthodontic patients is one of the great joys of dental practice, due to the satisfaction de-rived from rendering such a fine service to young children. To me at least, it is much more satisfying to shape a young child's face and mouth for a lifetime of service than to do patchwork and repair for the middle-aged.

One of the best ways to establish easy and friendly rapport with the adolescent is to listen to his inevitable questions. Answer them easily, explaining such details as are necessary. Do not oversell, but treat all details in a matter-of-fact manner. Assume that this child will act as well as all the other children in your practice. To assume that he will misbehave is to invite misbehavior.

Orthodontic treatment, as much as any other form of dental therapy, requires patient cooperation. Cooperation is best based on understanding. It is well to take time to discuss what you are attempting for the patient. Answer his questions simply and truthfully. Successful orthodontic treatment depends on a combination of child plus parent plus dentist working together. Explain this unusual relationship at the very start and assume that child and parents will play their roles as reliably as you will play yours.

b) *When Cooperation Fails*

At the first sign of lack of cooperation, talk the matter over quietly with the patient. Do not consult with the parents until you are convinced that you and the patient need their help. The ideal relationship is that of child and dentist working together, with the parents standing by for help only when needed. Such an understanding gives the child status and a feeling of responsibility, and he has respect for the dentist who has placed such confidence in him.

When the dentist fears that trouble may lie ahead, he should not attempt to shame the child into complying. Nor should there be threats, bribes or cajolery. All such approaches are degrading to the child. However, one may say something like this: "This appliance is very much like the one Fred Jones has been wearing for 6 months and we are getting nice results." The adolescent welcomes and respects responsibility if he understands why the responsibility is being given him. To treat a mentally healthy adolescent like an infant is to guarantee an infantile response. If the patient is uncooperative and persists in this spirit, even though the facts have been laid on the line before him, one should quietly bring the parents into the picture. However, all disciplining of the child should be left to the parents to do at home. It is their privilege and duty.

2. RELATIONSHIPS WITH PARENTS

a) Presenting the Treatment Plan

After completing the cursory examination of the patient and gathering the diagnostic records, try to avoid discussing the plan of treatment until another appointment. There are several good reasons for delaying the presentation to the parents: (1) it gives them time to think over the matter and discuss orthodontics with their friends; (2) it labels the problem as one that requires serious attention and study, not one to be treated with flippancy; (3) it gives you time to study the case, consult with others or read about similar problems. Parents often have less background knowledge of orthodontics than other phases of dentistry and thus need orientation. Take time to help them understand what you are proposing to do.

1) DESCRIBE THE CLINICAL PROBLEM.—Paint a verbal picture of the problem, filling in the parents' knowledge of growth. Photographs and casts of various stages of normal growth of occlusion help them to visualize the matter.

2) PROPOSE A SOLUTION.—First, state the purpose of treatment and then the suggested method of treatment. For example, the purpose might be to maintain the position of the first permanent molars lest they drift mesially, and the method might be the use of a fixed lingual archwire. Assign, in a casual manner, each person's task. "Johnnie's job will be to wear his appliance, keep his teeth clean and practice his exercises. Your job will be to see that he keeps his appointments. I will adjust the appliance and guide the development of his occlusion." Never guarantee orthodontic results; only promise that you will do your best to handle the problem.

3) DISCUSS FINANCIAL ARRANGEMENTS.—The methods of payment are best discussed at the visit during which the treatment plan is presented. Explain with care that all charges are for time, advice and services, not for appliances. Fees may be determined by the average rate for other services rendered in the office. It is logical to charge the same hourly income for orthodontics as for other services; to get less is unfair to you, to ask more is unfair to the patient. Many dentists have an initial fee that serves as a retainer and covers the greater amount of time spent in starting the case. It should never be said to be a fee for the appliance, for to do so is to place a higher premium on the wire or plastic than on your professional services. After the initial fee, charges may then be levied by the month, the quarter or the visit. For interceptive orthodontics in the general practitioner's office, charging per visit may be more practical. Unless one is very experienced in interceptive orthodontics, to quote a total fee is hazardous because of the difficulty in estimating the exact amount of office time needed to treat a given patient. Explain that broken appliances and broken appointments consume the dentist's time and therefore are chargeable.

After the oral presentation of the financial arrangements, send a letter to the parents stating the terms discussed in the office. The letter should be clear and straightforward, but friendly. It might include a sentence similar to this: "Unless I hear from you to the contrary, I shall assume that these arrangements are satisfactory."

4) MISCELLANEOUS.—When the treatment plan is presented, it is prudent to outline what might be done if the malocclusion does not respond to the suggested treatment. This can be done easily if the parents understand, for example, the difference between diagnosing and treating a carious lesion and diagnosing and treating a malocclusion. There seems to be no reason for hiding from them the fact that it is much easier, ordinarily, to plan treatment for a carious lesion than for a Class II malocclusion. Begin the treatment discussions with a frank, honest and professional approach and continue on that same high plane. It is best to leave "supersalesmanship" to the used-car dealer or real estate office.

"Shouldn't this work be done by an orthodontist?" When such an honest and straightforward question is posed, it might be answered in this fashion: "Mrs. Jones, I send many children to Doctor Brown, who is the orthodontist with whom I work. Betty's problem does not seem to be difficult enough to warrant referral. She has a type of problem I usually treat in my office. However, I will be happy to send Betty along to Doctor Brown for a consultation." Such an approach lets the parents know that your first concern is the child. Do not compete with the orthodontist in the parent's mind; you will always lose. Show the parents your role and the orthodontist's. You cannot do this honestly unless you are sure in your own mind of your role. If there is any doubt, refer the case to the orthodontist.

b) When Troubles Arise

Very few orthodontic cases are completed without encountering minor problems along the way. When trouble arises, label it, locate the person responsible and talk accordingly. Do not go over the child's head to the parent except when speaking to the child has failed to get results. Be firm, honest and patient. Remember that in most other types of dental and medical therapy the clinician does all the work. It may take a while for the child and parents to orient themselves to their roles in orthodontic treatment.

If you are certain of failure in the treatment, call in the parents alone for a talk. Review the history of the case for them, listing each problem that has arisen. Be fair, honest and candid. During this talk, it is a good plan to have all the records of the case on the desk for easy reference. If each missed appointment or appliance breakage is underlined in the case history in red, they are easily called to the parents' attention. After the review, ask for their reaction. If they suggest that you go ahead with the treatment, outline the new conditions under which you will proceed.

When such a conversation is necessary, two alternatives present themselves: (1) to proceed under improved conditions or (2) to refer the patient to a competent colleague who may have better success. If the latter course seems indicated, the idea might be presented in this fashion: "Doctor Johnson is a competent practitioner in whom I have confidence. Perhaps Mary will be better off with a fresh start." Always try to choose the course of action that will be best for the child, even though at this particular time you may have lost considerable respect for that child. Never continue treatment when you are sure that you cannot help.

There seems to be less difficulty in collecting payments for orthodontic services than for other dental services. Perhaps this is due to the usual method of installment payments; perhaps it is because the result is delivered in stages and not in a lump item, as is a denture or a bridge. It will be found that parents who are neglecting payments for their own dental work often will pay promptly for orthodontic work for their children.

3. Relationships with the Orthodontist

It is extremely difficult to do good interceptive orthodontics in a general practice without a firm relationship of mutual trust and confidence with an orthodontist. He should be the one to whom you refer problems that are too difficult for you. Consult him as is necessary and make it easy for him to say, "You are likely to get into trouble on this one. Why don't you just let me take it from the start?" It is wise to ask the orthodontist which records he would like you to keep, so that when referring a case to him you can provide the serial data of most use.

All orthodontists are not trained alike; therefore, they do varying amounts of interceptive orthodontics themselves. Although there has been a strong tendency toward increased amounts of early treatment in recent years, the orthodontist's most difficult and time-consuming job is still the correction of comprehensive problems in the young adult dentition.

Never leave the orthodontist with the idea that you are in competition with him; instead, give the impression that you are willing to do all the interceptive work your training and experience will permit. Most good orthodontists prefer that the family dentist be informed about facial growth, the development of occlusion and orthodontics in general. The general practitioner so informed is able to appraise better the work the orthodontist does for his patients. The skillful orthodontist is not afraid to have his work assessed; he wishes it, since his efforts are more likely to be appreciated. The well-informed general practitioner will treat more malocclusions in his own office and yet refer more comprehensive problems to the orthodontist.

The relationship between the family dentist and the orthodontist may break down if the general practitioner extends himself beyond his training and abilities. He cannot expect to be rescued repeatedly by the orthodontist for the same error in clinical judgment. One reason for the lack of enthusiasm shown by some orthodontists for treatment of malocclusions by the family dentist may be a previous experience with a general practitioner who tried to treat severe and complicated malocclusions without proper training. Any ethical dentist cannot help being upset when he sees a young child's mouth being harmed. However, many orthodontists who have had such experiences are easily won over when they see an attitude reflecting a sincere desire to serve the patient in an ethical manner.

4. RELATIONSHIPS WITH THE FAMILY PHYSICIAN

The average physician knows little concerning the field of orthodontics, but rarely knows how little he knows. In most medical schools, the students receive very little orientation in dentistry. The dentist should be just as patient in explaining the etiology of Class II malocclusion to the physician as he would want the physician to be were the discussion centered on acute infectious hepatitis. The physician often has difficulty understanding why dentists place such importance on the correction of orofacial pressure habits, since he has been well indoctrinated only in the psychologic aspects of the matter. It is well to listen and learn from him, since few dentists have the background to appreciate the immense field of child psychiatry. Whenever a patient whom you both are serving has nasorespiratory distress, thumb-sucking or similar problems involving both fields, a rare opportunity is presented. Use the case at hand to further the physician's knowledge of orthodontic objectives and to learn all you can concerning the medical aspects of the same problem. Make sure the physician understands that good orthodontics depends on excellent total health by inquiring about the condition of children who are his patients. The physician can be helpful on many occasions with orthodontic patients; make use of him. Orthodontics is one of the easiest places in dentistry to establish and maintain rapport with the physician.

5. RELATIONSHIPS WITH THE COMMERCIAL ORTHODONTIC LABORATORY

Special problems arise in assigning orthodontic appliance construction work to the laboratory. We are fortunate in the United States to have the services of many fine dental laboratories; however, not all of them are experienced in orthodontic appliance construction. Many dentists who can appraise regular dental laboratory work are not experienced enough to judge orthodontic laboratory work. A few suggestions are given here that may help establish good relationships with an orthodontic laboratory.

a) Deal only with a laboratory that you know to be ethical and whose orthodontic technicians are skilled workers. You may want to question a colleague who has used their services. The laboratories that advertise in the *American Journal of Orthodontics* usually have to provide good service to readers to make continued advertising worth while.

b) Never ask or permit a laboratory technician to make any part of the diagnosis. To expect a technician to make an adequate diagnosis from a set of casts alone is to ask of him the impossible. Beware of the laboratory that claims in its advertising to be able to render this service. It will be forever a mystery how some dentists have more faith in the judgment of a technician who has never seen the patient than they have in themselves. It is the dentist who has the legal, ethical and moral responsibilities to his patients; he cannot abrogate them. Nor should he ask a nondentist to assume his obligations. Any dentist who cannot diagnose a problem has no business trying to treat it.

c) Try, if possible, to work with a local laboratory in order to establish a personal relationship.

d) Always send a detailed prescription describing exactly what you want constructed.

e) Do as much work in your office as you can do efficiently and well. This means constructing as many appliances as possible directly in the mouth with prefabricated elements and making others in the office laboratory. Do not overlook the possibility of training one of your assistants to construct some orthodontic appliances.

In recent years, I have been called into consultation a disappointing number of times regarding malocclusions the treatment of which was undertaken by a well-meaning dentist who had utilized the "services" of one of the mail-order laboratories specializing in orthodontics. Frequently, the diagnosis, treatment plan and appliance have all been completed by the laboratory. A chapter of this book could easily be filled with pictures of the tragic results. Quite apart from the obvious ethical problem, it is proper to mention that it often is harder to complete a case begun wrong than it is to treat the same case from the start. Perhaps a good rule to follow is to shun those laboratories with the most flamboyant advertising and the wildest claims. All of us want to do good orthodontics for more children—but there is a right way and a wrong way to achieve that goal.

REFERENCES

1. Burlington Orthodontic Research Centre, Progress Report Series No. 6, 1960–1961, Division of Dental Research, Faculty of Dentistry, University of Toronto, 1961.
2. Fisk, R. O.: Physiological and sociophysiological significance of malocclusion, J. Canad. D. A. 29:635, 1963.
3. Grainger, R. M.: Orthodontic treatment priority index. Vital and Health Statistics Data Evaluation and Methods Research. Series 2, Number 25, NCHS, USPHS, 1967.
4. Summers, C. J.: A System for Identifying and Scoring Occlusal Disorders: The Occlusal Index. Doctoral thesis, School of Public Health, The University of Michigan, Ann Arbor, 1966.

SUGGESTED READINGS

Armstrong, C. J.: Orthodontics in the United Kingdom, Australian D. J. 10:78, 1965.
Bowden, J.: An outsider looks at orthodontics, Am. J. Orthodont. 53:858, 1967.
Knutson, J. W.: Status of orthodontics as a health service, J.A.D.A. 70:1204, 1965.

SOME TEXTBOOKS IN ORTHODONTICS OF USE TO THE FAMILY DENTIST

Adams, C. P.: *The Design and Construction of Removable Orthodontic Appliances* (3d ed.; Bristol: John Wright & Sons, Ltd., 1964).
Dickson, G. C.: *Orthodontics in General Dental Practice* (London: Pitman Publishing Co., Ltd., 1964).
Graber, T. M.: *Orthodontics: Principles and Practice* (3d ed.; Philadelphia: W. B. Saunders Company, 1972).
Gresham, H.: *A Manual of Orthodontics* (Christchurch, New Zealand: N. M. Peryer, 1957).
Horowitz, S. L., and Hixon, E. H.: *The Nature of Orthodontic Diagnosis* (St. Louis: The C. V. Mosby Company, 1966).
Hotz, R.: *Orthodontics in Everyday Practice* (Bern: Hans Huber, 1963).
Lundstrom, A.: *Introduction to Orthodontics* (New York: McGraw-Hill Book Company, Inc., 1961).
Salzman, J. A.: *Practice of Orthodontics* (Philadelphia: J. B. Lippincott Company, 1966).
Schwarz, A. M., and Gratzinger, M.: *Removable Orthodontic Appliances* (Philadelphia: W. B. Saunders Company, 1966).
Sassouni, V.: *Orthodontics in Dental Practice* (St. Louis: The C. V. Mosby Company, 1971).
Tulley, W. J.: *A Manual of Practical Orthodontics* (Baltimore: The Williams & Wilkins Company, 1960).
Walther, D. P.: *Orthodontic Notes* (Bristol: John Wright & Sons, Ltd., 1960).

XVII

Technics, Materials, Instruments

> Indeed, if a little knowledge is dangerous, where is the man
> who has so much as to be out of danger?—THOMAS HUXLEY,
> *Collected Essays*, Vol. III, *On Elemental Instruction
> in Physiology*

A. Basic laboratory technics

1. The bending of wire
2. Joining metals
   a) Soldering
      1) Essentials
      2) Soldering precious alloys
      3) Soldering stainless steel
   b) Spot-welding
3. Work casts
4. Record casts
5. Acrylic appliances

B. Basic clinical technics

1. Orthodontic impressions
2. Separation of teeth
3. Molar band formation
   a) Loop band (precious metal)
   b) Preformed bands
   c) Attachments for molar bands
      1) Buccal tubes
      2) Lingual sheaths
      3) Other attachments
4. Bands for incisors, cuspids and bicuspids
   a) General considerations
   b) Pinch type
   c) Preformed type
   d) Cuspid blanks
   e) Attachments for anterior bands
5. Overlays for primary molars
   a) Preformed
   b) Cast
6. Elastics

C. Fixed appliances

1. Lingual archwire
   a) Description
      1) Removable lingual archwire
      2) Fixed lingual archwire
   b) Construction
      1) When the bands are not cemented
      2) When the bands are cemented
      3) Forming the archwire
   c) Modifications
      1) Primary dentition
      2) Ellis loop lingual archwire
      3) Round post lingual archwire
      4) Horizontal lingual tube
      5) Porter lingual archwire
      6) Loop lingual archwire
   d) Attachments
      1) Auxiliary springs
      2) Lingual locks
2. Fixed space-maintainers
3. Palate-splitting devices
4. Simple labial archwires
   a) Light round labial archwire
      1) Description
      2) Indications
      3) Attachments and auxiliaries
   b) High labial archwire
      1) Description
      2) Indications
      3) Attachments, auxiliaries, modifications
   c) Lip-plumpers
5. Edgewise mechanism
   a) Description
   b) Repair and emergency adjustments
6. Light-wire appliances
   a) Description
   b) Repair and emergency adjustments
7. Twin-wire appliance
   a) Description
   b) Repair and emergency adjustments
8. Universal appliance
   a) Description
   b) Repair and emergency adjustments
9. The labiolingual appliance

D. Attached removable appliances

1. Hawley retainer
2. Bite planes
   a) Description
   b) Indications

    c) Types
      1) Maxillary flat bite plane
      2) Sved plate
      3) Sidlow hollow bite plane
      4) Mandibular inclined plane
  3. Multiple space-maintainers
  4. Space-regainers
  5. Stabilizing plates
  6. The Crozat appliance
    a) Description
    b) Advantages
    c) Disadvantages
  7. Extra-oral traction appliances
    a) Description
    b) Reasons for usage
  8. Jenkins' sliding plate

E. Loose removable appliances

  1. Oral shield
    a) Description
    b) Methods of handling plastic for oral shields
      1) Method 1
      2) Method 2
      3) Method 3
  2. Positioners
  3. Activator-type appliances (Andresen method, Norwegian system, Monobloc)
    a) Description
    b) Indications
  4. The Frankel appliance
    a) Description
    b) Application

F. Myotherapeutic exercises

  1. Purpose
  2. Limitations
  3. Principles
  4. Specific uses
    a) Orbicularis oris and circumoral muscles
    b) Mandibular posture
  5. Myofunctional appliances

G. Correction of deleterious oral habits

  1. Basic considerations
  2. Thumb-sucking (finger-sucking)
    a) Phase I: Normal and subclinically significant thumb-sucking
    b) Phase II: Clinically significant thumb-sucking
    c) Phase III: Intractable thumb-sucking
    d) Choice of appliance
  3. Tongue-thrusting
    a) Causes
    b) Diagnosis

c) Treatment
  1) Simple tongue-thrust
  2) Complex tongue-thrust
  3) Retained infantile swallow
4. Abnormal tongue posture
5. Lip-sucking and lip-biting
6. Fingernail-biting

H. Occlusal equilibration

1. Equilibration in the primary dentition
2. Equilibration in the permanent dentition
3. Equilibration in the mixed dentition

A. Basic Laboratory Technics

1. THE BENDING OF WIRE

All bends usually are placed in orthodontic wires by the fingers. Gentle bends may be made with the fingers alone. More acute bends require the use of pliers as well, but one should regard the pliers as a portable vise for holding the wire while making the bend (Fig. XVII-1).

Procedure

a) If possible, establish a fixed relationship of the wire before making any bends.

b) Place the wire in position and mark it with a wax pencil (a mascara eyebrow pencil works well) where the bend is to be made.

c) Grasp the wire in the pliers so that it may be bent downward by the fingers of the free hand against one beak (see Fig. XVII-1). Never bend a round wire over a sharp beak. Always use the rounded beak of the pliers to avoid nicking the wire. Pliers #118 and #137 are good for general wire bending.

d) Replace the wire in position to check the first bend made. Mark the location of the next bend and repeat the process.

e) Take care to make all bends at right angles to the long axis of the wire, unless a different angle is specifically required. It is much easier to control unwanted torque by keeping all bends in the same plane.

f) Never make a new bend until the last bend is perfect.

2. JOINING METALS

a) Soldering

Orthodontic soldering is more than the mere joining together of two pieces of metal; it is their union in a secure relationship to serve a specific purpose. Soldering should be done without appreciable alteration of the qualities of the metals being joined. Orthodontic soldering is best carried out with a small, specially designed orthodontic soldering burner or torch. Soldering also may be done by various electric devices, some of which are adjuncts to spot-welders. Electric soldering, for the most part, is less precise than the procedure described here.

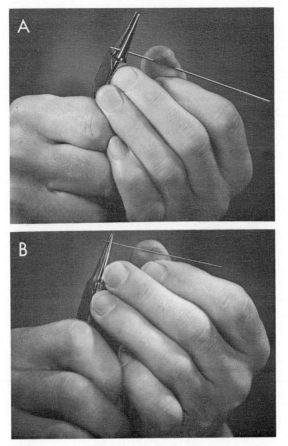

Fig. XVII-1.—Bending of wire for orthodontic appliances. **A,** correct way. Wire is near the hinge of the pliers, and the pliers are used as a portable vise. All force of application is done with the finger. **B,** improper way to bend wire.

Gas soldering

Before soldering, all necessary instruments and supplies should be at hand and the torch flame adjusted properly. A good flame for orthodontic soldering is 1 – 1½ high, with a well-defined point. When the flame is regulated properly, the burner will not give off a hissing sound. An examination of the flame will disclose three concentric cones: the inner, colorless cone of unburned gas, the middle, light blue reducing cone and the outer, dark blue oxidizing cone. It is easiest to solder when the metal is held just at the apex of the middle flame cone. The flame should not be in direct sunlight; a dark background is preferred.

The operator should be seated in a relaxed manner and have the torch so placed that during the soldering nothing will detract from his relaxed position. The

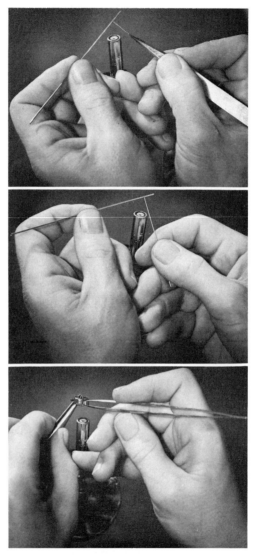

Fig. XVII-2.—Various methods of bracing fingers and hands to solder wires and attachments.

upper part of the arms from the shoulders to the elbows should rest closely to the body, with the arms bent at the elbows. Some operators prefer to brace the heels of the hands together, whereas others prefer to use the fingertips (Fig. XVII-2). Even this may vary with the particular soldering operation being performed. With the hands and arms in position holding the metal pieces in their correct relationship, the trunk of the body is bent forward to bring the appliance into the flame. The fingers, hands and arms remain braced as the body, bending at the hips, leans toward the flame. Some prefer to rotate the body to bring the wires into the flame. Whichever method is chosen, the operation is reversed when the soldering is completed.

1) ESSENTIALS

a) Orthodontic solders usually are supplied in wire form of various gauges and karats. The lower the karat designation the lower the melting point; also, the less resistance to discoloration in the mouth. 8K solder is not 8K gold. This designation means that the solder can be used with gold alloys as low as 8K. Orthodontic solder is available in other forms, e.g., disks, bars, etc., but the fine wire is most suited for general use.

b) When two soldering operations are in close proximity, the first should be done with higher-karat solder than the second. Soldering tweezers also may hold the piece with the beaks directly over the first solder joint to dissipate the heat in the region and protect the first soldered joint.

c) The solder's temperature should not be raised excessively above its melting point, as this destroys the properties of the solder.

d) When two objects of different size are to be soldered together, e.g., a large wire and a small wire, the heavier should be heated first. As it reaches the required temperature, the smaller wire may be brought into the flame.

e) After the solder has melted and the joint has been made, the components must be removed from the flame before overheating and without separating or jarring them before the solder has solidified.

f) Tweezers used in soldering should be kept in good shape, i.e., the points fine and clean.

2) SOLDERING PRECIOUS ALLOYS.—The flux used to solder precious alloys has a borax or boric acid base and either must be mixed with water to form a paste or can be purchased already mixed with petroleum jelly.

Procedure

The flux is applied to both parts at the point to be soldered, but the solder usually is applied only to the larger component being held in the fingers of the left hand, with the smaller being held in those of the right hand. The larger piece is introduced into the flame first, and as the solder begins to flow, the smaller one is applied. As the union is made, the operator reverses the movement of his body and removes the assembly from the flame. Until the solder cools below its melting point, the relationship of the components must not be disturbed. The solder flows readily when joining precious alloys, for a true solder union is formed; that is, some of the solder actually alloys with the parts being joined. The result is a firm and strong bond.

3) SOLDERING STAINLESS STEEL.—A fluoride flux is necessary for soldering stainless steel. It may be purchased, but the following formula provides an excellent product:

> 1 part potassium fluoride
> 1 part boric acid
>
> Grind well together in a mortar and add a few
> drops of water, if necessary, to form a paste.

The flux may be freshened by the addition of a crystal or two of potassium fluoride. This mixture is poisonous if ingested.

Procedure

Remove all grease and oxides from the metals to be soldered and apply a small amount of flux and solder to each part. The larger part, e.g., an archwire, is heated and the action of the flux observed closely. The flux will first fluff up and then subside. As the flux melts, it will take on the appearance of molten glass. At this point, the solder that has been fluxed should be applied to the archwire where the attachment is to be made. The other component, e.g., a spring, should have flux and solder applied in a like manner. The archwire is now held in the fingers of the left hand and the spring in the fingers of the right hand (see Fig. XVII-2). With the larger wire preceding, since it requires more heating, the two parts are brought into the flame. As the solder melts, the wires are touched and, without disturbing their relationship, removed. 8K gold solder is suggested for steel soldering, since it melts at a low temperature and does not oxidize quickly in the flame. Some advocate silver solder, but it is less satisfactory, for it oxidizes too quickly in the flame and tarnishes badly in the mouth. Many good solder alloys designed especially for stainless steel soldering are now on the market. Some are surprisingly efficient, flowing at a low temperature and standing up well in the mouth without tarnishing.

A true solder joint does not result when stainless steel and solder are joined; rather, there is an intimate mechanical union. With modern stainless steel alloys, however, surprising results may be obtained. Slightly more solder is needed and a slightly cooler flame than for soldering the gold alloys. The combination of low-karat solder and lower heat reduces the chances of harming the steel.

All steel auxiliary springs should be wrapped around the archwire at least twice to protect the solder joint and the annealed portion of the spring wire.

b) Spot-Welding

Spot-welding is the joining of two metal pieces by heating caused by a flow of electric current through the portions of the pieces in juxta-

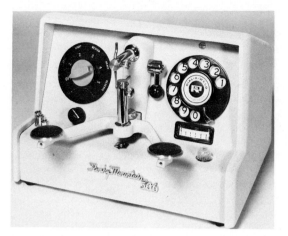

Fig. XVII-3.—Typical modern orthodontic spot-welder. (Courtesy of Rocky Mountain Metal Products Company.)

position. The parts to be joined are held together by electrodes. As the current passes through the electrodes and the metal pieces between them, resistance is built up within the metals to be welded. The heat generated is sufficient to cause a flowing together and union of the parts touching each other. A true weld is formed, and no solder or flux is used. The technic is used in orthodontics only with the stainless steel alloys, although in industry many different alloys are welded.

Apparatus

Several spot-welders that give satisfactory results are available to the dentist (Fig. XVII-3). All consist of an electrical circuit that permits variation of the current and the duration of the current flow through the electrodes holding the bits to be joined.

Fig. XVII-4.—Correct placement of band in the electrode for spot-welding.

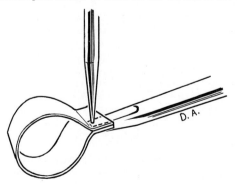

Technic

For best use, the welder points and the parts to be joined should be clean and dry. The parts should be held tightly together when the current is passed through them (Fig. XVII-4). Some welders exert considerable pressure at the time the weld is being made, which is said to produce a better joint. Avoid overheating, as this burns the metals and may even make a hole in a band. Never pass the current through unless the parts are close together, or a spark gap will be created that may burn the band or spring. Small auxiliary springs are "tacked" to the archwire in several places and wrapped around the archwire at least twice to protect the series of welds. Light auxiliary springs also may be held to archwires by wrapping a piece of anterior band material around the two wires and spot-welding the band material.

3. WORK CASTS

Work casts are those used for the construction of appliances. Accuracy is important, but it is not necessary to take time to make them pretty. Impressions for work casts usually are made of alginate, although when seating molar bands in the impression for construction of a lingual archwire, a combination compound-alginate impression is taken. The casts may be poured of laboratory plaster, stone or a combination of the two, according to need.

4. RECORD CASTS

Record casts are one of the most important sources of information for the dentist during treatment of the orthodontic case. The time required for their precise construction is time well spent.

After the impression has been removed from the mouth, the material should be handled in accordance with the manufacturer's directions. It is especially important to avoid prolonged exposure of the impression material to the air.

Procedure

Some prefer to pour the anatomic portion of the casts in white stone and the art portion or base in snow-white plaster. Although this makes more durable teeth on the casts, there will be a difference in color between the materials. Carefully made casts of a heavy mix of snow-white plaster will be strong enough for usual handling. Spatulate the plaster to a heavy mix, taking care to avoid entrapping bubbles. Place the plaster bowl over a vibrator and gently spatulate the mix to allow a maximum chance for the smaller bubbles to escape. Hold the impression tray atop the vibrator and start the flow of plaster into the impression at one heel. With a blunt instrument, gently tease the flowing plaster from one tooth's impression into the next. It is best to leave an excess of plaster in the impression.

A base is a necessity for proper orthodontic models. It aids in proper articulation of the teeth and protects the teeth against breakage. Bases

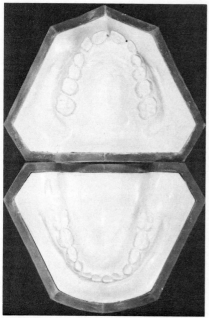

Fig. XVII-5.—Rubber base-formers.

are made in two ways—by the use of oriented base-formers or by means of a model-trimmer. If a model-trimmer is not available, suitable bases may be added by using rubber base-formers. Vibrate the base-former full of plaster and carefully seat into the moist plaster the anatomic portion taken from the impression. Use great care to place the dental arch symmetrically within the base-former (Fig. XVII-5). One may obtain flush posterior surfaces of the bases while the teeth are in occlusion by the following method: (1) Complete the base of one cast as described, preferably the upper. (2) Proceed with the lower in a similar fashion, but occlude the teeth with the wax bite or tie the anatomic part of the lower with dental floss or rubber bands to the completed upper in its base-former while placing the cast into the plaster in the lower base-former. (3) By keeping the bottom of the upper cast parallel with the bench top and the two bases flush against a surface at right angles to the bench top, the desired relationship is established. Usually, complete directions for this procedure are included with each set of rubber base-formers. This procedure takes some time, for one must wait between steps 1 and 2 while the plaster sets; nevertheless, it is a relatively simple method of obtaining adequate bases. Base-formers that are joined by a simple articulator may be purchased also.

Remove the casts from the base-formers and trim away all excess plaster. The casts may be polished by using a small Arkansas stone under running water or 000 waterproof carborundum paper. They are

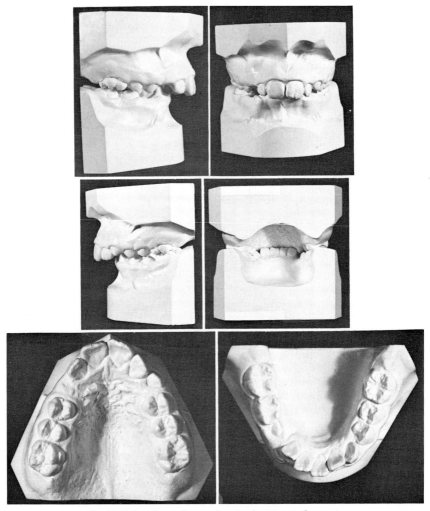

Fig. XVII-6.—A good set of orthodontic study casts.

then dried and polished by rubbing with talc or they are soaked in a soap solution. Make a concentrated solution of fine white soap by boiling. Allow the dry casts to remain in the solution for a few minutes only. After drying, a high luster may be achieved by polishing with a lint-free cotton rag. Commercial solutions for polishing casts also are available.

If the model-trimmer is to be used, the following method is satisfactory. Modern model-trimmers have devices attached to them that make trimming swift and easy.

a) After the anatomic portions have been poured and the plaster has achieved at least initial set, the cast is centered into large base-formers filled with plaster that is heavy and has just started to set.

b) After the base has set, remove the casts from the formers and grind the top of the base of the maxillary cast so that it is parallel to the occlusal plane.

c) The back of the maxillary cast is now ground at right angles to the median raphe and the base top prepared as in step *b*.

d) The sides are next trimmed symmetrically at right angles to the top of the maxillary base and roughly parallel to the line of the buccal cusps.

e) It is conventional to trim the anterior portion to a "V" shape with the apex coincident with the midline and the sides reflecting the arch form (Fig. XVII-6).

f) Now articulate the two casts by means of a wax bite and invert them so that the top of the maxillary cast is down on the model-trimmer plate. Move the articulated casts against the trimmer's wheel so that the mandibular cast's back side is ground flush with the previously prepared maxillary cast's back.

g) Place the mandibular cast upright on the posterior portion just prepared and grind away the bottom base, making it parallel to the maxillary base's top and the occlusal plane.

h) Prepare the sides of the mandibular cast parallel to the buccal segments (as in *d*) and perpendicular to the bottom of the base.

i) It is conventional to round off the front portion of the mandibular cast so that the curve approximates the dental arch itself (Fig. XVII-6).

j) Articulate the casts again, grinding off the posterior corners to form short segments, joining the sides and back by two obtuse angles (Fig. XVII-6).

k) With a vulcanite scraper and knife, clean out the lingual portion and any remaining excess plaster.

l) Dry, polish and label the casts (Fig. XVII-6).

Fig. XVII-7.—Right and wrong ways to trim acrylic resin when used in orthodontic appliances. Acrylic should not be festooned around the necks of teeth, for food will gather and Class V cavities may develop.

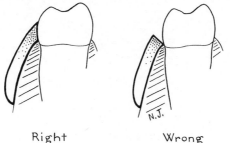

Right   Wrong

5. ACRYLIC APPLIANCES

Acrylic orthodontic appliances may be made by either the flask or quick-cure method. Appliances that are to be worn for some time probably should be made in the conventional flask manner. With either method, one common fault is seen in trimming and polishing the appliance. The plastic should fit snugly against the teeth so that saliva and food may empty easily from the embrasures and not collect around the necks of the teeth. In prosthetic appliances, the acrylic often is neatly trimmed and festooned around the necks of artificial teeth. This must not be done around natural teeth lest food accumulate in the groove formed by the festooning (Fig. XVII-7).

Retention of acrylic appliances during the mixed dentition stage often is a problem. The ordinary wrought wire clasp is of little use when the permanent teeth are not yet fully erupted. Several satisfactory clasps

Fig. XVII-8.—Some methods of retaining attached removable acrylic appliances. **A,** retaining eyelets. **B,** the Adams clasp. **C,** Duyzings clasp.

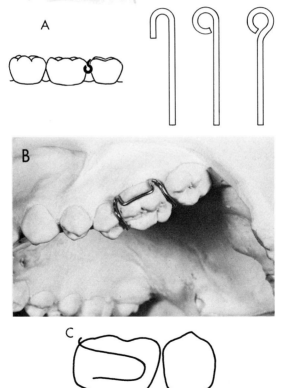

for acrylic orthodontic appliances are shown in Figure XVII-8. The Adams clasp is especially recommended.

B. Basic Clinical Technics

1. ORTHODONTIC IMPRESSIONS

A wide selection of trays should be kept on hand. From these, suitable ones may be chosen that, with a minimal amount of bending, will provide proper clearance from the teeth and soft tissues. Alginate impression material is satisfactory for orthodontic record casts.

When the teeth are in extreme malposition or the arch is abnormally shaped, it is useful to add soft wax to the impression tray. For example, it often is necessary to increase the palatal portion of the tray when the vault is narrow and high or wax may be added to the labial flange of the impression tray to carry the impression material well up into the vestibule in Class II, Division 1 cases (Fig. XVII-9). Figure XVII-10 shows a well-taken set of impressions. Note how the impression material was carried to the limits of the vestibule. The following points may aid in taking correct orthodontic impressions in children.

a) Always use the exact size of tray required.

b) Add wax where needed to ensure a complete impression of the supporting bony structures.

c) Mix the impression material in the proportions suggested by the manufacturer. Do not beat air into the impression material, as is done when mixing cake batter. Rather, smooth the material against the side of the bowl with the flat side of the spatula. Time the mixing.

d) Have the patient rinse his mouth well before taking the impression.

e) Seat the patient upright, with the eye-ear plane parallel to the floor.

f) When taking the upper impression, tip the tray up in the back to drive the excess material forward so that it is extruded into the labial vestibule and not down the throat. For the upper impression, stand behind the patient and hold the tray level with the occlusal plane.

Fig. XVII-9.—Soft wax adapted to an upper tray.

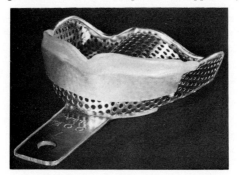

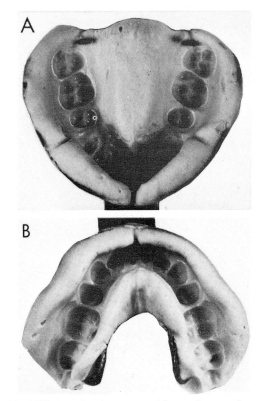

Fig. XVII-10.—Good upper and lower impressions.

g) When taking the lower impression, rotate the tray into the mouth, keeping the tray parallel with the occlusal plane. Have the patient extrude his tongue to push any excess impression material forward. Hold the tray in position by placing each index finger over the occlusal part of the tray and each thumb under the mandible.

It is less necessary when taking impressions for work casts to record the anatomy of the supporting structures high into the vestibule, but it is extremely important to preserve accurately the relationship of the appliance to the teeth. Impressions taken for the indirect construction of orthodontic appliances may be made in compound or a combination of compound and alginate. It is easier to replace bands and archwires into their proper sites with compound, but alginate is handier and more flexible. Sometimes it is helpful to put a bit of compound over a molar band and then take the alginate impression. Such a procedure combines the virtues of each material for a work cast.

2. SEPARATION OF TEETH

Often it is necessary to separate teeth before bands can be cemented. A length of .020-in. brass ligature wire is wrapped around a fountain pen or object of similar size (Fig. XVII-11, *A*). Remove the coil spring thus formed and cut it lengthwise, leaving a series of small rings. With #110 How pliers or #136 pliers, rotate the ring through the embrasure beneath the contact point but above the soft tissue (Fig. XVII-11, *B*). Twist the two loose ends and tuck them into the embrasure. When a series of separating wires is to be placed, put the wires through the embrasures and allow them to lie loosely before twisting the first one. Separation of the anterior teeth is better done with smaller wire, .010–.014 in. Stainless steel ligature wire is more sightly in the anterior region than is brass. Leave the separating wires in no longer than a few days, cut and remove by rotating the wire out of the embrasure just as it was inserted. Rarely is immediate separation indicated for orthodontic work. Other methods of separation are shown in Figure XVII-12.

Fig. XVII-11.—Method of separating teeth. **A,** soft brass separating wire wrapped around a fountain pen before cutting. **B,** individual loops left after cutting the spiral spring are rotated into position around the contact point.

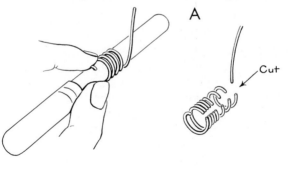

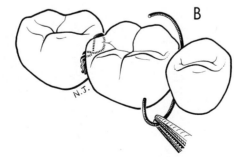

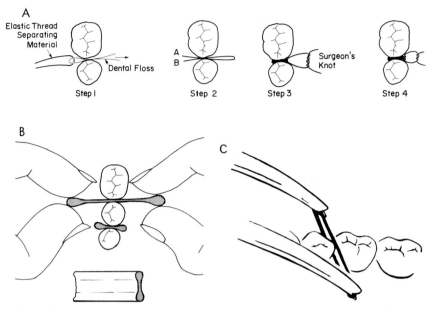

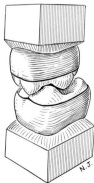

Fig. XVII-12.—Other methods of separation. **A,** elastic thread method. **B,** Maxian elastic separator. **C,** elastic separating loops.

3. Molar Band Formation

Molar bands may be made from precious or stainless steel material. A number of different methods are available so that bands may be made from (a) strip band material, (b) flat curved blanks, (c) contoured blanks, (d) cylinders, (e) loop bands or (f) preformed bands. Only the last two methods will be described here. Regardless of the material or method chosen, the finished band should be adapted closely to the contour of

Fig. XVII-13.—Upper and lower molar bands correctly contoured to avoid interference with intercuspation.

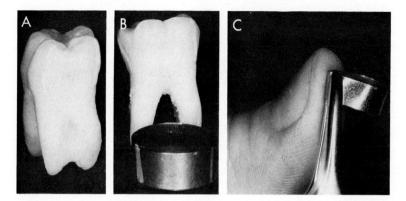

Fig. XVII-14.—A, a mandibular molar. Note how the buccal line angles are more curved than the lingual. Note, too, that the lingual cusps sit more vertically. **B,** a mandibular molar from the buccal view. Note that the distal and mesial angles converge markedly toward the cervix of the tooth. Contrast their angulation with the straight sides of the cylinder. **C,** the molar band must have placed in it the line angles of the tooth to which the band is to be fitted. Here, the operator is using a #114 pliers to place the line angles' contour into the band prior to squeezing the band on the tooth. This technic works particularly well with the loop molar band, since, by placing the line angles in the band before tightening, the force of tightening is utilized primarily for the niceties rather than the gross fitting.

the tooth, should be free of occlusion and should extend 0.5–1 mm. below the free margin of the gum (Fig. XVII-13). On the mesial and distal surfaces, the occlusal edge of the band should lie just at the marginal ridge. The gingival edge of the band should be festooned mesially and distally so that it will not cut into the transseptal periodontal fibers.

Before adapting a molar band, let us compare the anatomy of the upper and lower permanent molars. The crown of the upper molar usually is in line with the long axis of the root and presents lingual and buccal surfaces of approximately the same length occlusogingivally. In contrast, the crown of the lower molar has a lingual inclination from the long axis of the root and thus presents a longer buccal surface occlusogingivally (Fig. XVII-14). The path of insertion of the upper molar band is in line with the long axis of the tooth, whereas in the lower, the path of insertion is in line only with the crown. The problem is to get the rather flat metal form of the band to adapt to the contours of the tooth. Regardless of which banding technic is used, some contouring with pliers may be necessary.

a) Loop Band (Precious Metal)

A loop band is a cylinder with a small loop forming part of the cylinder (Fig. XVII-15). Such bands are contoured and are supplied in four sizes.

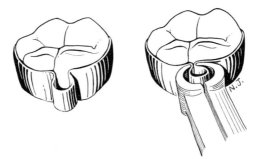

Fig. XVII-15.—Loop molar bands, available in four sizes, one of which can be adapted well to any molar. Special pliers (*right*) are needed for adaptation of this type of band.

By tightening the small loop, they can be fitted to many shapes and sizes of teeth. It is best to use a special pair of pliers for adaptation (Fig. XVII-15).

Steps in construction

(1) A size is selected that approximates the size of the molar to be banded. The band is slipped over the crown of the tooth and down to the gingival margin. The location of the line angles of the tooth will have been made in the band by this step. Now, with the #114 pliers, establish firmly the contour of all four of the line angles (see Fig. XVII-14). Reseat the band (Fig. XVII-16).

(2) The loop is closed with a pair of pliers made especially for this purpose, the band being drawn tightly around the tooth.

Fig. XVII-16.—Construction of maxillary molar bands. Note use of band driver.

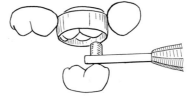

1. Seat the band by alternate pressure at the line angles

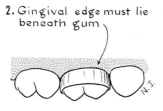

2. Gingival edge must lie beneath gum

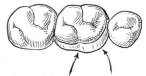

3. Burnish into grooves and against contours

(3) The band is removed and soldered with 18K solder along the seam made by pinching. It is important to use a high-karat solder, as the most convenient place to pinch this type of band is in the center of the buccal surface or on the mesiobuccal cusp. This, unfortunately, is where attachments are placed most frequently.

(4) Cut off the excess part of the loop and reseat the band until it is 0.5–1 mm. below the free margin of the gum lingually and bucally. It was not possible to do this previously without pinching the gum in the loop.

Although they are very handy and easy to use, some of the loop molar bands have the disadvantage of leaving a portion of the buccal surface of the crown exposed. This is undesirable in patients with poor oral hygiene. Loop bands have several advantages for the family dentist: (1) only a small supply of sizes is needed, (2) they are available in gold and hence a spot-welder is not needed, (3) they can be annealed and readapted easily and (4) they have scrap value. They are not made as quickly as the preformed band and they do have a soldered or spot-welded seam.

Several manufacturers now supply loop molar bands. Their products vary slightly, but the wider bands are preferred, since they permit the buccal surface to be covered more easily. The wider loop bands also are prefestooned on the proximal surfaces.

b) Preformed Bands (Fig. XVII-17)

Preformed bands are the most popular because they have been so perfected that one achieves a good fit routinely, they are easy to adapt quickly and their cost is low. They are made of stainless steel and come in a sufficiently large number of sizes to fit nearly all teeth. They are seated in the usual fashion (see Fig. XVII-16) and only occasionally require contouring. It is necessary to maintain a large inventory of such bands at all times. Attachments can be spot-welded to the bands by the manufacturer if that is desired.

c) Attachments for Molar Bands

1) BUCCAL TUBES.—Buccal tubes are used to hold labial archwires in position and for insertion of the inner bow of headgear appliances.

Fig. XVII-17.—Examples of preformed orthodontic bands. (Courtesy of Rocky Mountain Metal Products Company.)

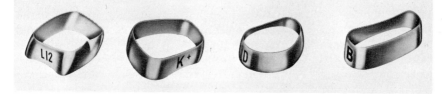

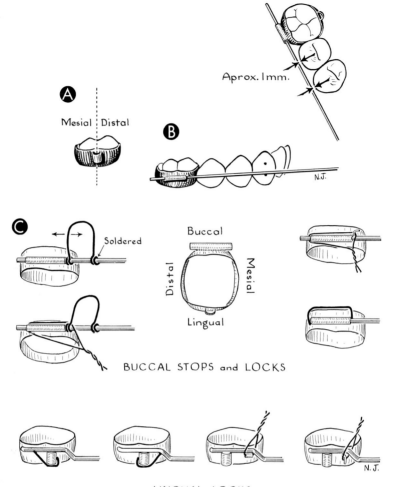

LINGUAL LOCKS

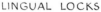

Fig. XVII-18.—Attachments to molar bands. **A,** lingual tube, which should be placed vertically at about the junction of the mesial and distal cusps. **B,** the relationship of the archwire to the buccal surfaces of the bicuspids when the buccal tube is placed correctly. **C,** types of buccal and lingual stops and locks used on molar bands.

They are soldered or spot-welded to the molar bands, usually at the junction of the middle and gingival thirds of the crown. The tube should be parallel to the occlusal surface of the tooth and in line with the buccal cusps (Fig. XVII-18, *A* and *B*), although this latter point may have to be compromised when the molar is rotated severely. Some methods

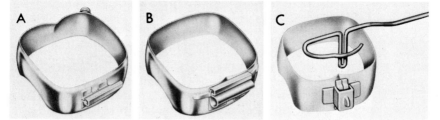

Fig. XVII-19.—Attachments for molar bands. **A,** single buccal tube and lingual button. **B,** a double buccal tube for the molar. **C,** the lingual tube, which receives the Ellis-type lingual archwire. (Courtesy of Rocky Mountain Metal Products Company.)

of stopping and locking archwires in buccal tubes are shown in Figure XVII-18, *C.* Each of the multibanded appliance systems has one or more special buccal tubes. When the second molars are erupted, they may receive the buccal tube, and brackets are placed on the first molar bands. Buccal tubes on lower molars must be checked carefully lest they interfere with the occlusion.

2) LINGUAL SHEATHS.—Lingual sheaths are placed on molar bands to receive and attach lingual archwires. Many variations of the lingual shaft and sheath are in current use; however, the standard specifications are 14-gauge half-round, 10 in. If cross-sectioned in the horizontal plane, the lumen is exactly a semicircle, hence the name "half-round" sheath. Other shapes are used, e.g., the Mershon, which has the shape of the letter D. Horizontal lingual sheaths also are used. Various locking methods are shown in Figure XVII-18, *C.*

Technic

The lingual sheath is placed on the molar band to receive the shaft soldered to the lingual archwire. The sheath should be placed in a vertical position in order to give the most stability to the lingual archwire (see Fig. XVII-18). The position of the sheath mesiodistally will vary with the method of securing the archwire to the molar band. If the standard soft wire lock is being used, the sheath should be placed at the center of the tooth in the region of the lingual groove (see Fig. XVII-18). Vertically, the sheath should be placed in the middle third of the tooth, leaving sufficient clearance gingivally for the lock wire. There must be enough room occlusally to permit clearance of the seated lingual archwire without interference with the bite.

Sheaths for Ellis lingual archwires are somewhat larger and are available in either stainless steel or precious alloy. Their use is discussed in the section on Lingual Archwire (p. 659).

3) OTHER ATTACHMENTS.—As the need arises, hooks, lugs, eyelets, buttons, etc., may be attached to the molar band (Fig. XVII-19).

4. Bands for Incisors, Cuspids and Bicuspids

a) General Considerations

Bands for the anterior teeth and the bicuspids may be made of precious metal or stainless steel and may be provided with a variety of attachments. Each of the several full-banded orthodontic appliances, for example, edgewise, twin-wire, universal, etc., has its own particular bracket designed for a specific technic. Although the complete use of these comprehensive orthodontic appliances is not discussed in this book, an introduction to certain of these appliances is given later and some of the brackets are discussed there.

Anterior bands are provided to give precise control of teeth during rotations and bodily movement. It is imperative that they be fitted accurately, placed at the correct height on the tooth and cemented well. Since the bands and brackets provide a means of joining several teeth together, one misplaced band or bracket affects the position of several teeth. The following measurements may be used to ensure correct placement of the bands.

Maxillary central incisors: middle third of the crown.
Maxillary lateral incisors: 1/64 in. incisally to the middle third of the crown. It is important to make this slight variation in placement to avoid extrusion of the lateral incisors.
Mandibular incisors: middle third of the crown.
Cuspids: 1/32 in. incisally to the middle third of the crown. Some judgment must be used for the maxillary cuspids, and it may be necessary to place them even a bit more incisally.
Mandibular first bicuspids: 1/32 in. gingivally to the middle third of the crown.
Other teeth: middle third of the crown.

A set of dividers may be used to compare placement of the bands from one tooth to another. A gadget for doing this more easily is available. Each band should be placed so that its bracket is perpendicular to the long axis of its tooth. If the bracket is malposed, it will be necessary to change its position later.

Anterior and bicuspid bands may be fashioned in several ways. The steps in construction, the advantages and the disadvantages of some of the more popular methods of construction are described here.

b) Pinch Type

Stainless steel: .125 × .003 in., with or without bracket
Precious:　　　.125 × .004 in., with or without bracket

The precious material for this type of band is supplied in 1¾ in. and 1 ft. lengths. The usual thickness is .004 in. The 1¾-in. strips are supplied with or without brackets attached. The steel is supplied in rolls and in 1¾-in. strips with the brackets spot-welded into place. The most popular thickness for stainless steel anterior bands is .003 in.

Steps in construction

(1) Secure separation, if necessary.

(2) A length of band material to permit some overlapping is adapted and pinched on the lingual surface (Fig. XVII-20, *A–C*). To ensure a snug fit, the band should be burnished well on the other surface. Take care during this step to hold the band at the correct incisogingival height.

(3) When the band has been fitted, it is removed from the tooth and soldered or spot-welded (Fig. XVII-20, *D* and *E*). While this is being done, the relationship of the pinched surfaces must be maintained with care. During soldering, the heat is applied from the lingual side of the band and the solder is flowed into the seam from the inside of the band (Fig. XVII-20, *D*). 18K solder is used for precious material and 8K solder if stainless steel is to be soldered. If the band is being spot-welded, follow the directions in Figure XVII-20, *E*.

(4) The excess material is trimmed off and the lingual surface of the band polished. If this step is not done properly, the band may become annoying to the tongue or interfere with the bite.

(5) Replace the band on the tooth and burnish it carefully. If this cannot be done without wrinkling, flow a small amount of *low-karat* solder over the inside of the lingual surface and reburnish. If this additional step does not provide a perfect fit, remake the band. This applies only to bands of precious material. If a steel band does not fit when burnished to the tooth, it is much easier to remake the entire band. Special pliers for pinching bands are available.

Fig. XVII-20.—Anterior band construction.

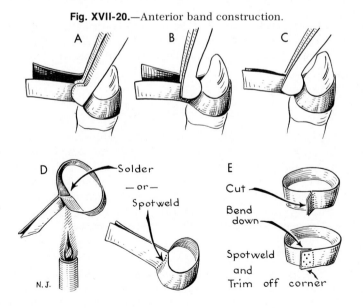

c) *Preformed Type*

Bands that are preformed to the shape of the tooth are available in a large selection of sizes. They are selected for size in much the same manner as described for the molars and adapted to the tooth by driving into position and burnishing. Preformed bands usually are supplied with brackets and lingual seating lugs attached. It is necessary to maintain a large inventory if preformed bands are to be used but they save much time and hence are cheaper.

d) *Cuspid Blanks*

Cuspid bands probably are the most difficult to make, owing to the high pitch of the labial surface of the crown. Furthermore, a wide variety of shapes and sizes of cuspid crowns is seen. The use of contoured cuspid blanks that are pinched to secure adaptation makes it much easier to secure a high-quality band than is possible with flat band material. Occasionally, they provide a better fit than preformed bands.

e) *Attachments for Anterior Bands*

There are many different types of brackets, each having its place in a particular technic (see Section C in this chapter). The bracket usually is placed on the band slot parallel with the incisal edge of the band. If the band has been placed correctly, the bracket is centered incisogingivally on the band. Mesiodistally, the bracket is placed in the center of the tooth.

Hooks and lingual buttons may be used in conjunction with brackets of various kinds to correct rotations of teeth. Eyelets are small rings that may be spot-welded or soldered onto a band to aid in rotating teeth.

5. Overlays for Primary Molars

a) *Preformed*

Preformed stainless steel overlays, also known as deciduous crown forms, are available in many sizes for the primary molars and cuspids. They are thin, light, inexpensive and easily and quickly adapted in the mouth. Unless the operator is unusually skilled in making bands, these preformed overlays will be found to give better retention than a band. Manufacturers provide good directions for their insertion, but the following method seems to be easier and more accurate.

Steps in construction

(1) With a set of dividers, measure the exact mesiodistal width of the tooth to be fitted. Select an overlay that is exactly this measurement.

(2) Contour the gingival margin of the overlay to reproduce exactly the con-

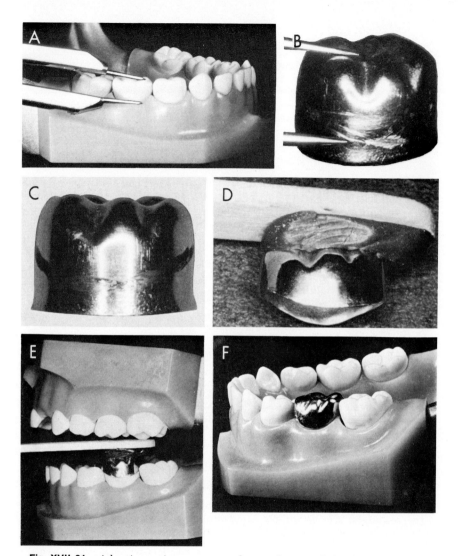

Fig. XVII-21.—Adapting primary crown forms. **A,** use of dividers to measure height of stainless steel crown forms. Dividers shown measuring height of tooth in mouth. Dividers are opened an extra 1 mm. so that measurement transferred to the crown form is the height of the cusp plus 1 mm., the excess 1 mm. to extend beneath the gingival margin. **B** and **C,** scratch marks made on crown forms. This process must be repeated around the tooth for each cusp. Scratches around the primary crown form are joined by a wax pencil mark to reproduce the exact gingival contour seen in the mouth. **D,** trimmed stainless steel crown form is inverted and placed into impression compound on end of tongue depressor. **E,** after compound has hardened, tongue depressor is carried to the mouth and patient bites down on it. Compound protects the occlusal surface of the crown form, and the force of the patient's bite easily drives the crown down onto the entire tooth and 1 mm. beneath the gingival margin around the whole circumference. **F,** completed stainless steel crown form.

tours seen in the mouth. This can be done best by using a finely pointed set of dividers. Take the dividers to the mouth or cast and set them so that one tip touches the point of any cusp of the molar to be fitted and the other tip lies on the gum 1 mm. lower than the gingival margin (Fig. XVII-21, *A*). With the dividers thus set, go to the corresponding cusp of the stainless steel overlay and scratch on its side the distance measured in the mouth (Fig. XVII-21, *B* and *C*). Repeat this procedure for all of the cusps. On the sides of the overlay will now appear scratch marks directly beneath each cusp. With crown and bridge shears, cut the overlay in a manner that will join the scratch marks and reproduce exactly the gingival contours seen in the mouth. The overlay now will be just 1 mm. higher than the height of the clinical crown. This procedure allows the overlay to fit accurately beneath the gum margin throughout its entire circumference. Up to this point, the overlay has not been placed on the tooth, yet it is completely festooned.

(3) Adapt the stainless steel crown to the tooth. Adaptation may be done best by using a tongue depressor. Invert the overlay and press its occlusal surface into the softened compound (Fig. XVII-21, *D*). Chill the compound. Now, as the stainless steel crown is placed on the tooth, the compound will protect the crown's cusps from damage during adaptation. Instruct the patient to bite gently on the tongue depressor, driving the overlay neatly into position on the tooth (Fig. XVII-21, *E*). The overlay should fit well and lie snugly beneath the entire gingival margin (Fig. XVII-21, *F*). When all goes well, it is necessary to try the crown on the tooth just this one time before cementation.

The entire fitting procedure is carried out directly in the mouth. The ease with which these crown forms, or overlays, may be adapted and their low cost make them exceedingly popular. Attachments may be either soldered or spot-welded into position after the overlay has been fitted.

b) Cast

In the past, cast gold inlays were used extensively, but they have been superseded by the stainless steel crown forms for most orthodontic purposes.

6. ELASTICS

A wide variety of sizes and strengths of rubber elastics are available that may be used in many ways to aid in tooth movements. An archwire that is brought to a bracket and held there by a steel ligature applies a single traumatic force to the periodontal membrane, but that force gradually decreases as the periodontal membrane recovers and bony adjustments take place. Light though they may seem, elastics apply a continual force to the periodontal membrane, making it more difficult for periodontal circulation to be re-established if too much force has been applied. For these reasons, less actual force must be used with elastics. A light continual force can be more damaging to the periodontal

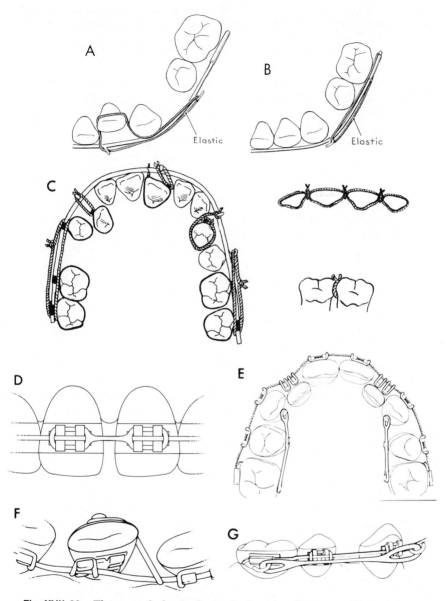

Fig. XVII-22.—The use of elastic force. **A,** the use of intramaxillary elastic to align the teeth and close the space in the line of arch. **B,** space closure. **C,** some uses for elastic thread (courtesy of Rocky Mountain Metal Products Company). **D–G,** the use of Alastics (courtesy of Unitek Corporation).

structures than a heavy single injury. Elastics are always attached to bands or archwires for their application of force to the teeth. *Never* should an elastic be placed around the naked teeth. Data usually are available from each manufacturer showing the actual forces in ounces for a given size of elastic as it is stretched over various distances.

Elastics are available as rubber bands, nylon-covered elastic thread and formed shapes for specific purposes (Fig. XVII-22). They are used to move teeth, to ligate archwires, for intermaxillary traction and for separation.

C. Fixed Appliances

1. LINGUAL ARCHWIRE

a) Description

The lingual archwire is a round wire (.032–.040 in. in diameter) closely adapted to the lingual surfaces of the teeth and attached to bands, usually on the first permanent molars (Fig. XVII-23). It is one of the most useful appliances, particularly during the mixed dentition. The archwire itself maintains the arch perimeter and auxiliary springs may be added to move teeth.

1) REMOVABLE LINGUAL ARCHWIRE.—The removable lingual archwire has precision fitting shafts that fit into corresponding sheaths in place on the lingual surface of the molar bands (see Fig. XVII-18). Various types of locks hold the appliance in position (see Fig. XVII-18, C). It is used as an active appliance or as a device to maintain the arch perimeter.

2) FIXED LINGUAL ARCHWIRE.—The fixed lingual archwire is soldered to the molar bands. It is used for the maintenance of arch length, for retention purposes and to supplement anchorage for tooth movements in the opposite denture. Its primary purpose is to maintain the arch perimeter, hence the reason it sometimes is called a holding arch.

b) Construction

1) WHEN THE BANDS ARE NOT CEMENTED.—The indirect construction of appliances may be done on work casts on which the molar bands are placed exactly as they will be in the mouth. The impression holds the molar bands while the casts are poured. Although any impression material may be used, a combination of compound and alginate seems the handiest.

Steps in procedure

(1) Place the molar bands firmly and precisely into position on their respective teeth (either with or without the buccal tubes and lingual sheaths soldered into place).

(2) Adapt a small ball of softened impression compound over the occlusal

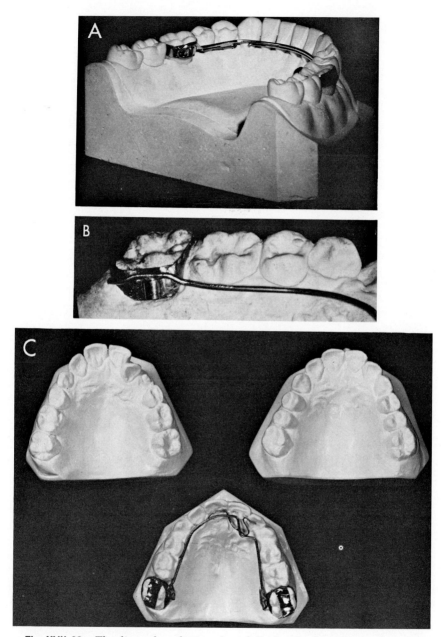

Fig. XVII-23.—The lingual archwire. **A** and **B,** detail of its adaptation to the gingival margin of the working cast. **C,** a lingual archwire with simple auxiliary spring.

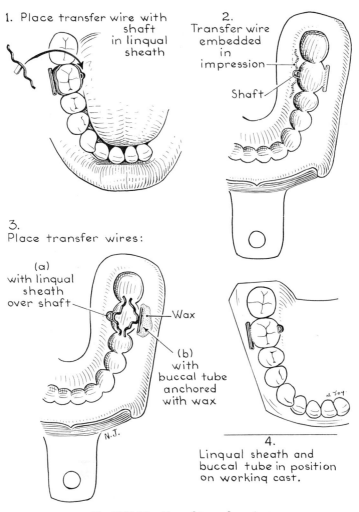

1. Place transfer wire with shaft in lingual sheath

2. Transfer wire embedded in impression—

Shaft

3. Place transfer wires:

(a) with lingual sheath over shaft—

—Wax

(b) with buccal tube anchored with wax

4. Lingual sheath and buccal tube in position on working cast.

Fig. XVII-24.—Use of transfer wires.

surfaces of the first molars and far enough lingually and bucally to engage the attachments.

(3) Secure an alginate impression in the usual manner, although it may be advantageous to use a bit less water than the directions call for. On removal of the tray from the mouth, there will be an indentation where the alginate has pulled around the compound.

(4) Gently remove the compound from the molars and seat the compound into place in the alginate impression. Occasionally, the molar bands are removed with the compound, but when made well they remain in the mouth.

(5) Remove the molar bands and seat firmly into place in the compound. It may be necessary to secure the bands to the compound or the compound to the alginate with a bit of sticky wax.

(6) A small staple or half of a paper clip is now stuck into the compound within each molar band. This bit of metal serves to reinforce the plaster or stone molar tooth during the repeated heating that occurs during several soldering procedures. If the attachments have not been in place and are to be soldered on the work cast, sometimes a small bit of utility wax placed on the inside of the band beneath the point where the tubes are to be attached will aid in heating the band during soldering.

(7) This work cast is, of course, destroyed when the bands are removed for cementation in the mouth.

2) WHEN THE BANDS ARE CEMENTED.—Occasionally, one will want to construct an appliance after the molar bands have been cemented to the teeth. It is possible to do this without removing the bands. The method involves the construction of transfer wires (Fig. XVII-24).

Steps in procedure

(1) One pair of transfer wires with half-round shafts, one pair with half-round sheaths and one pair with buccal tubes are needed for each dental arch. Transfer wires are simply a half-round shaft, sheath or buccal tube soldered in the middle of a .040-in. wire approximately 15 mm. in length. The wire is bent into a series of "wiggles" for securing a firmer grip within the alginate or plaster.

(2) Begin by placing the transfer wires with half-round shafts into position in the mouth. The shaft fits into the lingual sheath of the molar bands.

(3) When the impression (alginate alone, no compound) is removed from the mouth, it will unseat the transfer wire from the lingual sheath.

(4) Seat the buccal tube transfer wires into place within the impression material, securing the wires with wax.

(5) Place the lingual sheath transfer wires into position so that the sheaths fit over the shaft of the transfer wire held within the alginate impression material. It will now be seen that both of the latter two transfer wires will have their wiggled portions within the plaster crowns of the first molar teeth on the work casts. No bands will be used for the work casts, yet the relationship of the lingual sheaths and buccal tubes will have been established exactly as it was within the mouth.

3) FORMING THE ARCHWIRE

Steps in procedure

(1) File the end of a length of 14-guage half-round shafting square with the long axis and groove this squared end with a separation disk or file to a contour that will fit the round archwire to which it will be soldered. This permits more surface contact between shaft and archwire and hence a firmer soldered joint.

(2) Always attach one half-round shaft before attempting to bend the lingual archwire. Mark the desired point of attachment on a length of archwire, leaving a sufficient amount extending distally for attachment of the lock-

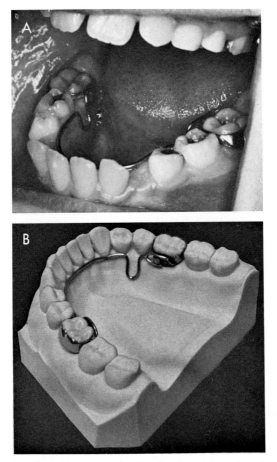

Fig. XVII-25.—The loop lingual archwire. **A,** a loop lingual archwire being used in a space supervision case. Note the relationship of the archwire to the gingival margin. **B,** a loop lingual archwire in place on a cast.

       wire. If control over the second molar is desired, a bit longer distal extension is necessary.

(3) Apply a very small amount of solder to the spot marked on the archwire. Since the shafting is precision drawn to fit the sheath, any excess solder will make it impossible to seat the shafting. Solder the shafting to the archwire. It is easier to buy the half-round shafting in 6-in. lengths that are segmented. After the solder joint is made, break the long length of shafting at the closest segment and trim the fractured end.

(4) Remove and polish excess solder from the shafting. If a neat fit cannot be obtained quickly, it is best to remove the shafting and solder a new one into place.

(5) When the shaft has been seated correctly into the sheath, make certain

that it does not extend through the gingival end of the tube. If it does, it will impinge on soft tissue and the lockwire cannot stabilize the archwire.

(6) Now remove the archwire and place the two "step" bends just mesial to the first molar (see Fig. XVII-23). These allow the archwire to maintain a level plane and lie stable. Shape the archwire to the general contour of the dental arch. The wire should lie just at the gingival margin and should be in a horizontal plane from the mesial portion of one first molar around the arch to the corresponding molar on the opposite side. The wire should be adapted to touch lightly all teeth except those badly malposed. It is not necessary to festoon the archwire elaborately to fit into all the embrasures. An upper lingual archwire must be adapted to prevent its being struck by the mandibular incisors. When the archwire is adapted around the arch to the first molar, another pair of "step" bends is placed to bring the wire back up to a height that will permit placement of the second half-round shaft. A vertical loop may be formed on each side just anterior to the first molar. Such a loop allows more flexibility in using the archwire (Fig. XVII-25). The archwire thus formed is called a loop lingual archwire.

(7) Suitable locks are attached (see Fig. XVII-18, C).

(8) After the archwire is formed and before the addition of auxiliary springs, it should be freed of all torque induced by the bending and soldering carried out thus far. This process is known as "killing" or "passivating" the wire.

Precious.—The archwire is seated on the working model with the lockwires adjusted to hold the half-round shafts in position. Hold the anterior portion of the wire snugly against the teeth with the butt end of a pair of soldering pliers or an old instrument and gently play a soft brush flame from the blowpipe over the appliance. This will remove the stresses and strains induced by working the wire, but care must be taken to avoid overheating the alloy. Always keep the temperature of the wire well below a red heat or the metal will lose its working properties.

Stainless steel.—The procedure is similar for steel, but greater care must be taken because the temper cannot be restored to steel once it is removed by overheating. Do not allow the wire to approach a red color. When a dull brownish appearance is noted and the metal emits a creaking sound, the correct temperature has been reached and must not be exceeded. Steel lingual archwires may be "passivated" very easily by attaching electric soldering electrodes to the archwire and building up heat within the wire as current is passed through it.

c) Modifications

1) **PRIMARY DENTITION.**—Lingual archwires may be attached to bands, overlays or primary crown forms on the primary molars with half-round shafts and sheaths as already described; however, the occlusogingival height sometimes is inadequate for vertical half-round shafts. The Porter lingual archwire is very useful in the primary dentition (see subsection 5 later in this section).

2) **ELLIS LOOP LINGUAL ARCHWIRE.**—The Ellis loop lingual archwire is designed to obviate the need to solder half-round shafts to the wire. By means of special loop-forming pliers, the archwire itself is bent to

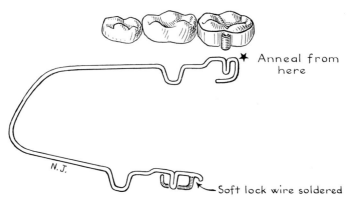

Fig. XVII-26.—Ellis loop lingual archwire. It does not require soldering of a half-round shaft. The shaft is made from the body of the wire with special pliers. Sheaths of special size for the molar band are obtainable also. Note the two different methods of locking. See also Figure XVII-19.

form a lug that is inserted into a special sheath on the molar band (Fig. XVII-26). Ellis attachments are available in both steel and precious alloys. It also is possible to buy the Ellis lingual archwires already formed in a variety of lengths.

Steps in technic

(1) With special pliers form a loop post in a .036-in. archwire.
(2) Fashion the anterior portion of the appliance as described for the regular lingual archwire. A U-bend placed vertically in the wire in the bicuspid region facilitates anteroposterior adjustments of the archwire and makes the adaptation of the second loop post much easier.
(3) When forming the second post, make the first bend 2–3 mm. distal to the position finally desired, since such an amount is used in forming the post.
(4) Two types of locks are shown in Figure XVII-26.
(5) The archwire may be "passivated" in the regular manner.

3) ROUND POST LINGUAL ARCHWIRE.—The lingual archwire may be bent to form the vertical post itself (Fig. XVII-27). This round post modification is useful when it is desired to rotate the molar to which the archwire is attached; for example, maxillary molars that drift mesially usually rotate lingually, and it may be advantageous to undo the process.

4) HORIZONTAL LINGUAL TUBE.—The lingual archwire may be constructed with one or two horizontal lingual tubes. Figure XVII-27 shows the use of a closed-end horizontal tube, a useful modification if the banded molar is to be tipped buccally, for example, to correct a crossbite. It is possible also to purchase a lingual molar attachment that accepts the archwire doubled on itself in the horizontal plane.

5) PORTER LINGUAL ARCHWIRE.—Another useful modification of the

lingual archwire is the Porter appliance (Fig. XVII-28). It is of use for correction of crossbites and in cleft palate cases. It utilizes true reciprocal anchorage and allows for precise differential tipping of the teeth buccally. It is easier to move different teeth different amounts with this appliance than with any other lingual archwire. It is one of the most useful of all appliances for therapy in the primary and mixed dentition. Note that it can be adjusted at the midline curve or at either curve as the wire comes forward to the half-round shaft. It is thus possible to move the buccal segment laterally in a parallel fashion. The first few times this wire is adjusted it is useful to trace its outline on a sheet of paper, make the adjustments thought necessary and retrace in order to see if they have been placed correctly.

6) LOOP LINGUAL ARCHWIRE.—This is a modification of the regular lingual archwire; however, it is so useful and important as to deserve special mention. It is shown in Figures XVII-25 and XVII-26. It may be made of round wire, preferably .032–.036 in. in diameter. The vertical loops may be adjusted to rotate molars, to upright molars and even to

Fig. XVII-27.—Variations in the lingual archwire. **A,** round post lingual archwire. **B,** horizontal tube lingual archwire. When the horizontal tube is used, its distal end usually is closed. **C,** position of the horizontal lingual tube. The archwire is doubled on itself and shaped with special pliers. The archwire remains in place within the tube by friction. **D,** an example of a maxillary lingual archwire using horizontal lingual tubes. (**C** and **D** courtesy of Dr. James McNamara.)

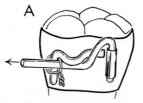
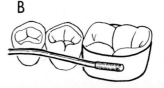
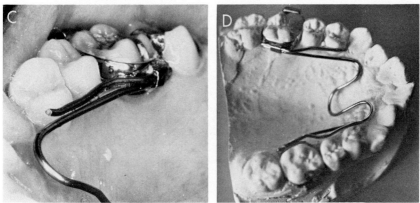

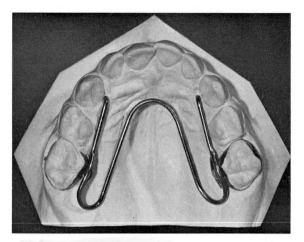

Fig. XVII-28.—The Porter lingual archwire. In this instance, the appliance was made for the correction of a functional crossbite in the primary dentition, one of the most frequent uses for the Porter appliance. This appliance utilizes true reciprocal anchorage. However, it can be adjusted to move the teeth on one side alone or to rotate molars.

move them distally a small amount. However, its best use comes when the buccal teeth are to be uprighted or tipped a bit buccally. As this movement ordinarily is done, the archwire moves buccally on an arc with its center of rotation at the midline-to-cuspid region; thus, the first molar moves a bit mesially as it goes buccally. By opening the loop slightly, the molars may go buccally without shortening the arch length.

d) Attachments

1) AUXILIARY SPRINGS.—These may be either precious alloy or stainless steel.

Steps in procedure

(1) The attachment of the auxiliary spring is made in an embrasure (Fig. XVII-29).
(2) Mark the archwire where the spring is to be and apply flux and a small amount of solder. With round-nosed pliers, shape the end of a length of .020–.024-in. spring wire in the form of a small shepherd's crook. If the spring is steel, add flux and a small amount of solder to this crook.
(3) Protect the spring wire with the archwire as they are brought into the flame. Solder the two wires together at right angles by slipping the crook over the archwire just as the solder melts.
(4) Smooth and polish the solder joint.
(5) Wrap the spring around the archwire two or three times in a direction such that the action of the spring against the teeth is one of uncoiling

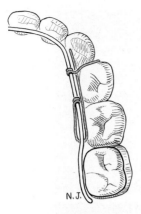

Fig. XVII-29.—Correct positioning of auxiliary springs.

(see Fig. XVII-29). The free end of the wrapped spring should lie closely to the linguo-inferior surface of the archwire. The spring is wrapped to protect that portion of the wire softened by the soldering. Having the spring wrapped around the wire also prevents its being swallowed should it become unsoldered.

(6) If the spring is to be spot-welded, similar precautions are taken.

2) LINGUAL LOCKS.—*Soft wire lock.*—The lockwire is of dead soft steel or precious alloy .024–.028 in. in diameter. The malleability of the lock-wire alloys permits repeated insertions and lockings without breaking. The usual place of attachment on the lingual archwire is 3–5 mm. distal to the half-round shafting. When the archwire is in place, the lockwire bends down and mesially to pass tightly beneath the gingival lumen of the half-round sheath. It may be bent sharply occlusally just at the mesial side of the sheath and terminated (see Fig. XVII-18, *C*). Leaving the free end mesially permits easier unlocking, although the position may be reversed if desired.

Tie lock.—The tie lock (see Fig. XVII-18, *C*) is used when patient cooperation is lacking.

2. FIXED SPACE-MAINTAINERS

Fixed space-maintainers may be made of cast overlays, preformed steel crown forms or bands with bars or wire projections to maintain space after premature loss of primary teeth. They are indicated when all other teeth can be repaired and the covered teeth will not be lost soon. The advantage of the fixed space-maintainers is their permanence; they are not easily lost or broken. Their disadvantages lie in difficulty of construction and their lack of adaptability to growth changes in the mouth. Sometimes two "simple" space-maintainers may be more diffi-cult to make and less satisfactory than one lingual archwire. Do not disregard the entire mouth and the developing occlusion simply be-cause one tooth is missing.

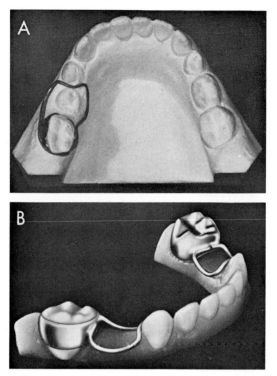

Fig. XVII-30.—A, band and loop space-maintainer. **B,** band and loop space-maintainer and a space-maintainer used with a primary crown form. (Courtesy of Rocky Mountain Metal Products Company.)

Fig. XVII-31.—A, a palate-splitting device in place in the arch. **B,** a radiograph of the same case after the palate has been split. Note the opening of the mid-palatal suture and the supernumerary teeth. This is the same case shown in Figure XV-36.

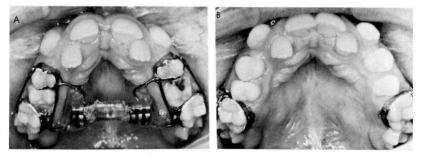

The fixed space-maintainer may attach to one or more primary crown forms or bands. A variety of ingenious space-maintainers have been suggested (Fig. XVII-30). Several types are available in prefabricated form.

3. PALATE-SPLITTING DEVICES

Rapid separation of the midpalatal suture in cases of maxillary insufficiency is obtained by means of screw devices soldered to bicuspid and molar bands (Fig. XVII-31, *A*). The suture is opened rather quickly (about 2–3 weeks) and the space created at the midline rapidly fills with bone (Fig. XVII-31, *B*).

4. SIMPLE LABIAL ARCHWIRES

a) *Light Round Labial Archwire*

1) DESCRIPTION.—The light round labial archwire usually is of steel with a diameter ranging from .012 to .022 in. The appliance, then, consists of molar bands with buccal tubes and a series of bands with brackets into which the light round labial archwire is ligated, the purpose of the archwire being to serve as a means of force application directly to the malposed teeth. Any of several brackets may be used, although the edgewise is the most versatile and hence the most popular (see Section B-4-e, Attachments for Anterior Bands, p. 650).

2) INDICATIONS.—This is a most satisfactory appliance for alignment and rotation of anterior teeth, since the teeth are brought into position by fitting the wire snugly into the brackets. It is an excellent appliance for alignment of the crowns of teeth, but difficulty usually is encountered in attempting alignment of the roots. Skillful use of rather complicated auxiliary attachments is required for en masse and bodily movements of teeth with this appliance. Fortunately, some malocclusions can be treated satisfactorily with just tipping movements. Every dentist must be able to align teeth for simple orthodontic procedures and to aid in restorative and prosthetic procedures. This appliance is most useful and versatile for many routine orthodontic tasks.

The appliance is constructed directly in the mouth after molar bands and the desired anterior and other bands have been made and cemented into position.

Construction

(1) Any size of round stainless steel wire may be used that will fit into the bracket slot. Sometimes a smaller wire is used to begin, followed by a slightly heavier wire. The standard edgewise brackets will receive wires up to .022 in. in diameter.

(2) One satisfactory method is to use .020-in. wire doubled on itself to fit snugly

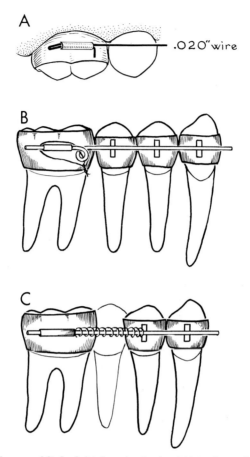

Fig. XVII-32.—A, use of light labial archwire in .040-in. buccal tube. **B,** method of tying back the archwire. **C,** use of compressed coil spring for opening space in the arch.

into .040-in. buccal tubes (Fig. XVII-32). The wire is shaped in an ideal fashion and inserted in the opposite buccal tube in a similar fashion. The free ends projecting mesially may be bent down to serve as stops determining the length of the archwire. The doubled end projecting distally may be bent a bit to serve as a friction retainer for the archwire within the buccal tube. Another method is to bend a complete running eyelet in the archwire a short distance ahead of the buccal tube. A ligature holds the archwire in position (Fig. XVII-32).

3) ATTACHMENTS AND AUXILIARIES.—Coil springs frequently are threaded onto the archwire to move the teeth into position (see Fig. XVII-32). The coil spring should be wound on an arbor of the same size as the archwire and should be wound from wire of no greater diameter

than .008 in. The novice is likely to utilize far too much force when using coil springs. It is wise to use coil springs of very small diameter wire (about .006 in.) and to compress the spring no more than one-fourth its relaxed length.

b) High Labial Archwire

1) DESCRIPTION.—The high labial archwire consists of a .040-in. round steel wire that is conventionally positioned in the posterior region but rises and lies above the necks of the anterior teeth (Fig. XVII-33) to utilize the muscular activity of the upper lip. Its principal disadvantage is the difficulty encountered in controlling individual teeth. Considerable skill is required, for example, to rotate anterior teeth with this appliance. Auxiliary springs are dropped from the main archwire to achieve individual tooth movements, but simple tipping is the only movement done with ease.

2) INDICATIONS.—Although this appliance is not as popular as it once was, a few still use it. I like to use it with extra-oral anchorage in the treatment of early Class II problems (Fig. XVII-33). It has the distinct advantage of continual force application to the molars. During the night, the headgear is attached, and during the day the archwire remains in the mouth so that the lips may act against it intermittently during function.

Fig. XVII-33.—**A,** high labial archwire. **B** and **C,** use of headgear with high labial archwire. **B,** intra-oral attachment. **C,** headgear and extra-oral attachment.

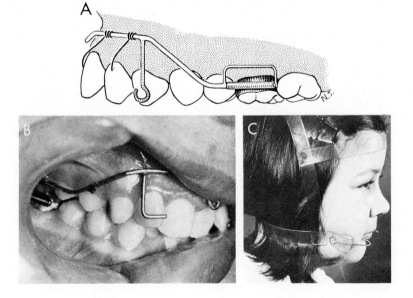

Construction

(1) Place a layer of adhesive tape on the work cast to cover all of the vestibular region from molar around to molar to provide a bit of space between the mucosa and the wire.

(2) The buccal tube alignment is the same as for the regular labial archwire, but it is most important to have a precision fit of the high labial archwire in the buccal tubes. Any play between wire and tube is magnified greatly in the anterior region and may cause irritation of the mucosa. It is almost impossible to use this appliance with success if it is not made with care and precision.

(3) Place a suitable stop (see Fig. XVII-18, C) on one end of a length of .040-in. steel wire and insert the wire in one of the buccal tubes on the work cast.

(4) With a grease pencil, mark the archwire in the region of the mesial surface of the second primary molar or second bicuspid. The archwire is now bent gingivally at this mark at an angle that will cause the wire to lie 5 mm. above the gingival margin at the cuspid-first bicuspid embrasure (see Fig. XVII-33). The high labial archwire should never touch the gingival tissues but should lie approximately 1 mm. away from them. As the alveolar bone curves to form the arch, so should the high labial archwire be curved.

(5) Mark the wire directly above the cuspid-first bicuspid embrasure and bend the wire to a horizontal plane. The wire should now lie 3–5 mm. above the gingival border of the incisors and be parallel to the buccal tubes.

(6) Between the cuspids, the height of the wire is constant except for a V-shaped notch bent into the wire to accommodate the labial frenum. It is extremely important to bend this notch with care so that the frenum is not irritated by the wire. The archwire between the cuspids lies 1 mm. away from the mucosa overlying the roots of the teeth and follows the general curvature of the alveolar arch. No attempt is made to shape the archwire to follow the convolutions in the alveolar process caused by any extreme labial positioning of the incisor roots.

(7) The process is reversed on the opposite side until the wire is bent down to insert into the buccal tube and is ready for the second stop. Before adding any auxiliary springs, make certain that the archwire lies passively in the buccal tubes and is equidistant from the soft tissues throughout.

(8) Hooks for the attachment of extra-oral anchorage (see Fig. XVII-33) are soldered to the wire in the cuspid region. Such hooks are best made of .030-in. stainless steel wire.

(9) Auxiliary finger springs for the movement of incisors or erupting cuspids may be added. They should be made from 0.14-in. or 0.16-in. stainless steel wire. The solder joint should be placed between the roots of the teeth to minimize the possibility of mucosal irritation. Each spring should be wrapped at least twice around the main archwire to protect the solder joint. The spring should be wrapped in a direction that will cause the spring to push the tooth lingually as unwinding occurs.

3) ATTACHMENTS, AUXILIARIES, MODIFICATIONS.—Attachments for use with elastic traction are shown in Figure XVII-33, as are the usual finger springs. This appliance is not recommended when alignment of maxillary incisors is a major problem.

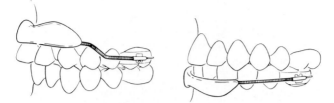

Fig. XVII-34.—Lip-plumping devices. (Courtesy of Rocky Mountain Metal Products Company.)

The high labial archwire may be used advantageously as a sectional archwire attached to an acrylic appliance (see Fig. XVII-49). The acrylic is cut away from the lingual surfaces of the incisors as they are moved lingually. It is best to maintain the position of such an appliance in the manner shown, with long spring arms that slip into place over buccal tubes on molar bands or with Adams clasps.

c) Lip-Plumpers

Lip-plumpers are heavy labial archwires inserted in buccal tubes of the molars and having a flange of acrylic added anteriorly to engage the lip (Fig. XVII-34). They are used to aid in correction of abnormal lip function, to help maintain the arch perimeter and even to move the molars distally a bit. They may be made or obtained prefabricated.

5. EDGEWISE MECHANISM

a) Description

The edgewise mechanism was the last and most advanced of the several appliances invented by Dr. Edward H. Angle. It is a multibanded precision appliance consisting of a rectangular labial archwire fitted and ligated into horizontal slots in brackets (Fig. XVII-35) on all the permanent teeth anterior to the second molars. The archwire terminates in rectangular tubes on the second molar bands. The archwire may be of stainless steel or precious alloy and originally was .022 × .028 in. The narrow (.022 in.) dimension lies against the labial and buccal surfaces of the teeth, hence the name. The appliance also may be made up of wires .022 × .025 in. or .022 × .022 in. Control in all directions is possible, and any individual tooth may be moved simultaneously in three directions; for example, an incisor may be moved lingually, distally and rotated around its long axis with one adjustment of the wire. Although the edgewise appliance does afford excellent and precise control of teeth, it is difficult to manipulate within the desired range of light forces. In recent years, the edgewise wire has been reduced by some to .018 in. in its narrow dimension.

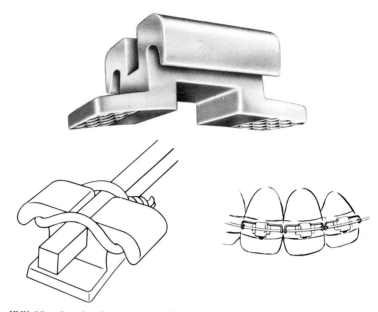

Fig. XVII-35.—One kind of edgewise bracket showing the method of ligation and the use of adjunct springs. (Courtesy of Rocky Mountain Metal Products Company.)

Fig. XVII-36.—An arch banded up with edgewise appliances, showing the use of rotating and aligning auxiliaries. (Courtesy of Rocky Mountain Metal Products Company.)

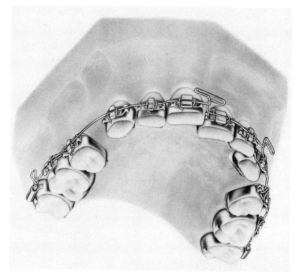

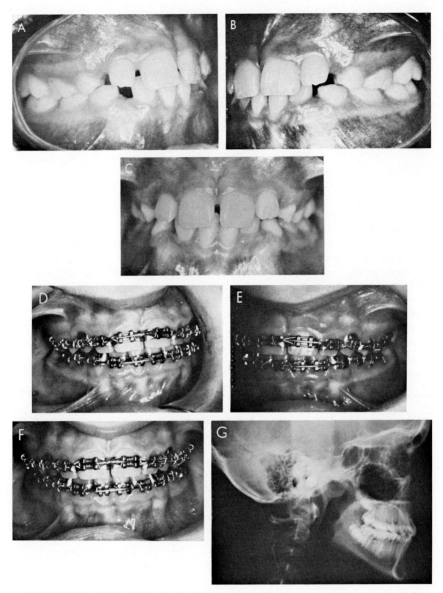

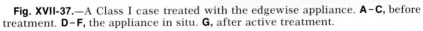

Fig. XVII-37.—A Class I case treated with the edgewise appliance. **A–C,** before treatment. **D–F,** the appliance in situ. **G,** after active treatment.

The edgewise bracket is useful, since it will accept any shape of wire up to .022 in. in diameter. Its versatility accounts for the many variations on the edgewise theme. A series of progressively larger light round wires are used initially to align, rotate and tip the teeth and to level the occlusal plane. This permits the greatest movements with light forces yet allows the precise finishing afforded by the mechanics of the rectangular wire. Many kinds of loops are incorporated into the wire to effect individual tooth movements, and the appliance is used in many, many ways. The modern edgewise mechanism is quite different from Angle's original appliance, for it has incorporated many ideas from other multibanded systems. Figure XVII-36 illustrates some of these edgewise appliances.

An important role in edgewise therapy is the concept of the ideal arch, which includes the idea that each tooth has an ideal position and angulation within an ideally shaped arch in order to achieve an ideal occlusal relationship with teeth of the opposing arch. Such a concept demands meticulously precise control of each tooth. Figure XVII-37 illustrates a case treated with the edgewise appliance.

The edgewise appliance is not particularly well suited for use during the mixed dentition and is difficult to use in the primary dentition. It finds its greatest application in the treatment of comprehensive malocclusions of the permanent dentition. The edgewise mechanism is one of the most difficult appliances to master, yet it is among the most popular in the United States because of its versatility in the permanent dentition. A description of its use is beyond the scope of this book; for detailed descriptions of its construction and manipulation consult the publications listed in the Suggested Readings at the end of this chapter.

b) Repair and Emergency Adjustments

If it is necessary to remove an appliance, do not cut the appliance itself but cut each ligature at the individual brackets (see Fig. XVII-35). Bands are recemented easily, but care must be taken to ensure the correct height of the bracket. Replace the band so that the bracket slots are the same height or extrusion will result. Before replacing the archwire, be certain that it has not been deformed. If you cannot repair and replace the archwire properly, remove it completely from the mouth and send it to the orthodontist in charge of the case.

6. LIGHT-WIRE APPLIANCES

a) Description

The so-called light-wire appliances were first designed and presented to the profession by P. R. Begg, an Australian orthodontist who introduced the idea of differential force control. Since some types of tooth movements evoke more tissue resistance than others, and some movements occur faster than others, Begg reasoned that by selectively choos-

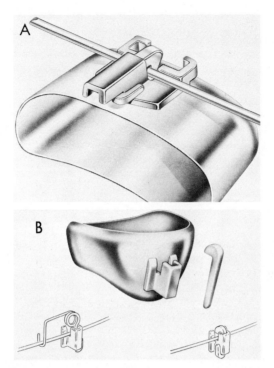

Fig. XVII-38.—A, some examples of modern light-wire brackets. **B,** the use of pins and root-aligning springs. (Courtesy of Rocky Mountain Metal Products Company.)

ing the movements required and relating the reciprocal reactions properly, all tooth movements might be carried out simultaneously. This could be done only if each movement were carried out within its ideal force range and as many movements as possible were mutually reciprocal and beneficial. Such ideas necessitated many changes in bracket and archwire design. The light-wire appliances are now several and varied from the original design, although all employ sophisticated concepts and theories of tooth movement and anchorage control. Standard light-wire therapy does not utilize extra-oral traction, frequently involves extraction of teeth and uses fewer auxiliaries than conventional edgewise therapy. Figure XVII-38 illustrates typical light-wire brackets and Figure XVII-39 illustrates a case treated by the light-wire method.

b) Repair and Emergency Adjustments

The labial arch is held in place by pins that must be cut for its removal. After the wire is removed, the patient should be advised to return

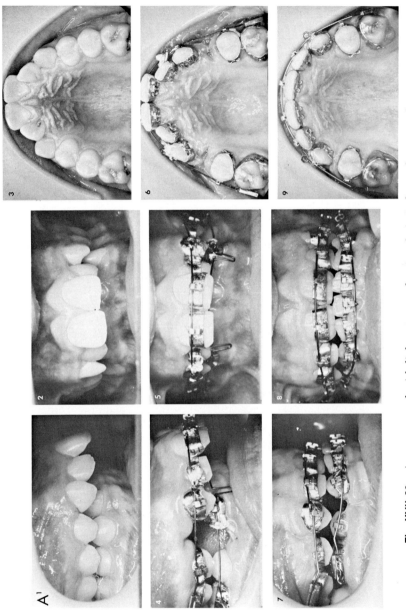

Fig. XVII-39.—A case treated with light-wire mechanics. **A,** **1–3,** the occlusion at the start of treatment; **4–6,** first-stage mechanics; **7–9,** second-stage mechanics. (*Continued.*)

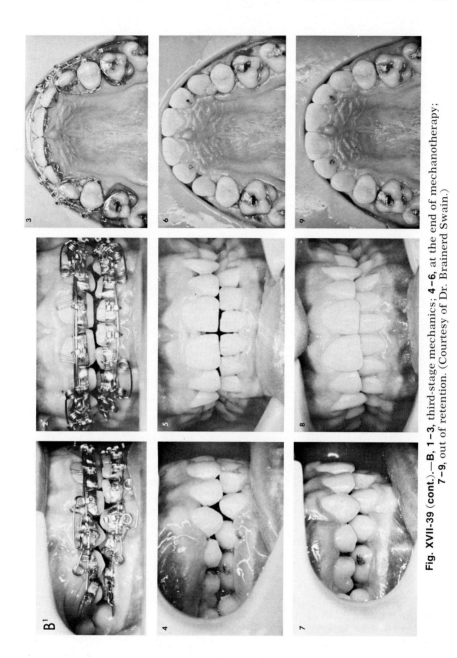

Fig. XVII-39 (cont.).—B, 1–3, third-stage mechanics; **4–6,** at the end of mechanotherapy; **7–9,** out of retention. (Courtesy of Dr. Brainerd Swain.)

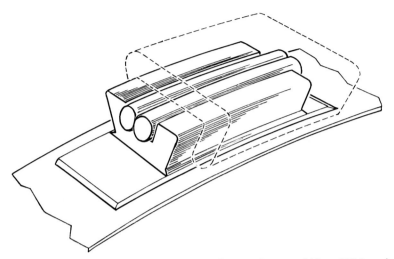

Fig. XVII-40.—Twin-wire bracket, machined to receive two .010 or .011 in. wires, held in place by a cap that slides over the bracket.

to the dentist treating the case as soon as possible. It is difficult—and often disadvantageous—to make temporizing adjustments to the appliance.

7. Twin-Wire Appliance

a) Description

The twin-wire appliance was invented by Dr. Joseph Johnson in an effort to design a mechanism that would offer precise control with light forces and minimal adjustments. It consists of a pair of stainless steel wires .010 or .011 in. in diameter fitted into stainless steel end tubes .022 in. inside diameter, .036 in. outside diameter and 1⅛ in. long. The end tubes fit into buccal tubes on the first molars. The twin wires in the anterior section fit precisely into a lock type of bracket consisting of two parts. One, welded to the band, has a precisely formed channel into which the wires fit. The other part is a covering cap that slides over the channel and is held in position by friction (Fig. XVII-40). Intermaxillary hooks are placed on the mesial end of the end tubes. The appliance is used with a lingual archwire when attempting buccal movements of teeth in the lateral segments or when extra anchorage is needed for intermaxillary traction. If control of the bicuspids is required, the end tubes may be shortened, although this makes the use of intermaxillary elastics difficult. Often a flat wire .011 × .022 in. is substituted for the twin wires. This appliance may be used with other types of brackets, for example, the edgewise (see Fig. XVII-35).

The twin-wire appliance has been popular in the United States because of its light, delicate action. Some difficulty is experienced, at least in my hands, in effecting bodily movement of teeth with this appliance. It is excellent for rotating and aligning anterior teeth. The twin-wire appliance has had a salutary effect on orthodontics, since it has shown how much can be done with light forces, with the result that the edgewise appliance is used far differently than when it was first introduced. The twin-wire appliance finds its greatest use in the late mixed and early permanent dentitions. Although it often is said to be an "automatic" appliance, it would seem to require almost as much adjustment as any other appliance if quality results are to be obtained. Furthermore, it is deceptively simple in appearance. The twin-wire appliance does not seem to be as popular today as it once was, perhaps because its primary advantages have been incorporated into the edgewise and light-wire systems. With both the edgewise and light-wire methods, it is easier to effect bodily tooth movements. A complete description of the construction and uses of the twin-wire appliance is beyond the scope of this book; however, a list of Suggested Readings is available at the end of this chapter.

Fig. XVII-41.—The twin arch bracket and sliding cap and a typical twin arch band-up. Note the end tubes, which fit into buccal tubes on the molars. From the end tubes the two small twin wires extrude to attach to the anteriors, which are banded. (Courtesy of Rocky Mountain Metal Products Company.)

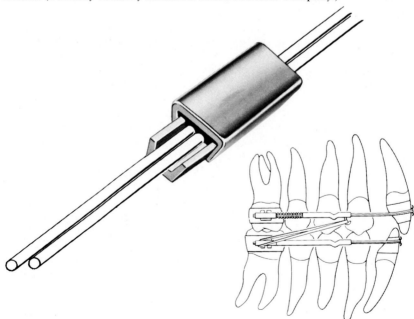

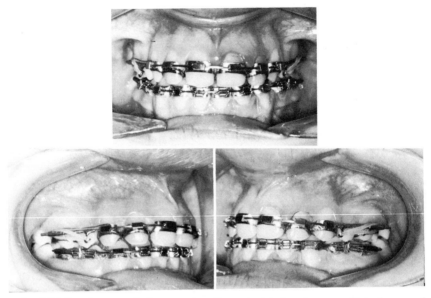

Fig. XVII-42.—Intra-oral photographs of a typical twin-wire case. Note the use of channel brackets in the upper arch but tie brackets on the lower incisors. (Courtesy of Dr. Faustin Weber.)

b) Repair and Emergency Adjustments

The most frequent repair problem with the twin-wire appliance is a lost cap lock. If none is available, a .010-in. ligature wire may be placed around the twin wires and threaded through a hole that is pierced in the bed of the bracket channel. A new band may be made using a different bracket, since the twin wires will fit well into any bracket with a .022-in. horizontal slot. If it is necessary to recement a band, remove the cap by sliding it sideways, recement the band and slide the cap back into place after the cement has set. If the appliance cannot be repaired properly, send all parts to the dentist treating the patient. Figure XVII-41 illustrates the appliance, Figure XVII-42 shows intra-oral photographs and Figure XVII-43 depicts a case treated in the typical way.

8. UNIVERSAL APPLIANCE

a) Description

The universal appliance is the design of Dr. Spencer Atkinson. It is a multibanded precision appliance consisting of one flat, .012 × .028 in., and one round, .014 in., wire used in combination (Fig. XVII-44). The flat wire is placed incisally. At different stages of treatment, various

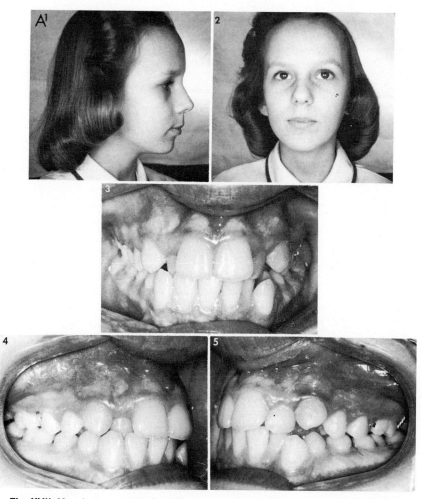

Fig. XVII-43.—A case treated with a twin-wire appliance. **A,** before treatment. (*Continued.*)

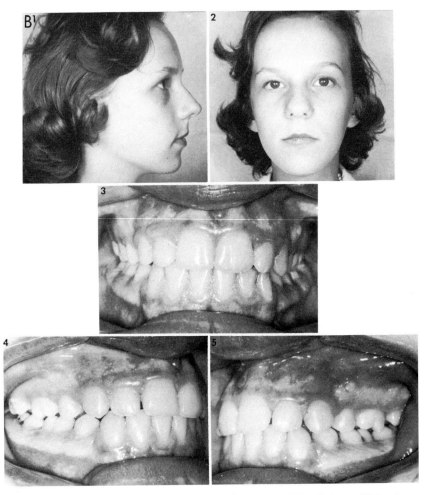

Fig. XVII-43 (cont.).—B, after treatment. (Courtesy of Dr. Faustin Weber.)

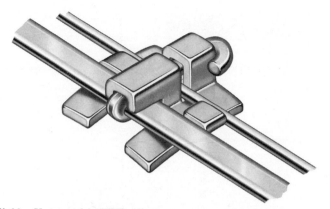

Fig. XVII-44.—Universal bracket. The two wires are held in place by lock pins. (Courtesy of Unitek Corporation.)

combinations of round and flat wires may be used, according to the type of movement desired. The wires are held in place by a small locking pin. Because of the many adjuncts used and the possible combinations of archwires, the appliance is very versatile. Its greatest advantage would seem to be its value in comprehensive malocclusions of the permanent dentition. Figure XVII-45 shows the steps in treatment of a case with the universal appliance. A complete description of the appliance and its method of use is not possible in a book of this type, but a list of Suggested Readings is placed at the end of this chapter.

b) Repair and Emergency Adjustments

The same general rules apply for the universal as for the edgewise and twin-wire appliances except that a locking pin is used instead of caps or ligatures. In the absence of such a pin, however, a ligature may be substituted.

9. THE LABIOLINGUAL APPLIANCE

DESCRIPTION.—The labiolingual appliance evolved from Mershon's lingual archwire and the heavy labial archwire. Although many men contributed to the refinement of the appliance, Dr. Oren Oliver probably did more to develop it than anyone else. The appliance consists of maxillary and mandibular labial and lingual archwires attached to molar bands. Auxiliary springs are primarily responsible for most tooth movements. A guideplane attached to the maxillary lingual archwire often is used in Class II treatment. Only occasionally are anterior teeth banded.

The appliance is very useful in the mixed dentition to preserve the arch perimeter and guide the erupting permanent teeth. It is less effi-

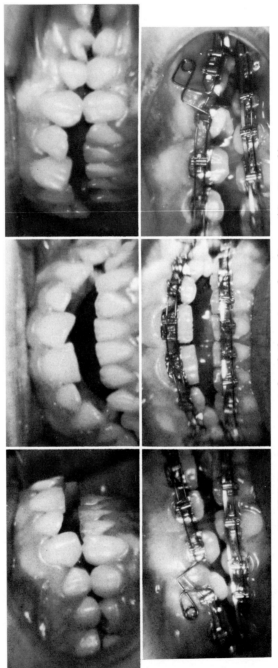

Fig. XVII-45.—A case treated with the universal appliance. (*Continued.*)

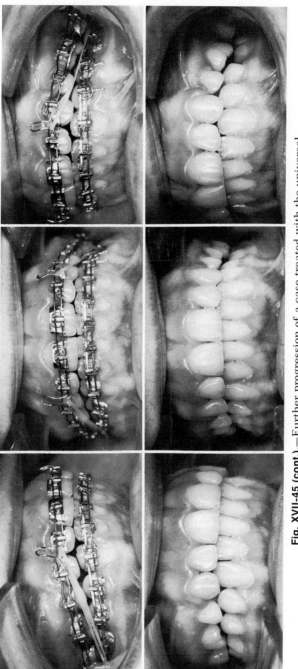

Fig. XVII-45 (cont.).—Further progression of a case treated with the universal appliance. (Courtesy of Dr. Jorge Fastlicht.)

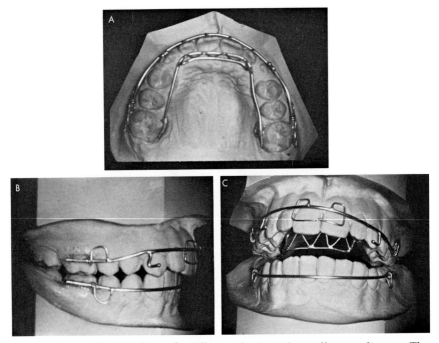

Fig. XVII-46.—The labiolingual appliance. **A,** view of maxillary appliances. The lingual arch should be constructed to be, as nearly as is possible, in one plane contacting the lingual surfaces of the incisors as near the cingulum as is possible. The labial also lies in one plane forming an ideal arch form in the incisor and cuspid regions, although it usually is not in contact with the bicuspids. Auxiliary springs may be added to either arch for individual tooth movements. **B,** side view of labial appliances. Note the relationship of the buccal tubes to the molars and the placement of auxiliary springs to align the incisors. **C,** front view. This view shows the guide plane, which also is seen in **A.** The guide plane is used in Class II, Division 1 treatment to reposition the mandible forward and to eliminate the intercuspation of the teeth. The forward positioning removes the deleterious action of the lower lip behind the upper incisors and makes possible flattening of the occlusal curve. Intermaxillary elastics (see Fig. XVII-47, **B**) aid in the distal movement of the maxillary molars.

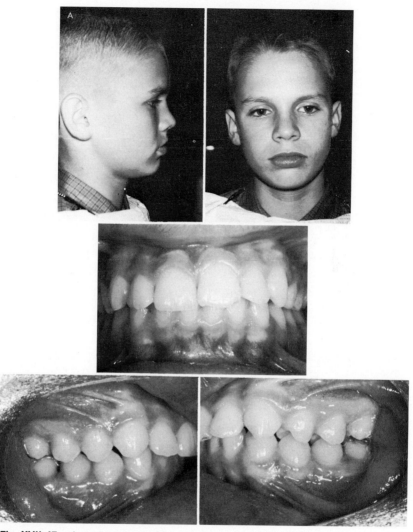

Fig. XVII-47.—A patient treated by means of a labiolingual appliance. **A,** views before treatment. (*Continued.*)

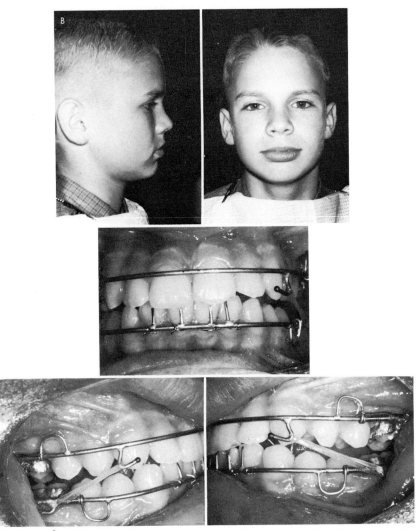

Fig. XVII-47 (cont.).—B, views immediately after placement of the occlusal guide plane and labial and lingual appliances. (*Continued.*)

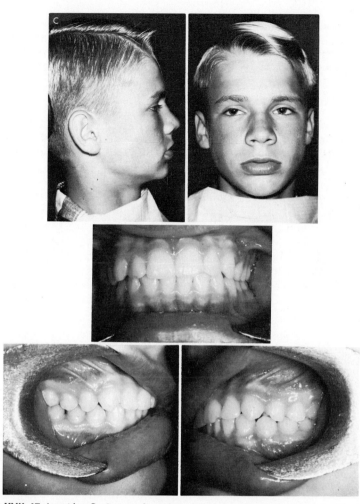

Fig. XVII-47 (cont.).—C, 6 months after removal of all appliances. The labio-lingual appliance often is used in conjunction with a bonded appliance, for example, the twin-wire appliance. However, this case was chosen because only the labiolingual appliance itself was used in the treatment. (Courtesy of Dr. William J. Oliver.)

cient when bodily movements of teeth or orthopedic effects on the craniofacial skeleton are required. As a complete system, it is much less popular than it once was, although parts of the labiolingual appliance are used by all orthodontists. Figure XVII-46 illustrates the appliance and Figure XVII-47 shows a case treated by this method.

D. Attached Removable Appliances

A removable appliance is one designed to be taken from the mouth by the patient. Removable appliances may be divided into two major classes—attached and loose. The rationale for the use of each class is different; therefore, they are discussed separately.

There are a number of different types of attached removable appliances with a variety of uses, such as moving teeth, guiding or directing growth and serving as retainers. Misunderstanding them arises largely from misuse, and they probably are overextended in usage by the inexperienced more than any other type of appliance. Only the Crozat appliance is considered a "system" of orthodontic therapy and it has several severe limitations for use by the average general practitioner. Attached removable appliances are useful as adjuncts or when assigned to specific limited roles. They have the following advantages over banded appliances:

> Good oral hygiene.
> Good appearance.
> More work is done by the laboratory.
> Adjustments can be made in less time.

They also have serious disadvantages:

> Most cannot effect precise tooth movements (some cannot effect any precisely).
> Patient cooperation often is a problem.
> They are deceptively simple in appearance.
> They often are more time-consuming than a simple banded appliance.
> They are very easy to misuse.

Generally, attached removable appliances should be used where they can do a more efficient job without compromising quality or stability of result. One should not think of them as alternatives to banded therapy, as so many do; each has its own place in the armamentarium of the modern dentist.

1. Hawley Retainer

The Hawley retainer is a removable plastic appliance used to retain new positions of teeth after active orthodontic therapy is completed (Fig. XVII-48). The name "Hawley appliance" often is misapplied to

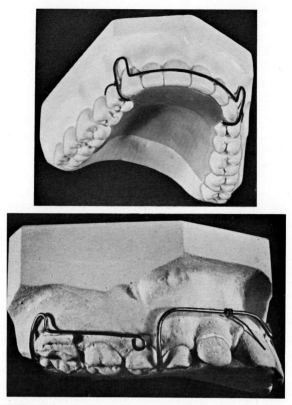

Fig. XVII-48 (top).—Maxillary Hawley appliance with flat bite plane.
Fig. XVII-49 (bottom).—High labial anterior section attached to maxillary Hawley appliance with bite plane. Note the long retaining spring lying above the buccal tube on the molar band and extending mesially for ease in removal.

a wide variety of removable appliances. Correctly, it should be used for the retaining appliance only. The maxillary appliance may or may not incorporate a bite plane. A wide variety of labial wires are used, the choice depending on the type of tooth movements that have been carried out. It is retained with molar clasps.

Construction

Ordinarily, the appliance is made of endothermic acrylic resin, although it may be flask-cured when a bite plane is used. The anterior labial section is made of .026-in. stainless steel wire. If a strip of adhesive tape is placed on the cast over the labial and buccal areas where the wire framework is to be constructed, the danger of irritating the soft tissues is minimized.

2. BITE PLANES

a) *Description*

Bite plane appliances are made of acrylic resin and include a shelf against which only certain teeth can occlude (see Fig. XVII-48). In the maxilla, this shelf lies behind the incisors and only the mandibular incisors meet it; all other teeth are kept from occlusion. Bite planes also are constructed to tip or deflect selected teeth out of position. In any bite plane, the mucosa as well as the other teeth supply the anchorage. A bite plane also may incorporate springs for movement of teeth (Figs. XVII-49 and XVII-50).

b) *Indications*

The bite plane is used when it is desired to cause the further eruption of posterior teeth, prevent further eruption of the incisors or deflect selected teeth that are erupting. Bite planes work best during the mixed dentition stage, when there is rapid growth of the alveolar process. They should be used with extreme discretion in adult dentitions, in which growth has ceased and the occlusal relationships have stabilized. There should always be a large freeway space or the musculature will not tolerate the appliance. The bite plane may be indicated (a) to treat excessive overbite in the mixed dentition stage, (b) to remove occlusal interlocking for the correction of crossbites or locked individual teeth, (c) as an aid in locating the ideal occlusal position, (d) for the temporary relief from temporomandibular joint pain when the joint symptoms are due to an eccentric occlusal relationship and (e) to aid in the control of bruxism. Several studies have shown that maxillary bite planes are far more likely to allow the eruption of posterior teeth than they are to intrude mandibular incisors; consequently, they probably are not indicated when the intrusion of incisors is the sole solution to the problem.

Construction

Bite planes may be constructed by the routine flasking method of acrylic curing or by the drip method used for endothermic acrylic resin. It is suggested that although other acrylic appliances may well be made of endothermic resin, it is better to use more conventional procedures for bite planes. Most bite planes incorporate a stainless steel framework for the movement of teeth or as an aid in retention. The detailed construction of each type of bite plane is given below.

c) *Types*

1) MAXILLARY FLAT BITE PLANE.—*Description and uses.*—The maxillary flat bite plane is used to remove tooth interferences and thus can serve as a diagnostic as well as a treatment appliance. Frequently it is

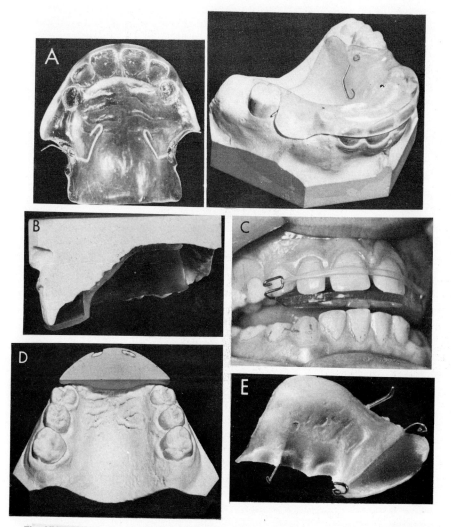

Fig. XVII-50.—A, the Sved plate. **B,** hollow incline maxillary appliance, suggested by Dr. Leonard Sidlow. This cross section shows fit in the mouth. Note the space behind the maxillary incisor. **C,** hollow incline appliance in the mouth. An extremely light elastic is worn on the labial surfaces of the upper incisors. **D,** method of constructing the hollow incline appliance. **E,** completed hollow incline appliance.

inserted as an adjunct in treatment of Class II malocclusions. It also aids in the treatment of excessive overbite during the mixed dentition stage. It may be used in conjunction with a labial section anteriorly to aid in the alignment of the maxillary incisors (see Fig. XVII-48), a high labial arch section may be used (see Fig. XVII-49) or a very light elastic strung around the incisors (see Fig. XVII-50).

Construction

The selected wire framework should be made first and held in position on the work casts during the curing of the acrylic resin. Any of the several retention devices illustrated may be used with the regular labial arch section. When using the high labial section, it is better to construct molar bands and utilize the long wire arms over buccal tubes, as shown in Figure XVII-49, or use Adams clasps. The bite plane should be absolutely flat. When trying the appliance in the mouth, use articulation paper between the mandibular incisors and the bite plane to assure yourself that all the incisors are striking evenly and can slide around easily on the polished flat plane. This appliance is not used to force the mandible to adopt a new position; rather, it is designed to remove tooth interferences so that the ideal position of the mandible may be made more visible.

As the posterior teeth come into occlusion or as the incisors abrade the bite plane, it may be necessary to resurface the bite plane.

2) Sved plate.—*Description.*—The Sved plate is a maxillary bite plane that covers the edges of the maxillary incisors (see Fig. XVII-50, *A*). The incisal covering provides a surprising amount of retention, especially during the late mixed dentition stage, when there are fewer posterior teeth to be clasped.

The Sved plate may be used for any of the purposes previously assigned to bite planes. In addition, it is particularly useful as an adjunct to headgear therapy. The plate may be worn during the day with light spring action against the upper molars and the posterior teeth separated by the plane. The appliance also is useful as a space-regainer.

It is not wise to insert a Sved plate at the time the maxillary cuspids are pressing tightly against the roots of the lateral incisors, since the crowns of the lateral incisors must be free to move away from the cuspids at this time. However, once the cuspids' path of eruption has changed and the crown is lying alongside the root of the lateral incisor, it is safe to insert this appliance.

Construction

It is best to construct the Sved plate by the orthodox flask-curing method, since a strong acrylic is needed. Ordinarily, it is made of clear acrylic resin, although the part on the labial portion of the incisors may be made of tooth color if desired.

3) Sidlow hollow bite plane.—*Description.*—This is a maxillary bite plane with an open space behind the maxillary incisors to facilitate

their retraction (see Fig. XVII-50). The hollow bite plane may be used when there is extreme labioversion of the maxillary anterior teeth either with or without a deep bite. The anchorage for the incisor movement is derived from the plate's contact with the palatal mucosa (see Fig. XVII-50, *B–E*).

Construction

The region just lingual to the incisors is built up on the maxillary work cast with a bit of stone or plaster to the incisal edges and extended backward for about 1 cm. (see Fig. XVII-50). The desired wire framework is now added to the altered work cast before curing the acrylic resin. The acrylic may be cured by either method, although the flasking technic is a bit better. The finished appliance fits the mouth as shown in Figure XVII-50.

The lingual inclined plane against which the maxillary incisors are retracted should slope slightly upward (see Fig. XVII-50). The hollow portion must not be extended too far posteriorly or the palatal anchorage will be lost. Failure to extend it far enough will cause the soft tissue to pile up lingual to the incisors. The incisors retract at a rapid rate with this appliance—so rapidly, in fact, that great care should be taken to use only the lightest of elastic forces. The labial edge of the appliance is ground off as the teeth move lingually up the hollow inclined plane.

4) MANDIBULAR INCLINED PLANE.—*Description.*—The mandibular inclined plane is an extension in plastic of mandibular teeth to engage and direct the eruption of one or more maxillary teeth or tip them into better positions (see Fig. XV-45). The mandibular inclined plane is used primarily to tip labially maxillary incisors that are locked in simple crossbite. It must be used only when there is sufficient space in the line of arch for the tooth in malposition. The mandibular inclined plane may be used posteriorly to deflect erupting posterior teeth out of crossed bite positions.

Construction

There are several ways to construct a mandibular inclined plane appliance.

The best method is to wax up a pattern on a work cast and make the appliance from flask-cured acrylic resin. One also can adapt a bit of self-curing acrylic resin directly to the mandibular incisors. After a few moments, it is removed and allowed to harden before polishing. The bevel on a mandibular inclined plane should be about 45 degrees to the long axis of the tooth and should be kept polished during use in the mouth. No excess plastic should extend onto the gingival mucosa. The anterior mandibular inclined plane should be cemented into place with temporary cement or a stiff mix of zinc oxide and eugenol. Leave it cemented in place no longer than about 2 weeks. If the crossbite has not been corrected in this time, the original diagnosis probably was in error and should be checked. The inclined plane is removed only after cutting the acrylic with a safe-side disk to the incisal edge. An instrument can then be inserted into the cut and twisted to fracture the plastic.

The posterior mandibular inclined plane is not cemented and is constructed and used much as a multiple acrylic space-maintainer (see below).

3. MULTIPLE SPACE-MAINTAINERS

DESCRIPTION AND USES.—Multiple space-maintainers are acrylic appliances covering the lingual mucosa and lingual surfaces of the teeth with plastic extending into the areas where primary teeth have been lost (Fig. XVII-51). They may be made in a wide variety of designs to fit individual needs. The plastic not only holds the space in the line of arch but is built up to engage the teeth of the opposite arch to maintain the plane of occlusion and prevent extrusion of opposing teeth.

Construction

Some have written of this appliance as if it were a partial denture for the primary dentition. However, one must be careful lest the prosthetic concepts of full and partial denture work for aged adults be carried over into the mixed dentition. Here, the primary purposes are to hold space in the line of arch

Fig. XVII-51.—**A,** acrylic multiple space-maintainer. **B,** acrylic space-maintainer with built-in regainer. The first permanent molar has not yet erupted and the first and second primary molars are lost. Sometimes the first molar tends to drift mesially before eruption. In this appliance, the saddle is constructed high enough to touch the occlusion. Often this is enough to keep the permanent molar distally. However, if it has tipped mesially, the saddle may be split and the appliance used as a space-regainer to tip the molar distally.

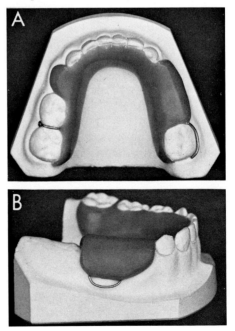

and prevent opposing teeth from extruding. Aesthetic considerations in the posterior region of the mixed dentition are only secondary, simply because the mixed dentition normally is not a complete and aesthetic stage of development. There is no reason to use acrylic teeth in the saddle areas or to take time to carve the saddle itself. A smooth saddle to the proper height will hold the vertical dimension, and opposing erupting teeth can move and slide into position with no danger of being locked by the carved occlusal pattern in the space-maintainer. Similarly, there is no reason to make a cast framework, as is done for the permanent type of partial denture inserted in adult mouths. The mixed dentition is a dynamic changing period, and appliances used with it must be capable of rapid adaptation. Finally, use of simple saddles and simple stainless steel retaining devices reduces markedly the cost of construction.

4. SPACE-REGAINERS

DESCRIPTION.—Space-regainers are appliances for regaining space lost in the line of the dental arch. They are used to tip to upright positions those teeth that have drifted after other teeth have been lost. Space-regainers find their greatest use in the mixed dentition after premature loss of primary molars and in positioning permanent teeth that are to be used as bridge abutments. The space-regainers are not to be used for *creating* space in the line of arch that was never there. Their sole purpose is to tip teeth and thus regain space that has been lost. Read Chapter XV, Section C-1-b for a discussion of the indications for use of these appliances.

Construction

Figure XV-23 shows a space-regainer used in the correction of ectopically erupting maxillary first permanent molars. The appliance shown also is of use for more routine space-regaining problems. It is simple and unusually efficient. A number of examples of space-regainers are shown in Figure XVII-52. Details of their construction and adjustment appear in the legends. In addition to these shown, the loop lingual archwire can be used for space regaining, as can lip-plumpers and extra-oral traction appliances.

5. STABILIZING PLATES

DESCRIPTION.—The stabilizing plate is a removable acrylic lingual appliance attached to molar bands by means of lingual shafts embedded in the plastic (Fig. XVII-53). The precise fit of the shaft within the sheath soldered to the molar band provides more stability than the regular acrylic lingual appliances described here. The stabilizing plate is used to maintain positively the molar position in difficult space management cases. It also provides supplemental anchorage when either intermaxillary or intramaxillary elastic traction is used. Anchorage is provided by all the teeth that it touches as well as the entire lingual mucosal area covered.

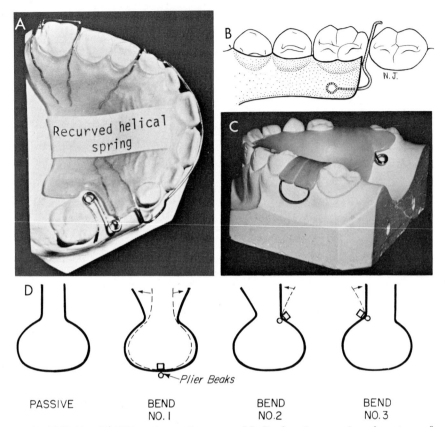

PASSIVE   BEND   BEND   BEND
                   NO. I   NO.2   NO.3

Fig. XVII-52.—Space-regainers. **A,** recurved helical spring regainer (courtesy of Dr. Fred DuPrai). Note the use of the Adams clasp on the opposite side. **B,** knee spring for use in tipping molars distally. **C,** split-saddle acrylic space-regainer, useful when greater distances must be regained than in **B.** Note another type of regainer spring on the opposite side of the arch. This is a coil spring lying beneath acrylic, yet acting against the first molar. **D,** method of adjusting the spring on the split-saddle regainer. (*Continued.*)

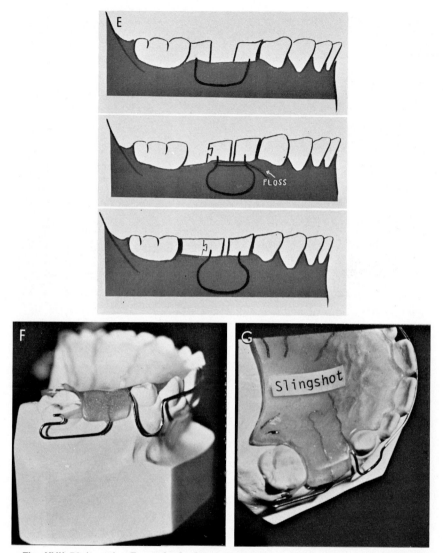

Fig. XVII-52 (cont.).—E, method of increasing the adjustment in a split-saddle regainer. As the molar moves distally, the appliance becomes more fragile. It is then possible to tie the distal portion forward with a piece of dental floss or stainless steel ligature and add acrylic posteriorly. In this fashion, the appliance is reactivated without adjusting the spring. **F** and **G,** slingshot regainer. Note the use of a light elastic joined to buccal lingual hooks (courtesy of Dr. Fred DuPrai). *(Continued.)*

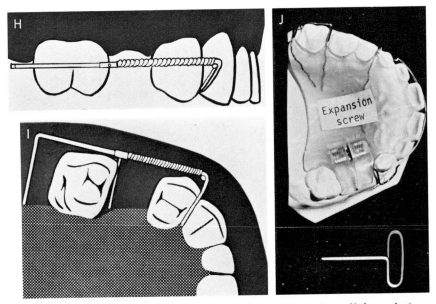

Fig. XVII-52 (cont.).—H and **I**, the sliding yoke space-regainer. **H**, buccal view. A .022-in. × .028-in. steel edgewise wire is used. A ball of solder is placed mesial to the cuspid bend of the wire. A coil spring is then threaded onto the wire, the sliding yoke is added and the wire is bent well distal to the molar to be moved. **I**, the sliding yoke is an edgewise buccal tube the inside diameter of which is exactly that of the wire. To the buccal tube is soldered at a right angle a small piece of stiff wire to engage the mesial of the molar. Note that the acrylic must be trimmed in a straight line on the lingual. This appliance is best anchored on the opposite side by an Adams clasp. It is more efficient in the maxillary than in the mandibular arch. **J**, the expansion screw regainer. These units are bought prefabricated and inserted into the acrylic appliance (courtesy of Dr. Fred DuPrai). *(Continued.)*

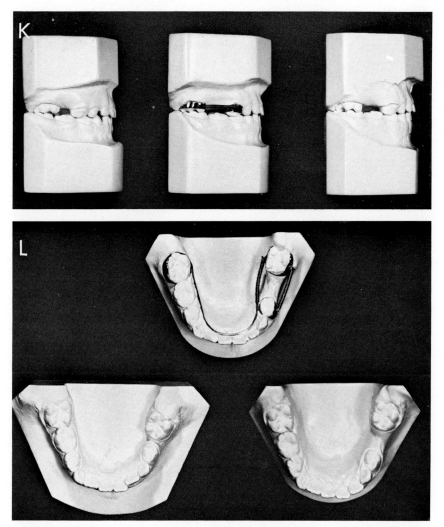

Fig. XVII-52 (cont.).—K and **L,** the double coil train regainer. This appliance consists of a lingual archwire soldered to a molar and cuspid band with buccal and lingual rings and compressed coil springs buccally and lingually against the molar to be moved distally. **K,** the use of the double coil train as a regainer in the upper arch; **L,** its use in the lower arch (courtesy of Dr. Fred Bruner).

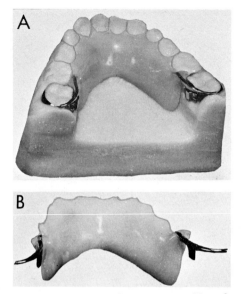

Fig. XVII-53.—Stabilizing plate. **A,** in place on a cast. Note that half-round shafts fit into the half-round sheaths on the molar bands, as in the lingual archwire. Attachments are available with stamped half-round shafts to eliminate soldering. **B,** the plate alone.

Construction

The plastic is cured over a wire framework holding a vertical half-round shaft on either side. A small framework on each side may be used or a regular lingual archwire constructed and the acrylic cured directly over it. In either case, the wire framework must lie far enough away from the soft tissues to allow the plastic to cover the wires completely. The vertical sheaths on the molar bands must be absolutely parallel. One of the best methods of making stabilizing plates is to use the Ellis sheath on the molar bands (see Fig. XVII-26). Since this receives a post made from the doubled archwire itself, the breakage of soldered joints is obviated.

6. THE CROZAT APPLIANCE

a) Description

The Crozat appliance is a removable appliance, usually made of precious alloy. It consists of body wires, lingual arms and a high labial archwire in the maxillary appliance (Fig. XVII-54). It is held in place by molar clasps.

b) Advantages

It is sightly; no bands are used.
It is clean because it is removable.

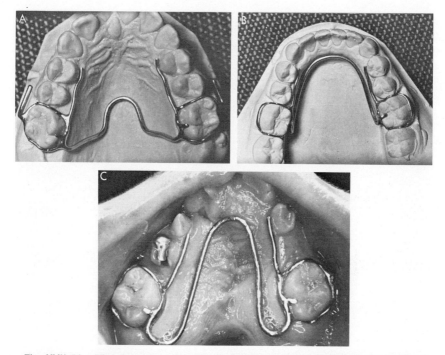

Fig. XVII-54.—The Crozat appliance. **A,** the basic upper appliance. **B,** the basic lower appliance. (**A** and **B** courtesy of Dr. Robert Smythe.) **C,** the appliance in place in a cleft palate patient (courtesy of Dr. S. D. Gore, Jr.).

It uses very light forces, since it will be removed by the patient if adjustments are painful.

The teeth remain in function throughout treatment.

It requires little time for adjustment.

The armamentarium of instruments and inventory of supplies are small.

c) Disadvantages

It demands a high degree of skill in fabrication.

It looks deceptively simple, whereas it is difficult to master.

It takes longer to effect results.

Closure of space after extractions is most difficult.

Maintenance of anchorage without loss requires great care and skill.

Few dental schools teach the use of the appliance, and it is not mastered in a 3-day lecture course.

The Crozat appliance is an old appliance that has been tried by many but mastered by few. It is indicated when caries is a factor, when results can be obtained without extractions and when aesthetics during treatment is essential.

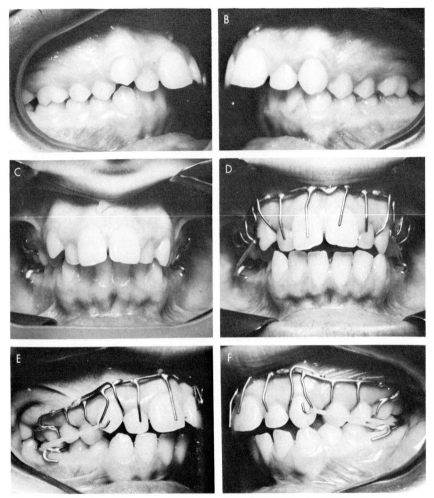

Fig. XVII-55.—A patient treated with the Crozat appliance. **A–C,** before therapy. **D–F,** the appliance in place. (*Continued.*)

Recently, there has been an increased interest in this appliance by family dentists and pedodontists, which is surprising, since many skilled and experienced orthodontists have rejected it after trial. It is a tried and proved appliance with limitations that seem to have gone unnoticed by some. Many ill-founded claims have been made for this appliance, which is unfortunate to those just learning and unfair to those who have taught its use and used it well for so many years. Figure XVII-55 illustrates a case treated with the Crozat appliance.

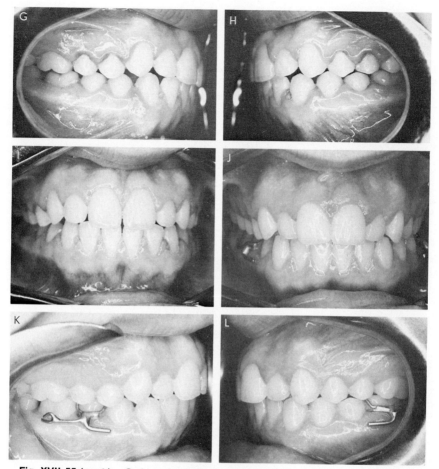

Fig. XVII-55 (cont.).—G-I, at the end of active therapy. **J-L,** at the end of upper arch retention. (Courtesy of Dr. S. D. Gore, Jr.)

7. Extra-Oral Traction Appliances

a) Description

For many years orthodontists have used extra-oral devices to apply force to the dentition in order to avoid some of the problems in anchorage control met within intermaxillary traction and to apply force in directions not otherwise possible.

b) Reasons for Usage

To move teeth—usually distally in the maxilla.
To reinforce anchorage of banded appliances.

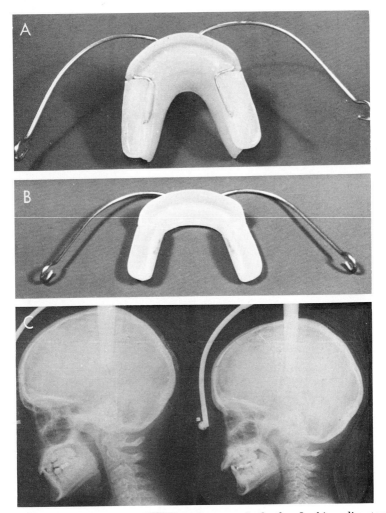

Fig. XVII-56.—Extra-oral traction appliances. **A–C,** the Jenkins director appliance, a combination modified activator and face bow. Note that the appliance
is made in three segments, which allows for easy adjustment of the buccal segments to various sizes of arches. **A,** an upper view. **B,** an underview. **C,** cephalograms, before and after, of a case treated with this appliance (courtesy of Dr.
D. Harvey Jenkins). **D,** simple neck strap, sometimes called cervical traction.
An elastic strap attaches to a face bow (see **F**). The inner smaller bow fits into
buccal tubes on molar bands; the outer bow attaches to the neck strap. **E,** straight-
pull headgear, which attaches to a face bow (see **F**). **F,** high-pull headgear (occipital traction) attached to a face bow. The high pull obviates extrusion of upper
molars. **G,** high-pull headgear with "J" hooks, which attach through the corner
of the mouth to an archwire ligated in brackets on bands cemented to the teeth.
H, combination high-pull and neck strap.

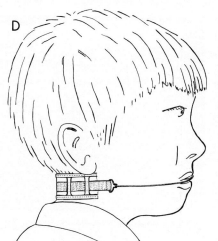

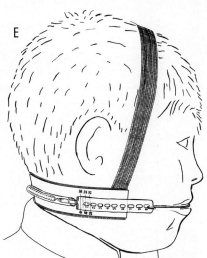

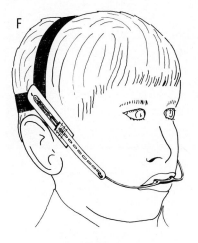

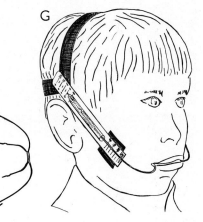

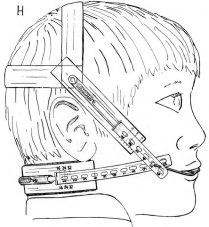

Fig. XVII-56.—See legend at foot of facing page.

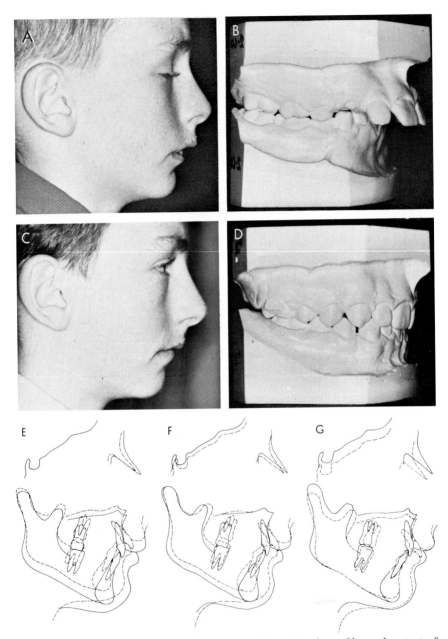

Fig. XVII-57.—A case treated with extra-oral traction. **A,** profile at the start of treatment. **B,** dental casts at the start of treatment. **C,** profile at the end of treatment. **D,** intra-oral casts at the end of treatment. The case was treated for a period with an activator to help aid skeletal growth, then extra-oral traction and, finally, a full-banded appliance. **E–G,** tracings before and after treatment.

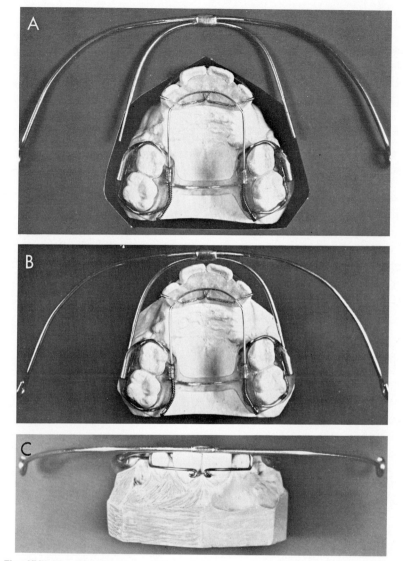

Fig. XVII-58.—The Jenkins sliding plate. **A,** the appliance disassembled. The metal framework fits tightly around the molars by means of an acrylic crib. Buccal tubes in the framework receive the face bow, which is worn in a high-pull fashion. The anterior segment is joined to the posterior by means of a wire that passes through lingual tubes. Tension is created by compressed coils. **B,** the assembled appliance. **C,** labial view. This appliance is used in skeletal Class II cases in combination with serial extraction procedures involving the loss of first bicuspids. (Courtesy of Dr. D. Harvey Jenkins.)

To restrain growth in the midface.
To effect orthopedic changes in the midface.
To alter the direction of growth of the mandible (see Fig. XV-49).

The mode of attachment and direction of force application vary with the task. Figure XVII-56 illustrates varieties of extra-oral traction appliances and uses. Figure XVII-57 shows the result of treatment with extra-oral force in typical cases.

8. Jenkins' Sliding Plate

Jenkins' sliding plate, a refinement of Heath's X-plate, is used to control arch development, the vertical dimension and the occlusal relationships when serial extractions are employed in severe discrepancy cases (Fig. XVII-58).

E. Loose Removable Appliances

Loose removable appliances are orthodontic devices that fit imprecisely in the mouth except during specific functions. They are contrived to:

Provide a more favorable muscular environment for the developing dentition and craniofacial skeleton.
Utilize muscular and/or mucosal anchorage.
Condition reflexes.
Stress bone to excite or direct its growth.
Move teeth.
Direct erupting teeth.

Loose removable appliances have all the advantages and disadvantages of attached removable appliances, but they have additional unique advantages:

They are controlled by the patient's own neuromuscular system, which acts as a servomechanism controlling the amount and direction of force application.
Their mode of action is directed primarily to the neuromusculature and only secondarily through the muscles to the teeth and bones.

1. Oral Shield
a) Description

The oral shield is a device fitting into the vestibule between the lips and the teeth for the purpose of retraining lip function. The oral shield effectively shuts off the ingress of air through the mouth and directs the contractions of the lips against any teeth in labioversion (Fig. XVII-59). It is used to retrain the lips, to correct simple labioversion of the maxillary anterior teeth and as a habit-correcting appliance (Fig. XVII-60). It is particularly good for strengthening the lip action and correcting mouth-breathing. It should never be inserted into a child's

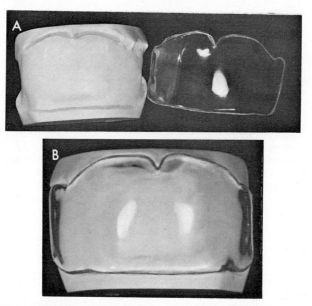

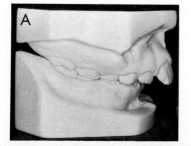

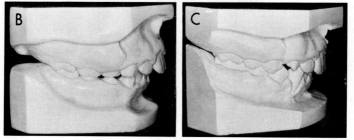

Fig. XVII-59 (above).—A, cast ready for construction of oral shield. A vestibular impression is taken and filled with plaster to the outline of the labial surfaces of the teeth. Plexiglas or acrylic is then fitted to the cast. **B,** cast with completed oral shield in place.

Fig. XVII-60 (below).—Treatment of Class I, type 2 malocclusion with the oral shield. **A,** at the start of treatment. **B,** after 3 months. **C,** after 6 months. Note the recession of gingival tissue around the neck of the mandibular cuspid. As incisor relationship improves, one must grind away the inside of the oral shield so that the shield itself does not cause traumatic occlusion of one of the teeth. Here, such clearance was not provided and of necessity the gingival margin had to recede.

mouth if the child has any kind of nasorespiratory distress or a nasal obstruction.

The oral shield should not be used for the correction of Class II malocclusions.

Construction

Take an accurate impression of the vestibule in compound, pour the impression in stone or plaster and separate. While the model is still wet, fill in with plaster the overjet, all embrasures, depressions and irregularities (see Fig. XVII-59). With a pencil, outline the periphery of the appliance on the model. The mark should lie approximately 2 mm. away from the mucobuccal fold and muscle attachments at all times and extend distally as far as the middle of the maxillary second molars. The cast now may be trimmed to a more workable size, but take care not to cut into the markings just made. Polish the labial aspects of the model and trim down any individual teeth in extreme labioversion if they are intended to be moved somewhat lingually.

b) Methods of Handling Plastic for Oral Shields

1) METHOD 1.—Adapt a sheet of tin foil or wax over the labial surface of the model and trim it to the penciled outline. Remove the tin foil and flatten it out on the paper covering of a sheet of Plexiglas 4 × 4 × ⅛ in. Trace the tin foil outline onto the paper and cut the Plexiglas, with the paper covering still in place, to the outlined form. Remove the paper covering from the Plexiglas, bevel and polish the cut edges of the plastic. Soften the Plexiglas in a gentle flame and adapt it to the work model so that the Plexiglas fits neatly the penciled outline. After it is fitted accurately, it should be polished before use.

2) METHOD 2.—A shorter method is identical up to the point of adapting the cut plastic to the model. At that time, take a heavy rubber band (like a cut section of an inner tube) and hold the Plexiglas in position

Fig. XVII-61.—A, teeth set up for construction of positioner. **B,** the positioner.

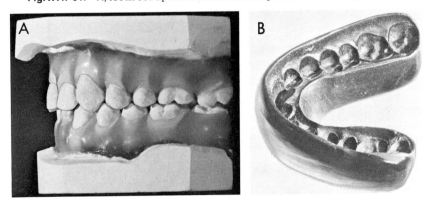

over the work model. Drop the model, Plexiglas and rubber holding them together into a pan of hot water. The heated water will soften the Plexiglas and the rubber's tension will mold the plastic to the cast. Remove from the water, cool, trim and polish.

3) METHOD 3.—In this method, endothermic acrylic resin is used as the plastic material. It may either be dripped on or made into a plastic dough and adapted with the fingers. The resulting appliance will not be transparent and will fit well.

Whichever method is used, the appliance must be accurate or the child cannot wear it. Sometimes he may tape his lips lightly with cellophane tape for a night or two while learning to hold the appliance in place. It should be worn as much as possible, including the entire night.

Some supply houses have a variety of preformed plastic blanks from which oral shields may be made more easily.

2. POSITIONERS

The positioner is a flexible appliance surrounding the crowns of all teeth in both jaws (Fig. XVII-61). It is used as a retainer and to complete the niceties of rotation and alignment after removal of appliances. It should not be used to attempt gross tooth movements, to direct the growth of the jaws or to reposition the mandible—nor is it a substitute for proper occlusal equilibration. The positioner is made of soft rubber or flexible plastic.

Construction

Two very accurate impressions are taken of each dental arch and poured in stone or plaster. A wax recording of the patient's retruded occlusal position is taken as well (see Chapter XI). One set of casts is mounted on an articulator, using the wax bite to secure the proper relationship. Cut off the teeth of the set of casts that are mounted and reset them into more ideal positions. If it is at all possible, leave two opposing molars in position. Care must be taken to keep each tooth as nearly in its original position as possible. This is the reason for not removing a molar in each arch if it can be avoided. Regard must be given to the alveolar conformation, arch shape and the ideal occlusal position (see Chapters V and XI). The waxed-up casts are now duplicated and the positioner made on them. Commercial laboratories will fabricate the positioner and also will do the setup of the teeth. If they are to do the latter, send along one of the wax bites and insist that the setting up be done on an articulator. The second set of casts serves as a record of the conditions at the time the positioner was inserted.

It is very easy to overextend this appliance. It is no substitute for proper manipulation of the archwires. Nor can the construction of this appliance be viewed with a sheerly mechanistic attitude. If the positioner is not constructed exactly to the patient's retruded occlusal position (and thus within accommodating limits of the ideal occlusal position) and at a tolerable vertical dimension, all of the strong contractions of the muscles of mastication are perverted to cause undue straining of the temporomandibular joint. An improperly made positioner can do harm.

3. ACTIVATOR-TYPE APPLIANCES (Andresen Method, Norwegian System, Monobloc)
a) Description

The activator is an appliance designed to alter the function of facial and jaw muscles in order to (1) provide a more favorable environment for the developing dentition and growing bones, (2) optimize the growth potential, (3) change the growth vectors, (4) inhibit growth in selected areas and (5) guide developing teeth into more favorable positions. It was originated by Prof. Viggo Andresen of Norway. His concepts were

Fig. XVII-62.—A, fit of the Andresen appliance inside the mouth. Here, the lower molar is permitted to erupt vertically, whereas the upper molar can erupt vertically but also slide buccally into correct interdigitation. **B,** method of grinding inside of the Andresen appliance. It is designed to fall into the mouth. The tongue lifts it during swallowing, and as the patient bites into the appliance during swallowing, the muscle forces are transmitted through the acrylic to come into contact with the mesial surface of each tooth, as shown. The wire spring is not active itself against the molar but rather is an adjustable point of contact for the molar. Force is applied by the muscles, not by the spring. **C,** method for trimming the acrylic around the incisors with an activator appliance. Note that the acrylic is removed lingually to the maxillary incisors. After they have been tipped somewhat, their incisal edge may be engaged in acrylic in order to prevent their extrusion. In the mandibular arch, the acrylic never touches the lingual of the crown of the mandibular incisor. It is very important not to move the mandibular denture mesially with the activator. Compare this drawing with the activator shown in Figure XVII-65, *F,* where it will be noted that both the incisors are stopped with the acrylic.

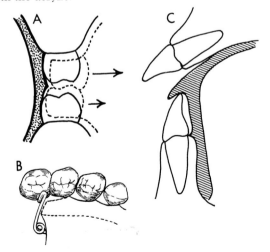

based on the idea that muscle activity can be used for the correction of malocclusion. Rogers' exercises and Andresen's "activator" have as their prime purpose the starting of new reflexes in the neuromusculature of the orofacial region. It is assumed that new neuromuscular reflexes can be directed to correct malocclusions. Andresen cited the differences between primitive people and those living on more highly refined diets. Primitive folk generally have better formed dento-alveolar arches, stronger musculature and keep their mouths closed while chewing. Keeping the mouth shut during function, Andresen believed, placed the tongue in a more advantageous position to aid in arch development. The Andresen activator is built to conform to the inside of the mouth with the teeth occluding against it (Fig. XVII-62). When the patient is relaxed and the jaws are apart, the appliance has no effect on the teeth but it does have an effect on the neuromusculature. The weight of the appliance, lying loose in the mouth, causes reflex closure of the mandible, bringing the teeth into contact with the appliance (Fig. XVII-62). The muscles themselves thus give the force application to the teeth through the appliance, and that application of force is, of course, under the reflex control of the patient's neuromuscular system. Herein lies the basic difference between the fixed and the loose removable appliances. The former move the teeth themselves, and the activator and other loose appliances train and direct the musculature to shape the occlusion. Some add springs to move certain teeth, but many who profess to use Andresen's method place more emphasis on the auxiliary springs than the basic concept of "functional jaw orthopedics." Since Andresen's definitive presentation there have been many misunderstandings, misconceptions, misusages and modifications of the original concept, yet it remains one of the most popular appliances throughout the world.

The appliance is worn at night only, although it is advantageous to wear it an hour or two before retiring during the learning period. The grinding described herein may be delayed to aid in adjusting to the appliance.

Construction

The appliance is constructed on casts placed in a more advantageous relationship than that existing in the maloccluded position (Fig. XVII-63). This new relationship is an arbitrary one, established first in a wax bite taken in the mouth and then kept in a plaster template (Fig. XVII-64) or an articulator. Steps in formation of the wire framework, adding acrylic and grinding are shown in Figure XVII-65. In Class II, for example, the mandible is brought down and forward from its former relationship with the maxillary dental arch. The appliance fits inside both dental arches like two Hawley appliances joined along the occlusal plane, but there the resemblance to the Hawley appliance ends.

The plastic between the teeth is ground away to direct the eruption of the teeth and alveolar growth to a more favorable final relationship (see Fig.

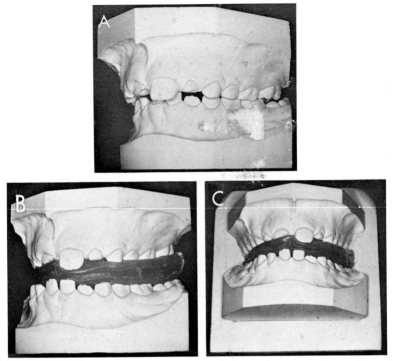

Fig. XVII-63.—A, casts before treatment with the Andresen appliance. **B,** method of the wax bite. **C,** casts with wax bite in place and construction of template.

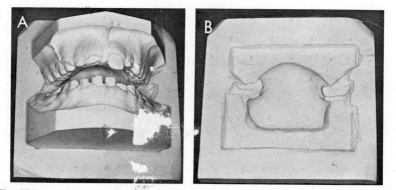

Fig. XVII-64.—A, template with casts in place and wax removed. **B,** finished template.

XVII-62). The muscles act against the teeth each time the patient swallows. Thus, the force comes reflexly from the muscles against the teeth by way of the inclined planes of the appliance.

There are two basically different ways to construct the appliance. Andresen suggested separating the teeth by about one-half the distance off the freeway space when establishing the wax record (Fig. XVII-66). Harvold, on the other hand, suggested establishing the wax bite record with the mandible positioned down and forward slightly past the postural position (Fig. XVII-66). Care must be taken to exceed the postural position, yet too much stretch may affect the gamma afferents adversely (see Chapter V). The modification is preferred, since it establishes a slight muscle tension, enabling a fixed position of the teeth and jaws against the appliance. The slight bit of stretching thus induced makes it easier to learn reflex control of the new position. Furthermore, it is easier to learn to wear the appliance, and the elastic effect of the muscles is advantageous.

Figures XVII-64 and XVII-65 illustrate the short method of construction. It also may be made by flasking a wax pattern and curing the acrylic in the ordinary manner, which results in an appliance of superior quality. Activators can be made by many commercial laboratories. Some modifications are shown in Figure XVII-67.

b) Indications

The activator is particularly suitable for modifying the degree of eruption and alveolar development in selected areas of the mouth, hence its indicated use for deep overbite. Its most frequent use is in the treatment of Class II in the primary or mixed dentitions (see Chapter XV, Section E). For Class II malocclusions, it is advocated as a means of changing mandibular growth (Fig. XVII-69). Finally, it is an excellent retaining device. Many orthodontists use the activator as the first part of diphasic treatment of severe Class II cases. They treat the skeleton with the activator and align the teeth later with fixed banded appli-

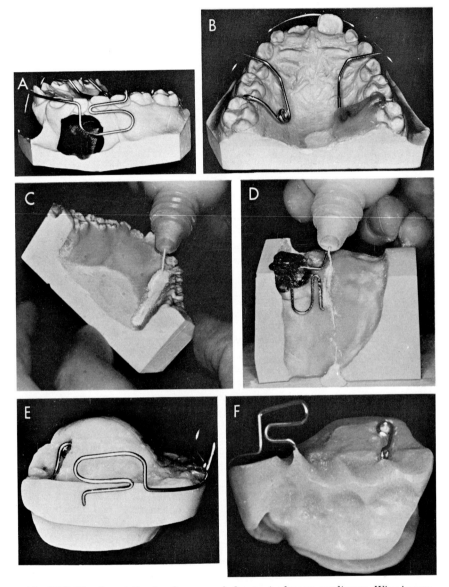

Fig. XVII-65.—A and **B,** wire framework for an Andresen appliance. Wire is constructed of .039-in. stainless steel. Note the wax covering the spring and holding the framework in position, and that the wire is free above the occlusion. **C,** quick-cure acrylic being applied to lower cast. **D,** joining the two casts with quick-cure acrylic. Note that the casts are seated well into the template. **E,** an Andresen appliance before trimming. Note the molar spring free, since it was covered with wax during curing of the acrylic. **F,** an Andresen appliance that has been adjusted and worn for some time. Note that the acrylic is ground in such a fashion that

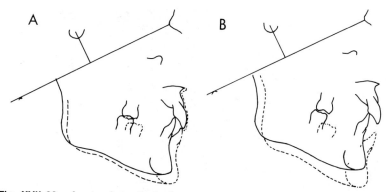

Fig. XVII-66.—A, usual method of constructing the Andresen appliance. Wax bite is constructed in this instance within the limits of the freeway space. **B,** Harvold's method. The mandible is held down and forward well past the freeway space.

Fig. XVII-67.—A, the open-front activator, occlusal view, with the appliance on the lower arch. Note that there are no acrylic stops for the incisors. This appliance may be worn during the day and it is possible to speak easily with it in place. **B,** an activator with a coffin spring. The appliance may be split in two for mild expansion forces or the coffin spring may be left in unactivated to teach a more superior tongue posture.

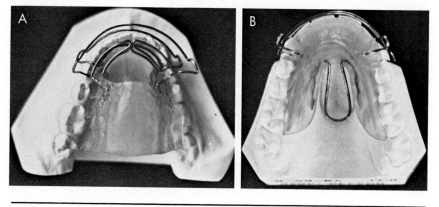

the maxillary teeth are guided distally as they erupt. The spring that engages the mesial of the maxillary first permanent molar is not intended to tip the tooth; rather, it serves as an adjustable guide plane down which the tooth erupts. In the mandibular arch, the acrylic is ground away to allow only the vertical eruption of the mandibular teeth. At no time must they be allowed to move mesially. Note in this instance that the acrylic has engaged the incisal edges of both the upper and lower incisors.

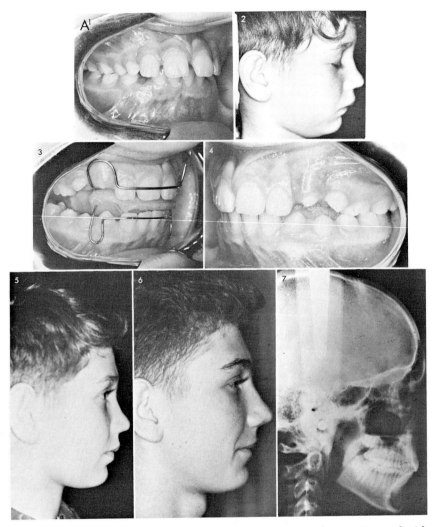

Fig. XVII-68.—Cases treated with the activator appliance. **A,** a case treated with activator alone. **1,** intra-oral view at the start of treatment. **2,** the facial profile at the start. **3,** the appliance in place in the mouth 1 year later. **4,** the occlusion 1 year later. Note the reduction of the overjet, the improvement in the open bite and the correction of the molar relationship as the cuspids and premolars erupt. **5,** the profile 1 year later. **6,** the profile at the end of treatment. **7,** cephalogram at the end of treatment. (*Continued.*)

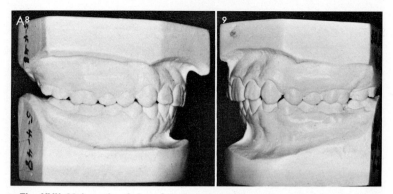

Fig. XVII-68 (cont.).—A-8 and **9,** the casts after retention. (*Continued.*)

Fig. XVII-68 (cont.).—A-10, cephalometric tracings: solid line—at the start of treatment; dotted line—at the end of active treatment; dashed line—at the end of the retention period. Cranial base orientation. **11,** same, oriented on palatal plane. **12,** same, oriented on mandibular plane and registered at the lingual symphysis. (*Continued.*)

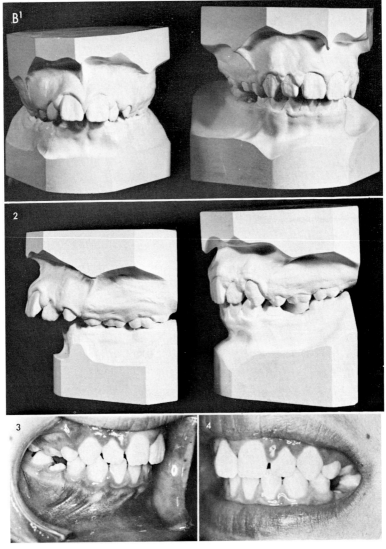

Fig. XVII-68 (cont.).—B, the use of the activator in diphasic orthodontic treatment. **1–2,** in each instance, the cast at the left is at the start of treatment and the cast at the right is at the end of activator therapy, although it will be necessary to place bands to complete the tooth movements in this case. In this instance, the activator was used to correct the gross malocclusion and the facial skeleton, but it is not a precise tooth-moving appliance. When tooth movements are needed to complete the case, bands must

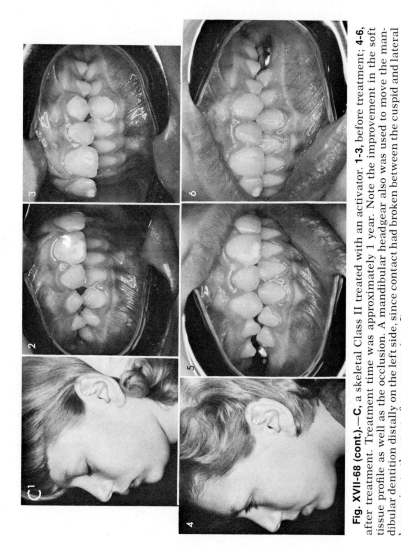

Fig. XVII-68 (cont.).—C, a skeletal Class II treated with an activator. **1-3,** before treatment; **4-6,** after treatment. Treatment time was approximately 1 year. Note the improvement in the soft tissue profile as well as the occlusion. A mandibular headgear also was used to move the mandibular dentition distally on the left side, since contact had broken between the cuspid and lateral here prior to the start of treatment (see **3**).

be added. **3** and **4,** intra-oral photographs after activator therapy. **5,** cephalograms at the start of treatment and 1 year later. (*Continued.*)

ances. The activator is not indicated when patient and parental cooperation and understanding are low, nor should it be used for definitive
tooth movements.

It seems a pity that the appliance is not more popular in the United
States, for clinical experience shows that it works well when used properly for indicated problems. A series of recent papers have revealed
much concerning the skeletal response to activator therapy, but the
details of the neuromuscular reactions are less well known (see Suggested Readings).

4. THE FRANKEL APPLIANCE

a) Description

Frankel combined the ideas of Kraus, who perfected the oral shield,
and Andresen to produce a new concept and a series of strange new

Fig. XVII-69.—The Frankel "Function Regulator" (type used for Class II). **A,** on
the upper cast. Note that the acrylic pads keep the buccal wall away from the
dental arch. **B,** in position on the cast. Note that the working bite is taken with
the incisors edge to edge. **C,** on the lower arch. **D,** in place in the mouth. This is
Rakosi's modification of the Frankel appliance. Note the acrylic between the
upper and lower teeth, as in the activator appliance, a modification much preferred by the author.

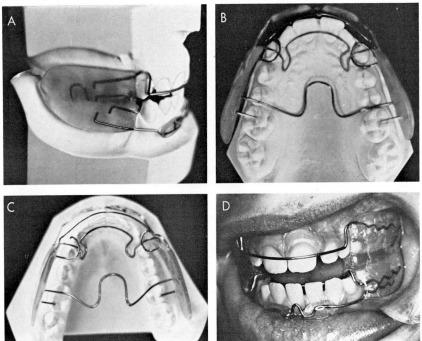

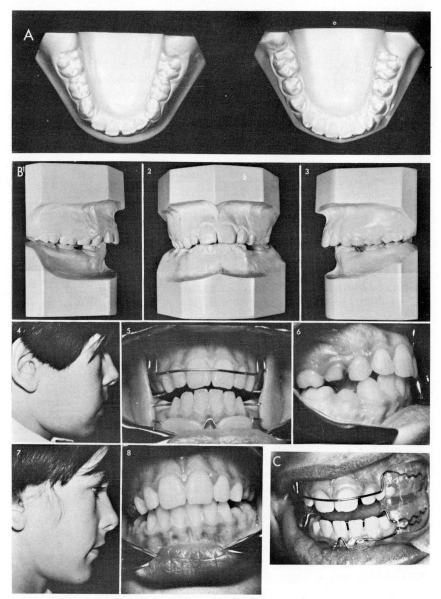

Fig. XVII-70.—The Frankel "Function Regulator." **A,** changes in the mandibular arch during treatment with the appliance. No expansive forces were used. **B,** treatment of a Class II malocclusion: **1–4,** before treatment; **5,** the appliance in place; **6–8,** after 17 months of treatment. Since this is a satisfactory improvement in molar occlusion and profile, the case required no precise tooth movements. (Courtesy of Dr. Fred Bruner.) **C,** Rakosi's modification of the Frankel "Function Regulator" in place. Compare with **B-5.** Note the buccal plastic pad, which restrains the cheek, and the lip-plumper, which removes the effects of excessive mentalis muscle activity.

723

appliances (Fig. XVII-69). The Frankel appliance usually does not touch the teeth; rather, it is constructed in such a way that the changed muscle balance and function effects the desired tooth movements and growth responses. The buccal musculature, in particular, is held away from the teeth, allowing the tongue to play a larger role in shaping the arch form and determining the position of the posterior teeth.

Construction

The appliance is constructed in a forward bite as is used for the activator, but Frankel places great stress on determining the amount of forward positioning by the resultant lip relationship. The elaborate wire framework shown in Figure XVII-69 is constructed and acrylic flanges and pads are provided to selectively alter lip and cheek positions.

b) Application

I have had only limited experience during the past 3 years with this appliance. It seems effective in Class II corrections of the type that respond well to activator therapy, but more care must be taken to avoid using the appliance when incisors in the lower arch are not perfectly upright. The Frankel appliance can take them off the base rather quickly. Sometimes it brings about remarkable changes in mandibular arch form. The vertical control of incisors and overbite and overjet correction are more difficult with the Frankel appliance than with the activator. Figure XVII-70 illustrates clinical results with the Frankel appliance.

F. Myotherapeutic Exercises

One person, more than any other, alerted American orthodontists to the relationship of muscles to malocclusion. As early as 1906, A. P. Rogers suggested that muscle exercises be used as an adjunct to mechanical correction of malocclusion. He described the role of muscle imbalance in the etiology of malocclusion and pictured the muscle environment of the teeth as "living orthodontic appliances." He also was careful to point out that although muscle exercises elsewhere in the body generally are used to increase the size or strength of the muscles, in the circumoral region the establishment of proper function and tonicity is paramount.

1. PURPOSE

The purpose of myotherapy is the creation of normal health and function in the orofacial musculature for the simple reason that they are important elements aiding growth and development of normal occlusion. Myotherapy is no substitute for mechanical appliances, nor can the appliances alone ensure a satisfactory retained result. They must be used together. Myotherapy is used to guide the development of the occlusion, to give the growth pattern an optimal chance to express itself and to provide the best retention possible for mechanically treated cases. Many who misunderstand the use of myotherapy would do well to reread some of Rogers' papers, for he stated the purposes clearly, even though others have misunderstood or misinterpreted.

2. LIMITATIONS

Muscle exercises will not greatly alter the bony growth pattern or perform heroic tooth movements. They can, however, aid in the unfolding of the inherent potential of the case and increase the chances for successful retention.

3. PRINCIPLES

(1) Establish early, with the minimum of mechanotherapy, the proper arch form and cuspal relationship. (2) Remove by occlusal equilibration any interferences in the primary dentition (see Section H later in this chapter). (3) Assign such muscle exercises as will best train the muscles to function normally, and continue their practice after the mechanotherapy to aid in the retention (Fig. XVII-71). Perhaps the most important principle of all is to study the possible role of muscle malfunction in the etiology of the malocclusion. A discussion of this matter before the insertion of the appliances establishes in the patient's and parents' minds the importance you place on the musculàture.

4. SPECIFIC USES

a) *Orbicularis Oris and Circumoral Muscles*

If the lips cannot seal because of procumbency of the incisors, it may be best to withhold the exercises until the incisors are retracted sufficiently for the lips to exert some effect against the teeth.

Usually it is the upper lip that is lazy and inefficient. It can be brought into better action by practicing stretching it over the lower lip in an attempt to touch the chin (see Fig. XVII-71).

A soft acrylic "plumper" may be made to fit inside the vestibule while the patient is doing the upper lip exercises.

Instruct the patient to fill his mouth with warm saline and forcibly squirt the solution between the teeth and back again.

Do not forget the role of musical instruments. Any brass instrument will soon produce fine lip tonicity. It is equally important to avoid the single-reed instruments, e.g., the clarinet, for patients with hypofunction of the maxillary lip and labioversion of the upper incisors.

If the patient's nasal passages are clear and he has no nasorespiratory distress, sometimes the placement of Scotch tape over the lips in the evening will help train them to remain sealed. During the day, the best

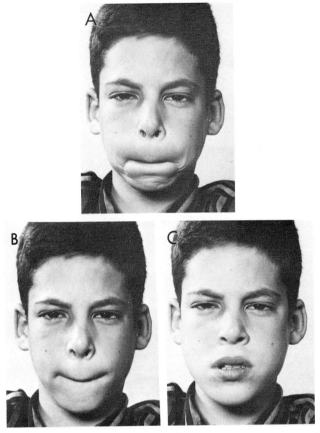

Fig. XVII-71.—A, myofunctional exercises to increase lip tonicity. **B,** another lip exercise. Here, the patient is trying to force the upper lip down to the chin. **C,** myofunctional exercise: the pterygoid. The patient is instructed to protrude the jaw as far as is possible, then relax it, and repeat until the pterygoid muscles are tired.

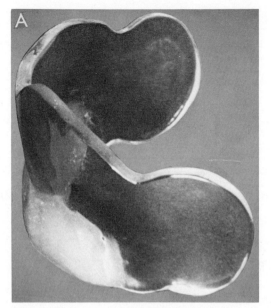

Fig. XVII-72.—The modified oral shield for training of the mentalis muscle. **A,** an oral shield is made in the usual fashion and base plate wax is added to the lower labial surface in sufficient quantity to inhibit the mentalis contraction on swallowing. Wax is added and contoured until the inhibition of the mentalis contraction is seen on the patient. Then the wax is converted to acrylic. (*Continued.*)

method is to make the patient very conscious of his lip posture.

The oral shield (see Section E-1) is an excellent device for stimulating circumoral function and teaching nasal breathing. It has the added advantage that it uses the muscle force generated to better the incisors' positions.

Baril, while studying lip and mentalis activity in the electromyographic laboratory at The University of Michigan, modified the oral shield as shown in Figure XVII-72 for the purpose of conditioning hyperactivity of the mentalis muscle.

b) Mandibular Posture

When a child has faulty body posture it is difficult for him to hold his mandible in its most advantageous position. When the spine is straight and the head is well placed over it with the eyes constantly looking ahead, the mandible is held in the best position of posture.

Simply having the patient walk upright with shoulders squared and eyes ahead sometimes produces startling effects in appearance. Also,

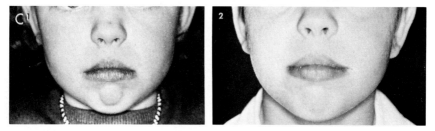

Fig. XVII-72 (cont.).—B, electromyograms of a patient before and immediately after insertion of the oral shield. Note the diminution of activity in the mentalis muscle. Usually it is necessary to wear the appliance for several months before the mentalis becomes quiescent. Then the labial plumper is gradually ground down before abandoning the appliances. For this usage, the oral shield is not inserted until the incisor correction has been obtained. **C-1,** face of a girl at the start of open bite treatment. **2,** the same face at the end of open bite treatment. Note the persistence of the hyperactive mentalis muscle. This is the kind of case on which the modified oral shield works very well.

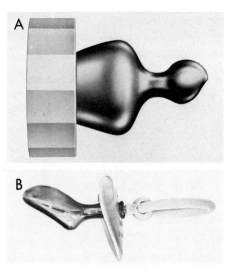

Fig. XVII-73.—A, the Nuk Sauger nipple. **B,** the Nuk Sauger exerciser. (Courtesy of Rocky Mountain Metal Products Company.)

Fig. XVII-74.—the mini-positioner. This appliance is purchased prefabricated in two sizes. It is made of soft white rubber and may be used as a functional guidance appliance in the primary and early mixed dentition. (Courtesy of Unitek Corporation.)

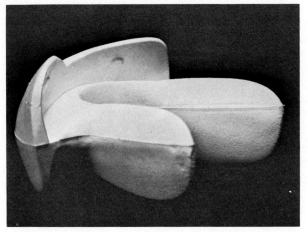

you may encourage some home exercises. One that is useful follows. Stand with the hands and arms relaxed at the side. Rise on the toes, inhale, pull back on the shoulders, turn the palms forward and protrude the mandible. Relax and repeat until tired. This will not make a bigger mandible or a better one, but it will help the child's posture and make him well aware of the relationship of muscles to all bone positions, including the jaw.

5. MYOFUNCTIONAL APPLIANCES

All of the loose removable appliances are devices to promote myotherapy. Others include the modified oral shield (see Fig. XVII-72) and the Nuk Sauger nipple and adjunctive exercisers (Fig. XVII-73). The nipple promotes mature swallows even in the infant, and the exerciser that is the same size as the nipple is an excellent pacifier or teething device. The larger exerciser has been found to be of little use.

The device shown in Figure XVII-74 is useful as an activator-like approach to Class II in the primary dentition. It is soft and a bit more readily accepted than the acrylic appliances.

G. Correction of Deleterious Oral Habits

Before attempting to control any suspected deleterious oral habit, it is important to bear in mind the role of the oral musculature in normal development of occlusion (Chapter V) and the mechanisms of habits in the etiology of malocclusion (Chapter VII). Usually there is no strong reason for plunging into a rigorous regimen of habit control; therefore, time can be taken to study the problem thoroughly. It would seem wise to concern ourselves with the control of oral habits that actually are deleterious to the occlusion; other undesirable oral habits may be treated best outside the dental profession. We dentists would do well to confine our efforts to the clinical problem we must treat—occlusion. Much silliness is written for the laity and profession alike by psychiatrists, psychologists and physicians—as well as by dentists. It is unfortunate that so much misinformation concerning this important subject appears in lay magazines. Much of the loose writing dealing with occlusion is not done by those who eventually must handle the problem.

One should define at the start that which is to be treated. Sometimes it is an open bite, sometimes a psychologic problem, sometimes a neuromuscular reflex. Always ask the questions: "What precisely is the habit to be controlled?" "Should any of the therapy be directed toward the parents?" The most common oral habits disruptive to occlusion are thumb-sucking, finger-sucking, tongue-thrusting, nail-biting, lip-biting and lip-sucking. Functional malocclusions also cause faulty habits deleterious to occlusal development. They are discussed in Chapter XV.

1. BASIC CONSIDERATIONS

Regardless of which oral habit is being corrected, two basic considerations apply:

(1) A reflex is involved. The problem is one of controlling a physiologic process; therefore, the rationale of therapy must be physiologic and not mechanical. The attempt always should be to alter the afferent arm of the reflex, and this alteration should be thought of in terms of muscle relearning. It follows that devices such as restraints, mitts and elbow braces, which supply little but mechanical interference, are to be shunned. The rationale of therapy is that of conditioning responses, not mechanics (see Chapter VII, Section D-5).

(2) It must be determined whether the malocclusion is of primary or secondary concern. We are dentists, and our minds and eyes are tuned to dental problems and dental solutions, but lingual archwires do not treat emotional disturbances.

2. THUMB-SUCKING (Finger-Sucking)

The term "thumb-sucking" has been used loosely to cover a wide variety of oral sucking habits. In this discussion we shall limit our remarks to the strictest interpretation of the term. Repeated forceful sucking of the thumb with associated strong buccal and lip contractions seems to be the type of sucking most likely to be related to malocclusion. The type of facial pattern makes some difference. A straight profile with a firm Class I occlusion seems to withstand the forces of thumb-sucking better than a typical Class II facial skeleton. Do not disregard the face in which the habit appears, for a mild habit in some faces is more detrimental than a severe one in others. Just as the factors that make up the habit vary, so do the faces. It is the combination of habit plus growing face that gives the clinical problem. The clinical aspects of the problem may be divided into three distinct phases of development.

a) Phase I: Normal and Subclinically Significant Thumb-Sucking

This phase extends from birth to about 3 years, depending on the child's social development. Most infants display a certain amount of thumb- and finger-sucking during this period, particularly at the time of weaning. Ordinarily, the sucking is naturally resolved toward the end of Phase I. However, should the infant show any tendencies to the "thumb-specific" type of vigorous sucking, a definite prophylactic approach should be taken because of possible occlusal harm. The use of a rubber pacifier toward the end of Phase I is much less harmful, at least from a dental point of view, than repeated vigorous thumb-sucking.

b) *Phase II: Clinically Significant Thumb-Sucking*

The second phase extends roughly from 3 to 6 or 7 years. Sucking practiced during this time deserves more serious attention from the dentist for two reasons: (1) it is an indication of possible clinically significant anxiety and (2) it is the best time to solve dental problems related to digital sucking. A firm and definite program of correction is indicated at this time (see below).

c) *Phase III: Intractable Thumb-Sucking*

Any thumb-sucking persisting after the fourth year presents the clinician with a difficult problem, for its persistence may be proof of problems other than simple malocclusion. A thumb-sucking habit seen during Phase III often requires forthright dental and psychologic therapy. Frequent consultation between dentist and psychologist or physician is indicated in order that an integrated approach may be made. Any thumb-sucking habit persisting until Phase III is likely to be but a symptom of a problem bigger than the resulting malocclusion.

Steps in treatment

(1) It is wise to begin with a discussion of the problem with the child, without the parent near. No threats or shaming should be used; instead, a calm, friendly attempt should be made to learn about the child and his attitudes toward the habit. Many children will say that they suck their thumbs only when they are asleep, and also declare that they want sincerely to be rid of the habit. One can use these statements to advantage by saying, "It's mighty difficult to control what you do while sleeping, isn't it?" "Would you like a little help to remind your thumb to stay out of your mouth when you are not awake to do so?" If the child can be brought along gently to give an honest and cooperative reply, it may be wise to suggest that such a reminder is available if he finds in the next 2 or 3 months that he cannot handle the problem alone. The child may be shown casts or photographs of mouths of children who have had detrimental sucking habits. Show the treated result, too, to establish in his mind what can be done with the dentist's help. In other words, use this first discussion to learn about the child and allow him to learn about the methods available for correction of the habit. Be gentle, for he may never have had a friendly discussion concerning the matter. Leave him with the idea that he is to do what he can by himself for 2 or 3 months, after which time you will discuss the situation again.

Excellent results have been obtained by use of a card that the child is given for scoring each morning to indicate whether the thumb was sucked during the night. It should not be a printed form, but rather a card with the child's name written on especially for him. Two columns are drawn labeled simply YES and NO. Make an appointment for the child to return in 2 weeks or less and bring the card. He has been instructed that he may suck his thumb if he wants to, but he must keep score for you so that you can learn about the severity of the habit. Do not encourage the disturbed, insecure child to lie to please you. Rather, teach him that one adult is interested in him and can discuss the thumb-sucking without scolding or shaming him. A surprising number of children will bring the habit under control themselves under this program. It may be varied a bit by prescribing Band-Aids to be placed on the thumb each night by the child to remind the thumb to stay out of his mouth. And even when it is necessary to resort to the appliance (see later in this discussion), the child is ready psychologically for it and the appliance serves merely to remind the thumb when he is asleep and cannot do so. A phonograph record is available to give the child to augment and reinforce this method of thumb-sucking control. Its script was written by me. It is available from Healthcare Records, 2132 Jefferson Avenue, Toledo, Ohio 43602.

(2) As the child enters the period of trying to control the habit himself, a talk should be had with one or both parents. Emphasize that no one should discuss the problem with the child nor should it be a subject for family discussion, since the dentist and the child will take care of it between them. Above all else, no disparaging remarks are to be made by anyone concerning the habit. Specifically ask the parents to watch the other children and grandparents within the family circle. The child thus loses the attention-getting aspects of the habit and is encouraged to work in a mature way with the dentist. A few children will cease the habit completely at this stage. Most will not, but will benefit greatly by the removal of family tensions centered on the thumb-sucking and will be prepared to work with the dentist.

(3) If the child is in Phase II, the next step is the insertion of a habit-correcting appliance (see below). If the child is in Phase III, the next step is consultation with the family physician, a competent clinical psychologist or a psychiatrist. Many school systems have such personnel who are conversant with this problem. After such consultative advice is sought, the therapy becomes a joint effort. Usually, appliances are not inserted until the child's over-all problems are defined and the thumb-sucking is seen in proper perspective.

d) Choice of Appliance

The ideal appliance to aid in the correction of a thumb-sucking habit would (1) offer no restraint whatever to normal muscular activity, (2) not require remembering to be used, (3) have no shame attached to its use and (4) not involve the parents. The oral shield can be used to aid in the correction of thumb-sucking (see Section E-1), but it requires an unusual amount of patient cooperation and is not used continually. Perhaps the best appliance is a lingual archwire with *short* spurs soldered at strategic locations to remind the thumb to keep out (Fig. XVII-75). This appliance is not a mechanical interference with the thumb and so should not take the form of a huge screen or so-called rake. It should be well adapted, out of the way of normal oral functioning and contain sufficient sharp, short spurs to provide mild afferent signals of discomfort each time the thumb is inserted. Note carefully the rationale of this appliance. A clear signal of discomfort or mild pain reminds the neuromuscular system, even when the child is asleep, that the thumb best not be inserted. At that point, the child knows he needs help to remind the thumb to keep out when he cannot do so, for example,

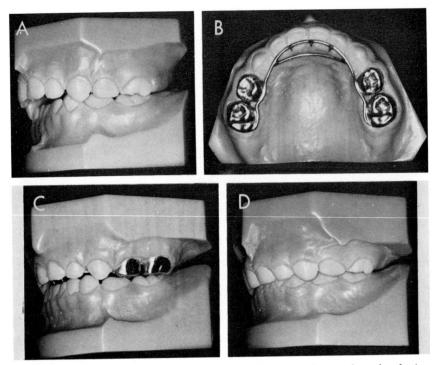

Fig. XVII-75.—Correction of thumb-sucking with an appliance. **A,** malocclusion before treatment. **B,** appliance in place on cast. It is made of .036-in. stainless steel wire soldered to four stainless steel primary crown forms. The spurs are very, very short, sharp and strategically placed. **C,** appliance in place and the teeth in occlusion. **D,** corrected malocclusion; time required was 4 months. The appliance did not correct the malocclusion, it treated the habit. The return of normal lip and tongue function closed the open bite and aligned the incisors.

when he is asleep. It is wrong to place any appliance as the first step in treatment, since the adjustment is likely to be too difficult. The permissive and more gradual approach outlined here is easier, takes less time, requires fewer appliances and provides better conditioning of responses than the traditional mechanistic approach.

Some of the huge and grotesque appliances suggested are mechanical deterrents only and thus provide nothing but frustration for the child. Thumb-suckers usually have that in abundance anyway. Advise the parents of the rationale and ask their help the first night or two. It is advisable for them to take time to quiet the child just before bedtime and give him an extra amount of attention and affection for a few days. Children in Phase III often will remove the appliance several times. It should always be recemented and the incident reported to the other clinician working on the problem.

3. TONGUE-THRUSTING

a) Causes

There are several causes of tongue-thrusting. It may be seen as a residuum of thumb-sucking or as a habit by itself. Frequently, it is learned early in life when there has been chronic tonsillitis or pharyngitis. Any chronic pain in the throat forces the tongue to be positioned forward, particularly during swallowing (see Chapters V and VII). If the throat condition remains, do not attempt correction of the tongue-thrust.

b) Diagnosis

Careful differentiation must be made of a simple tongue-thrust, a complex tongue-thrust, retention of an infantile swallowing pattern and faulty tongue posture (see Chapters V, VII and X). The prognosis for a simple tongue-thrust usually is excellent, good for a complex tongue-thrust and very poor for retained infantile swallowing patterns. Chapter X provides detailed procedures for examining orofacial muscular activities.

c) Treatment

1) SIMPLE TONGUE-THRUST.—The simple tongue-thrust is defined as a tongue-thrust with a teeth-together swallow. The malocclusion usually associated with it is a well-circumscribed open bite in the anterior region (Fig. XVII-76). Read Chapter X, Sections C and D for detailed descriptions of the procedures for examining the tongue and swallowing.

As mentioned above, the prognosis for a simple tongue-thrust usually

Fig. XVII-76.—An open bite due to a simple tongue-thrust. Note how circumscribed the open bite is.

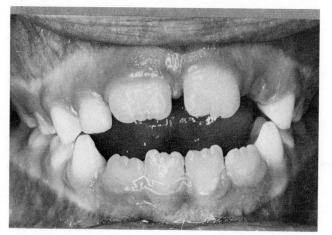

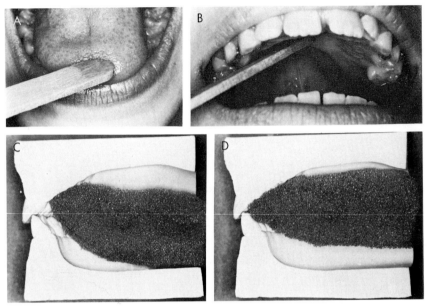

Fig. XVII-77.—A and **B,** the use of tactile signals to the tongue for teaching correct tongue position during swallowing. **C** and **D,** the use of visual signals for teaching correct tongue position during swallowing. These photographs show a set of casts cut in two and a soft red plastic sponge, which may be used to simulate tongue positions.

is excellent. If there is excessive labioversion of the maxillary incisors, treatment of the tongue-thrust should not begin until the incisors have been retracted. Many simple tongue-thrusts correct spontaneously during orthodontic therapy.

Steps in treatment

(1) Acquaint the patient with the abnormal swallow. This may be done by placing the index finger on the tip of the tongue and then on the junction of the

Fig. XVII-78.—The use of fruit drops to aid in tongue correction.

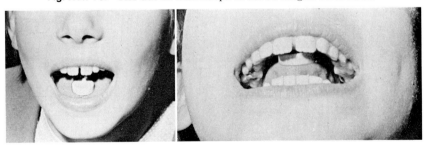

hard and soft palate and saying to the patient, "Most people swallow with this part of the tongue on this part of the palate. Now put your tongue tip up here, close your teeth, close your lips and swallow while holding the tongue in this position." The use of tactile signals helps the patient understand where his tongue should go (Fig. XVII-77). The patient should be instructed to practice, during the interval until the next appointment, correct swallowing at least 40 times a day and to record on a card the fact that he has done so. Practice may be with small amounts of water or a bite-size dry cereal. Very small orthodontic elastics can be held by the tongue tip against the palate during practice swallows. If the swallow is correct, the elastic will be retained; if it is incorrect, the elastic will be swallowed. This may best be spaced out over two or three practice sessions each day.

(2) When the new reflex has been learned on the conscious level, it is necessary to reinforce this reflex on the subconscious level. At the second appointment, the patient should be able to swallow correctly at will. However, he will demonstrate abnormal unconscious swallows. Flat sugarless fruit drops now can be used to reinforce the unconscious swallow. Preferred drops are biconcave and of some citric acid flavor such as lemon. The patient is instructed to place one of the fruit drops on the back of the tongue and to hold the fruit drop against the palate in the correct position until the candy has dissolved completely (Fig. XVII-78). In no circumstance is he to take a piece of the candy when it is not a part of the therapeutic program. Have the patient time himself, using a watch with a second hand (Fig. XVII-79). He should record on a card the time in minutes and seconds and then immediately replace the fruit drop in its correct place and start retiming. At first, he will be able to hold it in place but a few seconds but gradually he will learn. While he is learning, he is swallowing correctly unconsciously, since the timing procedure provides a bit of competition and he forgets about the swallows. This

Fig. XVII-79.—The distractive technic for correcting the unconscious swallow.

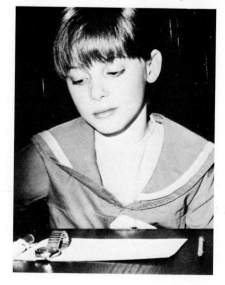

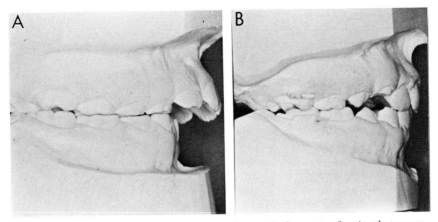

Fig. XVII-80.—A corrected simple tongue-thrust. **A,** the casts of a simple tongue-thrust in a mild Class II case at the start of extra-oral traction and space supervision therapy. **B,** after the molar relationship had been improved, the incisors retracted and the open bite spontaneously corrected by the orthodontic tooth movements.

combination of fruit drop and recorded timing is the best procedure I have devised yet for getting the reflex activity from the conscious to the unconscious levels. Usually, one practice session a day involving the dissolution of one fruit drop is satisfactory. It should be remembered that the timing procedure should not be omitted, since its distractive effects are most important. These two steps will correct a large percentage of all simple tongue-thrusts. However, one additional step sometimes is necessary.

(3) A soldered lingual archwire carefully adapted to the teeth and having attached to it *short* (2 mm.), sharp, strategically placed spurs can now be inserted. Protectively, the tongue is withdrawn from the abnormal position and placed properly during swallowing. Do not place such an appliance as the first step in therapy. It is much too traumatic to the patient and many patients will simply rip it out of the mouth. However, if steps 1 and 2 have been carried out properly, the patient can then accept the appliance. All simple tongue-thrusts should be correctable by these three sequential procedures. When one is not thus corrected, the condition has been misdiagnosed and is not truly a simple tongue-thrust.

To summarize, the treatment consists of three phases: the learning of a new reflex at the conscious level, the transferral to the subconscious level and the reinforcement of the new reflex. Figure XVII-80 illustrates a treated simple tongue-thrust problem.

Healthcare Records, 2132 Jefferson Avenue, Toledo, Ohio 43602 makes a phonograph record, script written by me, to augment and reinforce this tongue-training program at home.

2) **COMPLEX TONGUE-THRUST.**—This is defined as a tongue-thrust with a teeth-apart swallow. The malocclusion seen with a complex tongue-thrust has two distinguishing features: (1) there is a poor occlusal fit

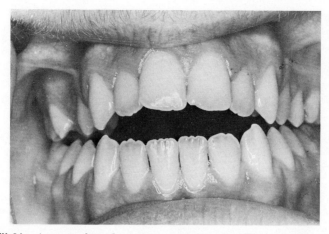

Fig. XVII-81.—An open bite due to a complex tongue-thrust. In this instance, the mandible dropped before the tongue-thrusts and the neat circumscribed area of the open bite as seen in the simple tongue-thrust is not observed.

prompting a slide into occlusion and (2) there is a generalized anterior open bite (Fig. XVII-81). One almost can diagnose a complex tongue-thrust from the casts alone. When the casts are taken in the hands and fitted together, there is uncertainty about what is precisely the patient's usual occlusal position. There is no stability of the intercuspation.

The prognosis for correction of a complex tongue-thrust is not as good as for a simple tongue-thrust, since there are two neuromuscular problems—an abnormal occlusal reflex and an abnormal swallow reflex. The patient's attention must be brought to the problem and the prognosis must be explained carefully at the start of therapy. Furthermore, much of the responsibility lies with the patient, who should know this at the very start of treatment.

Treatment

It is advisable, contrary to popular practice, to treat the occlusion first. After the orthodontic treatment is in its retentive stages, it is extremely important to do very careful occlusal equilibration. The muscle training follows the procedure for a simple tongue-thrust, with minor modifications. (1) When teaching the patient to swallow properly, great emphasis must be placed on keeping the teeth together, and step 1 of the treatment usually is prolonged with a complex tongue-thrust. (2) It always is necessary to use step 3, and some considerable time must be taken to reinforce the newly learned reflexes. A maxillary lingual archwire retainer may be used to which short, sharp spurs may be added. Even after the patient has mastered the new swallow and the abnormal actions of the lip and mentalis muscles are seen no longer, it is wise to leave the lingual archwire in a bit longer. Our present state of knowledge does not allow a 100% correction of cases of complex

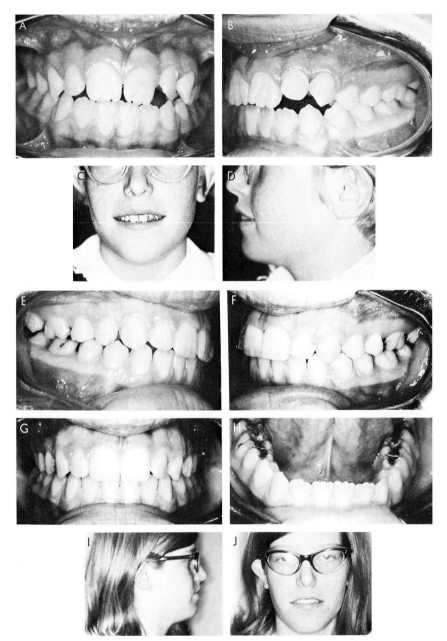

Fig. XVII-82.—A treated complex tongue-thrust. **A** and **B,** intra-oral views at the start of treatment. **C** and **D,** the soft tissue of the face before treatment. **E–G,** occlusal views at the end of treatment. This patient was treated orthodontically

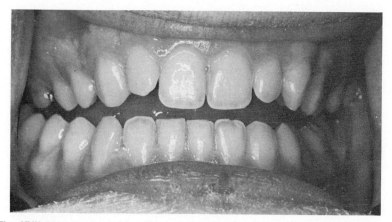

Fig. XVII-83.—An open bite due to a retained infantile swallow. Usually the teeth occlude on one molar in each quadrant. This patient was treated by a very competent orthodontist with full edgewise therapy. The photograph was taken 1 month after removal of the retainers.

tongue-thrust. Until we are wiser concerning these matters, it is very important to do meticulous tooth positioning, ultracareful equilibration and very patient myotherapy afterward. Despite the clinician's best efforts, there will be partial relapse in some cases (Fig. XVII-82).

3) RETAINED INFANTILE SWALLOW.—This is defined as the undue persistence of the infantile swallowing reflex. Very few people have a retained infantile swallow; those who do, ordinarily occlude on just one molar in each quadrant (Fig. XVII-83). Also, they demonstrate strong—almost violent—contractions of the VIIth cranial nerve muscles during swallowing while the tongue is protruded markedly and held between all of the teeth during the initial stages of the swallow. Such patients do not have expressive faces, since the VIIth nerve muscles are being used for the massive effort of stabilizing the mandible and not for the delicate facile movements of facial expression. Patients with a retained infantile swallow have serious difficulties in mastication and may have a very low gag threshold. Little is known concerning this severe clinical problem. Some believe that retained infantile swallowing is accompanied by infantile personality regression. Further, it is known that should these patients lose their teeth, satisfactory denture prosthesis is almost impossible. The prognosis for correction of the

---

twice previously before this correction was obtained. **H,** occlusal views at the end of retention. Note the persistence of the mamelons on the lower incisors, indicating that even yet there is not a full occlusal stop in the incisor region. **I** and **J,** facial soft tissue views at the end of treatment. Note some improvement in the posture of the lips at rest.

retained infantile swallow is very poor, since we have difficulty in conditioning such a primitive reflex as the infantile swallow.

At present, the role of the orthodontist is to impress on the patient the necessity for thorough, regular dental care, inasmuch as retention of the teeth is of paramount importance. It is hoped that current research will enlighten us sufficiently to provide better care for these individuals. Fortunately, the true retained infantile swallow is rare.

4. ABNORMAL TONGUE POSTURE

There are two forms of the protracted tongue posture: (1) the endogenous and (2) the acquired. Some patients, to maintain an airway, have an inherently abnormal tongue posture. During the arrival of the teeth, the tongue normally changes its posture and comes to rest inside the encircling dentition. In some children, the tip of the tongue persists in lying between the incisors. It is not known why this occurs, and it

Fig. XVII-84.—Open bite due to abnormal tongue posture. **A,** a Class II, Division 1 malocclusion 2 years out of retention. Note the return of a very mild open bite. This case was re-treated twice, returning each time to this relationship. **B,** a severe open bite due to abnormal tongue posture. There was no marked tongue-thrust on swallowing; rather, the tongue remained in this position most of the time.

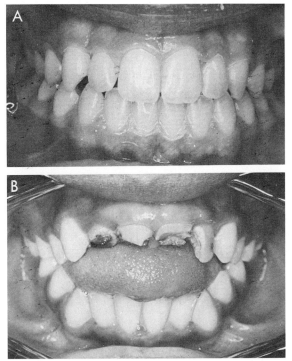

is very difficult to correct. Fortunately, the great majority of the endogenous protracted posture problems are not serious from an aesthetic standpoint and there is stability of the incisor relationship even though a mild open bite is seen (Fig. XVII-84, *A*). On rare occasions, quite serious open bites are present and have been present from the very first stages of eruption (Fig. XVII-84, *B*). The acquired protracted tongue posture is a more simple matter. Usually it is the result of chronic pharyngitis or tonsillitis or other nasorespiratory disturbance. It is best to refer the patient to an otolaryngologist for correction of the nasorespiratory problems before or coincidental with the orthodontic therapy. As long as the precipitating mechanism is present in the throat, the tongue will posture itself forward and repositioning of the incisors will not be stable. Many times the nasopharyngeal condition no longer exists but the tongue reflexly remains in a forward position. The posture in those circumstances usually can be induced to change by the simple expedient of leaving the anterior bands somewhat roughened on the lingual surfaces.

To summarize, there are two problems in abnormal posture of the tongue that have clinical significance: (1) the endogenous protracted tongue posture, for which the prognosis is poor and around which, unfortunately, the occlusion must be built, and (2) the acquired protracted tongue posture, which usually is correctable after the precipitating mechanisms in the throat have been removed.

5. LIP-SUCKING AND LIP-BITING

These habits are seen most frequently with an excessive overjet and/or overbite. In Class II, Division 1 cases, the lip habits frequently are severe and treatment should not be started until the incisors have been positioned correctly. Some lip habits are then self-correcting, but the hyperactive mentalis muscle remains. The oral shield, modified as shown in Figure XVII-72, is most useful. In Class I cases with labioversion, one occasionally can treat the incisal malposition and the habit simultaneously with an oral shield (see Fig. XVII-72).

6. FINGERNAIL-BITING

Nail-biting ordinarily is not seen until about the age of 3 or 4 years. Most psychologists seem to think that it is a reflection of anxiety or personality maladjustment. It reaches its peak of incidence during the teens. Children who bite their nails may have malocclusion, but it is not believed that any specific malocclusion is pathognomonic of nail-biting.

H. Occlusal Equilibration

Equilibrative procedures serve purposes in the primary and mixed dentitions different from those in the permanent dentition. Of necessity, the technics are different too. Before attempting any equilibrative

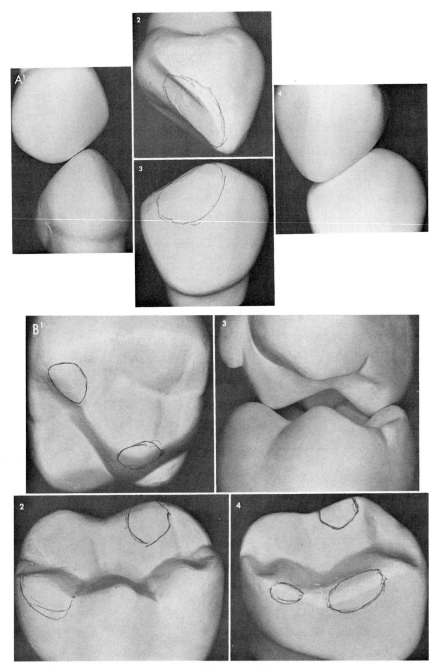

Fig. XVII-85.—See legend on facing page.

procedure, read thoroughly the section in Chapter XV pertaining to the particular clinical problem. Reread, also, Chapters V, X and Section E of Chapter XI. In Chapter XI, Section E, are given the procedures for taking a registration bite of the ideal occlusal position, the first step in equilibration in the primary dentition. One very good exercise is to try the equilibrative procedure on casts before attempting it in the mouth. Well-oriented casts may be marked with articulation paper and the plaster scraped away to simulate tooth grinding. Keeping a written record of the teeth and surfaces ground, and the order of the grinding, will be of value when actually doing the grinding in the mouth.

Cases treated by this procedure are illustrated in Chapter XV (e.g., Figs. XV-28, XV-29, XV-43, XV-46 and XV-47).

1. EQUILIBRATION IN THE PRIMARY DENTITION

The following articles and instruments are needed for equilibration in the primary dentition:

Articulation paper.
A small round or biscuit-shaped diamond point or stone.
A diamond disk (½ inch convex), with the abrasive on the convex side away from the handpiece.
Record casts.

It is useful to have an idea where the interferences are most likely to appear (Fig. XVII-85).

Procedure

(1) Teach the child to tap his teeth together with the midlines coinciding. Since this is the occlusal position they are reflexly avoiding, it requires some encouragement from the dentist. Place your thumbs beneath the mandible on either side, grasping it firmly while touching the gingivae in the cuspid region with the index fingers (Fig. XVII-86). Gently move the mandible to the desired position while giving verbal suggestions and tactile signals with the fingers on the gingivae. The initial occlusal interferences to be ground now will be seen clearly (Fig. XVII-87).
(2) Mark the midline interferences with articulating paper (Fig. XVII-88).

Fig. XVII-85.—A-1, the usual site of cuspid interference in the primary dentition. **2,** the area usually removed on the lingual of the maxillary cuspid. **3,** the area usually ground on the mandibular primary cuspid. **4,** the corrected primary cuspid relationship. **B-1,** the usual areas ground on the maxillary second primary molar. Note the relationship to the transverse ridge. **2,** the usual areas of interference and grinding on the mandibular second primary molar. **3,** the typical relationship of primary second molars when there is occlusal interference. **4,** the usual areas of interference on the mandibular first primary molar.

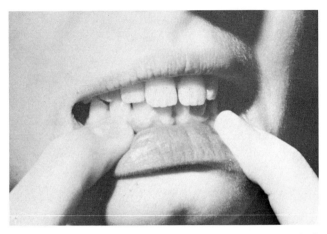

Fig. XVII-86.—Teaching the patient to tap his teeth together with the midlines coincident.

Fig. XVII-87.—**A,** typical interferences that appear when midlines are coincident. **B,** an atypical unilateral interference with the midlines together.

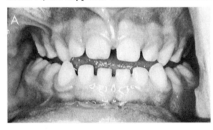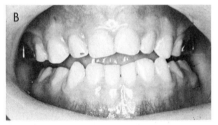

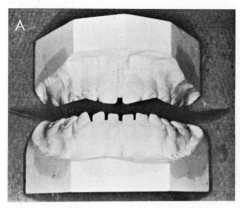

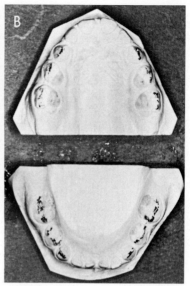

Fig. XVII-88.—Marking the interferences with articulation paper when the midlines are together. **A,** the correct position of the articulation paper, illustrated on casts. **B,** typical positions of midline interferences. Note that the markings persist on the lingual slopes of the buccal cusps in the upper arch. In a normal occlusion, these markings would be in the central fossae.

Fig. XVII-89.—Method of grinding the midline interferences. **A,** primary cuspid, lateral view. Note the areas of grinding and the change in relationship achieved by that grinding. **B,** primary molar. The method is similar to that for the cuspid.

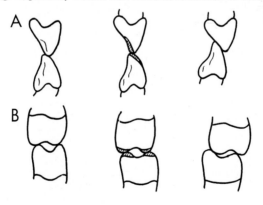

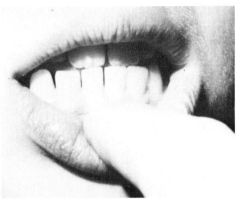

Fig. XVII-90.—Teaching the patient to protrude his jaw with the midlines coincident. The index finger is pushed against the gingiva in the lower central incisor region and the patient is instructed to advance the mandible, following the finger.

Fig. XVII-91.—The reasons for checking and grinding the protrusive interferences. These casts were taken after the midline interferences had been ground. By advancing the lower cast a very small amount (note that the incisors are not yet end to end), a typical interference is seen between the maxillary cuspid and the mesial marginal ridge of the mandibular first primary molar. Another interference seen frequently is between the lingual cusp of the maxillary first primary molar and the mesial marginal ridge of the mandibular second primary molar.

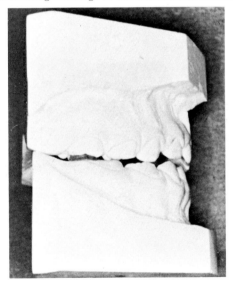

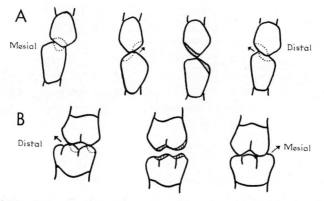

Fig. XVII-92.—Anteroposterior correction of functional malocclusion. **A**, primary cuspids. **B**, primary molars.

(3) Grind out the midline interferences as shown in Figure XVII-89. They usually are found first in the cuspids and perhaps later in the molars.

(4) Teach the child to protrude his jaw with the midlines together and the teeth touching. This may be done by placing your index finger against the gingivae at the mandibular midline and asking the child to follow your finger with his jaw as you gently withdraw your finger (Fig. XVII-90). The reason for this protrusive check of interferences is shown in Figure XVII-91.

(5) Mark the protrusive interferences with articulation paper.

(6) Grind away the protrusive interferences.

The effects of these equilibrative procedures on any functional aspects of Class II or Class III malocclusions are seen in Figure XVII-92.

2. EQUILIBRATION IN THE PERMANENT DENTITION

There are many reasons for equilibrating the permanent dentition. All completed orthodontic cases should be equilibrated when treatment has been undertaken in the permanent dentition. Equilibration of the permanent dentition ordinarily should not be undertaken without accurately mounted casts on an articulator for study and planning of the grinding procedure. What follows is the barest outline. The reader is referred to standard modern textbooks on periodontology for more complete technics. The method described has been adapted from the undergraduate notes of Ramfjord, but the terminology has been altered to be in keeping with that used in Chapters V, X and XI.

Equilibration is no substitute for meticulous positioning of teeth. It can, however, minimize the muscle's reaction to occlusal interferences, some of which cannot be removed with mechanotherapy.

Procedure

(1) If a cusp is making premature contact in the retruded occlusal position,

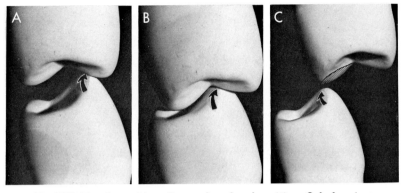

Fig. XVII-93.—A, working. **B,** usual occlusal position. **C,** balancing.

Fig. XVII-94.—A, working. **B.** usual occlusal position. **C,** balancing.

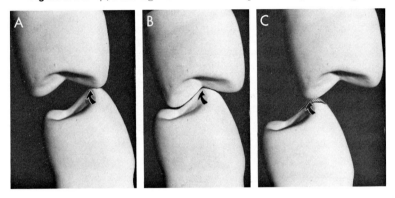

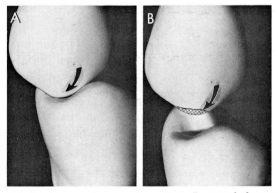

Fig. XVII-95.—A, usual occlusal position. **B,** retruded contact.

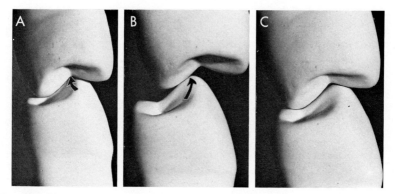

Fig. XVII-96.—A, usual occlusal position. **B,** retruded contact position. **C,** same after grinding.

the opposing groove or incline should be ground if the cusp interferes in only one or two functional key positions (Fig. XVII-93).

(2) The prematurely contacting cusps in the retruded occlusal position should be ground if there is interference in all of the three key positions (Fig. XVII-94).

(3) A forward slide into occlusion should be corrected by grinding on the interfering mesioclusal inclines of the upper teeth or the distoclusal inclines of the lower teeth. Occlusal stops should be maintained for premolars and molars without loss of vertical dimension (Fig. XVII-95).

(4) A lateral slide into occlusion should be corrected by widening of the central fossa at the level of the occlusal stop (Fig. XVII-96).

(5) If the lateral slide on the contacting teeth is away from the midline, grind as shown in Figure XVII-97.

(6) Adjust the working side on the guiding inclines, including the incisal edges and the buccal cusps of the upper teeth and the lingual cusps of the lower teeth (Fig. XVII-98).

Fig. XVII-97.—A, usual occlusal position. **B,** retruded contact position. **C,** same after grinding.

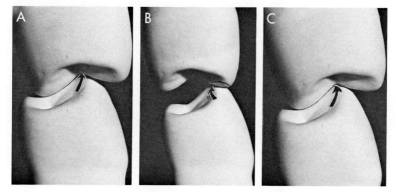

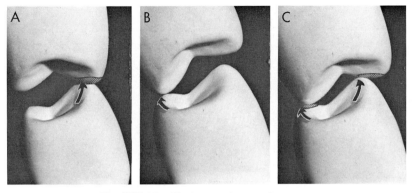

Fig. XVII-98.—Working side interference.

Fig. XVII-99.—**A,** usual occlusal position. **B,** protrusive contact. **C,** an unusual case.

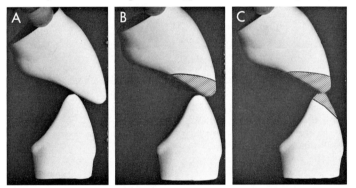

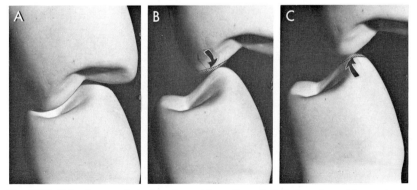

Fig. XVII-100.—**A,** usual occlusal position. **B** and **C,** balancing side contacts.

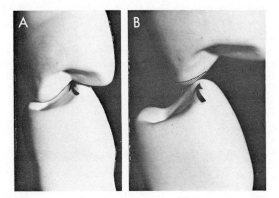

Fig. XVII-101.—A, usual occlusal position. **B,** balancing side contact.

(7) Adjust for protrusive contact on the incisal edges of the upper teeth, except in unusual cases (Fig. XVII-99).

(8) Do whole grinding on only one of two interfering cusps or inclines if they both serve as occlusal stops (Fig. XVII-100).

(9) If a cusp or incline that interferes in balance is out of occlusion in the usual position, grind on that cusp or incline (Fig. XVII-101).

(10) As a final procedure, remove any minor interferences that may remain between the retruded occlusal position and the ideal occlusal position.

3. Equilibration in the Mixed Dentition

Proceed in the mixed dentition as in the primary, grinding only primary teeth. Any permanent teeth that are interfering should be moved with appliances and not ground, since their position is likely to change many times before final adult occlusion is established.

Suggested Readings

Fixed Appliances

1. *Lingual Archwire*

Adams, P. E.: Labiolingual Technique, in Graber, T. M. (ed.), *Current Orthodontic Concepts and Techniques* (Philadelphia: W. B. Saunders Company, 1969), Chap. 5, pp. 275–346.
Tarpley, B. W.: *Technique and Treatment with the Labio-Lingual Appliance* (St. Louis: The C. V. Mosby Company, 1961).

2. *Fixed Space-Maintainers*

Proffitt, W. R., and Bennett, J. C.: Space maintenance serial extraction and the general practitioner, J. Am. Dent. A. 74:411, 1967.
Ryan, K. J.: Understanding and use of space maintenance procedures, J. Dent. Child. 31:22, 1964.
Zwemer, T. J.: Ten rules of the mixed dentition, J. Dent. Child. 35:298, 1968.

3. *Palate-Splitting Devices*

Haas, A. J.: The treatment of maxillary deficiency by opening the midpalatal suture, Angle Orthodont. 35:200, 1965.

Isaacson, R. J., Wood, J. L., and Ingram, A. H.: Forces produced by rapid maxillary expansion. I. Design of force measuring system, Angle Orthodont. 34:256, 1965.

4. *Simple Labial Archwires*

Adams, P. E.: Labiolingual Technique, in Graber, T. M. (ed.), *Current Orthodontic Concepts and Techniques* (Philadelphia: W. B. Saunders Company, 1969), Chap. 5, pp. 275–346.
Tarpley, B. W.: *Technique and Treatment with the Labio-Lingual Appliance* (St. Louis: The C. V. Mosby Company, 1961).

5. *Edgewise Mechanism*

Lindquist, J. T., and Stoner, M. M.: The Edgewise Appliance Today, in Graber, T. M. (ed.), *Current Orthodontic Concepts and Techniques* (Philadelphia: W. B. Saunders Company, 1969), Chap. 6, pp. 347–584.
Strang, R. H. W., and Thompson, W. M., Jr.: *A Textbook of Orthodontics* (Philadelphia: Lea & Febiger, 1958).
Thurow, R. C.: *Technique and Treatment with the Edgewise Appliance* (2d ed.; St. Louis: The C. V. Mosby Company, 1966).

6. *Light-Wire Appliances*

Begg, P. R.: *Begg Orthodontic Theory and Technique* (Philadelphia: W. B. Saunders Company, 1965).
Jarabak, J. R.: *Technique and Treatment with the Light Wire Appliance* (St. Louis: The C. V. Mosby Company, 1963).
Swain, B. F.: Begg Differential Light Forces Technic, in Graber, T. M. (ed.), *Current Orthodontic Concepts and Techniques* (Philadelphia: W. B. Saunders Company, 1969), Chap. 7, pp. 585–816.

7. *Twin-Wire Appliance*

Geoffrion, P.: *Clinical Application of the Twin-Wire Mechanism* (Paris: J. Prelat, 1962).
Shepard, E. E.: *Technique and Treatment with the Twin-Wire Appliance* (St. Louis: The C. V. Mosby Company, 1961).

8. *Universal Appliance*

Fastlicht, J.: The universal appliance today, J. Pract. Orthodont. Part I, 3:582; Part II, 3:639, 1969.
Fastlicht, J.: *Universal Appliance Technique* (Philadelphia: W. B. Saunders Company, 1972).
Stoller, A.: *The Universal Appliance* (St. Louis: The C. V. Mosby Company, 1971).

9. *The Labiolingual Appliance*

Adams, P. E.: Labiolingual Technique, in Graber, T. M. (ed.), *Current Orthodontic Concepts and Techniques* (Philadelphia: W. B. Saunders Company, 1969), Chap. 5, pp. 275–346.
Tarpley, B. W.: *Technique and Treatment with the Labio-Lingual Appliance* (St. Louis: The C. V. Mosby Company, 1961).

ATTACHED REMOVABLE APPLIANCES

Adams, C. P.: Removable appliances yesterday and today, Am. J. Orthodont. 55:748, 1969.
Adams, C. P.: *The Design and Construction of Removable Orthodontic Appliances* (4th ed.; Bristol: John Wright & Sons, Ltd., 1970).
Lamons, F. F.: The Crozat appliance, Am. J. Orthodont. 50:265, 1964.
Neumann, B.: Removable Appliances, in Graber, T. M. (ed.), *Current Orthodontic Concepts and Techniques* (Philadelphia: W. B. Saunders Company, 1969), Chap. 8, pp. 817–874.
Schwarz, A. M., and Gratzinger, M.: *Removable Orthodontic Appliances* (Philadelphia: W. B. Saunders Company, 1966).
Smythe, R. B.: Crozat removable appliance, Am. J. Orthodont. 55:739, 1969.

LOOSE REMOVABLE APPLIANCES

Adams, C. P.: *The Design and Construction of Removable Orthodontic Appliances* (4th ed.; Bristol: John Wright & Sons, Ltd., 1970).

Frankel, R.: Treatment of Class II, Division 1 malocclusion with functional correctors, Am. J. Orthodont. 55:265, 1969.
Gottlieb, E. L.: Success and failure with the positioner appliance, J. Pract. Orthodont. 2:506, 1968.
Grossman, W., and Moss, J. P.: Removable appliance therapy: Part I. Passive removable appliances, J. Pract. Orthodont. 2:28, 1968.
Harvold, E. P.: The role of function in the etiology and treatment of malocclusion, Am. J. Orthodont. 54:883, 1968.
Harvold, E. P., and Vargervick, K.: Morphogenetic response to activator treatment, Am. J. Orthodont. 60:478, 1971.
Moyers, R. E.: An American view of removable appliances, Dent. Pract. 15:117, 1964.
Neumann, B.: Removable Appliances, in Graber, T. M. (ed.), *Current Orthodontic Concepts and Techniques* (Philadelphia: W. B. Saunders Company, 1969), Chap. 8, pp. 817–874.
Schwarz, A. M., and Gratzinger, M.: *Removable Orthodontic Appliances* (Philadelphia: W. B. Saunders Company, 1966).
Symposium on Functional Therapy, Dent. Pract. 15:255, 1965.

CORRECTION OF DELETERIOUS ORAL HABITS

1. *Thumb-Sucking (Finger-Sucking)*

Davidson, P. O., Haryett, R. D., Sandilands, M., and Hanson, F. C.: Thumbsucking: Habit or symptom?, J. Dent. Child. 34:252, 1967.
Haryett, R. D., Hanson, F. C., Davidson, P. O., and Sandilands, M. L.: Chronic thumbsucking: The psychologic effects and the relative effectiveness of various methods of treatment, Am. J. Orthodont. 53:569, 1967.
Haryett, R. D., Sandilands, M. L., and Davidson, P. O.: Relative effectiveness of various methods of arresting thumbsucking, J. Canad. D. A. 34:5, 1968.
Haryett, R. D., Hanson, F. C., and Davidson, P. O.: Chronic thumbsucking, Am. J. Orthodont. 57:164, 1970.

2. *Tongue-Thrusting*

Moyers, R. E.: The Role of the Musculature in Orthodontic Diagnosis and Treatment Planning, in Kraus, B., and Riedel, R. (eds.), *Vistas in Orthodontics* (Philadelphia: Lea & Febiger, 1962), pp. 309–327.
Moyers, R. E.: Tongue problems and malocclusion, Dent. Clin. North America, p. 529, 1964.
Moyers, R. E.: Abnormal tongue function, Dentistry for the 70's Visu-Cassette Program, Health Information Systems, New York, 1971.

OCCLUSAL EQUILIBRATION

Ahlgren, J., and Posselt, U.: Need of functional analysis and selective grinding in orthodontics: A clinical and electromyographic study, Acta odont. scandinav. 21:187, 1963.
Ramfjord, S. P., and Ash, M. M.: *Occlusion* (2d ed.; Philadelphia: W. B. Saunders Company, 1971).

Index

A